Assessing Childhood Psychopathology and Developmental Disabilities

Assessing Childhood Psychopathology and Developmental Disabilities

Edited by

Johnny L. Matson
Louisiana State University, Baton Rouge, LA

Frank Andrasik
University of West Florida, Pensacola, FL

Michael L. Matson
Louisiana State University, Baton Rouge, LA

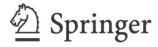 Springer

Editors

Johnny L. Matson
Department of Psychology
Louisiana State University
Baton Rouge, LA 70803
225-752-5924
johnmatson@aol.com

Frank Andrasik
Department of Psychology
University of West Florida
Pensacola, FL 32514-5751
fandrasik@uwf.edu

Michael L.Matson
Department of Psychology
Louisiana State University
Baton Rouge, LA 70803

ISBN: 978-0-387-09527-1   e-ISBN: 978-0-387-09528-8
DOI: 10.1007/978-0-387-09528-8

Library of Congress Control Number: 2008931166

Printed on acid-free paper

springer.com

Contents

List of Contributors

Frank Andrasik
Department of Psychology, University of West Florida,
Pensacola, FL 32514, fandrasik@uwf.edu

Scott P. Ardoin
Department of Psychology, University of South Carolina,
Columbia, SC, spardoin@sc.edu

Tammy D. Barry
Department of Psychology, The University of Southern Mississippi,
Hattiesburg, MS 39406, tammy.barry@usm.edu

Audrey Baumeister
Department of Psychology, Louisiana State University,
Baton Rouge, LA 70803

Jessica A. Boisjoli
Department of Psychology, Louisiana State University,
Baton Rouge, LA 70803

Carrie S.W. Borrero
Kennedy Krieger Institute Johns Hopkins University Medical School,
Baltimore, MD 21205

Stephanie Danner-Ogston
The Ohio State University, Columbus, OH 43210

Catherine Emily Durbin
WCAS Psychology, Northwestern University, Evanston, IL 60208,
edurbin@northwestern.edu

Dawn Eichen
Department of Psychiatry and Behavioral Sciences,
Duke University Medical Center, Durham, NC 27710

Camden Elliott
Department of Psychiatry and Behavioral Sciences,
Duke University Medical Center, Durham, NC 27710

Jack M. Fletcher
Department of Psychology, University of Houston,
Houston, TX 72204

Mary A. Fristad
Research & Psychological Services, Division of Child & Adolescent
Psychiatry, Department of Psychiatry, College of Medicine,
The Ohio State University, Columbus, OH 43210, fristad.1@osu.edu

Kristin A. Gansle
Department of Educational Theory, Policy, and Practice,
Louisiana State University, Baton Rouge, LA, kgansle@lsu.edu

Beth H. Garland
Baylor College of Medicine, Department of Psychology,
Texas A&M University, TX 77845, bhgarland@neo.tamu.edu

Drew Gouvier
Department of Psychology, Louisiana State University,
Baton Rouge, LA 70803, wgouvie@lsu.edu

Amie E. Grills-Taquechel
Department of Psychology, University of Houston, Houston, TX 72204,
aegrills@uh.edu

Rob Heffer
Department of Psychology, Texas A&M University, TX 778845,
Rob-Heffer@tamu.edu

Stephen D. A. Hupp
Department of Psychology, Southern Illinois University,
Edwardsville, IL 62026

Kola Ijaola
Department of Psychology, Louisiana State University,
Baton Rouge, LA 70803

Melissa F. Jackson
Department of Clinical and Forensic Psychology,
University of Alabama, Tuscaloosa, AL 35401, Melissa.jackson@ua.edu

Jeremy D. Jewell
Department of Psychology, Southern Illinois University,
Edwardsville, IL 62026, jejewel@siue.edu

R. W. Kamphaus
College of Education, Georgia State University, Atlanta, GA. 30302
rkamphaus@gsu.edu

Jennifer Lacy
Department of Psychology, Duke University Medical Center,
Durham, NC 27710

John E. Lochman
Department of Psychology, University of Alabama, Tuscaloosa, AL,
jlochman@gp.as.ua.edu

Johnny L. Matson
Department of Psychology, Louisiana State University,
Baton Rouge, LA 70803, Johnmatson@aol.com

Rhonda Merwin
Department of Psychiatry and Behavioral Sciences,
Duke University Medical Center, Durham, NC 27710

George H. Noell
Department of Psychology, Louisiana State University,
Baton Rouge, LA 70803, gnoell@lsu.edu

Cathleen C. Piazza
Munroe–Meyer Institute for Genetics and Rehabilitation,
University of Nebraska Medical Center, Omaha, NE 68198

Rosanna Polifroni
Department of Psychology, University of Houston, Houston, TX 72204

Andrew M. Pomerantz
Department of Psychology, Southern Illinois University,
Edwardsville, IL 62026

Nicole R. Powell
Department of Psychology, University of Alabama, Tuscaloosa, AL

Leslie Rescorla
Department of Psychology, Bryn Mawr College, Bryn Mawr, PA 19010,
lrescorl@brynmawr.edu

Cecil R. Reynolds
Texas A & M University, TX 78602, c-reynolds@tamu.edu

Carla Rime
Department of Psychology, University of West Florida,
Pensacola, FL 32514

Henry S. Roane
Munroe–Meyer Institute for Genetics and Rehabilitation,
University of Nebraska Medical Center, Omaha, NE 68198,
hroane@unmc.edu

Kimberly N. Sloman
Department of Psychology, University of Florida, Gainesville, FL 32611

Paula Sowerby
Department of Psychology, ADHD Research Clinic, University of Otago,
Dunedin, New Zealand, paula@psy.otago.ac.nz

Gail Tripp
Department of Psychology, University of Otago, Dunedin, New Zealand,
gtripp@psy.otago.ac.nz

Katie King Vogel
College of Education, University of Georgia, Athens, GA 30602.

Timothy R. Vollmer
Department of Psychology, University of Florida, Gainesville, FL 32611,
vollmera@ufl.edu

Sylia Wilson
WCAS Psychology, Northwestern University, Evanston, IL 60208

Anna Yaros
Center for the Prevention of Youth Behavior Problems,
Department of Psychology, University of Alabama, Tuscaloosa, AL

Matthew E. Young
The Ohio State University, Division of Child & Adolescent Psychiatry,
Columbus, OH 43210

Laura Young
Department of Psychology, University of Alabama, Tuscaloosa, AL

Nancy Zucker
Department of Psychiatry and Behavioral Sciences,
Duke University Medical Center, Durham, NC 27705,
Zucke001@mc.duke.edu

Part I

Introduction

1

History, Overview, and Trends in Child and Adolescent Psychological Assessment

ROBERT W. HEFFER, TAMMY D. BARRY, and BETH H. GARLAND

Systematically evaluating human performance and predicting important outcomes emerged in the far reaches of recorded history. For example, Gregory (2007) described that as early as 2200 BC Chinese emperors developed physical abilities, knowledge, and specific skill examinations for government officials and civil servants. However, assessment of children's abilities and behavior certainly predates even these distant instances of evaluation of adults.

We contend that child assessment has taken place as long as parents and other adults have observed and tracked changes in children's development. Parents notice changes over time within a given child and differences among children in abilities and responses to circumstances. This type of informal evaluation process certainly is a far cry from the empirically based, standardized methods of child and adolescent psychological assessment that have developed over the past 150 years or so, but it is foundational.

The current state-of-the-art of assessing childhood psychopathology and developmental disabilities is presented in this volume of a two-volume edited series. Each topic and issue covered includes a common core: adults have an interest in understanding, documenting, and predicting the capacities and experiences of children. In addition, these contributions to the literature have an applied slant: that is, interventions designed

ROBERT W. HEFFER, BETH H. GARLAND • Department of Psychology Texas A&M University, 4235 TAMU College Station, TX 778845-4235.
TAMMY D. BARRY • Department of Psychology, The University of Southern Mississippi, 118 College Drive, 5025 Hattiesburg, MS 39406.

J.L. Matson et al. (eds.), *Assessing Childhood Psychopathology and Developmental Disabilities*, DOI: 10.1007/978-0-387-09528-8,
© Springer Science+Business Media, LLC 2009

to influence outcomes emanate from competent assessment. Our psychological assessment approaches have become more sophisticated, but are linked historically to our predecessors' curiosity about how children grow and learn and what "to do" with this knowledge.

In this chapter, we use the words, "child" or "children" to refer to individuals whose chronological age ranges from birth to late adolescence. Otherwise, we note if a particular description applies specifically to an infant/toddler, preschool-aged young child, a school-aged child, or a teenager. First, we present an overview of some of the key historical events that have shaped child assessment today. We promise not to include every detail from Adam and Eve's parental observations of Cain, Abel, and Seth to the present! Next, we offer an overview of issues central to child assessment methods early in the 21st century. Finally, we suggest overarching trends that we believe are influencing directions for the field of child psychological assessment.

SYNOPSIS OF HISTORICAL EVENTS

Thorough and intriguing accounts of the historical underpinnings of psychological assessment and testing may be found in Gregory (2007), Kelley and Surbeck (2004), or Sattler (2008). From parental observations and assessment methods in antiquity, fast forward to the early 19th century, when Jean Marc Gaspard Itard, a physician and educator of children with deafness, wrote of his attempts to understand and intervene with Victor, the "Wild Boy of Aveyron" (Shattuck, 1994). Evidently, Victor lived on his own in the woods near Toulouse, France until perhaps age 12 years when he was discovered without verbal language and typical behavior. Itard's detailed record in 1807, *Reports on the Savage of Aveyron*, described systematic assessment and intervention methods to rehabilitate the social behavior and language development of this "feral child."

Edouard Seguin, who studied with Itard, established the first education program for mentally retarded children in 1837 (Gregory, 2007; Sattler, 2008). He later designed the *Seguin Form Board* and continued his innovative and pioneering work with developmentally disabled individuals when he emigrated to the United States. Also in France, Jean-Étienne Dominique Esquirol in 1838 distinguished written definitions of mental retardation (*idiocy*) versus mental illness (*dementia*) and proposed specific diagnostic criteria for levels of mental retardation (Gregory, 2007; Sattler, 2008).

Other trailblazers in psychology focused primarily on assessment of adult mental processes. For example, Wilhelm Wundt, who founded the first psychology laboratory in Leipzieg, Germany in 1879, and Sir Francis Galton in Great Britain established precise, systematic assessments of psychophysiological and sensory experiences. In the United States during the late 1800s and early 1900s, psychologists such James McKeen Catell and Robert M. Yerkes instituted research and assessment methods applied to adult mental and intellectual abilities (Gregory, 2007; Sattler, 2008). However, Lightner Witmer's "Psychological Clinic," founded at the University of Pennsylvania in 1896, featured intensive case studies of children—and some adults—from the Philadelphia community. Child clients were assessed and treated by a multidisciplinary team using clinical and research-based methods (Cellucci & Heffer, 2001; McReynolds, 1996). In addition, Granville Stanely Hall, founder of the American Psychological Association in 1892, established the "child study movement" in the United States (Fagan & Wise, 1994), laying the groundwork for the development of child assessment as a subspecialty area.

The work of Itard, Seguin, and Esquirol and the methods established by adult-focused psychologists—along with the concomitant social changes of the time (Habenstein & Olson, 2001)—set the stage for the invention of the first intelligence test, to be used with children, by Alfred Binet and his colleagues, published as the *Binet-Simon Scale* in 1905 (Gregory, 2007; Kelley & Surbeck, 2004). Due to laws regarding compulsory school attendance in both France and the United States, assessment methods were needed to identify levels of cognitive abilities and to predict success in various levels of education. In the United States in the early- to mid-1900s, psychologists such as Henry Herbert Goddard, E. L. Thorndike, Lewis M. Terman, Maud Merrill, Florence L. Goodenough, Arnold Gesell, Lucy Sprague Mitchell, and Psyche Cattell established scientific and practical aspects of child psychological assessment upon which current approaches are founded (Kelley & Surbeck, 2004; Sattler, 2008).

Following World War II, the evolution of standardized child assessment continued with the publishing in 1948 of R. G. Leiter's *Leiter International Performance Scale* and in 1949 of David Weschler's *Weschler Intelligence Test for Children* (Boake, 2002; Kelley & Surbeck, 2004). The *Leiter* was the first nonverbal, culturally fair test of intellectual abilities, most recently revised in 1997. Further readers will recognize that the *WISC* evidently "caught on," because as of 2003, it is in its fourth revision, the *WISC-IV*. Similarly in 2003, the *Simon-Binet Scale* of 1905 morphed into its fifth revision as the *Stanford-Binet Intelligence Scales-5*. Presently, the concept of intelligence in children and methods for evaluating cognitive functioning have diversified and become more intricate, reflecting the advance of child assessment regarding this complicated construct (Benson, 2003a,b,c; Sattler, 2008).

Based in part on developmental theorists' work (e.g., Piaget, 1970, 1971) "the emphasis [in child assessment in the mid-1900s]:shifted from intelligence testing to the study of personality, social, and motoric factors related to general functioning" (Kelley & Surbeck, 2004, p. 6). For example, in 1959 Anton Brenner published his *Brenner Developmental Gestalt Test of School Readiness* to evaluate children's preparedness for entering first grade. In 1961, the *Illinois Test of Psycholinguistic Ability*, in its third revision as of 2001, was published by S. A. Kirk and J. J. McCarthy as an individually administered test of language ability in children (Sattler, 2008). Over this time period, Edgar Doll (whose work spanned from 1912 to 1968) and colleagues used the *Vineland Social Maturity Scales*, first published in 1936 and revised in 2005 *as the Vineland Adaptive Behavior Scales-II*, to assess social, communication, and daily living skills in infants to older adults (Sattler, 2008).

Changes in education practices, United States federal laws, and society in general, gave rise from the 1960s to the 1980s to a range of standardized tests of child cognitive abilities and development (Kelley & Surbeck, 2004). For example, in 1967 David Weschler published his downward extension of the WISC, the *Weschler Preschool and Primary Scale of Intelligence (WPPSI)*. The WPPSI is in its third revision as of 2002. In 1969, Nancy Bayley published the *Bayley Scales of Infant Development*, which was revised as the *Bayley-III* in 2005. In addition, Dorothea McCarthy published her *McCarthy Scales of Children's Abilities (MSCA)* in 1970/1972 (Sattler, 2008). The MSCA is a hybrid of intelligence and developmental tests that evaluates verbal, perceptual-performance, quantitative memory, and motor abilities in young children.

Assessment of child behavioral, emotional, and personality functioning blossomed in the 1990s, from its humble beginnings with Florence Goodenough's *Draw A Man Test* in 1926 and subsequent permutations by John Buck in 1948 and Karen Machover in 1949. Specifically, in 1992 a version of the *Minnesota Multiphasic Personality Inventory* was designed and normed for 14- to 18-year-olds, the *MMPI-Adolescent*, by James Butcher and colleagues. Also in 1993, the *Millon Adolescent Clinical Inventory (MACI)* was published by Theodore Millon. Both the MMPI-A and the MACI continue to experience widespread use in research and applied settings as extensive, self-report measures of psychological functioning (Vance & Pumariega, 2001).

A welcome addition to the burgeoning body of literature on the *Personality Assessment Inventory (PAI*; Morey, 1991, 1996, 2003) is the *PAI-Adolescent* (Morey, 2007). Les Morey adapted the PAI-A for use with individuals aged 12 to 18 years and reported that it demonstrates comparable psychometric properties, practical strengths, and the solid theoretical foundation as its adult-normed predecessor. In addition, between 1998 and 2001, William Reynolds published a self-report measure for individuals aged 12 to 19 years, the *Adolescent Psychopathology Scale (APS)*, that provides multidimensional assessment across a range of psychopathology, personality, and social-emotional problems and competencies (Reynolds, 1998a,b, 2000, 2001). Also between 1995 and 2001, David Lachar and colleagues introduced their revision of the *Personality Inventory for Children (PIC-R)*, the *Personality Inventory for Youth (PIY)*, and the *Student Behavior Survey (SBS)* as a comprehensive assessment system of psychological functioning of children and adolescents, based on self-, parent-, and teacher-report (Lachar, 2004).

During the late 20th century to the present, Thomas Achenbach and colleagues developed the *Achenbach System of Empirically Based Assessment (ASEBA*; Achenbach & Rescorla, 2000, 2001) and Cecil Reynolds and Randy Kamphaus developed the *Behavior Assessment System for Children*, 2nd Edition (*BASC-2*; Reynolds & Kamphaus, 2004). The 2003 version of the ASEBA and the 2004 version of the BASC-2 are exemplars of multidomain, multimethod, multi-informant assessment systems (Kazdin, 2005) for assessing childhood psychopathology and other domains of behavioral, emotional, and school-related functioning (Heffer & Oxman, 2003). For continuity in life-span research and applications into adulthood, the BASC-2 offers norms for persons aged 2 through 25 years and the ASEBA includes norms on persons aged 1.5 to 59 years.

At present, myriad child assessment methods have sprouted to address almost any psychological process or construct that the reader can imagine (Sattler, 2006), as evidenced by the chapters in this volume. For example, researchers and practitioners alike may find ample resources regarding assessing and screening preschoolers (Campbell, 2002; Nuttal, Romero, & Kalesnik, 1992); interviewing children, parents, and teachers and conducting behavioral observations (LaGreca, Kuttler, & Stone, 2001; Sattler, 1998); using a "therapeutic assessment approach" with children and adolescents (Handler, 2007); family functioning (Heffer, Lane, & Snyder, 2003; Heffer & Snyder, 1998; Snyder, Cavell, Heffer, & Mangrum, 1995); psychopathy in adolescence (Edens & Cahill, 2007); and evaluating quality of life (Varni, Limbers, & Burwinkle, 2007a; 2007b) and other child health/pediatric psychology issues (Rodrigue, Geffken, & Streisand, 2000). Child assessors may focus on school-based assessments (D'Amato, Fletcher-Janzen, & Reynolds, 2005; House, 2002; Shapiro & Kratochwill, 2000; Sheridan, 2005) or primarily clinical diagnostic or categorical evaluations (Kamphaus & Campbell, 2006; Rapoport & Ismond, 1996; Shaffer, Lucas, & Richters, 1999). In fact, even "comprehensive assessment-to-intervention systems" are modeled for child assessors who intend to link assessment to intervention to process/outcome evaluation (Schroeder & Gordon, 2002).

Assessment of child psychopathology and developmental disabilities certainly has come a long way from informal parental observations and case studies of feral children. We turn your attention next to an overview of the current state-of the-art in child assessment and then to trends for future directions of the field. Where we have been, where we are, and where we are going are the themes.

OVERVIEW OF "STATE-OF-THE ART" IN CHILD ASSESSMENT

Ethical–legal issues and requirements of education laws demarcate child assessment from adult assessment. Of course, professional standards and guidelines generated to promote competent and ethical psychological assessment and research apply equally to evaluations conducted with individuals across the life-span. However, unique characteristics central to child assessment create interesting "twists" for psychologists (Lefaivre, Chambers, & Fernandez, 2007; Melton, Ehrenreich, & Lyons, 2001). Furthermore, as the field of clinical child psychology continues to grow, so does the number of assessment tools available (Mash & Hunsley, 2005). Many of these tools serve to advance research in the broader field of child and adolescent clinical psychology, whereas a large number also become available assessment methods for use by practitioners and researchers. In this section, we describe some of the ethical and legal challenges in child assessment and proffer suggestions for managing such conundrums. Then, we review six "state-of-the-art" approaches in child assessment, several major issues to be considered in the use of such approaches, and a few trends in the resultant outcomes of these approaches to child assessment.

Professional Standards and Guidelines

Each reader should be keenly aware that psychology as a profession has historically paid considerable attention to defining and promoting ethical behavior and standards for professional behavior (American Psychological Association, 1950, 1953, 1959; Hobbs, 1951). For example, the most recent version of "The Code," *Ethical Principles of Psychologists and Code of Conduct* (American Psychological Association, 2002a), provides aspirational goals and prescriptive directives regarding a range of research, assessment, intervention, teaching/training, consultation, and business activities of psychologists. Furthermore, the APA's *Record Keeping Guidelines* (American Psychological Association Committee on Professional Practice and Standards, 1993) have application to both child-focused and adult-focused practitioners and trainers of clinical, counseling, or school psychologists.

Other documents have been published specifically to guide professional activities and promote standards for psychological assessment and use of psychological tests. Examples of these documents include *Standards for Educational and Psychological Testing* (American Educational Research Association, American Psychological Association, and National Council on Measurement in Education, 1999), *Code for Fair Testing Practices* (American Psychological Association, 2003), *Code of Fair Testing Practices in Education* (National Council on Measurement in Education, 2004), and *Guidelines for Test User Qualifications* (American Psychological Association, 2000; Turner, DeMers, Fox, & Reed, 2001).

Similar documents elaborate on particular aspects of competent assessment such as *Guidelines for Computer-Based Test and Interpretations* (American Psychological Association, 1986), *Psychological Testing on the Internet* (Naglieri et al., 2004), *Guidelines for Providers of Psychological Services to Ethnic, Linguistic, and Culturally Diverse Populations* (American Psychological Association, 1990), *Guidelines on Multicultural Education, Training, Research, Practice, and Organizational Change for Psychologists* (American Psychological Association, 2002b), *Statement on Disclosure of Test Data* (American Psychological Association Committee on Psychological Tests and Assessment, 1996), and *Rights and Responsibilities of Test Takers: Guidelines and Expectations* (American Psychological Association Joint Committee on Testing Practices, 1998).

At least one professional guidelines document specific to child assessment is *Guidelines for Child Custody Evaluations in Divorce* (American Psychological Association Committee on Professional Practice and Standards, 1994). Additional information about psychological tests and testing as a practice and research enterprise may be viewed at http://www.apa.org/science/testing.html.

Interplay of Ethical and Legal/Forensic Issues

Most psychologists understand that ethical and competent professional behavior ideally is completely compatible with legal behavior. However, from time to time a dynamic tension erupts when a given state law, for example, creates a dilemma for a child assessor (Anderten, Staulcup, & Grisso, 2003). Evaluation of children evokes unique developmental, systems, and ethical issues that may inconsistently seem congruent with what a given law requires (Heffer & Oxman, 2003). The chronological age of the child, his or her developmental/cognitive capacity, the family, school, and/or medical system that is requesting the evaluation, and the purposes for which the evaluation will be used may evoke complicated problem-solving to balance ethical and legal expectations (Rae & Fournier, 1999). For example, issues of assent and consent for services, confidentiality of communications and records, consulting with extra-family systems (e.g., school or medical personnel), and state abuse reporting laws distinguish child assessment from adult assessment.

Ethical–legal challenges in child assessment abound, which make it such an exhilarating enterprise. Psychologists currently have resources to assist as they wrestle with ethical delimmas. Of course, we already have provided a number of references for professional standards and ethical behavior for psychologists. In addition, publications such as Bersoff (2003), Fisher (2003), and Nagy (2003) allow psychologists to "flesh out" issues that emanate from application of the *Ethical Principles of Psychologists and Code of Conduct* (American Psychological Association, 2002a). Furthermore, publications often exist that elucidate mental health laws specific to a given state. For example, Hays, Sutter, and McPherson (2002) and Shuman (2004) provide such references for psychologists in Texas.

For psychologists involved in service delivery roles, current information regarding the *Health Insurance Portability and Accountability Acts (HIPPA) of 1996* (Bersoff, 2003) may be viewed at http://www.apapractice. org/apo/hipaa/get_hipaa_compliant.html#. Effectively navigating child assessment activities in the schools vis-à-vis the *Individuals with Disabilities Education Improvement Act of 2004* (National Association of School Psychologists, 2007) may be facilitated by information at http://www. ed.gov/about/offices/list/osers/osep/index.html or http://nasponline. org/advocacy/IDEAinformation.aspx. Other resources are explicit to forensic evaluations of children or other evaluative activities that may interface with the legal system (American Psychological Association Committee on Psychological Tests and Assessment, 1996; Schacht, 2001; Schaffer, 2001).

Assessment Approaches

Although we do not include an exhaustive list of current and exemplary assessment approaches, we do highlight six recent and important advances in child assessment. First, the evolution of our understanding of brain and behavior relationships has been mirrored by growth in neuropsychological assessment (Williams & Boll, 1997). Once used primarily for understanding significant psychopathology and traumatic brain injury, neuropsychological assessment is now increasingly utilized to better disclose subtle differences in children presenting with a range of disorders, including Attention-Deficit/Hyperactivity Disorders (ADHD) and learning disabilities

(Williams & Boll, 1997). Neuropsychological assessment instruments are well suited to meet these increasing demands as the field of neuropsychology continues to assimilate knowledge from other disciplines, including those pertinent to child assessment, such as developmental psychology (Williams & Boll, 1997).

Furthermore, input from other fields has allowed the application of previously adult-oriented neuropsychological techniques to be more readily applied to child populations (Korkman, 1999), thus leading to the expansion of child-specific neuropsychological test batteries. Such batteries range from focusing on a circumscribed area of neuropsychological functioning, such as the *Children's Memory Scale* (Cohen, 1997), to encompassing a comprehensive neuropsychological examination that can be tailored to the client's needs, such as the *NEPSY-II* (Korkman, Kirk, & Kemp, 2007). A complete neuropsychological evaluation certainly is not implicated for every child referral.

However, the availability of these tools and the tremendous expansion of the subdiscipline of clinical neuropsychology (Heilbronner, 2007) provide abundant opportunities to employ these state-of-the-art approaches when indicated. Whereas neuropsychological assessment can provide information linking brain functioning and a child's behavior, conceptualizing the child within a broader, contextually based framework is imperative (Heffer, Lane, & Snyder, 2003). As such, a second progression in child assessment has been the inclusion of an ecological/systems approach in the process (Dishion & Stormshak, 2007; Mash & Hunsley, 2005).

Data from a broader perspective better informs assessment and can be integral to treatment planning. Thus, assessment approaches should seek an understanding of not only the individual child's functioning but also should assess domains of influence on the child, such as the parent–child dyad, broader family context, peer relations, school and academic functioning, and domains of influence on the family itself, such as life stress, community resources, or medical involvement (Brown, 2004; Dishion & Stormshak, 2007; Mash & Hunsley, 2005; Roberts, 2003). Although context affects functioning at any age, children are particularly dependent on external regulatory systems and are more strongly influenced by context than are adults (Carter, Briggs-Gowan, & Davis, 2004). Furthermore, parent–child interactions are often reciprocal in nature, with certain parenting behaviors and other characteristics of the parent serving as either risk or protective factors for the child's functioning (Carter et al., 2004). Hence, it is critical to understand the child's functioning within a contextual framework, especially given that such understanding can inform treatment decisions (Dishion & Stormshak, 2007).

Whereas both neuropsychological assessment and ecological/systems assessment broaden the amount of data gleaned about a child, a third trend in current assessment approaches allows for more specific, objective measurement in the assessment of individual childhood disorders (Mash & Hunsley, 2005). Fueled largely by the popularity of the use of time-efficient and cost-effective behavior rating scales in the assessment process (Kamphaus, Petoskey, & Rowe, 2000), this problem-focused assessment approach is particularly attractive to cost-focused healthcare systems that require practical symptom-based assessment, which lends itself to continuous monitoring of outcomes (Mash & Hunsley, 2005). Furthermore, a problem-focused approach to assessment fits cohesively with research on both assessment and treatment of disorders and can allow the practitioner or researcher to map symptoms directly on to *DSM-IV-TR* criteria (Mash & Hunsley, 2005). Indeed, although omnibus ratings scales, such as the *ASEBA* (Achenbach & Rescorla, 2000, 2001) and *BASC-2* (Reynolds & Kamphaus, 2004) will likely remain effective in years to come, tremendous growth in specialized or more problem-specific measures for childhood disorders is occurring. Both research and practice have moved toward the use of brief problem/disorder-specific measures and batteries (Mash & Hunsley, 2005).

Nevertheless, comorbidity in child functioning must be considered because target problems are often quite heterogeneous (Achenbach, 2005; Kazdin, 2005). A fourth approach to child assessment, building steadily over the past few decades, is multidomain, multimethod, multi-informant assessment techniques (Kazdin, 2005). Given the wide utility of assessment, the heterogeneity of functioning, and the rates of comorbidity among disorders, consideration of multiple domains in the assessment of child functioning is indispensable (Kazdin, 2005). Even if the presenting problem is specific and narrowly defined, evaluating multiple domains to ascertain a comprehensive representation of the child is important. Domains may include not only dysfunction, but also how well a child is performing in prosocial adaptive areas (Kazdin, 2005). Thus, any state-of-the-art assessment of a child should incorporate evaluation of multiple domains of functioning, based on multiple sources of information, using multiple assessment methods/measures (Kazdin, 2005).

Because any one measure likely fails to capture the entirety of a clinical concern, it is imperative that child assessment include multiple measures. In addition, even within the same mode of assessment (e.g., behavioral rating forms), practitioners and researchers may use various instruments to better gauge the complexities of a given problem. For example, a referral to evaluate for ADHD may include completion of parent, teacher, and child rating forms assessing for behavioral symptoms of inattention, hyperactivity, and impulsivity (e.g., *BASC-2*, Reynolds & Kamphaus, 2004), attentional difficulties (e.g., *Conner Rating Scales-Revised*, Conners, 2001a), and, at a more broad level, cognitive aspects of the problem (e.g., *Behavior Rating Inventory for Executive Function, BRIEF*; Gioia, Isquith, Guy, & Kenworthy, 2000). Likewise, different modes of assessment for the same clinical problem—such as use of a continuous performance test to measure sustained attention and behavior rating forms to assess "real life" attention problems—yield richer data than either mode alone.

Finally, assessment of a child's functioning based on multiple informants (e.g., parents, other caregivers, teachers, practitioners, self-report) is critical, given that each informant adds a unique perspective and captures variations across settings (Achenbach, 2005; Kazdin, 2005). The need for multi-informant assessment is underscored by a lack of uniform agreement commonly found among various raters of child social, emotional, and behavioral functioning (Kamphaus & Frick, 2005). In addition, some childhood disorders (e.g., ADHD) require documentation of impairment across more than one setting (American Psychiatric Association, 2000).

Fifth, functional assessment, including experimental functional analysis, has made robust advances in child assessment (Matson & Minshawi, 2007). These procedures, which allow antecedents, measurable actions, consequences, and contextual variables of child behavior to be evaluated in controlled settings, inform individualized interventions. Functional assessment and analysis approaches are becoming even more prevalent in applied settings (Horner, 1994; Matson & Minshawi, 2007), including homes (Moes & Frea, 2002), schools (Watson, Ray, Turner, & Logan, 1999), residential care settings (Field, Nash, Handwerk, Friman, 2004), and medical rehabilitation centers (Long, Blackman, Farrell, Smolkin, & Conaway, 2005), among others.

Through these procedures, environmental variables can be manipulated, which can further inform the practitioner of the function of target behaviors and, thus, identify what may be causing or maintaining an unwanted behavior (Watson et al., 1999). Furthermore, functional assessment and analysis link directly to intervention, which typically involves manipulation of environmental variables identified through the assessment (Watson et al., 1999). That is, the intervention can focus not only the behavior itself but also its function in an effort to improve treatment efficacy (Horner, 1994).

Functional assessment has widely been implemented with children with developmental disabilities, such as intellectual disabilities (Swender, Matson, Mayville, Gonzalez, & McDowell, 2006) and autism spectrum disorders (Moes & Frea, 2002). In addition, these procedures are increasingly used to assess children presenting with a range of other concerns, such as ADHD (Stahr, Cushing, Lane, & Fox, 2006), behavioral and academic problems (Kamps, Wendland, & Culpepper, 2006), and primary pediatric problems, for example, acquired brain injury (Long et al., 2005).

Sixth and finally, with progression in the field of child assessment and corresponding research, state-of-the-art assessment will need to embrace—or at least come to terms with—evidence-based practices. Whereas applied child psychology has long focused on evidence-based treatments (EBT) for childhood disorders, only recently has an emphasis been placed on evidence-based assessment (EBA; Mash & Hunsley, 2005). EBA is used to describe "assessment methods and processes that are based on empirical evidence in terms of both their reliability and validity as well as their clinical usefulness for prescribed populations and purposes" (Mash & Hunsley, 2005, p. 364).

In short, an EBA battery should be specific to the presenting problem and should provide incremental validity in measuring the presenting problem and its associated symptoms. That is, a measure included in an EBA battery should help predict the set of target behaviors and symptoms above and beyond that already assessed by other measures included in the battery (Mash & Hunsley, 2005).

Finally, EBAs should aid the practitioner in forming a case conceptualization, determining a *DSM–IV–TR* diagnosis, and generating subsequent treatment recommendations (Mash & Hunsley, 2005). These goals help to evaluate whether a given assessment meets the qualifications for EBA. That is, it is these purposes of assessment that distinguish EBA simply from a measure that demonstrates evidence of its psychometric properties and usefulness (Kazdin, 2005).

This final assessment approach is one that should sustain continued attention and interest for many years to come, because development of clear guidelines and policies to conduct EBA for specific disorders is greatly needed (Mash & Hunsley, 2005). It is complicated, however, in that no "gold standard" exists by which to validate assessments (Kazdin, 2005, p. 548). Efforts, however, have begun to establish EBA guidelines for myriad child and adolescent disorders, including anxiety (Silverman & Ollendick, 2005), depression (Klein, Dougherty, & Olino, 2005), bipolar disorder (Youngstrom, Findling, Youngstrom, & Calabrese, 2005), ADHD (Pelham, Fabiano, & Massetti, 2005), conduct problems (McMahon & Frick, 2005), and learning disabilities (Fletcher, Francis, & Morris, 2005), among others.

EBA should take into consideration key demographic characteristics of the child (e.g., gender, ethnicity, age) that may influence performance on a given measure, as well as to adequately evaluate both primary and secondary targets of assessment, particularly given the high rates of comorbidity among disorders (Kazdin, 2005; Mash & Hunsley, 2005).

Further development of EBA guidelines will need to balance being comprehensive but also flexible to meet the assortment of purposes of applied and research assessment, including case conceptualization, early identification, prognostic predictions, and treatment planning, monitoring, and evaluation (Kazdin, 2005; Mash & Hunsley, 2005). Likewise, other assessment parameters, such as the optimal amount and duration of assessment and the need for follow-up assessment, will require attention in future EBA research (Mash & Hunsley, 2005).

Issues in the Implementation of Child Assessment Approaches

When conducting child assessment, it is insufficient solely to implement a state-of-the-art approach. Child assessors must also consider important issues that influence the assessment process. Interpretations of assessment data must be filtered accordingly. Although an exhaustive list of implementation issues is beyond the scope of this chapter, four key issues are highlighted. First, an individual child must be assessed within the context of broader developmental theory, taking into account both the continuities and discontinuities of development (Achenbach, 2005). Indeed, the subdiscipline of developmental psychopathology has exerted tremendous influence in how a child assessor formulates child psychopathology and disability within a developmental framework (Yule, 1993).

A second contextual issue that may affect a given child's psychological functioning involves health and medical conditions. Increasingly since the late 1960s, psychologists with interests and training in working with children and families have developed innovative assessment and intervention strategies to serve families challenged by pediatric chronic illness and disability (Spirito & Kazak, 2006). Since Logan Wright's (1967) seminal article defined the pediatric psychologist as a unique subspecialty within applied psychology, the field of pediatric psychology or child health psychology has expanded to include greater numbers of scientist-practitioners, who are working in a larger variety of settings (Goreczny & Hersen, 1999).

Assessing children who experience acute illness, developmental delay or disability, or catastrophic, life-threatening injury or disease requires an appreciation for challenging life circumstances and a developmental and ecological/systems approach (Brown, 2004; Roberts, 2003). For example, understanding and operating effectively as a child assessor in a medical care system is a must for pediatric or child health psychologists (Drotar, 1995). Central features affecting the professional role of a pediatric psychologist include: (a) service provision and research depend strongly on collaboration among psychologists and physicians, (b) the families and children served typically are not psychiatrically disordered, and (c) assessment and intervention strategies are family-focused. Becoming familiar with the experiences of medically involved and developmentally disabled children and their families equips the savvy child assessor to place assessment data in its appropriate ecological context (Fletcher-Janzen & Reynolds, 2003; Graziano, 2002).

Third, throughout the assessment process, child practitioners and researchers must take into account the role of cultural and ethnicity variables (Achenbach, 2005). Many practical considerations of assessing a child from a different cultural and/or linguistic background are reviewed later in this chapter. However, at a broader level, individual differences within the context of cultural and ethnic diversity, even among subcultures within the United States, should be infused into every step of the assessment process (Canino & Spurlock, 2000; Gopaul-McNicol & Thomas-Presswood, 1998). It is also important to recognize that this process is especially intricate because "culture" is dynamic and often changes in response to other demands and needs for adaptation (Carter et al., 2004). The importance of considering diversity cannot be overstated; indeed, culture and ethnicity may not only be considered as possible subtle influences, but also may have major impact on assessment decisions, such as cut-points in EBA (Achenbach, 2005).

Fourth and lastly, improvements in assessment have resulted in earlier identification, and subsequent treatment, of problems in childhood (Carter et al., 2004). Early identification follows directly from advances in developmental psychopathology research, which allows us to understand the complexities of teasing apart psychopathology from typical developmental processes. Such research has also identified trajectories for various developmental processes and how early onset of problems differs from problems with a later onset. One example is the well-established differences between childhood-onset and adolescent-onset Conduct Disorder, the former of which is preceded by an early onset of aggression and irritability and often a previous diagnosis of Oppositional Defiant Disorder (Loeber, 1990). Early identification also has been aided by the expansion of standardized, norm-referenced measures for younger populations. Many child and adolescent instruments have been downwardly extended for use with younger ages and it is becoming common for newly developed measures to include a preschool version, such as the *BRIEF-Preschool Version* (*BRIEF-P*; Gioia et al., 2000).

Nevertheless, early identification of child psychopathology faces many challenges, including rapid developmental shifts in very young children's functioning and abilities, as well as the hesitance of many practitioners or parents to label young children with a psychological diagnosis (Carter et al., 2004). Yet, the preponderance of literature suggests that psychological problems in young children are typically not transient and are usually associated with a continuation of later problems, underscoring the importance of early identification (Briggs-Gowan, Carter, Bosson-Heenan, Guyer, & Horwitz, 2006).

Trends in Child Assessment

We have overviewed a historical perspective and issues germane to the current state-of-the art in child assessment. Now, we direct the reader to our peering into the "crystal ball" of the future for assessing children within their ecological context. Where will our Delorean take us … to new horizons or back to the future? We suggest three trends for the upcoming road-trip of child assessment: (a) the use of technology in assessment administration and scoring/interpretation, (b) the impact of taxometric statistical techniques on diagnoses, and (c) cultural/linguistic considerations.

Use of Technology in Child Assessment Administration

For the past few decades, computer technology has affected several aspects of assessment practices including test administration and scoring/interpretation of test results. With ever-changing and improving technology and security concerns, research has begun to consider these impacts on psychological assessment. Software has been developed for a number of assessment instruments to allow computerized self-administration. For example, the *Parenting Stress Index -3rd Edition* (*PSI-3*; Abidin, 1995), the *ASEBA* (Achenbach & Rescorla, 2000, 2001), and the *MMPI-A* (Butcher et al., 1992) are measures of emotional–behavioral functioning that can be answered at a computer by parents, children, or teachers. In addition, a majority of continuous performance tests for the diagnosis of problems with inattention and impulsivity are computerized, such as the C*onner's Kiddie Continuous Performance Test* (Conners, 2001b), the *Test of Variables of Attention* (*TOVA*; visual version) and *TOVA-A* (auditory version; Greenberg, Leark, Dupuy, Corman, & Kindschi, 2005), and the *Wisconsin Card Sorting Test: Computer version 4* (Heaton, 2005).

Several authors have discussed advantages of computerized administration, such as cost effectiveness (Rew, Horner, Riesch, & Caurin, 2004), increased speed of administration and scoring (Singleton, Horne, & Thomas, 1999), and precise response times for timed subtests (Luciana, 2003). From a data collection perspective of the practitioner or researcher Rew and colleagues (2004) suggested that computerized administration avoids certain assessment process problems possible with paper and pencil methods, such as marking two responses to an item or skipping an item in error. Computerized versions of tests of achievement, cognition, and comprehensive neuropsychological functioning are less common and likely will remain so (Camara, Nathan, & Puente, 2000; Mollica, Maruff, Collie, & Vance, 2005). Comprehensive and frequently used assessments, such as the *WISC-IV, WPPSI-III, NEPSY-II,* or the *Woodcock-Johnson Tests of Achievement* (Woodcock, McGrew, & Mather, 2007) are developed strictly for face-to-face administrations, replete with opportunities for informative behavioral observations.

Only a few studies have evaluated computerized measures of achievement, intellectual, and neuropsychological tasks. For example, Singleton et al. (1999) studied computerized assessment of mathematics ability and literacy and reported good psychometric properties of the computerized version as well as a moderate to good relation with literacy scores obtained by traditional methods 12 months later. Hargreaves, Shorrocks-Taylor, Swinnerton, Tait, and Threlfall (2004) likewise studied computerized assessment of children's mathematics ability and demonstrated similar scores on a computerized version and a traditional pencil and paper test. Luciana (2003) noted strong psychometric properties of the *Cambridge Neuropsychological Testing Automated Battery* (*CANTAB*; http://www.cantab.com) in a pediatric sample. Although Luciana (2003) stated that the use of the *CANTAB* does not replace a human assessor in neuropsychological testing, the use of the computerized assessment does allow for excellent standardization procedures that are not confounded by administrator influences.

Computer-Assisted Survey Interviewing (CASI) is a trendy application of computer administration for interviewing that may be applied to child assessment. CASI allows for presentation of all items in a measure or an altered presentation based on a decision tree formula to prompt follow-up information if a certain item is endorsed. Use of CASI provides a standardized presentation of items and preliminary background information and evaluation data, which then allows for face-to-face follow-up with a human assessor to refine the interview regarding specific areas of concern (McCullough & Miller, 2003).

CASI users report less embarrassment and discomfort with the computer-administered interviews compared to face-to-face interviews, especially if sensitive topics are covered, such as sexual behavior, drug/alcohol/substance use, or health-risk behaviors (McCullough & Miller, 2003; Newman, et al., 2002). Romer et al. (1997) demonstrated that adolescents reported more sexual experience and more favorable responses toward sex, after controlling for reported experience, on a computerized survey than when interviewed face-to-face. Davies and Morgan (2005) reported that the use of CASI designed for "vulnerable" youths in foster care provided a sense of empowerment and confidence to express their ideas, opinions, and concerns about foster home placements. In addition, Rew and colleagues (2004) used headphones to present an audio recording of items and also presented items visually in words on a computer screen, which allowed for non-English speakers and children with lower reading skills to participate. Valla, Bergeron, and Smolla (2000) also considered the issue of potential reading difficulty among young children and devised a diagnostic computerized interview with pictures and audio in different languages. They reported adequate to good psychometric properties for methods in which the interview was presented pictorially and aurally.

Several studies suggest that children prefer a computerized administration format over a face-to-face interview with an adult. In an evaluation of a program applied to forensic interviewing, children reported that they preferred the computerized interactive interview over the face-to-face interview (Powell, Wilson, & Hasty, 2002). Children may prefer the novel—or now more familiar to many children—medium to gather information. In particular, the use of animation and graphics may be a more entertaining method of collecting information relative to an adult interview.

Research findings do not, however, suggest universally positive outcomes of computerized administration of interviews. Connolly (2005) reported that face-to-face interviews elicited more statements that were also selected by participants for further discussion in later sessions. Although Connolly suggested that games and questionnaires often included in computer-assisted interviews might aid in increasing rapport, "They do not replace the need for direct communication with professionals" (p. 412).

Another CASI, designed to measure children's recall of a classroom event, found that most children reported correct responses on recall and were equally verbose in responses to the computer and to an adult interviewer (Donohue et al., 1999). This recall task also tested the children's reporting of a "secret" that occurred during the event. Children did not report the secret more frequently on the computer than with the adult, suggesting that the use of the computer may not create a more comfortable milieu in which to discuss sensitive or personal topics.

Use of Technology in Child Assessment Scoring and Interpretation

More frequently utilized by child assessors—compared to computer administration software—are desktop software or online scoring and interpretation services for many types of assessment (e.g., achievement, cognitive, neuropsychological, behavior, social–emotional). Computer-based test interpretation (CBTI) generally includes programs that use actuarial assessment programs, based on statistical equations, and automated assessment programs. CBTI reports are generated using an "if-then" formula by expert practitioners based on research and experience (Lichtenberger, 2006). Authors have recently noted several important benefits and limitations with CBTI, which predict a further expansion and adaptation of their use in the future.

One advantage of CBTI is the immediacy of receiving data both for individual clients as well as for group data used in research (Davies & Morgan, 2005). These software programs operate very quickly in comparison to personally calculating and looking up scores in tables and manuals. In addition to speed of data availability, the use of CBTI may increase divergent thinking about alternative assessment hypotheses and provide "virtual access to expert practitioners," who wrote the software reports (Harvey & Carlson, 2003, p. 99). In addition, Snyder (2000) offered a summary of benefits from existing literature, including reduction of errors in scoring, minimization of a practitioner's subjectivity or bias in an interpretation, and the ability to store entered information for later research use.

In spite of these benefits, authors have noted several important limitations to using CBTI. First, results produced by CBTI should be detailed enough to have already ruled out several hypotheses, but still be inclusive of possible hypotheses. In a review of several studies, Butcher, Perry, and Atlis (2000) concluded that CBTI reports are similar to results derived from a practitioner. However, CBTI reports should include a level of specificity and detail to avoid the Barnum Effect of giving overly generalizable descriptions that could apply to many people in general. This effect, they report, stems from a line of literature suggesting that people are more likely to report higher levels of accuracy with statements that are nonspecific, especially if those statements are given by an authority figure.

A second major limitation to the use of CBTI is variable validity and reliability evidence to support computer-generated interpretations. Garb (2000) noted that writers of the interpretive reports generated by computers do not always collect criterion information to empirically influence results. He argued that interpretations may come from clinical experience, rather than research findings, to make predictions about behavioral outcomes and generate hypotheses. Also, CBTI reports should be scrutinized for the validity of their report, for example, regarding the comparison group used by the software program and relevant demographic characteristics. Such demographic information may include cultural, linguistic, and economic variables, which are not always accounted for in the computer-generated interpretations (Butcher, et al., 2000, McCullough & Miller, 2003; Moreland, 1985; Snyder, 2000; Harvey & Carlson, 2003).

A lack of psychometric data for many CBTI applications calls into question the trustworthiness of the interpretation for some clinical or research uses. Therefore, proper caution and study is imperative before accepting the results of a given CBTI report. For a more detailed review of validity and reliability issues related to CBTI, please see Snyder (2000).

Both Garb (2000) and Lichtenberger (2006) provided recommendations for CBTI software. Garb (2000) asserted that computer-generated reports are not inappropriate to use, but suggested several recommendations to improve a system of CBTI. For example, information with the highest validity should be considered initially for statistical predictions. In addition, statistical-prediction rules can improve with more collection of criterion information, such as behavior sampling, other psychological testing, and structured interviewing. Lichtenberger (2006) suggested finding an optimal balance between practitioners' need for efficiency due to time limitations and their reliance on CBTI reports. She recommends four considerations for practitioners as they evaluate narrative summaries provided by CBTI to create a psychological report:

1. When evaluating all major hypotheses in a CBTI narrative consider additional data collected for evidence that might support or refute the CBTI hypothesis.
2. Consider alternate hypotheses in addition to those presented in the CBTI narrative. As in Step 1, determine if other evidence from the assessment supports or refutes hypotheses.
3. Review written notes from the assessment and clinical interview to avoid reliance on personal memory, which is subject to bias.

4. When available, use computer-based programs or other prediction formulas to evaluate additional data collected during the assessment that was not considered in the CBTI narrative (Lichtenberger, 2006, pp.27–28).

Lichtenberger (2006) adds that although computer-generated reports can provide important information, the human assessor must respect the uniqueness of the person being evaluated and her or his situation and consider all variables in generating—or concluding about—hypotheses.

Most research suggests a clear trend toward the use of CBTI and technological advances in computerized scoring and interpretation of data. Many potential benefits exist, but proper education about the validity and reliability of these programs is crucial to accurate assessment. In particular, compared to adult-focused assessment, even less is known about CBTI for frequently used child assessment measures. An important direction for future research will be the adaptation of computerized assessments with children and the continuing evaluation of the scoring and interpretation programs for child assessment measures.

Influence of Taxometric Statistical Techniques on Diagnoses

Taxometric research examines the discrete, rather than the continuous, nature of a trait or psychological disorder (Meehl, 1995). Meehl (1995) discovered a particular taxon, schizotaxia, which led to the diagnosis of schizophrenia in a certain subset of people evaluated.

Although Meehl's methods have experienced limited application in child assessment research, Beauchaine (2003) noted three important areas for future taxometric research. First, taxometrics could be useful in the early identification of children at risk for psychopathology. For example, studies have demonstrated links of family history of psychiatric symptoms and a temperament trait of behavioral reactivity as indicators of psychopathology later in childhood or adulthood.

For example, Woodward, Lenzenweger, Kagen, Snidman, and Arcus (2000) reported a High Reactivity (HR) taxon in young infants that showed qualitative differences measured by time spent crying, back arching, hyperextension of limbs, and leg movements. Later behavioral differences (e.g., smiling less, and less spontaneous comments to an unfamiliar adult) at 4.5 years were found for infants who were classified in the HR taxon. An empirical determination of these taxa could aid in early intervention techniques to target the onset and severity of a possible psychological disorder in a person's developmental history.

Second, taxometric research could aid in determining subtypes of current diagnoses, such as childhood-onset and adolescent-onset depression. Another example might involve the nature of Autistic Disorder, Pervasive Developmental Disorder, and Asperger's Disorder as discrete diagnoses versus a continuum known as Autism Spectrum Disorders with various subtypes. An additional example might include further empirical validation of the discreteness of the three subtypes of Attention-Deficit/Hyperactivity Disorder, in particular distinctions between ADHD, Combined Type and ADHD, Predominately Inattentive Type. Two groups of researchers have reported a rejection of a categorical representation of the core symptoms of ADHD (Frazier, Youngstrom, & Angle, 2007; Haslam, Williams, Prior, Haslam, Graetz, & Sawyer, 2006); however, further research is still needed to replicate these findings. Taxometric research may also clarify variations over the past several decades in the use of diagnoses such as childhood schizophrenia, childhood psychosis, and childhood bipolar disorder.

Lastly, Beauchaine (2003) noted that adult research has demonstrated discrete taxa for schizotypy, dissociative experiences, and psychopathology. However, he argued that currently the research literature is insufficient to determine the viability of a sensitive period when these traits first emerge. Although very few taxometric studies have been completed with children, two studies demonstrated the presence of taxa related to antisocial behavior based on self-report measures. These taxa indicated broad, long-term antisocial behavior as well as psychopathy (Skilling, Quinsey, & Craig, 2001; Vasey, Kotov, Frick, & Loney, 2005). Taxometic research could elucidate time periods in development for these emerging traits, with benefits being earlier, more effective, and more precisely tailored interventions.

Cultural/Linguistic Considerations in Child Assessment

An important trend in the best practices of assessment involves research and resources regarding assessment of a child who is bilingual and/or has limited English proficiency. One assessment approach with these children, especially those from different cultures or who speak English as a second language, has been to translate versions of the assessment instrument in a child's first language or to complete the English version assessment with an interpreter present. Valencia and Suzuki (2001) and Kamphaus (1993) argued these translations/interpretations may produce assessments that are not clear in the second language (poorly translated/ interpreted), may measure different constructs than the English version, and may not consider or provide appropriate regional dialects for various languages. Most importantly, newly constructed assessments—even if they are translations from English versions—should still be held to the rigor of psychometric evaluation. One may not assume that a translated version demonstrates the same psychometric properties of the English version. In addition, Fives and Flanagan (2002) asserted that although several of the well-studied, verbal intelligence tests have demonstrated limited test bias for special populations even in translated forms, intelligence testing with populations of limited communication abilities may yield more a measure of English proficiency than intelligence per se.

Current recommendations for assessing multilingual children are addressed by Ochoa (2003). For academic achievement assessment, child assessors are encouraged to use multiple methods of alternative assessment, such as school records, observations, performance assessments, and samples of the child's work or portfolio. For intellectual assessment, Ochoa (2003) suggests that current standardized measures of intelligence (e.g., *WISC-IV*; Wechsler, 2003), frequently given in English, should only be administered if the student demonstrates an acceptable Cognitive Academic Language Proficiency (CALP) in English.

Alternatives to verbally loaded intellectual assessment are tests of nonverbal intelligence, such as the *Universal Nonverbal Intelligence Test* (Bracken & McCallum, 1998) and the *Leiter International Performance Scale-Revised* (Roid & Miller, 2002), which focus on less verbally loaded, performance-based assessment. Proponents (e.g., Bracken & Naglieri, 2003; McCallum, Bracken, & Wasserman, 2001; Naglieri, 2003; Roid, Nellis, & McLellan 2003) of nonverbal measures of cognitive abilities argue that a de-emphasis on verbally loaded directions and items creates tests appropriate for special populations who may not understand spoken language or be able to use verbal communication. In addition, these assessments are judged to be less culturally weighted because they use universal pictorial images in items and universal signs of nonverbal communication (e.g., shaking head from side to side to indicate a negative response or "no") in directions.

However, a major weakness for some of these nonverbal tests is that although the participant may respond nonverbally to the task, the directions—and sometimes the items—are administered verbally, meaning receptive language is necessary for understanding the task. For children who have learned English as a second language or who are hearing- or speech-impaired, the validity of obtained scores may be questionable because the verbal directions were not clear to the child. Such assessment practices may result in misdiagnosis or inappropriate placement into certain service or education programs (Fives & Flanagan, 2002; McCallum et al., 2001; Valencia & Suzuki, 2001). In addition, some controversy exists regarding the nature of intellectual abilities measured by these nonverbal tests. Some researchers argue that these instruments measure a separate construct known as nonverbal intelligence or nonverbal abilities (Kamphaus, 1993; McCallum, et al., 2001). However, other researchers argue that whether tested verbally or nonverbally (or with both methods) measures of intelligence tap into the same general ability (Naglieri, 2003). This trend in intellectual assessment will likely continue in a controversial fashion.

Another trend in the assessment of bilingual children is the creation of the *Bilingual Verbal Ability Test* (*BVAT*; Munoz-Sandoval, Cummins, Alvarado, & Reuf, 1998). The BVAT incorporates three subtests of verbal ability that are first administered in English. Items answered incorrectly are later presented in the child's native language, with credit being earned if the child correctly answers the item. The combined score yields a measure of bilingual verbal ability. In addition to this score, the BVAT can be used to obtain a CALP and an aptitude score that can be compared to collected measures of achievement (Rhodes, Ochoa, & Ortiz, 2005). However, continued research regarding the psychometric properties of the *BVAT* is needed. Interested readers in this trend are encouraged to review Bracken (2004), Barona and Garcia (1990), Thomas and Grimes (1990), and Rhodes et al. (2005). Cultural competence of child assessors clearly will be emphasized for some time to come (Ecklund & Johnson, 2007)

EPILOGUE

Continuing research into the development of childhood disorders will shed light on future versions of the *Diagnostic and Statistical Manual–IV–TR* (American Psychiatric Association, 2000) and on less diagnosis-focused assessment (Kamphaus & Campbell, 2006). Of course a goal of such research will be to enhance the accuracy, utility, and predictive quality of assessment of child psychopathology and developmental disabilities. The future of child assessment seems bright, indeed. Certainly, the chapters that follow in this volume will shine and illuminate your path as a child assessor.

REFERENCES

Abidin, R. R. (1995). *Parenting stress index* (3rd ed.). Lutz, FL: Psychological Assessment Resources.

Achenbach, T. M. (2005). Advancing assessment of children and adolescents: Commentary on evidence-based assessment of child and adolescent disorders. *Journal of Clinical Child and Adolescent Psychology, 34,* 541–547.

Achenbach, T. M., & Rescorla, L. A. (2000). *Manual for the ASEBA Preschool Forms and Profiles: An integrated system for multi-informant assessemnt.* Burlington, VT: University of Vermont, Research Center for Children, Youth, and Families.

Achenbach, T. M., & Rescorla, L. A. (2001). *Manual for the ASEBA Preschool Forms and Profiles: An integrated system for multi-informant assessment.* Burlington, VT: University of Vermont, Research Center for Children, Youth, and Families.

American Educational Research Association, American Psychological Association, & National Council on Measurement in Education. (1999). *Standards for educational and psychological testing.* Washington, DC: American Educational Research Association.

American Psychiatric Association. (2000). Diagnostic and statistical manual of mental disorders: Text revision (DSM–IV–TR) (4th ed.). Washington, DC: Author.

American Psychological Association. (1950). Ethical standards for the distribution of psychological tests and diagnostic aids. *American Psychologist, 5,* 620–626.

American Psychological Association. (1953). *Ethical standards of psychologists.* Washington, DC: Author.

American Psychological Association. (1959). Ethical standards of psychologists. *American Psychologist, 14,* 279–282.

American Psychological Association. (1986). *Guidelines for computer-based tests and interpretations.* Washington, DC: Author.

American Psychological Association. (1990). *Guidelines for providers of psychological services to ethnic, linguistic, and culturally diverse populations.* Washington, DC: Author.

American Psychological Association. (1994). Guidelines for child custody evaluations in divorce. *American Psychologist, 49,* 677–680.

American Psychological Association (2000). *Report of the task force on test user qualifications.* Washington, DC: Author.

American Psychological Association. (2002a). Ethical principles of psychologists and code of conduct. *American Psychologist, 57,* 1060–1073.

American Psychological Association. (2002b). *Guidelines on multicultural education, training, research, practice, and organizational change for psychologists.* Washington, DC: Author.

American Psychological Association. (2003). *Code for fair testing practices.* Washington, DC: Author.

American Psychological Association Committee on Professional Practice and Standards. (1993). Record keeping guidelines. *American Psychologist, 48,* 984–986.

American Psychological Association Committee on Professional Practice and Standards. (1994). Guidelines for child custody evaluations in divorce proceedings. *American Psychologist, 49,* 677–680.

American Psychological Association Committee on Psychological Tests and Assessment. (1996). Statement on disclosure of test data. *American Psychologist, 51,* 644–668.

American Psychological Association Joint Committee on Testing Practices. (1998). The rights and responsibilities of test takers: Guidelines and expectations. Washington, DC: Author.

Anderten, P., Staulcup, V., Grisso, T. (2003). On being ethical in legal places. In D.N.Bersoff (Ed.). *Ethical conflicts in psychology* (3rd ed.) (pp. 512–513). Washington, DC: American Psychological Assoociation.

Barona, A., & Garcia, E. E. (1990). *Children at risk: Poverty, minority status, and other issues in educational equity.* Washington, DC: National Association of School Psychologists.

Beauchaine, T. P. (2003). Taxometrics and developmental psychopathology. *Development and Psychopathology, 15,* 501–527.

Benson, E. (2003a). Intelligent intelligence testing. *Monitor on Psychology, 24 (2),* 48–51.

Benson, E. (2003b). Breaking new ground. *Monitor on Psychology, 24 (2),* 52–54.

Benson, E. (2003c). Intelligence across cultures. *Monitor on Psychology, 24 (2),* 56–58.

Bersoff, D. N. (2003). HIPAA: Federal regulations of healthcare records. In D. N.Bersoff (Ed.). *Ethical conflicts in psychology* (3rd ed., pp. 526–528). Washington, DC: American Psychological Assoociation.

Boake, C. (2002). From the Binet–Simon to the Weschler–Bellevue: Tracing the history of intelligence testing. *Journal of Clinical and Experimental Neuropsychology, 42,* 383–405.

Bracken, B. (2004). *The psychoeducational assessment of preschool children* (3rd ed.). Mahwah, NJ: Lawrence Erlbaum.

Bracken, B. A., & McCallum, R. S. (1998). *Universal Nonverbal Intelligence Test.* Itasca, IL: Riverside.

Bracken, B. A., & Naglieri, J. A. (2003). Assessing diverse populations with nonverbal tests of general intelligence. In C. R. Reynolds & R. W. Kamphaus (Eds.), *Handbook of psychological & educational assessment of children: Intelligence, aptitude, and achievement* (pp. 243–274). New York: Guilford Press.

Briggs-Gowan, M. J., Carter, A. S., Bosson-Heenan, J., Guyer, A. E., & Horwitz, S. M. (2006). Are infant-toddler social-emotional and behavioral problems transient? *Journal of the American Academy of Child and Adolescent Psychiatry, 45,* 849–858.

Brown, R.T. (Ed.). (2004). *Handbook of pediatric psychology in school setting.* Cambridge, MA: Lawrence Erlbaum.

Butcher, J. N., Perry, J. N., & Atlis, M. M.(2000). Validity and utility of computer-based test interpretation. *Psychological Assessment, 12,* 6–18.

Butcher, J. N., Williams, C. L., Graham, J. R., Archer, R. P., Tellegen, A., & Ben-Porath, Y. S. (1992). *Minnesota Multiphasic Personality Inventory – Adolescent: Manual for administration, scoring, and interpretation.* Minneapolis: University of Minnesota Press.

Camara, W. J., Nathan, J. S., & Puente, A. E. (2000). Psychological test usage: Implications in professional psychology. *Professional Psychology: Research and Practice, 31,* 141–154.

Campbell, S. B. (2002). Behavior problems in preschool children: Clinical and developmental issues (2nd ed.). New York: Guilford Press.

Canino, I. A., & Spurlock, J. (2000). Culturally diverse children and adolescents: Assessment, diagnosis, and treatment (2nd ed.). New York: Guilford Press.

Carter, A. S., Briggs-Gowan, M. J., & Davis, N. O. (2004). Assessment of young children's social-emotional development and psychopathology: Recent advances and recommendations for practice. *Journal of Child Psychology and Psychiatry, 45,* 109–134.

Cellucci, A., & Heffer, R. W. (2001, August). *The role of training clinics in training ethical practices.* In R. Hawkins (Chair), Witmer's psychology clinic version 2001: Bridging science, practice & the community. *Symposium at the Continuing Education Workshop of the Association of Directors of Psychology Training Clinics,* San Francisco, CA.

Cohen, M. J. (1997). *Children's Memory Scale.* San Antonio, TX: The Psychological Corporation.

Conners, C. K. (2001a). *Conners Rating Scales-Revised; Technical manual.* New York: Mental Health Systems.

Conners, C. K. (2001b). *Conners' Kiddie Continuous Performance Test (K–CPT).* North Tonawanda, NY: MultiHealth Systems.

Connolly, P. (2005). Children, assessments, and computer-assisted interviewing. *Child Abuse Review, 14,* 407–414.

D'Amato, R. C., Fletcher-Janzen, E., & Reynolds, C. R. (Eds.). (2005). *Handbook of school psychology.* New York: John Wiley and Sons.

Davies, M., & Morgan, A. (2005). Using computer-assisted self-interviewing question-naires to facilitate consultation and participation with vulnerable young people. *Child Abuse Review, 14,* 389–406.

Dishion, T. J., & Stormshak, E. A. (2007). Ecological assessment. In T. J. Dishion & E. A. Stormshak (Eds.). *Intervening in children's lives: An ecological, family-centered approach to mental health care* (pp. 91–107). Washington, DC: American Psychological Association.

Donohue, A., Powell, M. B., & Wilson, J. C. (1999). The effects of computerised interview on children's recall of an event. *Computers in Human Behavior, 15,* 747–761.

Drotar, D. D. (1999). Consulting with pediatricians: Psychological perspectives. New York: Plenum Press.

Ecklund, K., & Johnson, W. B. (2007). The impact of a culture-sensitive intake assessment on the treatment of a depressed biracial child. *Clinical Case Studies, 6(6),* 468–482.

Edens, J. F., & Cahill, M. A. (2007). Psychopathy in adolescence and criminal recidivism in young adulthood. *Assessment,14,* 57–64.

Fagan, T. K. & Wise, P. S. (1994). *School psychology past, present, and future.* New York: Longman.

Field, C. E., Nash, H. M., Handwerk, M. L., & Friman, P. C. (2004). Using functional assessment and experimental functional analysis to individualize treatment for adolescents in a residential care setting. *Clinical Case Studies, 3,* 25–36.

Fisher, C. B. (2003), *Decoding the ethics code: A practical guide for psychologists.* Thousand Oaks, CA: Sage.

Fives, C. J., & Flanagan, R. (2002). A review of the universal nonverbal intelligence test (UNIT): An advance for evaluating youngsters with diverse needs. *School Psychology International, 23(4),* 425–448.

Fletcher, J. M., Francis, D. J., Morris, R. D., & Lyon, G. R. (2005). Evidence-based assessment of learning disabilities in children and adolescents. *Journal of Clinical Child and Adolescent Psychology, 34,* 506–522.

Fletcher-Fanzen, E., & Reynolds, C. R. (2003). *Childhood disorders diagnostic desk reference.* New York: John Wiley and Sons.

Frazier, T. W., Youngstrom, E. A., & Naugle, R. I. (2007). The latent structure of Attention Deficit/Hyperactivity Disorder in a clinic-referred sample. *Neuropsychology, 21,* 45–64.

Garb, H. N. (2000). Computers will become increasingly important for psychological assessment: Not that there's anything wrong with that! *Psychological Assessment, 12,* 31–39.

Gioia, G. A., Isquith, P. K., Guy, S. C., & Kenworthy, L. (2000). *Behavior rating inventory of executive function.* Lutz, FL: Psychological Assessment Resources.

Gopaul-McNicol, S., & Thomas-Presswood, T. (1998). Working with linguistically and culturally different children: Innovative clinical and educational approaches. Boston: Allyn and Bacon.

Goreczny, A. J., & Hersen, M. (1999). *Handbook of pediatric and adolescent health psychology.* Boston: Allyn and Bacon.

Graziano, A. M. (2002). Developmental disabilities: Introduction to a diverse field. Boston: Allyn and Bacon.

Greenberg, L. M., Leark, R. A., Dupuy, T. R., Corman, C. L., & Kinschi, C. L. (2005). *Test of Variables of Attention (TOVA/TOVA–A: Professional Manual.* Lutz, FL: Psychological Assessment Resources.

Gregory, R.J. (2007). Psychological testing: History, principles, and applications (5th ed.). Boston: Allyn and Bacon.

Habenstein, R., & Olson, R.A. (2001). Families and children in history. In C. E. Walker & M. C. Roberts (Eds.). *Handbook of clinical child psychology* (3rd ed., pp. 3–19). New York: John Wiley and Sons.

Handler, L. (2007). The use of therapeutic assessment with children and adolescents. In S. R. Smith & L. Handler (Eds). *The clinical assessment of children and adolescents: A practitioner handbook* (pp.53–72). Mahwah, NJ: Lawrence Erlbaum.

Hargreaves, M., Shorrocks-Taylor, D., Swinnerton, B., Tait, K., & Threlfall, J. (2004). Computer or paper? That is the question: Does the medium in which assessment questions are presented affect children's performance in mathematics? *Educational Research, 46,* 29–42.

Harvey, V. S., & Carlson, J. F. (2003). Ethical and professional issues with computer-related technology. *School Psychology Review, 32,* 92–107.

Haslam, N., Williams, B., Prior, M., Haslam, R., Graetz, B., & Sawyer, M. (2006). The latent structure of attention-deficit/hyperactivity disorder: A taxometric analysis. *Australian and New Zealand Journal of Psychiatry, 40,* 639–647.

Hays, J. R., Sutter, E. G., McPherson, R. H. (2002). *Texas mental health law: A sourcebook for mental health professionals.* Houston: Bayou.

Heaton, R.K. (2005). *The Wisconsin Card Sorting Test: Computer Version 4.* Lutz, FL: Psychological Assessment Resources.

Heffer, R. W., Lane, M. M., & Snyder, D. K. (2003). Therapeutic family assessment: A systems approach. In K. Jordan (Ed.), *Handbook of couple and family assessment* (pp. 21–47). New York: Prentice-Hall.

Heffer, R. W., & Oxman, D. L. (2003). A developmental-family systems approach to adolescent assessment. In K. Jordan (Ed.), *Handbook of couple and family assessment* (pp. 67–108). New York: Prentice-Hall.

Heffer, R. W., & Snyder, D. K. (1998). Comprehensive assessment of family functioning. In L. L'Abate (Ed.), *Family psychopathology: The relational roots of dysfunctional behavior* (pp. 207–235). New York: Guilford Press.

Heilbronner, R. L. (2007). American Academy of Clinical Neuropsychology (AACN) practice guidelines for neuropsychological assessment and consultation. *Clinical Neuropsychologist, 21,* 209–231.

Hobbs, N. (1951). Report of the American Psychological Association's Committee on Ethical Standards for Psychology to the Council of Representatives. Washington, DC: American Psychological Association.

Horner, R. H. (1994). Functional assessment: Contributions and future directions. *Journal of Applied Behavior Analysis, 27,* 401–404.

House, A.E. (1999). *DSM–IV diagnosis in the schools.* New York: Guilford Press.

Kamphaus, R.W. (1993). *Clinical assessment of children's intelligence.* Boston: Allyn and Bacon.

Kamphaus, R. W., & Campbell, J. M. (Eds.). (2006). *Psychodiagnostic assessment of children: Dimensional and categorical approaches.* New York: John Wiley and Sons.

Kamphaus, R. W., & Frick, P. J. (2005). *Clinical assessment of child and adolescent personality and behavior* (2nd ed.). New York: Springer Science-Business Media.

Kamphaus, R. W., Petoskey, M. D., & Rowe, E. W. (2000). Current trends in psychological testing of children. *Professional Psychology: Research and Practice, 31,* 155–164.

Kamps, D., Wendland, M., & Culpepper, M. (2006). Active teacher participation in functional behavior assessment for students with emotional and behavioral disorders risks in general education classrooms. *Behavioral Disorders, 31,* 128–146.

Kazdin, A. E. (2005). Evidence-based assessment for children and adolescents: Issues in measurement development and clinical application. *Journal of Clinical Child and Adolescent Psychology, 34,* 548–558.

Kelley, M. F., & Surbeck, E. (2004). History of preschool assessment. In B.A. Bracken (Ed.), *The psychoeducational assessment of preschool children* (3rd ed., pp. 1–18). Mahwah, NJ: Lawrence Erlbaum.

Klein, D. N., Dougherty, L. R., & Olino, T. M. (2005). Toward guidelines for evidence-based assessment of depression in children and adolescents. *Journal of Clinical Child and Adolescent Psychology, 34,* 412–432.

Korkman, M. (1999). Applying Luria's diagnostic principles in the neuropsychological assessment of children. *Neuropsychology Review, 9,* 89–105.

Korkman, S. L., Kirk, U., & Kemp, M. (2007). *NEPSY: A Developmental Neuropsychological Assessment* (2nd ed.). San Antonio, TX: Harcourt.

Lachar, D. (2004). The Personality Inventory for Children, Second Edition (PIC-2), the Personality Inventory for Youth (PIY), and the Student Behavior Survey (SBS*).* In M. Hersen (Ed.), *Comprehensive handbook of psychological assessment* (pp. 192–212). New York: John Wiley and Sons.

LaGreca, A. M., Kuttler, A. F., & Stone, W. L. (2001). Assessing children through interviews and behavioral observations. In C. E. Walker & M. C. Roberts (Eds.), *Handbook of clinical child psychology* (3rd ed., pp. 90–110). New York: John Wiley and Sons.

Lefaivre, M. J., Chambers, C. T., & Fernandez, C. V. (2007). Offering parents feedback on the results of psychological testing conducted for research purposes with children: Ethical issues and recommendations. *Journal of Clinical Child and Adolescent Psychology, 36,* 242–252.

Lichtenberger, E. O. (2006). Computer utilization and clinical judgment in psychological assessment reports. *Journal of Clinical Psychology, 62,* 19–32.

Loeber, R. (1990). Development and risk factors of juvenile antisocial behavior and delinquency. *Clinical Psychology Review, 10,* 1–42.

Long, C. E., Blackman, J. A., Farrell, W. J., Smolkin, M. E., & Conaway, M. R. (2005). A comparison of developmental versus functional assessment in the rehabilitation of young children. *Pediatric Rehabilitation, 8,* 156–161.

Luciana, M. (2003). Practitioner review: Computerized assessment of neuropsychological function in children: Clinical and research applications of the Cambridge Neuropsychological Testing Automated Battery (CANTAB). *Journal of Child Psychology and Psychiatry, 44,* 649–663.

Mash, E. J., & Hunsley, J. (2005). Evidence-based assessment of child and adolescent disorders: Issues and challenges. *Journal of Clinical Child and Adolescent Psychology, 34,* 362–379.

Matson, J. L., & Minshawi, N. F. (2007). Functional assessment of challenging behavior: Toward a strategy for applied settings. *Research in Developmental Disabilities, 28,* 353–361.

McCallum, S. (Ed.), *Handbook of nonverbal assessment.* (pp. 175–188). New York: Kluwer Academic Plenum.

McCallum, S., Bracken, B., & Wasserman, J. (2001) *Essentials of nonverbal assessment.* New York: John Wiley & Sons.

McCullough, C. S., & Miller, D. C. (2003). Computerized assessment. In C. R. Reynolds & R. W. Kamphaus (Eds.). *Handbook of psychological and educational assessment of children: Intelligence, aptitude, and achievement* (2nd ed., pp. 628–670). New York: Guilford Press.

McMahon, R. J., & Frick, P. J. (2005). Evidence-based assessment of conduct problems in children and adolescents. *Journal of Clinical Child and Adolescent Psychology, 34,* 477–505.

McReynolds, P. (1996). Lightner Witmer: A centennial tribute. *American Psychologist, 51,* 237–243.

Meehl, P. E. (1995). Bootstraps taxometrics: Solving the classification problem in psychopathology. *American Psychologist, 50,* 266–275.

Melton, G. B., Ehrenreich, N. S., & Lyons, P. M. (2001). Ethical and legal issues in mental health services to children. In C. E. Walker & M. C. Roberts (Eds.), *Handbook of clinical child psychology* (3rd ed., pp. 1074–1093). New York: John Wiley and Sons.

Moes, D. R., & Frea, W. D. (2002). Contextualized behavioral support in early intervention for children with autism and their families. *Journal of Autism and Developmental Disorders, 32,* 519–533.

Mollica, C. M., Maruff, P., Collie, A., & Vance, A. (2005). Repeated assessment of cognition in children and the measurement of performance change. *Child Neuropsychology, 11,* 303–310.

Moreland, K. L. (1985). Validation of computer-based test interpretations: Problems and prospects. *Journal of Consulting and Clinical Psychology, 53,* 816–825.

Morey, L. C. (1991). *Personality Assessment Inventory - Professional Manual*. Lutz, FL: Psychological Assessment Resources.

Morey, L. C. (1996). An interpretive guide to the Personality Assessment Inventory and the PAI Structural Summary Booklet. Lutz, FL: Psychological Assessment Resources.

Morey, L. C. (2003). *Essentials of PAI assessment*. New York: John Wiley & Sons.

Morey, L. C. (2007). Personality Assessment Inventory-Adolescent: Professional manual. New York: John Wiley & Sons.

Munoz-Sandoval, A. F., Cummins, J., Alvarado, C. G., & Reuf, M. L. (1998). *The bilingual verbal ability test*. Itasca, IL: Riverside.

Naglieri, J.A. (2003). Naglieri nonverbal ability tests: NNAT and MAT-EF. In R. S. McCallum (Ed.), *Handbook of nonverbal assessment* (pp. 241–258). New York: Kluwer Academic/Plenum.

Naglieri, J. A., Drasgow, F., Schmit, M., Handler, L., Prifitera, A., Margolis, A., & Velasquez, R. (2004). Psychological testing on the internet: New problems, old issues. *American Psychologist, 59*, 150–162.

Nagy, T. (2000). *Ethics in plain English: An illustrative casebook for psychologists*. New York: American Psychological Association.

National Association of School Psychologists. (2007). *NASP toolkit: Assessment alternatives under IDEA 2004*. Bethesda, MD: Author.

National Council on Measurement in Education. (2004.) *Code of fair testing practices in education*. Washington, DC: Joint Committee on Testing Practices.

Newman, J. C., Des Jarlais, D. C., Turner, C. F., Gribble, J., Cooley, P., & Paone, D. (2002). The differential effects of face-to-face and computer interview modes. *Research and Practice, 92*, 294–297.

Nuttal, E. V., Romero, I., & Kalesnik, J. (Eds.). (1992). *Assessing and screening preschoolers: Psychological and educational dimensions*. Boston: Allyn and Bacon.

Ochoa, S.H. (2003). Assessment of culturally and linguistically diverse children. In C. R. Reynolds & R. W. Kamphaus (Eds.). *Handbook of psychological and educational assessment of children: Intelligence, aptitude, and achievement* (2nd ed., pp. 563–583). New York: Guilford Press.

Pelham, W. E., Fabiano, G. A., & Massetti, G. M. (2005). Evidence-based assessment of attention deficit hyperactivity disorder in children and adolescents. *Journal of Clinical Child and Adolescent Psychology, 34*, 449–476.

Piaget, J. (1970). Piaget's theory. In P. H. Mussen (Ed.), *Manual of child psychology* (3rd ed., Vol. 1). New York: John Wiley and Sons.

Piaget, J. (1971). *The construction of reality in the child*. New York: Ballantine.

Powell, M. B., Wilson, J. C., & Hasty, M. K. (2002). Evaluation of the usefulness of 'Marvin'; A computerized assessment tool for investigative interviewers of children. *Computers in Human Behavior, 18*, 577–592.

Rae, W. A., & Fournier, C. J. (1999). Ethical and legal issues in the treatment of children and families. In S. W. Russ & T. H. Ollendick (Eds.), *Handbook of psychotherapies with children and families*. (pp. 67–83). New York: Kluwer Academic/Plenum.

Rapoport, J. L., & Ismond, D. R. (1996). *DSM–IV training guide for diagnosis of childhood disorders*. New York: Brunner/Mazel.

Rew, L., Horner, S. D., Riesch, L., & Cauvin, R. (2004). Computer-assisted survey interviewing of school-age children. *Advances in Nursing Science, 27(2)*, 129–137.

Reynolds, C. R., & Kamphaus, R. W. (2004). *Behavioral assessment system for children (BASC–2)*. Circle Pines, MN: AGS.

Reynolds, W. M. (1998a). Adolescent Psychopathology Scale: Administration and interpretation manual. Lutz, FL: Psychological Assessment Resources.

Reynolds, W. M. (1998b). *Adolescent Psychopathology Scale: Psychometric and technical manual*. Lutz, FL: Psychological Assessment Resources.

Reynolds, W. M. (2000). *Adolescent Psychopathology Scale-Short Form professional manual*. Lutz, FL: Psychological Assessment Resources.

Reynolds, W. M. (2001). Reynolds Adolescent Adjustment Screening Inventory professional manual. Lutz, FL: Psychological Assessment Resources.

Rhodes, R. L., Ochoa, S. H., & Ortiz, S. O. (2005). *Assessing culturally and linguistically diverse students: A practical guide*. New York: Guilford Press.

Roberts, M. C. (Ed.). (2003). *Handbook of pediatric psychology* (3rd ed.). New York: Guilford Press.

Rodrigue, J. R., Geffkin, G. R., Streisand, R. M. (2000). *Child health assessment: A handbook of measurement techniques.* Boston: Allyn and Bacon.

Roid, G. H., & Miller, L. J. (2002). *Leiter International Performance Scale-Revised.* Lutz, FL: Psychological Assessment Resources.

Roid, G., Nellis, L., & McLellan, M. (2003). Assessment with the Leiter International Performance Scale–Revised and the S-BIT. In R. S. McCallum (Ed.), *Handbook of nonverbal assessment.* (pp. 113–141). New York: Kluwer Academic/Plenum.

Romer, D., Hornki, R., Stanton, B., Black, M., Li, X., Ricardo, I., & Feigelman, S. (1997). "Talking" computers: A reliable and private method to conduct interviews on sensitive topics with children. *The Journal of Sex Research, 34,* 3–9.

Sattler, J. M. (1998). Clinical and forensic interviewing of children and families: Guidelines for the mental health, education, pediatric, and child maltreatment fields. San Diego: Jerome M. Sattler.

Sattler, J. M. (2006). *Assessment of children: Behavioral, social, and clinical foundations* (5th ed.). San Diego: Jerome M. Sattler.

Sattler, J. M. (2008). *Assessment of children: Cognitive applications* (5th ed.). San Diego: Jerome M. Sattler.

Schacht, T. E. (2001). Issues in the forensic evaluation of children and youth. In Vance, H. B., & Pumariega, A. J. (Eds.), *Clinical assessment of child and adolescent behavior* (pp. 98–119). New York: John Wiley and Sons.

Schaffer, A. B. (2001). Forensic evaluations of children and expert witness testimony. In C. E. Walker & M. C. Roberts (Eds.), *Handbook of clinical child psychology* (3rd ed., pp. 1094–1119). New York: John Wiley and Sons.

Schroeder, C. S., & Gordon, B. N. (2002). *Assessment and treatment of childhood problems: A clinician's guide* (2nd ed.). New York: Guilford Press.

Shaffer, D., Lucas, C. P., Ritchers, J. E. (Eds.). (1999). *Diagnostic assessment in child and adolescent psychopathology.* New York: Guilford Press.

Shapiro, E. S., & Kratochwill, T. R. (Eds.). (2000). *Conducting school-based assessments of child and adolescent behavior.* New York: Guilford Press.

Shattuck, R. (1994). *The forbidden experiment: The story of the wild boy of Aveyron.* New York: Kadansha International.

Sheridan, S. M. (2005). State of the art research in academic and behavioral assessment and intervention. *School Psychology Review, 34,* 1–8.

Shuman, D. W. (2004). *Law & mental health professionals: Texas.* Washington, DC: American Psychological Association.

Silverman, W. K., & Ollendick, T. H. (2005). Evidence-based assessment of anxiety and its disorders in children and adolescents. *Journal of Clinical Child and Adolescent Psychology, 34,* 380–411.

Singleton, C., Horne, J., & Thomas, K. (1999). Computerised baseline assessment of literacy. *Journal of Research in Reading, 22,* 67–80.

Skilling, T. A., Quinsey, V. L., & Craig, W. M. (2001). Evidence of a taxon underlying serious antisocial behavior in boys. *Criminal Justice and Behavior, 28,* 450–470.

Snyder, D. K. (2000). Computer-assisted judgment: Defining strengths and liabilities. *Psychological Assessment, 12,* 52–60.

Snyder, D. K., Cavell, T. A., Heffer, R. W., & Mangrum, L. F. (1995). Marital and family assessment: A multifaceted, multilevel approach. In R. H. Mikesell, D. D. Lusterman, & S. H. McDaniel (Eds.), *Family psychology and systems theory: A handbook* (pp. 163–182). Washington, DC: American Psychological Association.

Spirito, A., & Kazak, A. E. (2006). *Effective and emerging treatments in pediatric psychology.* New York: Oxford University Press.

Stahr, B., Cushing, D., Lane, K., & Fox, J. (2006). Efficacy of a function-based intervention in decreasing off-task behavior exhibited by a student with ADHD. *Journal of Positive Behavior Interventions, 8,* 201–211.

Swender, S. L., Matson, J. L., Mayville, S. B., Gonzalez, M. L., & McDowell, D. (2006). A functional assessment of handmouthing among persons with severe and profound intellectual disability. *Journal of Intellectual & Developmental Disability, 31,* 95–100.

Thomas, A., & Grimes, J. (1990). *Best practices in school psychology II.* Washington, DC: National Association of School Psychologists.

Turner, S. M., Demers, S. T., Fox, H. R., & Reed, G. M. (2001). APA's guidelines for test user qualifications. *American Psychologist, 56,* 1099–1113.

Valencia, R. R., Suzuki, L. A. (2001). Intelligence testing and minority students: foundations, performance factors, and assessment issues. Thousand Oaks: Sage.

Valla, J. P., Bergeron, L., & Smolla, N. (2000). The Dominic-R pictorial interview for 6- to 11-year-old children. *Journal of American Academy of Child and Adolescent Psychiatry, 39,* 85–93.

Vance, H. B., & Pumariega, A. J. (2001). *Clinical assessment of child and adolescent behavior.* New York: John Wiley and Sons.

Varni, J. W., Limbers, C. A., & Burwinkle, T. M. (2007a). Parent proxy-report of their children's health-related quality of life: An analysis of 13,878 parents' reliability and validity across age subgroups using the PedsQL™ 4.0 Generic Core Scales. *Health and Quality of Life Outcomes, 5(2),* 1–10.

Varni, J. W., Limbers, C. A., & Burwinkle, T. M. (2007b). Impaired health-related quality of life in children and adolescents with chronic conditions: A comparative analyses of 10 disease clusters and 33 disease categories/severities utilizing the PedsQL™ 4.0 Generic Core Scales. *Health and Quality of Life Outcomes, 5(43),* 1–15.

Vasey, M. W., Kotov, R., Frick, P. J., & Loney, B. R. (2005). The latent structure of psychopathy in youth: A taxometric investigation. *Journal of Abnormal Child Psychology, 33,* 411–429.

Watson, T. S., Ray, K. P., Turner, H. S., & Logan, P. (1999). Teacher-implemented functional analysis and treatment: A method for linking assessment to intervention. *School Psychology Review, 28,* 292–302.

Wechsler, D. (2003). *Wechsler Intelligence Scale for Children – fourth edition.* San Antonio, TX: Psychological Corporation.

Williams, M. A., & Boll, T. J. (1997). Recent advances in neuropsychological assessment of children. In G. Goldstein & T. M. Incagnoli (Eds.), *Contemporary approaches to neuropsychological assessment* (pp. 231–276). New York: Plenum Press.

Woodcock, R. W., McGrew, K. S., & Mather, N. (2007). *Woodcock Johnson Test of Achievement, 3rd edition, normative update.* Rolling Meadows, IL: Riverside.

Woodward, S. A., Lenzenweger, M. F., Kagen, J., Snidman, N., & Arcus, D. (2000). Taxonic structure of infant reactivity: Evidence from a taxometric perspective. *Psychological Science, 11,* 296–301.

Wright, L. (1967). The pediatric psychologist: A role model. *American Psychologist, 22,* 323–325.

Youngstrom, E. A., Findling, R. L., Youngstrom, J. K., & Calabrese, J. R. (2005). Toward an evidence-based assessment of pediatric bipolar disorder. *Journal of Clinical Child and Adolescent Psychology, 34,* 433–448.

Yule, W. (1993). *Developmental considerations in child assessment.* Needham Heights, MA: Allyn & Bacon.

2

Diagnostic Classification Systems

JEREMY D. JEWELL, STEPHEN D.A. HUPP, and ANDREW M. POMERANTZ

DEFINING MENTAL DISORDER

On the surface, the purpose of the *Diagnostic and Statistical Manual of Mental Disorders, 4th Edition, Text Revision* (*DSM–IV–TR*; American Psychiatric Association, 2000) is straightforward. Contemporary practice requires a standard "catalogue" of mental disorders, with each disorder defined conceptually, and criteria for formal diagnosis set forth. This chapter explores the development of the *DSM–IV–TR*, the history of the *DSM* including previous versions, advantages and disadvantages of the current model of classification, and possible revisions for future editions of the *DSM*. To begin, however, one must understand that the concept of "mental disorder" is complicated by many issues, including the idea that mental disorders are rooted in societal norms as well as the context of history.

The origin of the concept of mental illness may date back to prehistoric man. That is, it is likely that prehistoric man had some understanding of the "mind", and that surgery to the skull might relieve symptoms of illness due to head injury (Liu & Apuzzo, 2003). As human society has progressed, however, the concept of mental illness has both expanded as well as become more complex. Consider, for example, the mental disorder of depression. In the case where a person may suffer a personal loss and experience grief, at what point in time does that grief become psychopathological depression? In this case, culture and society must somehow draw the line between the normal grieving process and psychopathology. The distinction must be made in terms of the specific behaviors exhibited (frequent fatigue or suicidal ideation) as well as the duration of the pathological behavior (one week

JEREMY D. JEWELL, STEPHEN D. A. HUPP, and ANDREW M. POMERANTZ • Southern Illinois University Edwardsville, Diagnostic Classification Systems

J.L. Matson et al. (eds.), *Assessing Childhood Psychopathology and Developmental Disabilities*, DOI: 10.1007/978-0-387-09528-8, © Springer Science+Business Media, LLC 2009

31

versus one year). Also consider schizophrenia. Typical symptoms of this disorder include the presence of delusions. However, if one were to admit that she believed in a spiritual world or the afterlife, she would probably not be labeled "delusional" despite the fact that there is no supporting scientific evidence for an afterlife. Therefore, even mental disorders with the greatest amount of research in some sense are founded on society's assumption of what is, and is not, normal.

Similarly, society's historical context has often affected our understanding of mental disorder. For example, homosexuality was included as a diagnosable mental disorder in the first two editions of the *DSM* (APA, 1952, 1968). Society's view of homosexuality as a defect in one's character was at that time reflected in the *DSM–I* and *DSM–II* classification of homosexuality (Sexual Orientation Disturbance) as a mental disorder. As society's view on homosexuality has changed, however, so has the classification of homosexuality as a mental disorder. Therefore, although scientists conduct research on various forms of mental illness, one must acknowledge that this academic exercise occurs in the context of both sociocultural norms to some extent, as well as the context of history.

Understanding this, what can we say is a mental disorder? The current *DSM–IV–TR* defines a mental disorder as

> ... a clinically significant behavioral or psychological syndrome or pattern that occurs in an individual and that is associated with present distress (e.g., a painful symptom) or disability (i.e., impairment in one or more important areas of functioning) or with a significantly increased risk of suffering death, pain, disability, or an important loss of freedom. (APA, 2000, p. xxxi)

One should note that there are several important components to this definition, including the concept that the individual must be experiencing some sort of pain (presently or in the future) or impairment due to the symptoms of the disorder. The advantage of a broad definition such as this, is that it allows clinicians to include a host of disorders in cases where patients themselves may either not recognize their own symptomology as reflecting a disorder (e.g., during a psychotic episode) or even when patients may resign themselves to a longstanding period of suffering (e.g., dysthymia).

Because changing societal norms have continued to shape the definition of mental disorders over time, it is important to take a closer look at the development of the *DSM* and other classification systems.

HISTORY OF DIAGNOSTIC CLASSIFICATION SYSTEMS

Pre-*DSM*

Until the publication of the original *DSM* in 1952, the history of diagnostic classification systems for mental disorders in the United States was characterized by a lack of unification. Some of the early efforts were motivated by statistical, rather than clinical, factors. When the U.S. census was conducted in 1840, it included a single category of mental illness ("idiocy/insanity") to describe portions of the American populace. This was the first time that data were systematically collected via the census for this purpose. In the 1880 census, seven categories of mental illness were included in the census materials, many of which were labeled with terms that now seem antiquated (e.g., monomania, dipsomania, melancholia). Soon, a committee within the American Psychiatric Association began to collaborate with the census bureau in order to gather more extensive data. However, the emphasis remained primarily statistical rather than clinical (APA, 1952, 2000).

Formal diagnostic categorization of mental disorders for clinical purposes was uncommon prior to the approach of the twentieth century. By 1900, many large hospitals and training centers had developed their own systems of labeling and record-keeping for mental illness. These systems were idiosyncratic, having been created solely to meet the needs of the home institution. As increasing numbers of these individualized systems appeared, communication between mental health professionals and agencies was restricted by the lack of a common language describing mental disorders (APA, 1952, 2000; Langenbucher & Nathan, 2006).

In the late 1920s, efforts emerged to create a standardized nomenclature, although it would take decades to attain this goal. Some of the individualized systems of diagnostic classification were adopted widely, including systems created by the U.S. Army and the Veteran's Administration hospitals. These few systems remained in competition with each other until the original *DSM* effectively replaced them in 1952 (APA, 1952, APA, 2000).

DSM–I—DSM–III–R

The first edition of the *DSM*, published by the American Psychiatric Association in 1952, was essentially a modified version of the International Classification of Diseases (ICD, published by the World Health Organization). The ICD was in its sixth edition at the time, and it was the first time in which that manual included a category for mental illnesses (APA, 2000). The *DSM–I* was followed by a revision, *DSM–II*, in 1968. These two editions are similar to each other and also quite different from any of the subsequent *DSM* revisions. The language included in the *DSM–I* and *DSM–II* indicates a very strong psychoanalytic emphasis; indeed, the psychoanalytic approach was prominent in all areas of clinical work at that time. It is also noteworthy that the first two editions of the *DSM* lacked specific diagnostic criteria; that is, each disorder was described in a brief paragraph or two. The absence of specific criteria to determine whether an individual qualified for a disorder made the first two editions of the *DSM* less clinically useful than they could have been. The *DSM–I* included very few disorders specifically characterizing pathology in children or adolescents, and they were placed within a larger category with many "transient" adult disorders. For example, the *DSM–II* included a category of disorders entitled "Behavioral Disorders of Childhood and Adolescence," which included only six specific disorders.

The publication of the *DSM–III* represented a significant change in the *DSM* classification system (Widiger & Trull, 2007). The *DSM–III* was quite different from its predecessors in a variety of ways, most obvious of which was greatly increased size and scope. The *DSM–III* was much more extensive than the *DSM–I* and the *DSM–II*; it included a great deal more text and a far greater number of disorders, including a sizeable number of newly defined disorders for children and adolescents (Houts, 2002). The authors of the *DSM–III* also made an explicit effort to use empirical data as the basis for diagnostic categories, an emphasis that was not present in the first two editions. The *DSM–III* also shed the psychoanalytic language and any influence that it might reflect, endorsing instead a more atheoretical approach to mental illness. Unlike the first two editions, the *DSM–III* included specific criteria and thresholds to define disorders. Additionally, the *DSM–III* marked the first appearance of a multiaxial system, including Axis I (most clinical disorders), Axis II (e.g., developmental disorders and personality disorders), Axis III (relevant medical conditions), Axis IV (relevant psychosocial and environmental factors), and Axis V (Global Assessment of Functioning on a scale from 0 to 100). Collectively, the changes evident in the *DSM–III* resulted in a more inclusive and clinically useful manual than the first two editions of the *DSM*.

The *DSM–III* was followed by the publication of the *DSM–III–R* in 1987. As its edition number indicates (with "R" standing for "revised"), the *DSM–III–R* did not represent an overhaul of the *DSM–III*. Instead, it was a relatively minor revision intended to clear up some inconsistent and ambiguous aspects of the *DSM–III* (APA, 2000). Thus, the *DSM–III–R* was quite similar in structure, format, and length to the *DSM–III*. In fact, all subsequent revisions of the *DSM* have remained consistent with the general structure, format, and length of the *DSM–III*.

DEVELOPMENT OF *DSM–IV*

In 1994, the American Psychiatric Association published the fourth edition of the *DSM* (*DSM–IV*; APA, 1994a). In 2000, another edition was published, entitled *DSM–IV–TR*, with "TR" standing for "text revision." The term "text revision" refers to the fact that only the text describing the diagnoses—not the diagnostic criteria—differs between the *DSM–IV* and the term *DSM–IV–TR*. That is, the *DSM–IV–TR* contains exactly the same diagnostic criteria as the *DSM–IV*, and they are officially defined in exactly the same way. The essential difference between the *DSM–IV–TR* and the *DSM–IV* is the addition of new text in the *DSM–IV–TR* to describe recent findings relevant to existing disorders. For the sake of simplicity, this chapter simply uses the term the *DSM–IV* to refer to both the *DSM–IV* and the *DSM–IV–TR*.

The creation of the *DSM–IV* was a massive effort, involving the collaborative work of over 1,000 people and a period of time greater than five years (APA, 1994b). It was overseen by a coordinating Task Force and 13 independent Work Groups, each of which focused on a particular category of psychopathology (e.g., Child and Adolescent Disorders, Anxiety Disorders, Mood Disorders, Personality Disorders). Throughout its development, its authors emphasized that empirical evidence was the cornerstone on which the *DSM–IV* was built, and was also the primary requirement for any changes from the previous edition of the *DSM* (APA, 1994b). The process of creating the *DSM–IV* included three primary phases: literature reviews, reanalysis of existing datasets, and focused field trials (each of these three phases is described in more detail below.) After these three phases were completed, the *DSM–IV* Draft Criteria were released, with which the *DSM–IV* creators hoped to elicit feedback from the professional community, including any problems they could foresee before the draft criteria were made official (APA, 1994b). Incorporating this feedback, *DSM–IV* was published in 1994.

Literature Reviews

Especially since the publication of the *DSM–III* in 1980, a significant body of empirical literature has accumulated regarding specific disorders. Much of this literature is pertinent to the revision of the manual, so a primary task of the *DSM–IV* authors was to undertake a large-scale review. Each Work Group was instructed to ascertain the most important issues for their category of diagnoses, and then to conduct a systematic comprehensive review of the literature to address those issues. Selected parts of the results of these literature reviews are included in the *DSM–IV* text, and the results are included more extensively in the separate *DSM* Sourcebook (APA, 1994b, 2000).

The literature review conducted by each Work Group focused exclusively on their category of diagnoses, and followed the same six-step format (APA, 1994b; 2000).

1. *Statement of the Issues*. In this section, the researchers identified the most important issues within their category that were to be addressed by the literature review.
2. *Significance of the Issues*. Here, the researchers explained some possible diagnostic or clinical ramifications of the issues identified in the previous section.
3. *Methods*. The researchers described how many studies it examined, how it went about searching for and finding the studies, why certain studies were included or excluded from the review, and other aspects of the literature review methods.
4. *Results*. Here, the researchers presented the findings of their literature review. They were instructed to produce results that were objective, thorough, and concise.
5. *Discussion*. This section features consideration of the implications of the results, including multiple options for resolving the issues described in the first two sections.
6. *Recommendations*. Here, the researchers selected the option or options (among those listed in the previous section) that, based on the review of the literature, they believed were most viable.

Data Reanalyses

In some cases, the literature review process revealed areas in which insufficient research existed to address important diagnostic issues for various work groups. In these situations, the researchers often obtained existing datasets and reanalyzed them utilizing new methods (APA 1994b, 2000). By doing so, they were able to address gaps in the published literature on diagnostic and clinical issues. A total of 40 data reanalyses were conducted for the *DSM–IV*, usually via collaboration with researchers at different sites. Typically, the data used in these reanalyses were originally collected for epidemiological purposes or to examine treatment methods, but in this context, the focus was diagnostic (APA, 2000).

Field Trials

The overall purpose of the field trials was to determine how well the proposed *DSM–IV* criteria actually functioned in applied settings that represented the kinds of sites where *DSM–IV* criteria might actually be used. In total, there were 12 field trials involving over 70 separate sites and over 6,000 subjects. The sites selected, as well as the subjects served there, represented a diverse range of cultural and ethnic backgrounds. Thus, the cross-cultural generalizability of proposed diagnostic criteria was addressed (APA, 2000).

A primary goal of the field trials was to investigate the extent to which the proposed revisions would affect the reliability and validity of the diagnostic criteria. Diagnostic criteria were considered both in sets (i.e., the full list of criteria for Generalized Anxiety Disorder, including requirements regarding thresholds and combinations of criteria) and individually (i.e., each specific criterion listed for Generalized Anxiety). Additionally, the field trials allowed the *DSM–IV* authors to appreciate the impact that the proposed diagnostic revisions might have on the day-to-day practice of clinicians who rely on the *DSM–IV*. One way in which these questions were explored was to compare the criteria for mental disorders directly according to various sources. In other words, at a field trial site, the investigators might have utilized both *DSM–III–R* and various proposed *DSM–IV* criteria sets, and then compared the outcome of the use of each to the other (APA, 1994b; 2000).

Throughout the process of creating the *DSM–IV*, its authors emphasized that any revisions would need to be justified by empirical research: "The threshold for making revisions in *DSM–IV* was set higher than that for *DSM–III* and *DSM–III–R*. Decisions had to be substantiated by explicit statements of rationale and by the systematic review of relevant empirical data" (APA, 2000, p. xxviii). There were a number of potential new diagnoses that the *DSM–IV* authors considered; many of those that were not added as new categories appear in an appendix of the manual entitled "Criteria Sets and Axes Provided for Further Study." One purpose of including them in an appendix is to stimulate research among interested researchers. Among the proposed disorders included in this appendix are Premenstrual Dysphoric Disorder, Binge-Eating Disorder,

Minor Depressive Disorder, Recurrent Brief Depressive Disorder, and Passive-Aggressive Personality Disorder.

It is also notable that the *DSM–IV* is the first edition of the manual to contain an appendix devoted to issues of culture. This appendix includes an "outline for cultural formulation," which is intended to encourage mental health professionals performing diagnoses to consider such factors as the individual's cultural identity and ways in which cultural factors may influence the psychosocial environment and the relationship between the individual and the professional (APA, 2000).

Creation of the *DSM–IV* was an immense task, and although its authors explain the significant efforts taken to ensure maximum reliability, validity, and clinical utility, they also realize that our understanding of mental illness will continue to improve: "The advance of fundamental understanding of mental disorders will undoubtedly provide much clearer (and probably often very different) answers to the questions raised [by the *DSM–IV* review process]" (APA, 1994b, p. xxi).

FORMAT OF THE *DSM–IV*

In this section, the major topics and the format of the *DSM–IV* (2000) are described. The text of the *DSM–IV* begins with the typical acknowledgments and broad statements on the purposes, use, and development of the *DSM–IV*. The authors proceed to describe the multiaxial system and how to derive a multiaxial diagnosis. Within this, the authors provide the Global Assessment of Functioning (GAF). Beginning on page 39, disorders are catalogued and described based on broader sections. Examples of these broad sections include Mood Disorders, Anxiety Disorders, as well as Disorders Usually First Diagnosed in Infancy, Childhood, or Adolescence.

Within each section, each disorder is described in a uniform manner. First, the "diagnostic features" of the disorder are described. These features are described and conceptualized rather broadly, and are not a simple list of symptoms or diagnostic criteria. For example, the diagnostic features of Conduct Disorder are described as "... a repetitive and persistent pattern of behavior in which the basic rights of others or major age-appropriate societal norms or rules are violated (Criterion A)" (p. 93). Next, the "subtypes and/or specifiers" heading refers to any particular subtypes that may be appropriate to the diagnosis (e.g., for Conduct Disorder, Childhood Onset Type or Adolescent Onset Type can be specified). Additionally, appropriate specifiers, such as mild, moderate, or severe, are listed and described. Other types of specifiers may exist as well, such as the specifier "chronic" for Major Depressive Disorder. If subtypes or specifiers do not exist for a particular disorder, this section is not included in that disorder description. Any special instructions for the recording of the diagnosis, including the relationship between the *DSM–IV* diagnosis and ICD–9 diagnosis, are then noted in the "recording procedures" section.

The next broad section for each disorder is "associated features and disorders," which is usually divided into the following three sections: associated descriptive features and mental disorders, associated laboratory

findings, and associated physical examination findings and general medical conditions. "Associated descriptive features and mental disorders"
include those features that have been associated with the disorder to a
lesser extent, and in some cases these features were not found to contribute significantly to the sensitivity or specificity of the diagnosis in the field
trials. "Associated laboratory findings" refers to particular laboratory findings that are either considered diagnostic of the disorder, associated with
the disorder, or are perhaps a secondary effect of the disorder.

Next, the *DSM–IV* provides several sections that give further description to the disorder. First, "specific culture, age, and gender features"
describes any differences that may occur in the expression, initiation, or
maintenance of the disorder based on these demographic characteristics
of the patient. Next, the "prevalence" section gives some broad range of
the prevalence of the disorder based on the existing research. "Course"
refers to research findings on the onset of the disorder, course of the disorder, duration, and other similar concepts. The "familial pattern" section
summarizes research on the presumed heritability of the disorder based
on current research findings. The heritability of other related disorders
may also be described (e.g., the familial pattern of any mood disorder in
patients with Major Depressive Disorder). In the "differential diagnosis"
section, the *DSM–IV* authors describe how other similar disorders may be
differentiated from the disorder in question. This information is critical
when one considers that many disorders have the same or similar criteria
when compared to other disorders. Finally, the *DSM–IV* provides the specific diagnostic criteria required for the particular disorder.

The *DSM–IV* ends with a number of useful appendices. For example, "decision trees for differential diagnoses" and "criteria sets and axes
provided for further study" are provided. Additionally, other appendices
provide for an analysis of the compatibility of a particular diagnosis with
ICD–10 diagnoses.

ICD–10 CLASSIFICATION OF MENTAL
AND BEHAVIORAL DISORDERS

The tenth edition of the *International Statistical Classification of Diseases and Health Related Problems* (ICD–10; World Health Organization,
1992, 1993) is a broad diagnostic system including all diseases and other
problems related to health. The first edition, the *International List of Causes
of Death* was adopted in the late 1800s and was originally developed to
represent a list of possible causes of death to be used internationally. The
World Health Organization (WHO) began publishing the sixth edition of the
ICD in 1948, and this revision was the first to broaden the scope of the
classification system to include mental disorders. By comparison, the first
edition of the *DSM* was published soon thereafter in 1952.

The *ICD–7* was published in 1955; however, there were no changes to
the mental disorders. In the late 1960s, when the *ICD–8* and *DSM–II* were
published, some effort was made to increase the compatibility of these
systems. At this time, both systems received criticism regarding the lack

of empirical support for the reliability and validity of their diagnoses (Widiger, 2005). The *ICD–9* was published in 1977, and in an effort to increase reliability it included a glossary with more detailed descriptions of disorders. Published soon thereafter, the *DSM–III* also continued to develop the descriptions of disorders. The *DSM–III* also had other innovations (e.g., explicit sets of criteria) that made it less compatible with the *ICD–9*, and this decrease in compatibility was counter to the ultimate goal of facilitating communication between professionals (Widiger, 2005). The *ICD–10* and the *DSM–IV* were both published in the early 1990s with an increased effort at improving compatibility.

The fifth chapter of the *ICD–10* is the Classification of Mental and Behavioral Disorders. There are two different versions of this chapter, and the first published version was the Clinical Descriptions and Diagnostic Guidelines (CDDG; WHO, 1992) used by clinicians. This version includes narrative descriptions of disorders. The WHO also subsequently derived the Diagnostic Criteria for Research (DCR, WHO, 1993) from the clinical version. Although the clinical and research versions are very similar, there are some differences. Specifically, the research version leaves out some of the descriptive information for each disorder. More importantly, the research version is more restrictive than the clinical version by delineating clear and highly specified criteria and lists of symptoms. The clinical and research versions combined are similar to the scope of information included in the *DSM–IV*.

Overall, the *ICD–10* continued to move away from vague descriptions and the inclusion of unsupported etiologies, and toward clear operational definitions with improved reliability (Bertelsen, 1999). Separate field trials were conducted for both the clinical and research versions in over 30 countries. For both versions, 2,400 patients were assessed by at least two clinicians, and both yielded high interrater reliability for diagnoses (Üstün, Chatterji, & Andrews, 2002). Alternatively, however, the more difficult question of validity and clinical utility of the diagnostic categories continued to be raised.

Although there is considerable overlap between the *ICD–10* and *DSM–IV–TR*, the ICD–10 is most commonly used in Europe, Asia, and Africa, whereas the *DSM–IV* is more commonly used in the Americas (Jablensky & Kendell, 2002). Having both a clinical and a research version of the *ICD–10* Classification of Mental and Behavioral Disorders makes comparison between the *ICD–10* and *DSM–IV* both more complicated and difficult, and has led to confusion about which version of the *ICD–10* is being used during comparisons (First & Pincus, 1999).

Generally speaking, the most significant difference between these two classification systems is that the *ICD–10* is a more comprehensive system including the wide range of diseases and other medical problems, whereas the *DSM–IV* focuses only on psychological disorders. Even within the psychological disorders, the *ICD–10* has a greater emphasis on distinguishing between "organic" disorders and other types of disorders. The multiaxial approach is another general difference between the two systems. The *DSM–IV* includes a five-axis approach, whereas the WHO did not publish a multiaxial system (WHO, 1996) until a few years after the original publication of the *ICD–10*. There are also some differences between the specific axes.

The majority of the psychological disorders in both the *DSM–IV* and *ICD–10* are highly similar, but there are some significant differences between the two systems. These systems can be directly compared by using another book, *Cross-walks ICD–10–DSM–IV–TR: A Synopsis of Classifications of Mental Disorders* (Schulte-Markwort, Marutt, & Riedesser, 2003). Focusing on *ICD–DSM* comparisons that most directly affect children, the *ICD–10* has substantially more disorders for children in several ways. First, the *ICD–10* sometimes allows for separate disorders for children (e.g., Social Anxiety Disorder of Childhood) and adults (e.g., Social Phobias), whereas the *DSM–IV* uses the same diagnosis for both (i.e., Social Anxiety Disorder). Second, the *ICD–10* has some "mixed" disorders that are not included in the *DSM–IV*, and examples of these include Depressive Conduct Disorder and Hyperkinetic Conduct Disorder. Finally, for many of the types of disorders diagnosed in childhood, the *ICD–10* divides them into more possible diagnoses. For example, whereas the *DSM–IV* has five types of Pervasive Developmental Disorders, the *ICD–10* describes additional disorders including both Atypical Autism as well as Overactive Disorder Associated with Mental Retardation. Also, compared to Conduct Disorder in the *DSM–IV*, the *ICD–10* provides three separate disorders (i.e., Conduct Disorder Confined to the Family Context, Unsocialized Conduct Disorder, and Socialized Conduct Disorder).

Although many of the disorders are similar between the two systems, they still differ somewhat in label and symptoms. For example, the *DSM–IV* uses the label Attention-Deficit/Hyperactivity Disorder, and the ICD–10 includes a few Hyperkinetic Disorders (e.g., Disturbance of Activity and Attention) with slightly different criteria. Also, both Attention-Deficit/Hyperactivity Disorder (in the *DSM–IV*) and Disturbance of Activity and Attention (in the *ICD–10*) have many similar symptoms (sometimes with slight wording differences); however, the *ICD–10* has an increased distinction between hyperactivity and impulsivity.

As psychology journals continue to have greater international contributions, having two different major classification systems creates more confusion regarding diagnoses. This confusion is somewhat tempered by the fact that the *DSM–IV* is used more internationally with researchers than with clinicians; however, this increases the gap between international research and practice. Having two different versions of the *ICD–10* also adds to the possible confusion. The existence of different major systems for cataloguing mental disorders also emphasizes that the current diagnostic categories are not static and are subject to change. In fact new editions of the *DSM* and *ICD* will likely be published within the next few years. Jablensky and Kendell (2002) suggest that the next revision of the *DSM* is more likely to have radical changes because the *ICD* is more constrained by coordinating the efforts of many more countries. Although some view the omission of unsupported etiologies in the *ICD–10* as a step in the right direction, some have called for revisiting inclusion of supported etiological theories in the next revision of the *ICD* (Üstün, Chatteri, & Andrews, 2002).

THE PURPOSES AND USES OF A DIAGNOSTIC CLASSIFICATION SYSTEM

In a generic sense, a nosological system is simply a system of classifying disease or pathology. Therefore, most would agree that the *DSM–IV*, as well as all previous versions of the *DSM*, can be understood as nosological in nature. However, as the *DSM* has evolved from its first edition to the current one, the primary purpose of this classification system has drastically changed. Specifically, the first two versions of the *DSM* were known as primarily an explanatory nosological system that was rooted almost exclusively in psychoanalytic theory. Therefore, the primary purpose of the system was to explain the etiology of particular disorders from this theoretical framework.

With the introduction of the *DSM–III*, however, the nosological system became more descriptive or typological (Bertelsen, 1999). The *DSM–III* drifted away from explaining the etiology of particular disorders, and a great deal of attention was paid to specifically and accurately describing the symptoms of each disorder in the hopes of elevating the reliability of the diagnostic system. Another implication of this evolution of the diagnostic model is that the *DSM–III* and *DSM–IV* are relatively atheoretical. Although an atheoretical nosological system allows it to be more broadly applied to a variety of disorders as well as clinicians with a variety of theoretical backgrounds and training, these advantages come at a cost. In particular, an atheoretical nosological system may lack explanatory power as to the etiology of particular disorders, thus affecting patient treatment (Frances & Egger, 1999). Subsequent sections of this chapter continue to come back to this issue of an explanatory versus descriptive nosological system.

Given that the current *DSM–IV* is primarily descriptive in nature, one must consider the strengths and multiple purposes of such a system. The primary motivating force in moving the *DSM* to a descriptive classification system was to increase the reliability of the diagnostic system. Specifically, many clinicians in the field became concerned regarding the lack of standard practice in diagnosis that existed prior to the *DSM–III*. At a more fundamental level, however, a diagnostic system is critical so that those within the profession can communicate with each other using a universal nomenclature. One can imagine the chaos and confusion that would prevail if hundreds of professionals attempted to describe groups of similar patients or existing constructs without any agreed-upon system that defined these groups. Therefore, a foundational prerequisite to any diagnostic classification system is that it must allow for clinicians to come to the same diagnostic conclusion given information gathered from a patient that reflects a particular set of symptoms.

Related to this, previous research using the *DSM–II* indicated that diagnostic reliability between clinicians ranged from poor to fair on almost all of the diagnostic categories (Spitzer & Fleiss, 1974). With regard to diagnostic reliability, researchers publishing on the *DSM–IV* indicate that there is increasing reliability compared to previous versions of the *DSM*, although there are a number of diagnoses where diagnostic reliability continues to be problematic (APA, 1998).

Another purpose of a diagnostic classification system such as the *DSM–IV* is the need to conduct clinical research on particular populations. Again, a reliable diagnostic system is a fundamental prerequisite needed to conduct such research. For example, imagine that a group of researchers wanted to test the efficacy of a new antidepressant drug. In order to do so, they would need to administer the drug to a group of persons suffering from depression, while also administering a placebo to a similar group of persons with depression. In order to draw accurate conclusions regarding the efficacy of the new drug, it is critical that both groups of people diagnosed with Major Depressive Disorder are highly similar in the symptoms, as well as the level of impairment they exhibit. Another obvious reason for a reliable diagnostic classification symptom is that the efficacy of this new antidepressant drug presumes that there are symptoms of depression that exist in the person so that a change can be noted by researchers. If someone who was not clinically depressed were to be included in the experimental research group, the results might underestimate the effects of this antidepressant as there were no symptoms of depression to decrease or eliminate in that particular person.

A recent meta-analysis of inpatient psychotherapy effectiveness by Kösters, Burlingame, Nachtigall, and Strauss (2006) provides another example of the need for reliable diagnostic categories for research purposes. The results of the meta-analysis indicated that the strength of improvement that could be attributed to inpatient psychotherapy treatment differed as a function of the patient's diagnosis. Specifically, patients with mood and anxiety disorders improved to a greater extent when compared to patients with other disorders such as Schizophrenia (Kösters et al., 2006). Understanding this, the field of psychology can now examine the treatments for persons with these various diagnoses and attempt to improve those treatments that are relatively less successful. Again, important research such as this can only be conducted when a reliable diagnostic classification system exists.

Similarly, there has been a general movement in clinical psychology toward specifically detailed interventions that are both standardized and manualized. In fact, Division 12 of the American Psychological Association has begun establishing a list of treatments that researchers support for particular diagnoses (American Psychological Association, Division 12 Society of Clinical Psychology, n.d.). These empirically supported treatments (ESTs) are catalogued and matched by disorder, rather than endorsing a particular treatment wholesale. Treatment planning based on a particular diagnosis is not necessarily new to psychology, yet it is the specificity of the particular treatment intervention matched with a very specifically diagnosed disorder that is somewhat novel. Again, reliable diagnosis is a fundamental prerequisite to this move toward choosing an empirically supported treatment based on a particular diagnosis.

Another use of the DSM diagnostic classification system is that there are many other public institutions that rely on an accurate diagnosis. For example, in the United States, the Social Security Administration policy on disability determination partially relies on criteria for Mental Retardation to determine social security disability benefits for that disability status. These criteria are closely related to the criteria set forth in the *DSM–IV*.

This example is just one where a mental disorder may qualify someone for government support. Similarly, the Individuals with Disabilities Education Act (IDEA; Department of Education, 2005) allows for children with a diagnosis of Attention-Deficit/Hyperactivity Disorder (ADHD) to be eligible for special education services in the public schools through the category of Other Health Impaired (OHI). However, the IDEA legislation itself does not specify the criteria for ADHD. Rather, IDEA relies on the symptom criteria as outlined in the *DSM–IV*, as part of the criteria necessary for a child to be determined as Other Health Impaired (Department of Education, 2005).

A final use of the *DSM* diagnostic classification system, and perhaps the most controversial, is to allow for third-party payment for psychological services. Specifically, a significant portion of the population in the United States has private health insurance coverage. These health insurers usually require a formal diagnosis, using either the *DSM–IV* or *ICD-10*, in order to reimburse the provider. This situation has generated a great deal of debate, most especially concerning the rights of the insured and privacy of medical records (for a detailed review of similar issues see Newman & Bricklin, 1991). Given the direct relationship between a categorical diagnostic system such as the *DSM–IV* and reimbursement for mental health services, persons who suffer from a mental illness but at a subthreshold level may be denied services from their insurance provider. Again, this is not an explicitly stated purpose of the *DSM–IV* by its authors, but merely an undesirable effect of the healthcare system that has evolved over time.

As can be seen, there are numerous purposes for a nosological classification system such as the *DSM–IV*. These purposes all rely on the reliable and accurate diagnosis of mental disorders. As the *DSM–IV* has moved from an explanatory to a descriptive classification system, proponents would argue that this shift has resulted in an increase in diagnostic reliability. On the other hand, some critics would also argue that because of this shift, the utility and validity of the *DSM* has suffered considerably in order to gain this increase in reliability (Widiger & Clark, 2000).

DISADVANTAGES OF THE *DSM–IV*

Since the first edition of the *DSM* in 1952, there have been numerous critics of this classification system, and the *ICD–10* is subject to the same types of criticisms. Most recently, criticism has been focused on the *DSM–IV* because of its increasing adherence to the "medical model" of mental illness (Widiger & Clark, 2000). Although there is some variation as to how experts define this medical model, some possibilities are outlined below as well and an explanation is provided as to how the medical model affects our understanding of mental illness.

The Medical Model of Mental Illness

The medical model of mental illness can be understood as having similarities with the medical community's understanding of physical illness (Cloninger, 1999). The assumptions of the medical model as they apply to mental illness are threefold. First, it is assumed that the concept of a disease exists, and that persons can be placed into two categories, those who are diseased and those who are healthy and without disease. This categorical way of conceptualizing mental illness, as opposed to placing persons along a continuum of disease and health (also known as a dimensional model), are discussed in more detail in further sections. The second assumption of the medical model is that the disease, or mental illness, resides within the individual (as opposed to the individual's circumstances, context, relationships, etc.). The third assumption is that any treatment to alleviate this disease must occur at the level of the individual as well. When one understands these assumptions that are implicit in the medical model, coupled with the descriptive and atheoretical nature of the *DSM–IV* as previously described, a type of tautological circular reasoning can arise. Specifically, one might ask, "Why is this child often truant, cruel to people, and cruel to animals," which would be answered "Because he has Conduct Disorder." The next question is, "Why does this child have Conduct Disorder," to which might come the answer, "Because he is often truant, he is cruel to people, and is cruel to animals." This error in reasoning is often referred to as "reifying" disorders, and many have urged clinicians and researchers to formulate mental disorders as simplified descriptions of behavior clusters rather than actual entities (Knapp & Jensen, 2006).

Another related disadvantage of the medical model of mental illness is that the model in and of itself lends credibility to a biological etiology of mental illness, when in fact such an exclusive etiology may not necessarily exist. For example, when working within a nosological system that assumes that disease lies within the individual, resulting research will most likely examine the disease at the individual level, neglecting other facets of the human experience that contribute to the mental disorder. This process of scientific inquiry, if allowed to proceed in this fashion, could then build a research literature that describes mental disorders as biological in origin (neglecting other avenues of research).

Acknowledging the Environmental Context

The question as to the etiology of mental disorders leads to another important concept related to the medical model, which is the relative importance of environmental variables in understanding mental illness. Bronfenbrenner (1979) first discussed what he described as the ecological model of psychological functioning. This model changed the internal process of the "disease" of mental illness to one wherein an individual's internal characteristics do not fit within his environmental context. Bronfenbrenner (1979) theorized that each child is surrounded by a complex ecology or environment with which he or she interacts. This environment consists of relationships and systems proximal to the child, such as other family members. Additionally, however, the child is both directly and indirectly affected by other systems in the environment, including the school environment, religious and other community organizations, and other broader cultural variables.

Therefore, the ecological model would view the aggressive behaviors of an individual child within their social context. Whether these aggressive behaviors might be indicative of a mental disorder depends on whether they are adaptive and fit within the child's context. If this particular child lives in a home where violence is both modeled and expected, and within a high crime neighborhood that exposes the child to daily threats, then aggressive behavior may in fact be adaptive and may not necessarily be indicative of a mental disorder. On the other hand, if that same child lives in a safe environment where aggression is punished, then repeated displays of aggression would be maladaptive. This aggression could lead to impairment of the child's functioning, and could be viewed as a symptom of a mental disorder.

The Categorical Nature of the *DSM–IV*

Another disadvantage, or weakness, of the *DSM–IV* is the categorical view of mental illness. Again, this concept is related to the medical model of mental disorders as persons are either considered as having a mental disorder, or not having a disorder. Many argue that this view of psychological functioning ignores the reality of the human existence (Widiger & Trull, 2007). In fact, the authors of the *DSM–IV* were themselves concerned with what might be perceived as an absolutist view of the categorical nature of the classification system, and they address this issue in the preface of the text. Specifically, they state the following.

> In *DSM–IV*, there is no assumption that each category of mental disorder is a completely discrete entity with absolute boundaries dividing it from other mental disorders or from no mental disorder. There is also no assumption that all individuals described as having the same mental disorder are alike in all important ways. (APA, 2000, p. xxxi).

However, although this point is acknowledged in the *DSM–IV*, the reality is that the current *DSM* lays out a specific diagnostic classification system that for the most part does not allow the diagnosis of any disorder falling below the threshold. Specifically, clinicians must simply judge whether a patient does or does not have a particular mental disorder. Again, the authors (APA, 2000) of the *DSM–IV* go on to justify and rationalize the categorical nature of the *DSM–IV* when stating:

> Although dimensional systems increase reliability and communicate more clinical information (because they report clinical attributes that might be subthreshold in a categorical system), they have serious limitations and thus far have been less useful than categorical systems in clinical practice and in stimulating research. (APA, 2000, p. xxxii).

Given this, there are two caveats to understanding the *DSM–IV* as a purely categorical diagnostic system. First, some *DSM–IV* disorders allow for a "Not Otherwise Specified" (NOS) diagnosis. For example, a NOS diagnosis might apply if the clinician cannot establish the required time frame for impairment required to formally diagnose a particular disorder. Thus, this system does allow for some flexibility in diagnosing individuals when clinical judgment determines that a disorder exists but that a lack of information regarding the patient's functioning does not allow that patient to qualify for a particular diagnosis. Secondly, some disorders require clinicians to specify the level of impairment as mild, moderate, or severe. This qualifier of severity usually depends on the number of symptoms displayed by the patient as well as the qualitatively judged severity of those symptoms. Again, qualifiers of impairment and severity lend a somewhat dimensional quality to the *DSM–IV*, allowing clinicians to distinguish patients to some extent within a diagnostic category.

Many would argue that the rigidity of the current categorical system is unfortunate, but is also necessary in a system that has been highly operationalized in an attempt to maximize diagnostic reliability. However, researchers in the field also maintain that many more persons suffer from psychological distress that could be considered a subthreshold disorder compared to those who meet the full criteria for a mental disorder (Helmchen & Linden, 2000). Given this, the current system of diagnosis may not accurately reflect the true broad continuum of psychological functioning.

A final point related to this is the fact that the *DSM–IV* is not a classification system that measures or classifies health or adaptive psychological functioning. Rather, all of the diagnoses that are catalogued in this diagnostic system are considered illnesses. For clinicians in fields such as positive psychology and health psychology, this fact may be somewhat frustrating. Although related topics in human resiliency are important and have begun to garner more research attention (Greene, Galambos, & Lee, 2003), this view of adaptive psychological functioning is not captured or described in the current diagnostic system (Cloninger, 1999). Again, there are two exceptions to this within the *DSM–IV* itself. First, the *DSM–IV* provides the Global Assessment of Functioning (GAF) scale that allows clinicians to rate client functioning (from 1 to 100). The GAF is estimated on Axis V and is part of a standard multiaxial diagnosis. An important component of the GAF related to resiliency is the scale between 91 and 100 that allows clinicians to identify patients who have "superior functioning" relative to typical nondisordered individuals (p. 34).

Another component of the *DSM–IV–TR* that allows for the description and assessment of psychological health and adaptation is the Defensive Functioning Scale (DFS), located on p. 807 of the manual. The DFS follows from psychoanalytic theory by describing psychological defenses that are available to a person as they attempt to cope with either internal or external stressors. Many of these defenses are maladaptive in nature (e.g., psychotic denial), however, other defenses are catalogued that would reflect an optimal and perhaps even superior level of functioning. Such defense mechanisms include affiliation, altruism, and humor (APA, 2000). Currently, the DFS is only included in the *DSM–IV* as a possible consideration for future versions of the DSM so that clinicians may estimate and describe psychological defenses that are at a client's disposal. Although the DFS is merely a possibility for use in future versions of the DSM, some researchers and theorists in the field have encouraged continued examination of this scale and the constructs measured (Blais, Conboy, Wilcox, & Norman, 1996).

ALTERNATIVE THOUGHTS ON CLASSIFICATION

The *DSM–IV* enjoys widespread use as the most utilized diagnostic classification system in both clinical and research settings. However, critics of the system abound, and several conceptual alternatives to the *DSM–IV* have been put forward. Some of these alternatives are limited to a particular diagnostic class (e.g., personality disorders), or are in the beginning stage of their theoretical and conceptual construction, whereas other alternatives such as the Psychodynamic Diagnostic Manual (Alliance of Psychoanalytic Organizations, 2006; PDM) and the Diagnostic Classification of Mental Health and Developmental Disorders of Infancy and Early Childhood (Zero to Three: National Center for Infants, Toddlers, and Families, 1994) are currently in print and exist as either competitors or adjuncts to the *DSM–IV*, depending on one's view.

The PDM is a product of the collaboration of five psychoanalytic associations (Packard, 2007). The primary impetus for the creation of the PDM was the complaint from clinicians that although the *DSM–IV* easily separates diagnostic groups for research purposes, it also neglects to include a theoretical foundation that serves to inform treatment planning. The PDM, on the other hand, relies on the foundation of psychoanalytic theory to explain mental health as well as dysfunction. The manual describes three axes: the P axis describes personality variables, the M axis describes mental functioning, and the S axis describes symptom patterns. The authors of the PDM emphasize that the manual is not necessarily a direct competitor to the *DSM–IV*, but can be used as an adjunct for the purpose of increasing clinician effectiveness (Packard, 2007).

The Diagnostic Classification: 0–3 (Zero to Three: National Center for Infants, Toddlers, and Families, 1994) is essentially a diagnostic classification system that has been specifically derived for classifying mental illness and developmental disorders in very young children and infants. Again, given that the *DSM–IV* provides a limited number of diagnostic categories that apply to children from birth to age three, one could consider this manual as more of a complement to the *DSM–IV* rather than a direct competitor in all cases. The Diagnostic Classification: 0–3 (1994) describes a multiaxial system of diagnosis very similar to the *DSM–IV*, except that clinicians note Relationship Classification for Axis II, as opposed to typical Axis II disorders in the *DSM–IV* that largely include personality disorders.

Besides the PDM and Diagnostic Classification: 0–3, which can be used as standalone diagnostic manuals, other researchers and theorists have begun to describe alternative models of classification. For example, Cloninger (1999) has proposed an alternative to the *DSM–IV* that draws from a number of theoretical origins. The author describes a "psychobiologically based paradigm" that acknowledges the importance of certain innate personality characteristics that exist. Cloninger uses evolutionary theory to explain the development of these characteristics as well as their continuous variability within the human race.

These characteristics are purported to be measured by the Temperament and Character Inventory (TCI). Data gathered from the TCI on a clinical population relates these broader temperament and character constructs to both the existence of mental health as well as dysfunction. Some of the differences between this paradigm and the *DSM–IV* as noted by the author include a more developmental perspective on human functioning, and an equal emphasis on mental health. Although Cloninger (1999) alludes to the interaction of neurological processes and the psychological development of the individual, others (Hollander, 2006) have also relied on neurological research to both explain and categorize particular mental disorders.

Specifically, Hollander (2006) calls on future conceptualizations of substance use and impulse control disorders as well as Obsessive-Compulsive Disorder to consider neurological functioning and related laboratory findings in their clinical diagnosis. With continued research in neuroimaging that relates neurological functioning to behavioral and emotional dysfunction, a more physiological and neurological classification system of mental illness is being called on by some in the field (Charney, Barlow, Botteron, Cohen, Goldman, Gur et al., 2002).

Another alternative to the current *DSM–IV* classification of mental illness is the underlying conceptual structure of particular rating scales. Lahey, Applegate, Waldman, Loft, Hankin, and Rick (2004) discuss how particular diagnostic categories such as ADHD are conceptualized differently between the *DSM–IV* and the subscale scores (and the items that derive them) provided on particular rating scales.

Given this, the authors developed an interview covering many of the diagnosable disorders in childhood and adolescence. In examining data from 1,358 participants, the authors tested several taxonomic classifications of psychopathology through both exploratory and confirmatory factor analysis. The authors then describe how the current *DSM–IV* criteria and related categories both agree and differ with the factors derived from their data. For example, these authors describe a factor that describes both hyperactive/impulsive as well as oppositional defiant criteria, thus combining two separate *DSM–IV* diagnoses (Oppositional Defiant Disorder and Attention-Deficit/Hyperactivity Disorder Hyperactive Impulsive Subtype) into a single category of psychopathology. Thus these authors argue for an alternative taxonomy that relies on an empirical investigation of both self and caretaker reports of symptomology (Lahey et al., 2004). For a similar study using empirical methods to derive and confirm personality diagnoses in adolescence, see Westen, Shedler, Durrett, Glass, and Martens (2003).

Jensen, Knapp, and Mrazek (2006a) present an evolutionary perspective of psychological disorders, and this perspective sets the stage for a new way of thinking about diagnoses. Overall, they suggest that the *DSM–IV* considers disorders, by definition, to be maladaptive. However, they add that the symptoms contributing to most disorders are only maladaptive in most modern-day settings. That is, many clusters of symptoms may have actually been adaptive in the evolutionary history of humans. Jensen et al. (2006a) provide evolutionary theories for several disorders that are common in children and adolescents.

For example, the authors apply evolutionary theory to ADHD. That is, inattention, hyperactivity, and impulsivity (i.e., some of the criteria for ADHD) are often maladaptive in modern homes and classrooms. However, there may have been a time in the evolutionary history of humans when these behaviors served an important function. In fact, Jensen, Mrazek et al. (2006) suggest that being too focused on a task may actually be maladaptive in settings that have a high likelihood of danger (e.g., attack from wild animals). Thus, being easily distracted by small changes on the horizon may actually help a person survive. What has been termed "inattention" in the *DSM* is labeled "scanning" behavior in this theory. Also, "hyperactivity" may also be adaptive at times, particularly in settings with few resources. That is, very active behavior may include exploring an environment for scarce resources. Active behavior may also help stimulate muscle development and motor skills. Lastly, in this theory, impulsive behavior may make the difference between success and failure when pouncing on a prey or defending against an attacker. Jensen et al. (2006b) use the term "response-ready" as an alternative to the label ADHD, suggesting that response-ready behavior has been very adaptive in the evolutionary history of humans in some environments.

Similar evolutionary theories for other disorders have also been presented. For example, social anxiety may represent an adaptive sensitivity to social hostility, and panic attacks sometimes alert organisms to actual dangers, such as potential suffocation (Pine & Shapiro, 2006). In a similar vein, depressive behavior may be adaptive in the sense that it ensures the loser of a battle gives up fighting in order to survive (Pfeffer, 2006). Finally, behaviors associated with Conduct Disorder, such as aggression and cunning, also clearly have some survival value in certain environments (Kruesi & Schowalter, 2006). If nothing else, evolutionary theory forces one to consider the context within which behaviors occur, and that context often determines if the behavior is adaptive or maladaptive.

THOUGHTS ON THE *DSM–V*

With the publication of the *DSM–IV* in 1994, well over a decade has now passed with no significant changes made to the diagnostic classification system itself. However, preparatory work on the *DSM–V* has been ongoing for the past several years (Widiger & Simonsen, 2005). A series of white papers, developed by the *DSM–V* Research Planning Work Group, was recently published as an edited book entitled *Research Agenda for DSM–V* (APA, 2002). This source outlined the current research on several fundamental areas of diagnostic classification, including neuroimaging research, animal models, understanding psychopathology within a developmental context, the diagnosis of personality disorders, and other related topics. Additional white papers have been published more recently regarding similar topics.

A website, entitled the *DSM–V Prelude Project* (http://dsm5.org/index.cfm), has been created to both inform professionals in the field regarding the revision process as well as solicit feedback (First, Regier, & Narrow, n.d.).

The most recent work toward the *DSM–V* includes a series of ongoing NIH-sponsored conferences, whose purpose is to lay out a framework for the research agenda that will guide the revision process (Sirovatka, 2004). The next step in the revision process was the appointment of work groups, which occurred in 2008. Therefore, according to the current timeline the publication of the *DSM–V* is anticipated to be May of 2012 (First, Regier, & Narrow, n.d.).

Given that a great deal of preliminary discussion has already taken place regarding the next *DSM*, a few patterns have begun to emerge. First, there is building consensus for a dimensional model of personality disorder as opposed to the current categorical model in the *DSM–IV* (Widiger & Trull, 2007). These authors argue that the current categorical model provides a number of diagnostic problems, including criteria overlap between diagnostic categories and heterogeneity within diagnostic categories. Additionally, they posit that a dimensional model of personality dysfunction, possibly based on the Five Factor Model, would alleviate many of these current diagnostic issues. In fact, others in the field advocate for a dimensional model (as opposed to a categorical one) for many of the other disorders (e.g., mood disorders) listed in the *DSM–IV* (Widiger & Clark, 2000).

Although many behaviorists have proposed replacing the DSM with other systems altogether, Scotti, Morris, McNeil, and Hawkins (1996) suggest improvements for future revisions of the *DSM*. Specifically, they propose revisions to the multiaxial approach that include a focus on the function of behavior. Scotti et al. suggest the diagnostic categories in the *DSM* already give clinicians a starting point with which to begin a functional analysis. A diagnosis describes people with a similar set of behaviors, making it easier for the clinician to start hypothesizing about etiology and potential treatments. However, diagnostic categories typically represent fairly heterogeneous groups of people, thus there remains a need for ideographic assessment, and this could be better reflected in the multiaxial approach of the *DSM*. Goals of the *DSM* include improving diagnosis, communication, research, and treatment. These authors argue that the *DSM* is effective at these first three goals, but that it falls significantly short in helping with treatment planning.

To improve the multiaxial system, Scotti et al. (1996) propose changes to Axis III and Axis IV, with the other axes remaining unchanged. In the *DSM–IV–TR*, Axis III is reserved for General Medical Conditions, and Axis IV is for Psychosocial and Environmental Problems. In the Scotti et al. proposal the medical problems axis would be significantly expanded and relabeled "Ideographic Case Analysis". Part of this axis would include medical conditions that affect the diagnosis, but it would also be expanded to include antecedents and consequences of the primary symptoms. The Psychosocial and Environmental Problems axis would also be expanded and relabeled "Psychosocial and Environmental Resources and Deficits". Although it would continue to include similar problems to those in the current system, it would also have a significant increased focus on resources and client strengths that can be used and built upon to improve treatment outcome. In a later summary of this proposal, Reitman and Hupp (2002) also emphasized the importance of improving Axis V, Global Assessment of Functioning, to include scores from assessment tools with empirical support (e.g., questionnaires) rather than the very broad and generic rating used in the current *DSM*.

Although critics of the *DSM–IV* look to make substantial changes in the upcoming *DSM–V* through the revision process, there are others in the field that continue to defend at least aspects of current practice using the *DSM–IV* as the most empirically supported (Hiller, 2006). Since the publication of the *DSM–III*, the DSM has served as an atheoretical classification system that strives for universal applicability, cutting across both theoretical lines as well as investigations into the etiology of disorders. History, perhaps, will judge whether the *DSM–III*, *DSM–III–R*, and *DSM–IV* have been successful in this endeavor. Perhaps the future of psychiatric diagnosis lies in the integration of theory, rather than the removal of theory. In the words of Banzato (2004), this future would rely on "the combination of sophisticated conceptual framework, methodological pluralism and sound scientific empirical evidence" (p. 500).

REFERENCES

Alliance of Psychoanalytic Organizations. (2006). *Psychodynamic diagnostic manual.* Silver Spring, MD: Author.

American Psychiatric Association. (1952). *Diagnostic and statistical manual of mental disorders.* Washington, DC: Author.

American Psychiatric Association. (1968). *Diagnostic and statistical manual of mental disorders* (2nd ed.). Washington, DC: Author.

American Psychiatric Association. (1980). *Diagnostic and statistical manual of mental disorders* (3rd ed.). Washington, DC: Author.

American Psychiatric Association. (1987). *Diagnostic and statistical manual of mental disorders* (3rd ed., rev.). Washington, DC: Author.

American Psychiatric Association. (1994a). *Diagnostic and statistical manual of mental disorders* (4th ed.). Washington, DC: Author.

American Psychiatric Association. (1994b). *DSM–IV sourcebook: Volume 1.* Washington, DC: Author.

American Psychiatric Association. (1998). *DSM–IV sourcebook: Volume 4.* Washington, DC: Author.

American Psychiatric Association. (2000). *Diagnostic and statistical manual of mental disorders* (4th ed., text revision). Washington, DC: Author.

American Psychiatric Association. (2002). A *research agenda for DSM–V.* Washington, DC: Author.

American Psychological Association, Division 12 Society of Clinical Psychology. (n.d.). *A guide to beneficial psychotherapy.* Retrieved March 7, 2007, from http://www.apa.org/divisions/div12/cppi.html.

Banzato, C. (2004). Classification in psychiatry: The move towards ICD–11 and DSM–V. *Current Opinion in Psychiatry, 17,* 497–501.

Bertelsen, A. (1999). Reflections on the clinical utility of the ICD–10 and DSM–IV classifications and their diagnostic criteria. *Australian and New Zealand Journal of Psychiatry, 33,* 166–173.

Blais, M. A., Conboy, C. A., Wilcox, N., & Norman, D. K. (1996). An empirical study of the DSM–IV defensive functioning scale in personality disordered patients. *Comprehensive Psychiatry, 37,* 435–440.

Bronfenbrenner, U. (1979). *The ecology of human development.* Cambridge, MA: Harvard University Press.

Charney, D., Barlow, D., Botteron, K., Cohen, J., Goldman, D., Gur, R., Lin, K., et al., (2002). Neuroscience research agenda to guide development of a pathophysiologically based classification system. In D.J. Kupfer, M. B. First, & D. A. Regier (Eds.), *A research agenda for DSM–V*. Washington, DC: American Psychiatric Association.

Cloninger, C. R. (1999). A new conceptual paradigm from genetics and psychobiology for the science of mental health. *Australian and New Zealand Journal of Psychiatry, 33,* 174–186.

Department of Education. (2005). 34 CFR Parts 300, 301 and 304 Federal Register June 21, 2005.

First, M. B., & Pincus, H. A. (1999). Classification in psychiatry: ICD–10 v. DSM–IV: A response. *British Journal of Psychiatry, 175,* 205–209.

First, M. B., Regier, D. A., & Narrow, W. (n.d.). *DSM–V prelude project: Research and outreach.* Retrieved March 1, 2007, from DSM–V Prelude Project Web site: http://dsm5.org/index.cfm.

Frances, A. J. & Egger, H. L. (1999). Whither psychiatric diagnosis. *Australian and New Zealand Journal of Psychiatry, 33,* 161–165.

Greene, R. R., Galambos, C., & Lee, Youjung, (2003). Resilience theory: Theoretical and professional conceptualizations. *Journal of Human Behavior in the Social Environment, 8,* 75–91.

Helmchen, H., & Linden, M. (2000). Subthreshold disorders in psychiatry: Clinical reality, methodological artifact, and the double-threshold problem. *Comprehensive Psychiatry, 41,* 1–7.

Hiller, W. (2006). Don't change a winning horse. *Journal of Psychosomatic Research, 60,* 345–347.

Hollander, E. (2006). Behavioral and substance addictions: A new proposed DSM–V category characterized by impulsive choice, reward sensitivity, and fronto-striatal circuit impairment. *CNS Spectrums, 11,* 814–822.

Houts, A. C. (2002). Discovery, invention, and the expansion of the modern *Diagnostic and Statistical Manuals of Mental Disorders.* In L. E. Beutler & M. L. Malik (Eds.), *Rethinking the DSM: A psychological perspective.* Washington, DC: American Psychological Association.

Jablensky, A., & Kendell, R. E. (2002). Criteria for assessing a classification in psychiatry. In M. Maj, W. Gaebel, J. J. López-Ibor, & N. Sartorius (Eds.), *Psychiatric diagnosis and classification* (pp. 1–24). New York: John Wiley & Sons.

Jensen, P. S., Knapp, P., & Mrazek, D. A. (2006a). *Toward a new diagnostic system for child psychopathology: Moving beyond the DSM.* New York: Guilford Press.

Jensen, P. S., Mrazek, D. A., Knapp, P., Steinberg, L., Pfeffer, C. R., Schowalter, J., & Shapiro, T. (2006b). Application of evolutionary models to Attention Deficit/Hyperactivity Disorder. In P. Jensen, P. Knapp, & D. A. Mrazek (Eds.), *Toward a new diagnostic system for child psychopathology: Moving beyond the DSM* (pp. 96–110). New York: Guilford Press.

Knapp, P., & Jensen, P. S. (2006). Recommendations for the DSM–V. In P. Jensen, P. Knapp, & D. A. Mrazek (Eds.), Toward a new diagnostic system for child *psychopathology: Moving beyond the DSM* (pp. 111–130). New York: Guilford Press.

Kösters, M., Burlingame, G. M., Nachtigall, C., & Strauss, B. (2006). A meta-analytic review of the effectiveness of inpatient group therapy. *Group Dynamics: Theory, Research, and Practice, 10,* 146–163.

Kruesi, M., & Schowalter (2006). Conduct disorder and evolutionary biology. In P. Jensen, P. Knapp, & D. A. Mrazek (Eds.), *Toward a new diagnostic system for child psychopathology: Moving beyond the DSM* (pp. 111–130). New York: Guilford Press.

Lahey, B. B., Applegate, B., Waldman, I. D., Loft, J. D., Hankin, B. L., & Rick, J. (2004). The structure of child and adolescent psychopathology: Generating new hypotheses. *Journal of Abnormal Psychology, 113,* 358–385.

Langenbucher, J. & Nathan, P. E. (2006). Diagnosis and classification. In M. Hersen & J. C. Thomas (Eds.), *Comprehensive handbook of personality and psychopathology: Volume 2,* pp 3–20. Hoboken, NJ: Wiley.

Liu, C. Y. & Apuzzo, M. L. J. (2003). The genesis of neurosurgery and the evolution of the neurosurgical operative environment: Part I – prehistory to 2003. *Neurosurgery, 52,* 3–19.

Newman, R. & Bricklin, P. M. (1991). Parameters of managed mental health care: Legal, ethical, and professional guidelines. *Professional Psychology: Research and Practice, 22,* 26–35.

Packard, E. (2007). A new tool for psychotherapists. *Monitor on Psychology, 38,* 30–32.

Pfeffer, C. R. (2006). An evolutionary perspective on childhood depression. In P. Jensen, P. Knapp, & D. A. Mrazek (Eds.), *Toward a new diagnostic system for child psychopathology: Moving beyond the DSM* (pp. 78–95). New York: Guilford Press.

Pine, D. S., & Shapiro, T. (2006). A developmental evolutionary perspective on two anxiety disorders. In P. Jensen, P. Knapp, & D. A. Mrazek (Eds.), *Toward a new diagnostic system for child psychopathology: Moving beyond the DSM* (pp. 58–77). New York: Guilford Press.

Reitman, D., & Hupp, S. D. A. (2002). Behavior problems in the school setting: Synthesizing structural and functional assessment. In M. L. Kelley, G. H. Noell, and D. Reitman (Eds.), *Practitioner's guide to empirically based measures of school behavior.* New York: Plenum.

Schulte-Markwort, M., Marutt, K., & Riedesser, P. (2003). *Cross-walks ICD–10 – DSM–IV–TR: A synopsis of classifications of mental disorders.* Cambridge, MA: Hogrefe & Huber.

Scotti, J. R., Morris, T. L., McNeil, C. B., & Hawkins, R. P. (1996). *DSM–IV* and disorders of childhood and adolescence: Can structural criteria be functional? *Journal of Consulting and Clinical Psychology, 64,* 1177–1191.

Sirovatka, P. (2004, Winter). DSM research planning. *Psychiatric Research Report, 20,* 1–3.

Spitzer, R. L. & Fleiss, J. L. (1974). A re-analysis of the reliability of psychiatric diagnosis. *British Journal of Psychiatry, 125,* 341–347.

Üstün, T. B., Chatterji, S., & Andrews, G. (2002). International classifications and the diagnosis of mental disorders: Strengths, limitations and future perspectives. In M. Maj, W. Gaebel, J. J. López-Ibor, & N. Sartorius (Eds.), *Psychiatric diagnosis and classification* (pp. 25–46). New York: John Wiley & Sons.

Westen, D., Shedler, J., Durrett, C., Glass, S., & Martens, A. (2003). Personality diagnoses in adolescence: *DSM–IV* Axis II diagnoses and an empirically derived alternative. *American Journal of Psychiatry, 160,* 952–966.

Widiger, T. A. (2005). Classification and diagnosis: Historical development and contemporary issues. In J. E. Maddux, & B. A. Winstead (Eds), *Psychopathology: Foundations for a contemporary understanding* (pp. 63–83). Mahwah, NJ: Lawrence Erlbaum.

Widiger, T. A. & Clark, L. A. (2000). Toward DSM–V and the classification of psychopathology. *Psychological Bulletin, 126,* 946–963.

Widiger, T. A. & Simonsen, E. (2005). Introduction to the special section: The American Psychiatric Association's research agenda for the *DSM–V. Journal of Personality Disorders, 19,* 103–109.

Widiger, T. A., & Trull, T. J. (2007). Plate tectonics in the classification of personality disorder: Shifting to a dimensional model. *American Psychologist, 62,* 71–83.

World Health Organization (1992). *International classification of diseases classification of mental and behavioral disorders: Clinical descriptions and diagnostic guidelines* (10th revision). Geneva: Author.

World Health Organization (1993). *International classification of diseases classification of mental and behavioral disorders: Diagnostic criteria for research* (10th revision). Geneva: Author.

World Health Organization (1996). *Multiaxial classification of child and adolescent psychiatric disorders: The ICD–10 classification of mental and behavioural disorders in children and adolescents.* Geneva: Author.

Zero to Three: National Center for Infants, Toddlers, and Families. (1994). *Diagnostic classification of mental health and developmental disorders of infancy and early childhood: Diagnostic classification: 0–3.* Washington, DC: Author.

3

Interview and Report Writing

AMIE E. GRILLS-TAQUECHEL, ROSANNA POLIFRONI, and JACK M. FLETCHER

The interview is a critical component of the psychological assessment of a child. In addition to the standard unstructured interview, several structured interviews have been developed for use with children and their parents/caregivers.[1] This chapter is designed to introduce and familiarize the reader with not only which interviews are available for use when assessing children, but also with techniques appropriate and effective for use during interviews when a child is the identified client. We discuss considerations in using interview procedures with children who have disabilities as well as other factors related to the use of interviews, such as language dominance. Considerations for basic report writing are also described.

INTERVIEWS FOR CHILDREN

Interviews are often the most comprehensive assessment tools for clinicians, allowing for the evaluation and observation of both behavioral and emotional functioning. Historically, reliance was given to parental reports and any information given by the child was considered secondary. In fact, children were rarely included in the interview process due to beliefs that they lacked the cognitive capabilities to give accurate statements about their feelings and behaviors (Edelbrock & Costello, 1990; Herjanic, Herjanic, Brown, & Wheatt, 1975). The seminal work of Lapouse and Monk

---

[1] Note: Although interviews are intended to be conducted with any primary caregiver as informant (e.g., parents, grandparents, stepparents, guardian ad litem, etc.), use of the term "parent" is employed from this point forward for reading ease.

AMIE E. GRILLS-TAQUECHEL, ROSANNA POLIFRONI, and JACK M. FLETCHER •
Department of Psychology, University of Houston, Tx 72204-5022.

J.L. Matson et al. (eds.), *Assessing Childhood Psychopathology and Developmental Disabilities*, DOI: 10.1007/978-0-387-09528-8,
© Springer Science+Business Media, LLC 2009

(1958), as well as Rutter and colleagues (Rutter & Graham, 1968; Rutter, Tizard, & Whitmore, 1970; Rutter, Tizard, Yule, Graham, & Whitmore, 1976; Rutter, Tizard, Yule, Graham, & Whitmore, 1977), altered the manner in which the reports of youth were considered by demonstrating psychometric soundness for child structured interviews. Thus, currently most clinicians consider the child to be an essential informant in the interview process (Chambers et al., 1985; De Los Reyes & Kazdin, 2005; Edelbrock, Costello, Dulcan, Kalas, & Conover, 1985; Grills & Ollendick, 2002; Kazdin, French, & Unis, 1983; Moretti, Fine, Haley, & Marriage, 1985; Ollendick & Hersen, 1993; Verhulst, Althaus, & Berden, 1987). Consequently, numerous parent/child interview measures and techniques have been developed. At a basic level, interviews can be differentiated by the amount of structure utilized to elicit responses, with most falling into the categories of unstructured, semi-structured, and highly structured.

Unstructured Interviews

An unstructured interview is conducted as part of most, if not all, evaluations and is commonly the first significant contact the family has with the clinician. Most clinicians begin their assessment with some form of unstructured interview, with variations occurring in the depth, breadth, and participants (i.e., child, caregivers, siblings, etc.) included. A particular strength of the unstructured interview format is the individualized nature, which allows for significant clinician freedom and judgment. Apart from the typically included demographic (e.g., age of child, level of acculturation) and introductory (e.g., "What brings you in today") information, there are no required/standard question sets, which allows for flexibility in pursuing ambiguous responses or gathering greater details. However, unstructured diagnostic interviews should not be mistaken as an opportunity to simply engage in conversation with the client. In order to collect sufficient information, preparation and organization are required to direct discussion toward topics that are relevant to the problem at hand, and that will aid in eventual diagnostic and/or treatment decisions.

Unstructured interviews are perhaps best suited for the more experienced clinician, who would be better equipped with the skills necessary for asking the "right" questions (Sattler & Hoge, 2006). For example, a trained clinician is more likely to know which questions elicit the most useful and relevant information from the child, whereas a lay interviewer may spend too much time in general conversation or asking irrelevant questions that could inhibit the eventual diagnostic or treatment formulation (Sattler & Hoge, 2006). Of course, a less experienced clinician can become more experienced through practice sessions and supervised unstructured interview administrations. In addition, newer clinicians may benefit from gradually moving from a structured to unstructured format. For example, becoming familiar with the probe and follow-up questions typically included in more structured interviews, as well as areas of differential diagnosis (e.g., *DSM-IV-TR*, American Psychiatric Association, 2000), may help establish a flowing questioning style while remaining comprehensive in the scope of inquiries.

Structured Interviews

Structured diagnostic interviews were designed to increase the reliability of diagnoses by standardizing the method used to elicit responses. This, in turn, is expected to have the effect of increasing the reliability of the responses and eliminating potential biases (e.g., making decisions prior to the collection of all the information, only collecting confirming or disconfirming evidence) associated with clinical judgment (Angold, 2002). Structured interviews formally examine particular problem areas with several expectations, including that the interviews: (1) are internally consistent, (2) have specific rules regarding the content and order of the questions asked (e.g., asking whether depressed mood is present prior to asking the possible effects of the depressed mood) as well as the manner of recording responses, and (3) have some degree of guidance provided for arriving at final diagnostic decisions (Weiss, 1993).

Structured interviews are generally geared toward gathering information about specific *DSM* criteria and are therefore typically ideal for assessing psychiatric symptoms and formulating diagnoses. Furthermore, structured interviews are commonly used because they include a standard set of questions designed to cover the range of topics necessary for obtaining relevant information about the interviewee's presenting problems. The degree to which the interview fits with these expectations and the amount of latitude allotted to the examiner result in classifications of semi-structured or highly structured.

For the most part, the format of (semi/highly) structured parent and child companion interviews is similar. The typical layout is: (1) an introductory section designed to help build rapport with the informant (e.g., demographics, school, psychological history) and elicit initial information regarding presenting problems and history; (2) disorder-specific sections targeting symptom presence, frequency, intensity, duration, and interference; (3) diagnostic formulations based on preset algorithms and/or clinical judgments. All of the interviews can be used in either research or clinical settings and typically require one to three hours to complete. In addition, for most interview sets, the parent version contains additional diagnostic categories (e.g., the child version of the ADIS does not contain the enuresis section whereas the parent version does) and can be used alone when the child is too young to complete his or her respective version. In addition, most structured interviews are comprised of questions that are asked in a branching manner. For each diagnostic category, there are screener or core questions that must be administered. Secondary questions are then asked only if the child/parent endorsed the initial screener questions. However, if the initial questions are not endorsed, the interview proceeds to the next diagnostic category.

Highly structured interviews are more restrictive in the amount of freedom allotted to the interviewer. With these interviews, it is generally expected that examiners ask all questions in the same manner and order, as well as record all responses in a prespecified manner. Given the rigid format, clinical judgment is reduced and specific and/or extensive training is usually not required. In fact, highly structured interviews are commonly administered by laypersons (e.g., individuals without a formal degree in psychology, psychiatry, or social work) and several have been converted to computer-based formats. Two of the more commonly utilized highly structured interviews are described below and summarized in Table 3.1.

   The Diagnostic Interview Schedule for Children (DISC; Shaffer, Fisher, Lucas, Dulcan, & Schwab-Stone, 2000) was designed to assess *DSM-IV/*

Table 3.1. Summary of Commonly Utilizzed Structured Diagnostic Interviews

Interview	Type	~Length/ interview	Age Range	Cost Range	Interviewer	Informant and Specifications
DISC-IV	Highly structured	1–2 hours	9–17 (child version) 6–17 (parent version)	$150 to $2000	Trained Lay Interviewers	Child and parent
ChIPS	Highly structured	40 min.	6–18 (child/ parent versions)	$115	Highly Trained Lay Interviewer	Child and Parent
CAPA	Interviewer/ glossary-based	1 hour	9–17 (child version)	$2650 for information packet/ training	Highly Trained/ Experienced Lay Interviewer	Child and Parent
ADIS-IV	Semi-structured	3 hours	7–17 (child/ parent versions)	$26 for manual and parent/ child interview	Highly Trained Lay Interviewers	Child and Parent Interviewed Separately
DICA-IV	Semi-structured	1 to 2 hours	6–12 (child version) 13–18 (adolescent version) 6–18 (parent version)	$1000 for computer Paper/ pencil cost varies	Highly Trained Lay Interviewer	Same Clinician Child and Parent
KSADS-IV	Semi-structured	1.25–1.5 hours	6–18 (child/ parent versions)	E- $75; P/L- Online; P-IVR- Free	Trained Clinicians	Parent (1st) and Child Interviewed Separately Same Clinician
ISCA	Semi-structured	45 min.– 2.5 hours	8–17 (child/ parent versions)	Obtain from developer	Trained Clinicians	Parent (1st) and Child Interviewed Separately Same Clinician

ICD-10 psychiatric disorders that can be identified in children and adolescents (see Table 3.2). The DISC-IV evaluates symptoms from the past year, as well as recent (last month) symptoms for any areas endorsed. The DISC utilizes "gate" questions that allow the interviewer to skip sections of the interview that are irrelevant to the individual without hindering the reliability of the examination. Given the highly structured format, little training is required for the administration of the DISC. Indeed, lay interviewers and computer administration (C-DISC-4.0) are common inasmuch as questions are read verbatim following a specified order and diagnoses

Table 3.2. Summary of Possible Diagnoses Covered by the Structured Interviews Reviewed

	K-SADS	ADIS-IV	DISC-IV	DICA	CAPA	ISCA	ChIPS
Major depression	Y	Y	Y	Y	Y	Y	Y
Dysthymia	Y	Y	Y	Y	Y	Y	Y
Bipolar Disorder	Y	N	Y	Y	Y	Y	Y
Mania	Y	N	Y	Y	Y	Y	Y
Hypomania	Y	N	Y	Y	Y	Y	Y
Cyclothymia	Y	N	N	N	Y	Y	N
Somatization Disorder	N	N	N	Y	Y	Y	N
Anorexia Nervosa	Y	Y[b]	Y	Y	Y	Y	Y
Bulimia Nervosa	Y	Y[b]	Y	Y	Y	Y	Y
PICA	N	N	Y	N	N	N	N
Enuresis	Y[a]	Y[c]	Y	N	Y	Y	Y
Encopresis	Y[a]	N	Y	N	Y	Y	Y
Sleep Disorders	N	N	N	N	Y	Y	N
Tic Disorders	Y[a]	N	Y	Y	Y	N	N
Trichotillomania	N	N	Y	N	Y	N	N
Schizophrenia	Y	N	Y	N	Y	N	Y
Schizoaffective	Y	N	N	N	Y	N	N
Delusional Disorder	N	N	Y	N	Y	N	N
Generalized Anxiety Disorder	Y	Y	Y	Y	Y	Y	Y
Separation Anxiety Disorder	Y	Y	Y	Y	Y	Y	Y
Obsessive-Compulsive Disorder	Y	Y	Y	Y	Y	Y	Y
Simple Phobia	Y	Y	Y	Y	Y	Y	Y
Social Phobia	Y	Y	Y	Y	Y	Y	Y
Agoraphobia	Y	Y	Y	N	N	N	N
Panic Disorder	Y	Y	Y	Y	Y	Y	N
Selective Mutism	Y	N	Y	N	Y	N	N
Posttraumatic Stress Disorder	Y	Y	Y	Y	Y	N	Y
Acute Stress Disorder	N	N	N	N	-	-	Y
Adjustment Disorder	N	N	N	N	Y	Y	N
Oppositional Defiant Disorder	Y	Y[c]	Y	Y	Y	Y	Y
Attention Deficit Hyperactivity Disorder	Y	Y	Y	Y	Y[c]	Y	Y
Conduct Disorder	Y	Y[c]	Y	Y	Y	Y	Y
Substance Disorders	Y	Y	Y	Y	Y	Y	Y
Personality Disorders	Y	N	N	N	N	Y	N
Gender Identity Disorder	N	N	Y	Y	N	N	N

[a] K-SADS-E & K-SADS-P/L versions only.
[b] screens for these disorders only.
[c] parent version only.

are computer generated. The DISC has been extensively researched and several additional versions (e.g., Spanish, Teacher) have also been developed (Shaffer et al., 2000). A sample item from the DISC-IV, Parent Version is provided as an illustration of this highly structured interview (see Figure 3.1).

The Children's Interview for Psychiatric Syndromes (ChIPS; Weller, Weller, Fristad, Rooney, & Schecter, 2000; Weller, Weller, Teare, & Fristad, 1999) is also considered a highly structured interview and was designed to cater to younger children. It is shorter than other structured interviews and it incorporates concise sentence structure and simple language to ensure comprehension. The ChIPS for *DSM-IV* includes 20 sections that assess Axis I diagnoses (see Table 3.2) and two sections that examine psychosocial stressors. Lay interviewers can be trained in the administration of the ChIPS, with a scoring manual used to record and summarize responses according to *DSM-IV* criteria. Extensive studies have been conducted and published on the development of the ChIPS (Fristad et al., 1998a; Fristad et al., 1998b; Fristad, Teare, Weller, Weller, & Salmon, 1998c; Teare, Fristad, Weller, Weller, & Salmon, 1998a, 1998b).

Although highly structured formats allow for more confidence in the exactness of the interview's administration and perhaps more reliable findings, the rigidity of the interview may also make it seem impersonal, hinder the establishment of rapport, and interfere with reliability and validity by not providing the interviewee the opportunity to report all difficulties or to explore them in full depth (Breton et al., 1995; LaGreca & Stone, 1992; Verhulst et al., 1987). As a result, the use of highly structured interviews may result in unanswered questions for the clinician that might have been addressed in a less structured format (e.g., knowing a child feels sad most days does not answer questions of potential precipitants, etiological factors, or responses by others in the child's environment). Another area of critique of structured interviews is their heavy emphasis on diagnosis generation. That is, structured interviews leave little room for assessing the context of the behavior, as well as how developmental stages may dictate stage-specific behavior for which a diagnosis may be unwarranted.

A combination of structured and unstructured interview formats, semi-structured interviews include a suggested order and configuration like that of highly structured interviews; however, there is also more opportunity to follow up on certain questions, and flexibility on the phrasing and recording of questions and responses. Emphasis is placed on obtaining consistent and reliable information, so that extensive training is generally required for administration of semi-structured interviews to ensure that clinical discretion will be applied judiciously. Although not an exhaustive list, several of the more commonly utilized semi-structured interviews for *DSM-IV* are described below and summarized in Table 3.1.

The Schedule for Affective Disorders and Schizophrenia for School-Age Children (K-SADS) has a primary focus on affective disorders, however, several additional psychiatric disorders are also examined (see Table 3.2). The three most current and widely used versions of the K-SADS are: Present State (P-IVR; Ambrosini & Dixon, 1996), Epidemiological (E-Version 5;

0=NO 1=SOMETIMES/SOMEWHAT 2=YES 7,77=REFUSE TO ANSWER 8,88=NOT APPLICABLE 9,99=DON'T KNOW

Some [children/young people] get very upset or nervous when they are not with their parents or with the grown-ups who usually look after them. I am going to ask you some questions about that.

1. In the last year—that is, since [[NAME EVENT]/[NAME CURRENT MONTH]   0 2 7 9 [16]
   of last year]—was there a time when ____often wanted to stay at home and
   not go (to [school/work] or other) places without you

   IF YES, A. Were there several weeks in a row when [he/she] seemed   0 2 7 9 [17]
         nervous or afraid about being away from you or away from home?

         B. Now, what about the <u>last four weeks</u>?   0 2 7 9 [18]
         Since [[NAME EVENT]//the beginning of/the middle of/the end of
         [LAST MONTH]], has [he/she] wanted to stay home because [he/she]
         was worried about going (to [school/work] or other) places without you

Figure 3.1. Separation Anxiety Disorder Sample Question from a Highly Structured Interview (DISC-IV)

Orvaschel, 1995), and Present/Lifetime (P/L; Kaufman et al., 1997). Each of these interviews has child and parent companion versions that differ primarily in regard to the diagnostic time frame examined. For example, the K-SADS-P-IVR examines disorders from the past 12 months and most recent episode, whereas the K-SADS-E and P/L focus on current and lifetime disorders.

In general, the K-SADS parent version is administered before the child version, with discrepancies addressed in a subsequent joint interview. Following the interviews and consideration of all reports (e.g., parent, child, school, clinicians), the clinician determines summary severity scores and diagnoses are made based on criteria checklists of symptom severity (i.e., Research Diagnostic Criteria). Other KSADS sections include behavioral observations, global impressions, and reliability and completeness of the interview. Clinically trained interviewers familiar with *KSADS* are required for administering this semi-structured interview and training costs are noted to vary by version (Ambrosini, 2000). A sample item from the *KSADS-P-IVR* is provided as an illustration of this semi-structured interview (see Figure 3.2).

The Child and Adolescent Psychiatric Assessment (CAPA; Angold, Prendergast, Cox, & Harrington, 1995; Angold & Costello, 2000) is a semi-structured interview designed to generate *DSM-IV* diagnoses. The CAPA has been referred to as "glossary based" because it includes an interview glossary that has detailed definitions of each symptom, which then provides the basis for client response interpretation (Angold & Fisher, 1999). The diagnostic section of the interview is given first and includes evaluation of symptoms and functional impairment followed by the assessment of family structure, functioning, and resources. Each diagnostic section includes a brief description of the symptom being assessed, as well as

SEPARATION ANXIETY

Refers to feelings of <u>excessive anxiety</u> (butterflies in stomach, nervousness, scary feelings) <u>in context of separation</u> from mother or major attachment figure. Younger child may exhibit a pattern of discomfort when traveling alone, or refusal/homesickness when attending camp or sleep-overs. They may show demanding, intrusive behavior, needing constant attention, or show an unusually conscientious, comforting, or eager to please behavioral pattern. Older children or adolescents may begin refusing school, worry about leaving for college, and/or avoid situations involving separations. Symptoms frequently accompanying separation anxiety are listed below. DSM-III-R identified Distress with Separation as anticipatory distress or separation distress. DSM-IV collapses these two symptoms.

FIRST SCORE THE SYMPTOMS LISTED BELOW, THEN RATE **OVERALL SEVERITY**.

SCHOOL REFUSAL

	No Info	No	Slight	Mild/ Moderate	Severe/ Extreme
Reluctance to go to school. Differentiate from Truancy and loss of interest in school because Child can't perform from Depressive Disorder.	0	1	2	3	4

- Have you been going to school?
- Missed any days? What happened? (If sick)
  What kind of sickness did you have?   2-Occasionally.
- Did you take medicine, have a fever,   3-Sometimes/Often.
  see the doctor?   4-Most of the time/
- Did just staying at home make you better?   Almost all the time.
- Do you have any worries about
  being in school?
- Do you get any scary feelings about
  going to school, when you're getting ready
  to go, or on your way there?
- Does having these worries make
  you feel like this?
  One day, most days, every school day?
- Have you ever left school before it's over?
  What's happened? Where did you go?

WHAT ABOUT THE LAST WEEK?   LAST WEEK: 0 1 2 3 4

Figure 3.2. Separation Anxiety Disorder Sample Question from a Semi-Structured Interview (KSADS-P-IVR)

screening questions, which must be asked verbatim unless modified wording is required for child comprehension.

Optional follow-up questions are also provided for the clinician to use if clarification of previous responses is necessary. Additionally, coding rules are applied for rating symptoms in terms of intensity, setting, and timing, as applicable. After the interview, the examiner completes a series of questions based on behavioral observations (i.e., motor behavior, level of activity, apparent mood, and social interaction). Interviewers must have at least a bachelor's degree and receive extensive training in CAPA administration by a qualified *CAPA* trainer over the course of approximately one month.

The Diagnostic Interview for Children and Adolescents (DICA; Reich, 1998; 2000) is a semi-structured interview designed to examine a wide range of youth psychiatric disorders (see Table 3.2). There are two separate youth versions (for ages 6–12 and 13–17 years) and a corresponding parent version. The DICA begins with a joint parent/child interview of demographics, school, and psychiatric and medical histories. This is followed by separately conducted diagnostic sections of the parent and youth interviews. In addition, the parent version also includes inquiries of psychosocial stressors, risk/protective factors, perinatal, delivery, and early child development. The DICA includes structured probes to allow the clinician to clarify interviewee responses when warranted (Silverman, 1994; Ollendick, King, & Yule, 1994).

Following completion of the interview, the interviewer pursues problematic areas which are then resolved by consultation with the DICA manual and/or discussion with more experienced clinicians or primary investigators. A highly structured computerized version of the DICA is also available for administration by trained interviewers or the informant alone. Interviewers must hold at least a bachelor's degree and require approximately two to four weeks of training in the DICA. The focus of the interviewer is on rating each symptom and not ruling upon the presence or absence of diagnoses (Reich, 2000).

The Interview Schedule for Children and Adolescents (ISCA; Kovacs, 1997; Sherrill & Kovacs, 2000) is a semi-structured, symptom-oriented interview that allows for the generation of several diagnoses by mapping symptoms onto the *DSM-IV* disorders (see Table 3.2). The ISCA contains five sections: signs and symptoms (e.g., anxiety, dysregulated behavior), mental status (i.e., orientation), behavioral observations (i.e., nonverbal expression), clinical impressions (i.e., social maturity), and developmental milestones (i.e., dating). There is also one item that examines the child's global functioning and social impairment. The ISCA assesses current symptoms; however, separate current/lifetime and current/interim (i.e., since last assessment) versions are also available.

The ISCA is usually administered by the same clinician to the parent(s) first and then the child separately. Although all questions (roughly 105) are asked of each informant, the interviewer can decide upon the order of administration. At the end of the assessment the interviewer combines the ratings from both the parent and child to establish an overall symptom rating. A diagnosis is made based on correspondence between established criteria (e.g., *DSM*) and the clinical significance and temporal sequence of the overall symptom ratings. Clinically relevant experience with semi-structured interviews and diagnostic system(s) is requisite for ISCA administration.

The Anxiety Disorders Interview Schedule for DSM-IV, Child and Parent Versions (ADIS-IV:C/P; Silverman & Albano, 1996) is a semi-structured interview that permits diagnoses of all anxiety disorders, as well as several other disorders of childhood and adolescence (e.g., Attention-Deficit/ Hyperactivity Disorder, Dysthymia) from the *DSM-IV* (see Table 3.2). The parent and child versions overlap considerably; however, the parent version contains several additional disorders (e.g., Conduct Disorder, Oppositional Defiant Disorder, Enuresis) as well as requires greater detail regarding the history and consequences of problems. The child version probes for more in-depth descriptions of symptoms and phenomenology, while providing a simpler format and wordings (Silverman & Nelles, 1988).

During the interview, respondents are first asked to answer "yes" or "no" to several screener questions. If the child or parent responds affirmatively to the screener, the clinician continues to assess symptoms within that section as well as obtain frequency, intensity, and interference ratings as appropriate. These ratings (e.g., symptom count and interference rating) assist the clinician in identifying which diagnostic criteria are met for the child. Following the interview, clinicians assign severity ratings for each diagnosis met based on their subjective interpretation from the child and parent reports. ADIS training is required prior to administration and it is recommended that the same clinician interview the child and subsequently the parent(s) (Albano & Silverman, 1996).

PSYCHOMETRICS OF INTERVIEW PROCEDURES

Psychometric studies have been conducted for each of the above-described interviews. In general, researchers have been concerned with demonstrating the reliability (i.e., consistency of measurement), validity (i.e., degree it assesses what it purports to measure), and clinical utility of these interviews. Overall, consistent findings have been reported across the various structured interviews for which reliability data is available (cf., ADIS: Albano & Silverman, 1996; Weems, Silverman, Saavedra, Pina, & Lumpkin, 1999; Wood, Piacentini, Bergman, McCracken, & Barrios. 2002; CAPA: Angold & Costello, 2000; ChIPS: Weller et al., 2000; DICA: Reich, 1998; 2000; DISC: Costello, Edelbrock, & Costello, 1985; Shaffer et al., 2000; ISCA: Sherrill & Kovacs, 2000; KSADS: Ambrosini, 2000). Acceptable test–retest and interrater reliability estimates have been documented for each of the structured interviews (Angold, 2002; Grills-Taquechel & Ollendick, 2002, 2007). In contrast, findings for multiple-informant reliability (e.g., parent–child agreement) have been more varied (Angold, 2002; De Los Reyes & Kazdin, 2005; Grills-Taquechel & Ollendick, 2002, 2007), a result also commonly reported for behavior rating scales (Achenbach, Dumenci, & Rescorla, 2002; Achenbach, McConaughy, & Howell, 1987; De Los Reyes & Kazdin, 2005; DiBartolo & Grills, 2006).

Attempts to understand informant discordance have been made at the interview (e.g., order effects, length, structure), interviewer (e.g., experience level, site differences, biases), and interviewee (e.g., age, gender, disorder type, motivation) levels with generally inconsistent results (Grills-Taquechel & Ollendick, 2002, 2007). Thus, the broad consensus in the youth assessment area is that parent(s) and children should both be involved in the assessment of youth symptoms and diagnoses (Jensen et al., 1999; Silverman & Ollendick, 2005, 2008). Moreover, teacher and school reports are also important with child cases, as the child may behave differently in academic settings and/or the parent may be unaware of the child's school behaviors (Karver, 2006; Tripp, Schaughency, & Clarke, 2006). Thus, despite potential disagreements, inclusion of multiple informants is imperative for acquiring the most comprehensive and accurate account of the child's presenting problems, particularly given the situation-specific nature of some child behaviors (e.g., inattention at school but not when watching television). Therefore, rather than searching for the "correct" answer among multiple informants, it has been recommended that clinicians consider all sources of information and allow discrepancies to be interpreted as informative, not problematic (Boyle et al., 1996; Schwab-Stone et al., 1996).

Varied results have also been presented for the validity of structured interviews. For example, studies have reported positive results regarding construct and/or criterion-related validity (Ambrosini, 2000; Angold & Costello, 2000; Boyle et al., 1996; Cohen, O'Connor, Lewis, Velez, & Malachowski, 1987; Fristad, Cummins, et al., 1998; Fristad, Teare, et al., 1998; Hodges, McKnew, Burbach, & Roebuck, 1987; Kaufman et al., 1997; Piacentini et al., 1993; Reich, 2000; Schwab-Stone et al., 1996; Teare et al., 1998a; Wood et al., 2002). However, concordance for diagnoses generated by structured interviews and "real world" clinicians has often been poor (Jensen & Weisz, 2002; Jewell, Handwerk, Almquist, & Lucas, 2004; Lewcyz, Garland, Hurlburt, Gearity, & Hough, 2003). To illustrate, studies have shown poor validity when diagnoses obtained from diagnostic interviews are compared to clinician diagnoses at outpatient clinics (Ezpeleta, de la Osa, Doménech, Navarro, & Losilla, 1997), inpatient clinics (Pellegrino, Singh, & Carmanico, 1999; Vitiello, Malone, Buschle, & Delaney, 1990), and on admission (Weinstein, Stone, Noam, & Grimes, 1989) and discharge (Aronen, Noam, & Weinstein, 1993; Welner, Reich, Herjanic, Jung, & Amado, 1987) from these settings.

Nonetheless, establishing the validity of diagnoses based on diagnostic interviews is difficult because there is no "gold standard" with which to compare the findings. That is, no definitive standard exists to compare the accuracy of diagnoses generated from structured and unstructured clinician interviews, and numerous factors could influence either side (Jensen & Weisz, 2002). Finally, it is important to note that structured interviews must be considered within the context of the diagnostic system upon which they are based. If diagnostic criteria are not presented in a manner that allows for their adequate assessment, this will be reflected in the interviews as well. Thus, problems with diagnostic interviews may speak to the need for further alterations or amendments to the diagnostic system itself (Achenbach, 2005).

The clinical utility of structured interviews has also received discussion. For example, as the selection and course of psychological treatments often follow from the particular diagnosis received (Silverman & Ollendick, 2008), interview problems can translate into inappropriate case conceptualization and treatment planning. Likewise, researchers often use structured interviews in studies designed to further understanding of child psychopathology and treatment. However, if the findings resulting from these interviews are unreliable, then the information cannot be translated to meaningful clinical practice. In addition, the boundary between normal and pathological problems will be more blurred than usual given the dimensional nature of most disorders affecting children, and interviewers may have increased difficulty making reliable diagnostic decisions. Thus, incorporating functional assessments into structured interviews or including a separate functional analysis interview (e.g., Questions About Behavioral Function; Matson, Bamburg, Cherry, & Paclawskyj, 1999) may help alleviate these problems by examining information at a more idiographic level (Scotti, Morris, McNeil, & Hawkins, 1996). Likewise, a "prescriptive" approach of matching endorsed symptoms with appropriate treatment strategies has recently gained attention as a manner of increasing the clinical meaningfulness of interview information (Chorpita, 2007; Eisen & Silverman, 1993, 1998; Ollendick, 1995; Ollendick, Hagopian, & Huntzinger, 1991).

Selecting Interview Procedures

In addition to consideration of psychometric issues, numerous other factors may guide selection among the various structured diagnostic interviews. For example, the rating system used to score responses and compile information, required training for administration, and costs of interviews vary widely (see Table 3.1). In addition, the setting in which the interview will take place can be influential. For instance, research, epidemiological, or clinical trial settings will likely involve more in-depth and lengthier interview (and overall assessment) processes. Within these settings a complete structured interview might be given to the parent and child (along with other assessments). Conversely, in a typical practice setting the clinician would be less likely to engage in a complete interview, due to issues such as cost, lengthiness, and relevance. Rather, in these cases, clinicians often select to engage in unstructured interviewing alone, or in combination with the most relevant modules of a structured interview. As noted in Table 3.2, not all interviews cover the same diagnostic categories; thus, the primary area of study or presenting problem may also guide the selection of an interview.

The child's age may also help determine the type of interview to select. For example, only a subset of the structured interviews are purported to assess younger children (less than eight years of age; see Table 3.1). Furthermore, the more structured an interview is, the more difficulty younger children may experience, particularly without the benefit of clinician clarifications and/or elaborations. Indeed, some researchers believe the information contained in structured interviews can be too complex or beyond young children's cognitive capabilities (Breton et al., 1995; Brunshaw & Szatmari, 1988; Edelbrock et al., 1985; Ezpeleta et al., 1997; Herjanic & Reich, 1982; Piacentini et al., 1993; Schwab-Stone, Fallon, Briggs, & Crowther, 1994; Valla, Bergeron, Berube, Gaudet, & St Georges, 1994; Welner et al., 1987; Young, O'Brien, Gutterman, & Cohen, 1987).

The attention spans of younger children are shorter than adolescents and adults, which could also be problematic with lengthier interviews. This is not meant to imply that younger children's input is not valued, but rather that appropriate strategies should be selected based on the developmental level of the child. To illustrate, the more flexible, semi-structured format has been recommended for younger children because multiple examples, visual aids, and explanations can be utilized (Sattler & Hoge, 2006). Furthermore, the use of pictorial aids has been recommended and incorporated into interviews designed for younger children (cf., Scott, Short, Singer, Russ, & Minnes, 2006; Valla, Bergeron, & Smolla, 2000). Nevertheless, given the similarities among interviews, most often the clinician or researcher's discretion or preference guides the final selection. In fact, Hodges (1994) suggested that there is not one "best" interview, but rather, that researchers and clinicians should determine which interview to use based on the sample and focus of their endeavor.

INTERVIEW PROCESS

Regardless of whether unstructured or structured interview formats will dominate the assessment, oftentimes the first interview that occurs is conducted with both the parent(s) and child present. During this interview, basic clinic policies can be covered (e.g., confidentiality procedures), and a general understanding of the concerns that led to the assessment can be discussed. Ideally, this joint session is followed by time spent individually with the child and parent(s) to obtain each perspective unhindered by the others' presence. Even the views and perceptions of younger children are often invaluable and observation of parent–child interactions and/or family dynamics can also be highly informative (e.g., is the parent paying attention to the child? Does the parent interact with the child or engage the child in discussion?). During the interview the clinician will also have the opportunity to observe and make inferences about the child's thoughts, feelings, and behaviors (e.g., does the child separate easily from the parent? Does the child have labels and understanding of diverse emotions?).

The primary goal of this initial interview is generally to gather as much information as possible about the child's history, presenting problems, and the environment in which these difficulties exist. Many clinicians find use of a comprehensive developmental history form, completed prior to the first meeting, to be helpful (see Appendix A for an example). This form can then be reviewed by the clinician with subsequent questions asked for clarification as needed. In addition, parent and teacher forms (e.g., Child Behavior Checklists, Achenbach, 2001; Swanson, Nolan, and Pelham Questionnaire, Swanson et al., 2001) can be included in a preinterview packet completed before the clinic visit and examined for noted areas of concern for follow-up during the interview.

Rapport with the clinician is of utmost importance as the nature of this relationship will set the tone for the rest of the interview, assessment, and/or therapy contact. Preschool children tend to warm up quickly and respond well to an interviewer who is friendly and supportive (Bierman &

Schwartz, 1986). Children in grade school may be more intimidated by the interview experience and may need to be eased into the process. This can be accomplished by inviting the child to explore the toys in the room or discussing "fun topics" (e.g., friends, sports, hobbies) rather than immediately sitting down and commencing with the interview. Adolescents may appear more stand-offish and are generally more responsive to open communication and honesty (LaGreca, 1990). In addition, adolescents typically ask more questions about confidentiality issues that should be clarified with all parties prior to continuing the assessment (LaGreca, 1990).

The clinician should prepare by making sure the setup of the room where the interview will take place is "child friendly" (e.g., smaller chairs for young children, appropriate decorations and toys/activities), as the room is often the first impression the child and his or her parents will have of the assessment experience. The room should feel welcoming to the family without too much clutter or bright/noisy objects that can be tempting distractions, particularly for a child who is restless or hyperactive (Thompson & Rudolph, 2000), and could hinder successful interview completion. The ability of the child to feel comfortable in the environment can improve rapport and ease him or her into the assessment process.

Once adequate rapport has been established, the goal becomes investigation of the child's presenting problems. Although any one interview type might be sufficient, intermixing is also common. For example, an unstructured interview format could be used to determine specific diagnostic considerations and modules from a structured interview could then follow as needed. Conversely, a highly structured interview could be conducted to screen for potential psychopathology with an unstructured interview subsequently conducted for clarifications and to gather additional information (e.g., on the course of the disorder).

As previously noted, with structured interviews, the questions asked are primarily diagnostic. If the interview format is unstructured, the topics of discussion pertain to factors that appear to be relevant and immediate to the child. Generally, topics discussed here include, but are not limited to, symptom presentation, severity of symptoms, duration and onset of problems, somatic concerns, stressors, as well as individual and environmental strengths (Greenspan & Greenspan, 2003). During this discussion the clinician should be attune to the child's temperament, attitude, willingness to cooperate, language difficulties, observable emotional change during topic transitions, and nonverbal behaviors suggestive of distress (Sattler & Hoge, 2006).

When interviewing younger children the clinician should try to keep the questions as simple and as open-ended as possible. This is more difficult when using structured interviews because the questions are fixed and responses are limited. Furthermore, the clinician should be aware of normative developmental domains (e.g., language, cognitive, and social; Bierman & Schwartz, 1986; Greenspan & Greenspan, 2003; Herba, Landau, Russell, Ecker, & Phillips, 2006; Wareham & Salmon, 2006), in order to accurately distinguish between what is severely deviant from normal and what is maladaptive at a stage-specific level and can be self corrected with age (Sattler & Hoge, 2006). This will also assist the clinician in determining areas in need of further evaluation.

Suggested communication skills that help maintain rapport and facilitate discussion are verbal and nonverbal acknowledgments of the child's thoughts or feelings, descriptive statements that are nonevaluative, reflective statements, statements of positive evaluation, questions, and summary statements which indicate to the child that you have been listening and paying attention (Sattler & Hodges, 2006). The interviewer can also ascertain the child's level of understanding by asking for summarizations of the questions being asked in the child's own words. Avoidance of critical statements and use of praise for the client's discussion can also be used to maintain good rapport and cooperation. Although similar communication approaches are also appropriate during parent interviews, parents frequently require less prompting as they have often sought the assessment.

For children experiencing difficulty sustaining focus or cooperation during the interview process, Sattler and Hoge (2006) also recommend summarizing the discussion up to the point of withdrawal and then rephrasing the question, using hypothetical questions and scenarios, or presenting acceptable alternatives. Techniques such as these have been found to be most effective with younger children who are either not willing to participate or are showing difficulty communicating their experiences (Wesson & Salmon, 2001). Depending on the developmental level of the child, play-oriented interview techniques can also be introduced at these times. For example, therapy games (e.g., thinking, feeling doing), drawing activities (e.g., draw a story about your (family, school, friends) and tell a story about it), stories (e.g., told to solve hypothetical problems), and use of toys (e.g., dolls whose actions the therapist can ask the child to describe) can be introduced (Bierman & Schwartz, 1986; Priestley & Pipe, 1997; Salmon, 2006; Wesson & Salmon, 2001). Similarly, the therapist can engage the child in conversation while also participating in parallel play (e.g., shooting baskets on a mini hoop, building with blocks).

These techniques can also be used when sensitive and painful topics become the focus of the interview. If the child begins to experience distress, the clinician should not necessarily move away from the topic, but rather could try utilizing a different interview tool or discussing the distress (depending on the child's developmental level). Indeed, experienced clinicians become adept at identifying and subtly probing areas of distress, and then helping the child reconstitute. An interview should not be confused with a therapeutic effort, and could compromise (or enhance) the clinician's ability to subsequently engage in intervention with a child. All of these alternative activities allow the child to express his or her thoughts and feelings in reaction to given situations. The clinician should use clinical judgment when interpreting responses or artistic creations, as these will primarily be used to generate conversation and in conjunction with semi-structured and unstructured interviews. In addition, the inclusion of breaks can be useful for regaining/refocusing attention. However, these techniques are more difficult with structured interviews because of their established guidelines and rigid format.

The clinician should end the interview with a summary of the main points discussed regarding the presenting problems and other relevant material offered by the interviewee. This is an opportunity for the clinician to ask any final questions or clarify any ambiguous responses. The parent/child should also be given an opportunity to ask any questions or express any concerns not discussed previously.

CONSIDERATIONS FOR CHILDREN WITH DISABILITIES AND ALTERNATIVE LANGUAGE BACKGROUNDS

Modifications of Procedures

In conducting any kind of an interview with a child who has a disability, modifications may be necessary. For example, if the child has an oral language disorder that interferes with comprehension of speech, it may be necessary to simplify the language of an unstructured or semi-structured interview so that the vocabulary level is appropriate for the child. Furthermore, it may be more difficult to utilize a structured interview with someone who has a comprehension problem because the language is less modifiable. Similarly, reading problems are common in children (and in adults). If the highly structured interview is administered on a computer that requires significant reading, this may be frustrating to the child (or to the parent) and it may be necessary to read the items to the interviewee.

There are other considerations that may be relevant depending on the presenting problem and these should always be considered in selecting and administering a semi-structured or highly structured interview. It is always important to ensure that the interview is appropriate for the participant. Children with mental retardation or with autism may not be able to provide adequate self-reports and it will be important to rely on third-party observers for these children. Most scales are only designed for English speakers and are not translated to other languages and/or have little normative data for non-English speakers. Translations are questionable procedures inasmuch as language conventions also vary. If a scale must be administered in another language, the items should be adapted beforehand and great caution exercised in interpreting the results. For an unstructured interview, it is easier for a clinician to adapt and modify his or her interaction style according to the language and disability of the participant.

Adaptive Behavior Assessments

An important consideration for evaluating children with developmental disabilities is the need to assess adaptive behavior. Adaptive behavior assessments are particularly important for individuals with mental retardation because the definition of mental retardation requires evidence of intellectual and adaptive behavior functions that are two standard deviations below average (American Association of Mental Retardation; AAMR, 2002). Because they rely on third-party informants and address everyday functioning in social and other domains, adaptive behavior assessments can be helpful in evaluating children with autism and pervasive developmental disorders as well.

In addition, many adaptive behavior scales have separate maladaptive behavior domains that are not computed as part of the adaptive behavior quotient, but are very helpful in evaluating children where social function is a major consideration. For instance, although assessments of adaptive behavior are less frequently used for children who have learning disabilities, they can be helpful with other high-incidence disabilities when language or attention is a factor (e.g., ADHD), because they are based on the reports of others. For children who have significant language problems, an assessment of adaptive behavior can be helpful in terms of differentiating cognitive problems that interfere with performance on a cognitive test versus the child's capacity for habitual everyday functioning.

Adaptive behavior is formally defined as "the collection of conceptual, social, and practical skills that have been learned by people in order to function in their everyday lives" (AAMR, 2002, p. 14). The AAMR (2002) goes on to indicate that "for the diagnosis of mental retardation, significant limitations in adaptive behavior should be established through the use of standardized measures normed on the general population including people with disabilities and people without disabilities." On these standardized measures, significant limitations in adaptive behavior are operationally defined as performance that is at least two standard deviations below the mean on either (a) one or more of the following three types of adaptive behavior: conceptual, social, and practical; or (b) an overall score on a standardized measure of conceptual, social, and practical skills (p. 14).

To illustrate the assessment of adaptive behavior, we briefly summarize three different assessments that vary in their administration characteristics. All three measures share an emphasis on the importance of multiple informants who are familiar with the person who is the identified evaluatee. This means that adequate assessments of adaptive behavior involve more than just one person. In addition, because of the cognitive limitations of many people who are the subject of adaptive behavior assessments, third-party observers (caretakers, parents, etc.) are critical informants and are often regarded as more reliable than the person herself. Certainly, it is possible to use adaptive behavior scales to support decisions about vocational abilities, aptitude and judgment, level of independence, and so on, particularly in adults. Here it may be more reasonable to complete self-reports based on adaptive behavior scales, but individuals with cognitive impairments are often not reliable informants and may tend to deny their adaptive behavior limitations.

Vineland Adaptive Behavior Scales-2 (Vineland; Sparrow, Cicchetti, & Balla, 2005) The second edition of the Vineland assesses adaptive behavior in four domains: communication, daily living skills, socialization, and motor skills. It yields a standardized score (M = 100; SD = 15) in each domain, a composite score, and an optional maladaptive behavior index. Within each of the domains/index, there are subdomains that permit a more refined grouping of items. Although containing different names, the domains of the Vineland line up with the domains recognized in the AAMR (2002) definition. There are three forms of the Vineland that are available, including a survey interview form, parent/caregiver form, and expanded interview form, all with norms from birth through 90 years of age, and a teacher rating form for individuals from 3 to 22 years of age. The Vineland is different from other adaptive behavior instruments in that it is administered through a semi-structured interview. Vineland items are scored on a 0–2 scale indicating the degree to which a person habitually performs that described item. The interviewer uses a starting point in each of the domains to initiate an interview with a caregiver. For example, in discussing language, the interviewer might say, "Tell me about the kinds of words that Billy uses around the house." From there, additional questions would be asked that would refine the caregiver responses and used to score the Vineland according to the basal and ceiling rules. Because of the focus on the semi-structured interview, the Vineland is never given as a self-report.

The Vineland is standardized on a nationally represented sample of 3,687 individuals who range in age from birth to 90 years and is aligned with the 2000 census. The internal consistency reliability is very high (>.90) for the four primary domains and most of the subdomains have reliabilities above .80. Test–re-test reliability for domains ranges from .92–.98. Interviewer reliability in younger children is more variable (.48–.92 across subdomains), but .70–.74 for older children. There is good control for measurement bias by virtue of gender and ethnicity. The manual also presents evidence for concurrent validity relative to other assessments of adaptive behavior. Importantly, the correlations with intellectual assessments are low, which is important because there should be some independence of IQ and adaptive behavior assessments.

Scales of Independent Behavior: Revised (SIB-R; Bruniniks, Woodcock, Weatherman, & Hill, 1996) In contrast to the Vineland, the SIB-R is a highly structured interview that assesses adaptive behavior in motor, social interaction/communication, personal living, and community living domains. It also has a problem behavior assessment that is independent of the adaptive behavior assessment. It yields standardized scores in each domain and a composite score (*M* = 100; *SD* = 15). The SIB-R covers the age range from infancy to about 80 years. It has a long form that takes about an hour to administer and a short form that takes about 20 minutes to administer. As with the Vineland, the SIB-R is typically done with an informant, although with high-functioning individuals it can be done as a self-report. In contrast to the Vineland, the items are read to the respondent and then scored by the interviewer.

The SIB-R was normed on a sample of over 2,000 individuals from about 3 months to 90 years of age. It is lined up with the 1990 census data. Internal consistency coefficients are generally high for the Full Scale and somewhat lower for the short form. The split reliabilities are above .88 for the four cluster scores and the manual reports good correlations of the SIB-R with other assessments of adaptive behavior. It has also been highly correlated with the cognitive ability index from the Woodcock–Johnson Cognitive Battery.

Adaptive Behavior Assessment System-2 (ABAS-2; Harrison & Oakland, 2005) The ABAS-2 has been designed specifically to conform to the AAMR (2002) definitions of adaptive behavior. It is administered in a highly structured format and usually with multiple third-party informants. The ABAS-2 includes a teacher form, a parent form, and an adult form. The parent form has components from birth to 5–21 years; the teacher form is for 2–5 years and for 5–21 years; and the adult form is for 16–89 years. In addition to assessing the conceptual, social, and practical domains outlined by the AAMR, it also breaks into 10 specific adaptive skill areas that underline these constructs and provides a composite score ($M = 100$; $SD = 15$). The respondent completes each on a 0–3 scoring rubric that indicates how often the identified patient correctly performs a behavior without help when behavior is expected to be displayed. Each of the infant–preschool, school-age, and adult forms has been designed for at least two different respondents. For each of these forms, the standardization samples range from 750–1690 tied to the 2000 census.

The ABAS-2 has strong psychometric characteristics, with good reliability. The reliability coefficients for the overall composite range from .97–.99 and .91–.98 for the adaptive domains. Because, among the adaptive behavior measures, the ABAS-2 is more likely to be used for self-report purposes, it is important to attend to the reading level required, with Sattler (2002) specifically noting that the reading level required for the ABAS may be as high as seventh grade. The ABAS has also been found to correlate with an older version of the Vineland at .82. The manual indicates that it can be completed with "high functioning" individuals and gives examples of the use of the *ABAS-2* for vocational decisions with individuals who do not have cognitive impairment. However, the manual is also ambiguous as to the definition of "high functioning," and there are no reliability or validity data presented for self-reports with individuals who have mental retardation. The reliability coefficients for adults with neurological disorders, such as Alzheimer's, are also weak. The construct validity information on the ABAS-2 does not support its ability to identify ten separate domains of adaptive behavior; however, there is some evidence that it may measure three separate domains and the best fitting models identify adaptive behavior as a unitary construct.

These examples of adaptive behavior scales can be used to extend the results of an interview assessment. As with any other interview procedure, it is important to take into account factors that influence how a person is able to demonstrate adaptive behaviors. Level of education, the nature of the disability, language dominance factors, and other issues should always be factored into the determination of adaptive behavior level, particularly for a high-stakes clinical diagnosis such as mental retardation. Moreover, the use of multiple responders is critical for adaptive behavior assessments, because they are largely based on third parties.

REPORT WRITING

Many novice clinicians find report writing to be a challenge; likely in part due to inexperience and in part due to differing styles and expectations among supervisors and colleagues. It is important for report writers to develop a standard template, particularly when they are learning to write reports. A standard template that lays out the different parts of the report helps consolidate the data and the different types of interpretations. In addition, it helps the novice report writer deal with the biggest problem in writing reports, which is how to organize the data, which can be voluminous.

Organization can also be useful as there is a tendency for report writers to include data that extend beyond the comprehension of nonpsychological consumers and to often write reports that are longer than really necessary. Nonetheless, psychological reports should include all the data that are available. Interviews are often given in the context of other procedures, such as assessments of cognitive function. It is important to integrate the interview information and report it at a construct level, as opposed to individual responses or even detailed discussions of specific scores. A report is always an opinion by a psychologist that utilizes the test data, but is tempered by clinical judgment that is informed by the data, behavioral observations, and relevant history.

To help develop a template, consider a report that includes the following sections: Referral Information, Procedures Employed, Relevant Background Information, Behavioral Observations, Assessment Results and Interpretations, Clinical Formulation/Conclusions, and Recommendations. The Referral Information section should be a brief summary that provides pertinent demographics, identifying the name, age, and ethnicity of the child. Usually a clinician would include information about the referral source, any specific concerns that led to the referral, and the primary assessment question. Oftentimes this information can be obtained from an intake form or interview

The Procedures section is simply a list of all the instruments, interviews, and other tools used to collect data. The information in the Relevant Background section can come from many sources, including previous evaluations, medical records, unstructured interviews of the child, parent and teacher rating scales, and other sources. Care should be given in revealing personal information, family conflicts, and other information that may need confidentiality if a report is going to a school or at some point could involve a forensic situation. In addition, it is important to apply scrupulous judgment in determining the accuracy of different reports about the child. The clinician does not need to demonstrate his thought processes in summarizing this information, but simply provide the most reasonable summary and indicate whether there are consistencies or inconsistencies across different sources.

The Behavioral Observations section typically entails a brief mental status examination of the child that includes appearance, affect, mood, speech, attention, and any other behaviors that are relevant to understanding the child's presentation and the adequacy of the evaluation. This section should always conclude with a statement about whether the results appropriately estimate the child's current level of functioning.

Test Results and Interpretations is the data section of the report. The areas covered in this section will vary depending on what measures have been administered. In a typical comprehensive child evaluation, this section is divided into four different sections: Intelligence, Cognitive Assessment, Academic Achievement, and Behavioral Adjustment. A review of the components of the first three sections is beyond the scope of this chapter, but helps put interview information in context. Information derived from an interview would typically be summarized in the Behavioral section. Focus is on relevant constructs, particularly because different tests may have complementary information and the job of the clinician is to integrate the data into a coherent statement (e.g., about the child's intellectual or behavioral level). In dealing with the interview, we would typically organize different interviews by the procedure and discuss the specific results of each interview. This is largely because we have selected interviews for specific purposes. If the interview yields data, we will typically refer to significant elevations, although it is not likely that we would discuss every single scale. Rather, there would be an effort to provide a coherent accounting of the results of the interview.

The Clinical Formulation/Conclusions section is a precise formulation of the overall results of the assessment. It should be short and concise, highlighting the essential components of the findings, while also tying all relevant pieces of information together. If a diagnostic impression is generated, this will be identified at the end of the Conclusions. Sometimes a justification of different classifications (diagnosis) is also provided. The Conclusions section should specifically address the referral question. Recommendations follow and are often listed as consecutive numbers that are tied to the formulation. In general, it is important for the recommendations to be flexible and to take into account the resources that are available to the family. It should address all the different dimensions covered in the report.

It is important to write reports that are clear and appropriate for the person who will be a consumer. For example, many physicians are not interested in the thought processes of the psychologist and essentially focus on the Conclusion section. More concise reports are more likely to be read in full. Other psychologists may wish to actually see more of the data. In this case, a consent form should be signed and the data could actually be delivered to another psychologist when appropriate and allowed by state laws. Most state rules as well as the rules of publishers prohibit the release of raw data to nonpsychologists. The most important component of a report is the Recommendations. The purpose of doing an evaluation is to determine interventions that would be helpful to the child and to the family. The report should be written in a way that supports the recommendations and makes clear the direction recommended by the clinician who conducted the evaluation.

SUMMARY

As illustrated throughout this chapter, the interview is a critical element of the psychological assessment of a child, allowing for the evaluation and observation of behavioral and emotional functioning. Unstructured interviews are conducted as part of most clinical evaluations, however, (semi- or highly) structured interviews are often preferable for diagnostic and research purposes. The standardization of structured interviews allows for increased diagnostic reliability and the rigid format permits administration by laypersons or computers, as well as clinicians. On the other hand, the strict format may also interfere with reliability and validity, as it may not provide the interviewee with the opportunity to report all difficulties or explore them in greater depth. As a result, the clinician using the structured interview may have unanswered questions that need to be addressed in a less-structured format. Another reason clinicians may choose to use a less-structured format is to allow for the establishment of good rapport with the child. As this is one of the most important factors of successful interview administration with children, clinicians should not immediately commence with an inflexible format as the impersonal nature may hinder rapport.

The typical layout of structured parent–child interviews is as follows: an introductory section to gather basic information regarding presenting problems and history; a disorder-specific section that focuses on symptom presence, frequency, intensity, duration, interference, and diagnostic formulations. Two of the most commonly utilized highly structured interviews include the DISC and ChIPS, whereas the K-SADS, CAPA, DICA, ISCA, and ADIS are frequently utilized semi-structured interviews. Each of these allows for assessment of *DSM-IV* psychiatric disorders, with varying diagnoses and age ranges covered, completion times, costs, and training levels required for administration. Psychometric studies of these interviews suggest acceptable test–retest and interrater reliability estimates for each. Multiple informant reliability is typically poorer, likely due to myriad influences, and further illustrates the importance of interviewing multiple informants and interpreting conflicting depictions as informative rather than problematic. Likewise, results for the validity of these structured interviews indicate adequate construct and/or criterion-related validity, but poor concordance for diagnoses generated by diagnostic interviews and clinicians in other settings.

Once an interview is chosen, the process by which it is given is similar regardless of whether the format is unstructured or structured. For example, the first interview is usually conducted as a joint session with the parent and child followed by time individually to account for any hindrance the other's presence may have had upon the informant. Thereafter the primary goal becomes the exploration of the child's presenting problems. Topics discussed will include symptom presentation, severity, duration, and so on. Other things to consider when administering child interviews include the setup of the room, age, developmental level, and the appropriateness of the use of play-oriented interview techniques.

When interviewing children with disabilities, modifications to the aforementioned interview process and format are usually required. For example, using a structured interview with someone who has a comprehension, reading, or language problem is more difficult because the rigid format does not allow for modification. Therefore, in most cases, unstructured interviews are preferable for children with disabilities. It is also useful to include assessment of the child's adaptive behaviors in instances when the child has, or is suspected to have, a developmental disability (e.g., Mental Retardation). Interviews of adaptive behaviors are typically conducted with the child's parents, and may be of semi-structured (e.g., Vineland-2) or highly structured (e.g., SIB-R, ABAS-2) format.

Finally, the discussion of report writing is included as this is the best way to gather and organize all the data collected during the interview (and any additional assessment measures given). Recommendations for report writing were reviewed in this chapter. In addition, a suggested report template was discussed and included the following sections: Referral Information, Procedures Employed, Relevant Background Information, Behavioral Observations, Assessment Results and Interpretations, Clinical Formulation/Conclusions, and Recommendations. The recommendations made at the end of the report are crucial as the purpose of doing an evaluation is to determine helpful interventions for the child and family. The inclusion of all of the sec-

APPENDIX A

Sample Developmental History Questionnaire

Child's Name:		Date of Birth:	Age:
Adopted? ❑ Yes ❑ No			

Form Completed by:	Date:

Parent's Name:			Parent's Name:		
Address:	:		Address		
City:	State:	Zip:	City:	State:	Zip:
Home Phone:			Home Phone:		
Work Phone:			Work Phone:		

I. FAMILY INFORMATION

A. Parents

Father:	Age:	Occupation:
	Years of Education:	Highest Degree:
	Year Married:	If Divorced, Year:
Mother:	Age:	Occupation:
	Years of Education:	Highest Degree:
	Year Married:	If Divorced, Year:
Custodial Agreement:		

B. Brothers and Sisters

Name	Sex	Age	Grade	Where living,	Relationship (full, half, step)

C. Family History

	Relationship to Child
1. Attention Deficit Disorder	
2. Learning Disability	
3. Speech/Language Problems	
4. Epilepsy	
5. Slow Learner	
6. Anxiety	
7. Depression	
8. Bipolar Disorder	
9. Conduct Problems	
10. Alcohol Abuse	
11. Substance Abuse	
12. Mental Retardation	
13. Schizophrenia	

II.   PREGNANCY INFORMATION

A. Medical Condition

Type	Yes/No	Month of Pregnancy	Description
Illness			
Hypertension			
Bleeding			
Diabetes			
Exposure to toxic substance			
Exposure to x-rays			
Medications			

B. Labor and Delivery

Was labor normal? _____	Labor lasted _____ hours.
Full Term? ❏ Yes ❏ No	
If no, premature delivery occurred at _____ months of pregnancy.	
Delivery was: _____ Vaginal _____ Head first _____ Breech _____ C-Section	
Birth Weight: _____ lbs. _____ ozs.	Length: _____ inches

C. Baby

	Yes	No	
Was normal at birth?			
Cried immediately following birth?			
Needed help breathing?			For how long? _____
Needed oxygen?			For how long? _____
Needed blood transfusion?			
Had jaundice during first week?			
Was discharged from newborn nursery at			_____ days of life.

D. Developmental History

How old (months) was your child when he/she:			
Crawled?	Stood?	Sat?	Walked?
Spoke in simple phrases?	Said first words?		
Did your child ever have difficulty speaking? ❏ No ❏ Yes - Age? _____			
Completed toilet training?			

III. MEDICAL HISTORY OF CHILD

A. Illnesses

	Yes/No	Age (yrs.)	Complications
Chickenpox			
Measles			
German Measles			
Rheumatic Fever			
Pneumonia			
Meningitis			
Encephalitis			
Head Injury			
Recurrent Strep Throat			
Sinus/Ear Infections			
Asthma			
Allergies			
Other Illnesses			
Other Injuries			

B. Operations

Type	Year	Complications/ Results	

IV. EDUCATIONAL HISTORY

Current School:			
Address:			
City:	State:	Zip:	
Phone:		Fax:	
Principal:		Main Teacher:	
What kinds of grades is your child currently getting in school?			
Has your child's school performance changed from prior years?			

Please complete below, beginning with kindergarten.

**Type of Class. Please indicate whether your child was in Regular, Gifted/Talented, Special Education, 504, or Other (please explain).

School Year	Grade	Age	School Name	Pass (Y/N)	Type of Class**
	K				
	1				
	2				
	3				
	4				
	5				
	6				
	7				
	8				
	9				
	10				
	11				
	12				

Has your child been diagnosed with:

Diagnosis	Year	Treatment
ADD/ADHD		
Learning Disabilities		
Speech or Language Delay		
Developmental Delay		
Fine or Gross Motor Delay		
Pervasive Developmental Delay		
Autism		
Tourette's Syndrome		
Seizure Disorder		
Traumatic Brain Injury		
Headaches		
Visual Problems		

Has your child had any of these behavioral problems? (Please circle)

Short Attention Span	Yes	No
Clumsy	Yes	No
Truancy	Yes	No
Overly Active	Yes	No
Fighting	Yes	No
Underachieving	Yes	No
Anxiety/Fearfulness	Yes	No

What is your child's current sleeping habits/schedule (e.g., Bedtime, Time child wakes up in the morning, Nightmares/Sleep Problems)

Abuse History-To your knowledge has your child ever been physically/sexually abused?

V. MEDICATION HISTORY List prescription medication child has taken on a regular basis (i.E., Stimulants, antidepressants, anticonvulsants):

Medication	Dose	Reason for Medication	Age

VI. FAMILY STRESSORS List any stressors that your child-family has experienced in the past two years (e.g., death ofpet, death/illness of family members, school performance issues, financial stresses):

tions provided will provide a comprehensive report of the child's behavioral and emotional functioning as evidenced from the given assessment.

REFERENCES

Achenbach, T. (2005). Advancing assessment of children and adolescents: Commentary on evidence-based assessment of child and adolescent disorders. *Journal of Clinical Child and Adolescent Psychology, 34,* 541–547.

Achenbach, T. H. (2001). Manuals for the Child Behavior Checklist and Caregiver/ Teacher *Report Forms / 1½–5, 6–18.* Burlington, VT: ASEBA.

Achenbach, T. M., Dumenci, L., & Rescorla, L. A. (2002). Ten-year comparisons of problems and competencies for national samples of youth: Self, parent and teacher reports. *Journal of Emotional and Behavioral Disorders, 10,* 194–203.

Achenbach, T. M., McConaughy, S. H., & Howell, C. T. (1987). Child/adolescent behavioral and emotional problems: Implications of cross-informant correlations for situational specificity. *Psychological Bulletin, 101,* 213–232.

Albano, A. M., & Silverman, W. K. (1996). *The Anxiety Disorders Interview Schedule for Children for DSM–IV: Clinician manual (child and parent versions).* New York: Oxford Press.

Ambrosini, P. J. (2000). Historical development and present status of the Schedule for Affective Disorders and Schizophrenia for School-Age Children (K-SADS). *Journal of the American Academy of Child and Adolescent Psychiatry, 39,* 49–58.

Ambrosini, P. J., & Dixon, J. F. (1996). *Schedule for Affective Disorders and Schizophrenia for School-Age Children (K–SADS–IVR)-Present State and Epidemiological Version.* Medical College of Pennsylvania and Hahneman University.

American Association on Mental Retardation (2002). *Mental retardation: Definition,* classification, and systems of support (10th ed.). Washington DC: Author.

American Psychiatric Association. (2000). *Diagnostic and statistical manual of mental disorders* (4th ed., text revision). Washington, DC: Allen Frances.

Angold, A. (2002). Diagnostic interviews with parents and children. In M. Rutter & E. Taylor (Eds.), *Child and adolescent psychiatry: Modern approaches* (4th ed., 32–51). Oxford, UK: Blackwell.

Angold, A., & Costello, E. (2000). The Child and Adolescent Psychiatric Assessment (CAPA). *Journal of the American Academy of Child & Adolescent Psychiatry, 39,* 39–48.

Angold, A., & Fisher, P. (1999). Interviewer-based interviews. *Diagnostic assessment in child and adolescent psychopathology* (pp. 34–64). New York: Guilford Press.

Angold, A., Prendergast, M., Cox, A., & Harrington, R. (1995). The Child and Adolescent Psychiatric Assessment (CAPA). *Psychological Medicine, 25,* 739–753.

Aronen, E., Noam, G., & Weinstein, S. (1993). Structured diagnostic interviews and clinicians' discharge diagnoses in hospitalized adolescents. *Journal of the American Academy of Child & Adolescent Psychiatry, 32,* 674–681.

Bierman, K., & Schwartz, L. (1986). Clinical child interviews: Approaches and developmental considerations. *Journal of Child & Adolescent Psychotherapy, 3,* 267–278.

Boyle, M. H., Offord, D. R., Racine, Y. A., Szatmari, P., Sanford, M., & Fleming, J. E. (1996). Interviews versus checklists: Adequacy for classifying childhood psychiatric disorder based on adolescent reports. *International Journal of Methods in Psychiatric Research, 6,* 309–319.

Breton, J., Bergeron, L., Valla, J., Lepine, S., Houde, L., & Gaudet, N. (1995). Do children aged 9 through 11 years understand the DISC version 2.25 questions? *Journal of the American Academy of Child and Adolescent Psychiatry, 34,* 946–956.

Bruininks, R., Woodcock, R., Weatherman, R. & Hill, B. (1996). *Scales of Independent Behavior–Revised.* Itasca, IL: Riverside.

Brunshaw, J. M., & Szatmari, P. (1988). The agreement between behaviour checklists and structured psychiatric interviews for children. *Canadian Journal of Psychiatry, 33,* 474–481.

Chambers, W. J., Puig-Antich, J., Hirsch, M., Paez, P., Ambrosini, P. J., Tabrizi, M. A., & Davies, M. (1985). The assessment of affective disorders in children and adolescents by semistructured interview: Test-retest reliability of the schedule for affective disorders and schizophrenia for school-age children, present episode version. *Archives of General Psychiatry, 42*, 696–702.

Chorpita, B. F. (2007). *Modular cognitive-behavioral therapy for childhood anxiety disorders.* New York: Guilford Press.

Cohen, P., O'Connor, P., Lewis, S., Velez, C. N., & Malachowski, B. (1987). Comparison of DISC and K–SADS–P interviews of an epidemiological sample of children. *Journal of the American Academy of Child and Adolescent Psychiatry, 26*, 662–667.

Costello, E., Edelbrock, C., & Costello, A. (1985). Validity of the NIMH Diagnostic Interview Schedule for Children: A comparison between psychiatric and pediatric referrals. *Journal of Abnormal Child Psychology, 13*, 579–595.

De Los Reyes, A., & Kazdin, A. E. (2005). Informant discrepancies in the assessment of childhood psychopathology: A critical review, theoretical framework, and recommendations for further study. *Psychological Bulletin, 131*, 483–509.

DiBartolo, P., & Grills, A. (2006). Who is best at predicting children's anxiety in response to a social evaluative task? A comparison of child, parent, and teacher reports. *Journal of Anxiety Disorders, 20*, 630–645.

Edelbrock, C., & Costello, A. J. (1990). Structured interviews for children and adolescents. In G. Goldstein & M. Hersen (Eds.), *Handbook of psychological assessment. Pergamon general psychology series* (Vol. 131, pp. 308–323). New York: Pergamon Press.

Edelbrock, C., Costello, A. J., Dulcan, M. K., Kalas, R., & Conover, N. C. (1985). Age differences in the reliability of the psychiatric interview of the child. *Child Development, 56*, 265–275.

Eisen, A.R., & Silverman, W.K. (1993). Should I relax or change my thoughts? A preliminary study of the treatment of Overanxious Disorder in children. *Journal of Cognitive Psychotherapy, 7*, 265–280.

Eisen, A. R., & Silverman, W. K. (1998). Prescriptive treatment for generalized anxiety disorder in children. *Behavior Therapy, 29*, 105–121.

Ezpeleta, L., de la Osa, N., Doménech, J. M., Navarro, J. B., & Losilla, J. M. (1997). Diagnostic agreement between clinicians and the diagnostic interview for children and adolescents–DICA–R–in an outpatient sample. *Journal of Child Psychology and Psychiatry and Allied Disciplines, 38*, 431–440.

Fristad, M. A., Cummins, J., Verducci, J. S., Teare, M., Weller, E. B., & Weller, R. A. (1998a). Study IV: Concurrent validity of the *DSM–IV* revised Children's Interview for Psychiatric Syndromes (ChIPS). *Journal of Child and Adolescent Psychopharmacology, 8*, 227–236.

Fristad, M. A., Glickman, A. R., Verducci, J. S., Teare, M., Weller, E. B., & Weller, R. A. (1998b). Study V: Children's Interview for Psychiatric Syndromes (ChIPS): Psychometrics in two community samples. *Journal of Child and Adolescent Psychopharmacology*, 8, 237–245.

Fristad, M. A., Teare, M., Weller, E. B., Weller, R. A., & Salmon, P. (1998c). Study III: Development and concurrent validity of the Children's Interview for Psychiatric Syndromes (ChIPS). *Journal of Child and Adolescent Psychopharmacology, 8*, 221–226.

Greenspan, S., & Greenspan, N. (2003). *The clinical interview of the child* (3rd ed). Washington DC: American Psychiatric Publishing.

Grills-Taquechel, A. E., & Ollendick, T. H. (2007). Diagnostic interviewing. In M. Hersen and A. M. Gross (Eds.), *Handbook of clinical psychology (Volume 2): Children and adolescents.* New York: John Wiley & Sons

Grills, A. E., & Ollendick, T. H. (2002). Issues in parent-child agreement: The case of structured diagnostic interviews. *Clinical Child and Family Psychology Review, 5*, 57–83.

Harrison, P. L., & Oakland, T. (2003). *Adaptive behavior assessment system* (2nd ed.). San Antonio, TX: PsychCorp.

Herba, C., Landau, S., Russell, T., Ecker, C., & Phillips, M. (2006). The development of emotion-processing in children: Effects of age, emotion, and intensity. *Journal of Child Psychology and Psychiatry, 47*, 1098–1106.

Herjanic, B., Herjanic, M., Brown, F., & Wheatt, T. (1975). Are children reliable reporters? *Journal of Abnormal Child Psychology, 3*, 41–48.

Herjanic, B., & Reich, W. (1982). Development of a structured psychiatric interview for children: Agreement between child and parent on individual symptoms. *Journal of Abnormal Child Psychology, 10,* 307–324.

Hodges, K. (1994). Debate and argument: Reply to David Shaffer: Structured interviews for assessing children. *Journal of Child Psychology and Psychiatry and Allied Disciplines, 35,* 785–787.

Hodges, K., Kline, J., Stern, L., Cytryn, L., & McKnew, D. (1982). The development of a child assessment interview for research and clinical use. *Journal of Abnormal Child Psychology, 10,* 173–189.

Hodges, K., McKnew, D., Burbach, D.J., & Roebuck, L. (1987). Diagnostic concordance between the Child Assessment Schedule (CAS) and the Schedule for Affective Disorders and Schizophrenia for School-Age Children (K-SADS) in an outpatient sample using lay interviewers. *Journal of the American Academy of Child and Adolescent Psychiatry, 26,* 654–661.

Jensen, P. S., Rubio-Stipec, M., Canino, G., Bird, H. R., Dulcan, M. K., Schwab-Stone, M. E., & Lahey, B. B. (1999). Parent and child contributions to diagnosis of mental disorder: Are both informants always necessary? *Journal of the American Academy of Child and Adolescent Psychiatry, 38,* 1569–1579.

Jensen, A., & Weisz, J. (2002). Assessing match and mismatch between practitioner-generated and standardized interview-generated diagnoses for clinic-referred children and adolescents. *Journal of Consulting and Clinical Psychology, 70,* 158–168.

Jewell, J., Handwerk, M., Almquist, J., & Lucas, C. (2004). Comparing the validity of clinician-generated diagnosis of conduct disorder to the Diagnostic Interview Schedule for Children. *Journal of Clinical Child and Adolescent Psychology, 33,* 536–546.

Karver, M. S. (2006). Determinants of multipleinformant agreement on child and adolescent behavior. *Journal of Abnormal Child Psychology, 34,* 251–262.

Kaufman, J., Birmaher, B., Brent, D., Rao, U., Flynn, C., Moreci, P., Williamson, D., & Ryan, N. (1997). Schedule for Affective Disorders and Schizophrenia for School-Age Children-Present and Lifetime version (K–SADS–PL): Initial reliability and validity data. *Journal of the American Academy of Child and Adolescent Psychiatry, 36,* 980–988.

Kazdin, A. E., French, N. H., & Unis, A. S. (1983). Child, mother, and father evaluations of depression in psychiatric inpatient children. *Journal of Abnormal Child Psychology, 11,* 167–180.

Kovacs, M. (1997). The Interview Schedule for Children and Adolescents (ISCA); Current and Lifetime (ISCA–C & L) and Current and Interim (ISCA–C & I) Versions. Pittsburgh, PA: Western Psychiatric Institute and Clinic.

LaGreca, A. M. (1990). *Through the eyes of the child: Obtaining self-reports from children and adolescents.* Needham Heights, MA: Allyn & Bacon.

LaGreca, A. M., & Stone, W. L. (1992). Assessing children through interviews and behavioral observations. In C. E. Walker and M. C. Roberts (Eds.), *Handbook of clinical child psychology* (2nd ed., pp. 63–83). New York: Wiley Interscience.

Lapouse, R., & Monk, M. A. (1958). An epidemiologic study of behavior characteristics of children. *American Journal of Public Health, 48,* 1134–1144.

Lewczyk, C., Garland, A., Hurlburt, M., Gearity, J., & Hough, R. (2003). Comparing DISC-IV and clinician diagnoses among youths receiving public mental health services. *Journal of the American Academy of Child & Adolescent Psychiatry, 42,* 349–356.

Matson, J., Bamburg, J., Cherry, K., & Paclawskyj, T. (1999). A validity study on the Questions About Behavioral Function (QABF) scale: Predicting treatment success for self-injury, aggression, and stereotypies. *Research in Developmental Disabilities, 20,* 163–175.

Moretti, M. M., Fine, S., Haley, G., & Marriage, K. (1985). Childhood and adolescent depression: Child-report versus parent-report information. *Journal of the American Academy of Child Psychiatry, 24,* 298–302.

Ollendick, T. (1995). Cognitive behavioral treatment of panic disorder with agoraphobia in adolescents: A multiple baseline design analysis. *Behavior Therapy, 26,* 517–531.

Ollendick, T. H., & Hersen, M. (1993). (Eds.) *Handbook of child and adolescent assessment.* Boston, MA: Allyn and Bacon.

Ollendick, T., Hagopian, L., & Huntzinger, R. (1991). Cognitive-behavior therapy with nighttime fearful children. *Journal of Behavior Therapy and Experimental Psychiatry, 22,* 113–121.

Ollendick, T., King, N., & Yule, W. (1994). *International handbook of phobic and anxiety disorders in children and adolescents.* New York: Plenum Press.

Orvaschel, H. (1995). *Schedule for Affective Disorders and Schizophrenia for School-Age Children Epidemiologic Version-5.* Ft. Lauderdale, FL: Center for Psychological Studies, Nova Southeastern University.

Pellegrino, J., Singh, N., & Carmanico, S. (1999). Concordance among three diagnostic procedures for identifying depression in children and adolescents with EBD. *Journal of Emotional and Behavioral Disorders, 7,* 118–127.

Piacentini, J., Shaffer, D., Fisher, P., Schwab-Stone, M., Davies, M., & Gioia, P. (1993). The diagnostic interview schedule for children-revised version (DISC–R): III. Concurrent Criterion Validity. *Journal of the American Academy of Child and Adolescent Psychiatry, 32,* 658–665.

Priestley, G., & Pipe, M. E. (1997). Using toys and models in interviews with young children. *Applied Cognitive Psychology, 11,* 69–87.

Reich, W. (1998). *The Diagnostic Interview for Children and Adolescents (DICA): DSM–IV version.* St. Louis, MO: Washington University School of Medicine.

Reich, W. (2000). Diagnostic interview for children and adolescents (DICA). *Journal of the American Academy of Child and Adolescent Psychiatry, 39,* 59–66.

Rutter, M., & Graham, P. (1968). The reliability and validity of the psychiatric assessment of the child: I. Interview with the child. *British Journal of Psychiatry, 114,* 563–579.

Rutter, M., Tizard, J., & Whitmore, K. (1970). *Education, health, and behavior.* London, England: Longmans.

Rutter, M., Tizard, J., Yule, W., Graham, P., & Whitmore, K. (1976). Isle of Wright studies 1964–1974. *Psychological Medicine, 6,* 313–332.

Rutter, M., Tizard, J., Yule, W., Graham, P., & Whitmore, K. (1977). Isle of Wright studies 1964–1974. In S. Chess, & A. Thomas (Eds.), *Annual progress in child psychiatry and child development* (pp. 359–392). New York: Brunner/Mazel.

Salmon, K. (2006). Toys in clinical interviews with children: Review and implications for practice. *Clinical Psychologist, 10,* 54–59.

Sattler, J. (2002). *Assessment of children: Behavioral and clinical applications* (4th ed.). San Diego, CA: Author.

Sattler, J. M., & Hoge, R. (2006). *Assessment of children: Behavioral and clinical applications* (5th ed.). San Diego, CA: Author.

Schwab–Stone, M., Fallon, T., Briggs, M., & Crowther, B. (1994). Reliability of diagnostic reporting for children aged 6–11 years: A test-retest study of the Diagnostic Interview Schedule for Children-Revised. *American Journal of Psychiatry, 151,* 1048–1054.

Schwab–Stone, M. E., Shaffer, D., Dulcan, M. K., Jensen, P. S., Fisher, P., Bird, H. R., Goodman, S. H., Lahey, B. B., Lichtman, J. H., Canino, G., Rubio–Stipec, M., & Rae, D. S. (1996). Criterion validity of the NIMH Diagnostic Interview Schedule for Children Version 2.3 (DISC–2.3). *Journal of the American Academy of Child and Adolescent Psychiatry, 35,* 878–888.

Scott, T., Short, E., Singer, L., Russ, S., & Minnes, S. (2006). Psychometric properties of the dominic interactive assessment: A computerized self-report for children. *Assessment, 13,* 16–26.

Scotti, J., Morris, T., McNeil, C., & Hawkins, R. (1996). *DSM–IV* and disorders of childhood and adolescence: Can structural criteria be functional?. *Journal of Consulting and Clinical Psychology, 64,* 1177–1191.

Shaffer, D., Fisher, P., Lucas, C.P., Dulcan, M. K., & Schwab–Stone, M. E. (2000). NIMH Diagnostic Interview Schedule for Children Version IV (NIMH DISC–IV): Description, differences from previous versions, and reliability of some common diagnoses. *Journal of the American Academy of Child and Adolescent Psychiatry, 39,* 28–38.

Sherrill, J., & Kovacs, M. (2000). Interview Schedule for Children and Adolescents (ISCA). *Journal of the American Academy of Child & Adolescent Psychiatry, 39,* 67–75.

Silverman, W. (1994). Structured diagnostic interviews. *International handbook of phobic* and anxiety disorders in children and adolescents (pp. 293–315). New York: Plenum Press.

Silverman, W. K. & Albano, A. M. (1996). *Anxiety Disorders Interview Schedule, Parent/Child Version.* New York: Oxford University Press.

Silverman, W. K., & Nelles, W. B. (1988). The Anxiety Disorders Interview Schedule for Children. *Journal of the American Academy of Child and Adolescent Psychiatry, 27,* 772–778.

Silverman, W. K., & Ollendick, T. H. (2005). Evidence-based assessment of anxiety and its disorders in children and adolescents. *Journal of Clinical Child and Adolescent Psychology, 34,* 380–411.

Silverman, W. K., & Ollendick, T. H. (2008). Assessment of child and adolescent anxiety disorders. In J. Hunsley & E. Mash (Eds.), *A guide to assessments that work.* New York: Oxford University Press.

Sparrow, S. S., Cicchetti, D. V., & Balla, D. A. (2005). *Vineland–II: Vineland Adaptive Behavior Scales* (2nd ed.). Circle Pines, MN: AGS.

Swanson, J. M., Kraemer, H. C., Hinshaw, S. P., Arnold, L. E., Conners, C. K., Abikoff, H. B., et al. (2001). Clinical relevance of the primary findings of the MTA: Success rates based on severity of ADHD and ODD symptoms at the end of treatment. *Journal of the American Academy of Child and Adolescent Psychiatry, 40,* 168–179.

Teare, M., Fristad, M. A., Weller, E. B., Weller, R. A., & Salmon, P. (1998a). Study I: Development and criterion validity of the Children's Interview for Psychiatric Syndromes. *Journal of Child and Adolescent Psychopharmacology, 8,* 205–211.

Teare, M., Fristad, M. A., Weller, E. B., Weller, R. A., & Salmon, P. (1998b). Study II: Concurrent validity of the DSM–III–R Children's Interview for Psychiatric Syndromes. *Journal of Child and Adolescent Psychopharmacology, 8,* 213–219.

Thompson, C. L. & Rudolph, L. B. (2000). *Counseling children* (5th ed.). Belmont, CA: Wadsworth/Thompson Learning.

Tripp, G., Schaughency, E., & Clarke, B. (2006). Parent and teacher rating scales in the evaluation of attention-deficit hyperactivity disorder: Contribution to diagnosis and differential diagnosis in clinically referred children. *Journal of Developmental & Behavioral Pediatrics, 27,* 209–218.

Valla, J. P., Bergeron, L., Berube, H., Gaudet, N., & St Georges, M. (1994). A structured pictoral questionnaire to assess DSM–III–R based diagnoses in children (6–11 years): Development, validity, and reliability. *Journal of Abnormal Child Psychology, 22,* 403–423.

Valla, J., Bergeron, L., & Smolla, N. (2000). The Dominic-R: A pictorial interview for 6- to 11-year-old children. *Journal of the American Academy of Child & Adolescent Psychiatry, 39,* 85–93.

Verhulst, F. C., Althaus, M., & Berden, G.F. (1987). The Child Assessment Schedule: Parent-child agreement and validity measures. *Journal of Child Psychology and Psychiatry and Allied Disciplines, 28,* 455–466.

Vitiello, B., Malone, R., Buschle, P., & Delaney, M. (1990). Reliability of DSM–III diagnoses of hospitalized children. *Hospital & Community Psychiatry, 41,* 63–67.

Wareham, P., & Salmon, K. (2006). Mother-child reminiscing about everyday experiences: Implications for psychological interventions in the preschool years. *Clinical Psychology Review, 26,* 535–554.

Weems, C., Silverman, W., Saavedra, L., Pina, A., & Lumpkin, P. (1999). The discrimination of children's phobias using the Revised Fear Survey Schedule for Children. *Journal of Child Psychology and Psychiatry, 40,* 941–952.

Weinstein, S., Stone, K., Noam, G., & Grimes, K. (1989). Comparison of DISC with clinicians' DSM–III diagnoses in psychiatric inpatients. *Journal of the American Academy of Child & Adolescent Psychiatry, 28,* 53–60.

Weiss, D.S. (1993). Structured clinical interview techniques. In J. P. Wilson, & R. Beverley (Eds.), International handbook of traumatic stress syndromes (pp. 179–187). New York: Plenum Press.

Weller, E. B., Weller, R. A., Fristad, M. A., Rooney, M. T., & Schecter, J. (2000). Children's Interview for Psychiatric Syndromes (ChIPS). *Journal of the American Academy of Child and Adolescent Psychiatry, 39,* 76–84.

Weller, E. B., Weller, R. A., Teare, M., & Fristad, M. A. (1999). *Children's Interview for Psychiatric Syndromes (ChIPS).* Washington DC: American Psychiatric Press.

Welner, Z., Reich, W., Herjanic, B., Jung, K. G., & Amado, H. (1987). Reliability, validity, and parent child agreement studies of the diagnostic interview for children and adolescents (DICA). *Journal of the American Academy of Child and Adolescent Psychiatry, 26,* 649–653.

Wesson, M., & Salmon, K. (2001). Drawing and showing: Helping children to report emotionally laden events. *Applied Cognitive Psychology, 15,* 301–320

Wood, J., Piacentini, J., Bergman, R., McCracken, J., & Barrios, V. (2002). Concurrent validity of the anxiety disorders section of the Anxiety Disorders Interview Schedule for DSM–IV: Child and Parent Versions. *Journal of Clinical Child and Adolescent Psychology, 31,* 335–342.

Young, J. G., O'Brien, J. D., Gutterman, E. M., & Cohen, P. (1987). Research on the clinical interview. *Journal of the American Academy of Child and Adolescent Psychiatry, 30,* 613–620.

Part II

Assessment of Specific Problems

.

4

Intelligence Testing

R.W. KAMPHAUS, CECIL R. REYNOLDS, and KATIE KING VOGEL

Much has changed in intelligence testing technology and application since the time of Binet's (1905) breakthrough. Prior to Wechsler's innovation of measuring verbal and "performance" abilities on a common test, intelligence tests of the first half of the 20th century typically offered one composite score and focused on assessment of the general intelligence construct. Edgar Doll (1953) identified the problem of overapplication and limitations of intelligence testing for the therapeutic programming for individuals with developmental disabilities in the 1930s and gave us the first measure of adaptive behavior, the Vineland Social Maturity Scales (Doll, 1935), to act as adjunct information more allied with day-to-day living skills than provided by formal assessment of intellectual functions.

During the latter half of the 20th century, intelligence tests began to offer an increasing array of composite or "part" scores intended to produce a more comprehensive evaluation of individual cognitive strengths and challenges. Consequently, interpretation focused more on patterns of abilities within individuals (ipsative test score interpretation) as opposed to just considering deviance from normative standards (Kamphaus, in press. At the outset of the 21st century the pendulum is returning to mid-swing with the concept of general intelligence gathering renewed favor in test interpretation, due in part to problems with new test overfactoring that has produced an ever-increasing array of composite scores of dubious clinical or scientific value (Frazier & Youngstrom, 2007).

These trends have significant implications for the cognitive assessment of individuals with developmental disabilities. Although some concepts and principals such as general intelligence are largely unchanged, the

R. W. KAMPHAUS • Georgia State University, Atlanta, GA. 30302 rkamphaus@gsu.edu
CECIL R. REYNOLDS • Texas A & M University.
KATIE KING VOGEL • University of Georgia.

J.L. Matson et al. (eds.), *Assessing Childhood Psychopathology and Developmental Disabilities*, DOI: 10.1007/978-0-387-09528-8,
© Springer Science+Business Media, LLC 2009

tests themselves and interpretive practices and their uses have changed dramatically. This continuity and change is the focus of this chapter.

THE TESTS

The status of the available intelligence testing technology is vastly improved over previous generations. In fact, intelligence tests could now be considered a relatively "mature" technology in that virtually every test does a good job of measuring the core constructs of interest, namely general, verbal, and spatial cognitive abilities (see Table 4.1). Metaphorically speaking, intelligence tests are mature in the same sense that Magnetic Resonance Imaging (MRI) scanners all work on the same basic principles regardless of the manufacturer (i.e., Phillips, General Electric, or other manufacturers).

The maturation of intelligence testing technology is made possible by the emergence of unifying theories of cognitive abilities based on hundreds of factor analytic studies of various tests, both experimental and commercial ones. We propose Carroll's (1993) as the most important unifying theory available today because it incorporates general intelligence into the model while at the same time accounting for the influence of more discrete cognitive abilities. Other popular models, such as the Cattell–Horn approach (McGrew, 2005) include virtually identical specific abilities but eschew the existence of an overarching general intelligence, a construct that is supported by thousands of investigations and one hundred years of science (Jensen, 1998; Kamphaus, in press). To understand the abilities assessed by the newer tests it is important first to give an executive summary of Carroll's theory.

John B. Carroll's tome represents one of the most ambitious undertakings in the history of factor analytic research. Carroll (1993) gathered hundreds of sets of correlational data for cognitive tests, both experimental and clinical, and reanalyzed the data using factor analysis. This compilation of factor analytic findings is of such breadth and depth that no distillation of his findings will suffice, including that which follows. There is no substitute for reading his original text in its entirety.

In its simplest form, the three-stratum theory derives from data, not clinical or theoretical musings. The data used to generate the theory are the results of over 400 hierarchical factor analyses that yielded three "strata" of factors. The first "narrow" stratum consists of factors that measure relatively discrete cognitive abilities such as Piagetian reasoning, lexical knowledge, spelling ability, visual memory, spatial scanning, speech sound discrimination, ideational fluency, rate of test taking, and simple reaction time. The second "broad" stratum in the hierarchy represents measures of traits that are combinations of stratum-one measures. The stratum-two construct of crystallized intelligence, for example, is produced by measuring first-stratum traits such as tests of language development, verbal language comprehension, and lexical knowledge. The complete list of second-stratum traits hypothesized by Carroll includes fluid intelligence, crystallized intelligence, general memory and learning, broad visual perception, broad auditory perception, broad retrieval ability,

Table 4.1. Three Statum Theory (Carroll, 1993) Cognitive Abilities Hypothesized to Be Assessed by the Composite Scores of Modern Popular Intelligence Tests

	General Intelligence	Fluid Intelligence	Crystalized Intelligence	Memory & Learning	Broad Visual Perception	Broad Auditory Perception	Broad Retr Ability	Broad Cog Speediness	Processing Speed
WISC–IV									
FS	X								
VCI			X						
PRI		X			X				
WMI				X					
PSI								X	
RIAS									
CIX	X								
VIX			X						
NIX					X				
CMX				X					
KABC–II									
FCI	X								
Gsm				X					
Gv					X				
Glr							X		
Gf		X							
Gc			X						
S–Binet 5									
FSIQ	X								
VIQ			X						
NVIQ					X				
FR		X							
KN			X						
QR		X							
VS					X				
WM				X					

(continued)

Table 4.1. (continued)

	General Intelligence	Fluid Intelligence	Crystalized Intelligence	Memory & Learning	Broad Visual Perception	Broad Auditory Perception	Broad Retr Ability	Broad Cog Speediness	Processing Speed
WJ–III									
Gc			X						
Glr							X		
Gv					X				
Ga						X			
Gf		X							
Gs								X	X
Gsm				X					
DAS–II									
VA			X						
NVA		X							
SA					X				
WM				X					
PS									X
SR									
SNC									
GCA	X								

broad cognitive speediness, and processing speed (i.e., reaction time decision speed) (See Table 4.1). He found equivocal evidence for the existence of a quantitative reasoning ability factor.

Stratum three represents the concept of general intelligence, the basic premise of which has been supported in thousands of empirical investigations for nearly eight decades (e.g., see Jensen, 1998). It can be said that the invention of the correlation coefficient by Charles Spearman (1927) set the stage for the development of the construct of general intelligence (g). Spearman made the insightful observation that cognitive tests tended to positively correlate with one another, a finding well confirmed by Carroll (1993) among many other researchers. This positive manifold, as it is sometimes called, suggested to Spearman that performance on cognitive tests was in large part determined by a common latent trait that causes all cognitive (or intelligence) tests to correlate. He identified this central trait as g and theorized that the observed positive manifold supports the idea that this is the most important intellectual trait (also see Jensen, 1998; Kamphaus, in press; Schmidt & Hunter, 2004).

The exact nature of this latent trait called g is yet to be determined, thus causing some criticism of the construct. Some work of the last decade, however, purports to have made progress toward understanding this latent trait and the reason for the observed positive manifold. A couple of the hypotheses offered to explain psychometric g include reasoning ability and working memory (Gustafsson, 1999). Reasoning ability is best represented by measures of fluid ability (discussed later). Working memory capacity has also been cited as a central mechanism of g (Kyllonen, 1996). Both hypotheses have some empirical support suggesting that progress will continue to be made.

The important message communicated by the data in Table 4.1 is that all major modern tests measure general intelligence, crystallized, spatial, and memory abilities to some extent, and most measure fluid abilities. Differentiation begins to occur with the remaining abilities in stratum II, abilities that are less highly correlated with general intelligence, academic achievement, and important life outcomes. And, it could very well be that these latter factors are not actually measured well by modern intelligence tests.

Buttressing this point, Frazier and Youngstrom (2007) conducted a study in which they examined the factor structure of several tests of cognitive ability using minimum average partial (MAP) analysis and Horn's parallel analysis (HPA). They examined tests dating from 1949 to tests currently in use. The purpose of their study was to identify the number of factors per test using MAP and HPA, and compare that number to the number of factors purportedly measured by each test. Their results indicated that the number of factors identified through HPA and MAP analyses were significantly less than the number of purported factors, suggesting that overfactoring is indeed occurring. Also, there was a significant increase in the purported number of factors measured from past to current tests. Finally, although test length increased marginally, the number of purported factors increased exponentially.

Frazier and Youngstrom proposed several possible causal factors for overfactoring. First, they suggested that increasingly complex theories of intelligence, those with a hierarchical order and multiple strata, for example, may be driving the test authors to try to measure these additional abilities. Second, they point to test publishers and their desire to provide more clinically useful instruments. Measuring additional abilities can provide greater interpretative value and lead to more useful recommendations. The authors also suggest that the publishers are including measures of additional factors, which may not be clinically useful, to appeal to researchers. Publishers are also driven continually to provide new versions of tests that are bigger and better (i.e., measure more constructs) than previous tests. Third, they proposed that overfactoring may be occurring due to the application of "liberal" statistical criteria and theoretically driven statistical methods associated with principal component analysis (PCA), confirmatory factor analysis (CFA), and exploratory factor analysis (EFA) that can lead to the retention of too many factors.

In order to remedy the growing problem of overfactoring, Frazier and Youngstrom recommended either (1) increasing test length to measure the additional purported abilities or (2) simply measuring g with briefer measures of ability. Furthermore, they recommended that if publishers choose to increase test length, they should increase the number of subtests per factor, to four in some cases, to increase internal consistency reliability to an acceptable level. This thorough analysis of factor-analytic procedures as applied to intelligence test development has many implications, one of them being that interpretation methods should focus on the well-worn factors assessed by virtually all intelligence tests (if internal consistency reliability is excellent at about .90 and above), with less emphasis placed on occasionally offered composites with fewer indicators, that have less reliability and criterion-related validity evidence. These points are elucidated in the following section.

INTERPRETATION ISSUES

Profile Analysis

The term profile analysis means interpreting the varying elevations (i.e., profile) of subtest and index scores on an intelligence test in an effort to determine cognitive strengths and weaknesses. Many intelligence tests, such as the Wechsler scales, became popular tools of profile analysis. Pfeiffer, Reddy, Kletzel, Schmelzer, and Boyer (2000) found that clinicians often interpret individual subtest scores on measures of intelligence as cognitive strengths and weaknesses. Although popular among clinicians, the practice of profile analysis has fallen out of favor with researchers.

In order to conduct a subtest level profile analysis, one must first derive an ipsative profile, which involves finding the mean subtest scaled score for an individual examinee. Then, the mean subtest score is subtracted from each subtest scaled score, resulting in a difference score (see Kaufman, 1994). Because difference scores are relatively unreliable

(Kamphaus, in press), a significance test is used to determine whether the obtained difference is statistically different from zero (usually $p \leq .05$). If the difference score exceeds the required value, the subtest can be considered a cognitive strength or weakness, depending on the direction of the difference. For example, if a client scores significantly higher on the Matrix Reasoning subtest of the WISC-IV than any other subtest, a clinician might say that that client has a relative strength in logical reasoning and the ability to recognize patterns. Likewise, if a client scores significantly lower on the Coding subtest of the WISC-IV, a clinician might conclude that the client has a relative weakness in the ability to work quickly and accurately with simple novel stimuli.

As illustrated by these examples, it is somewhat imprecise to make generalizations about cognitive functioning based upon one subtest score. Reynolds and Kamphaus (2003) furthered this argument and provided an efficacious solution by creating a new test, the Reynolds Intellectual Assessment Scales (RIAS) which emphasized the measurement of general intelligence accompanied by two broad stratum II factors, crystallized and fluid intelligence. Reynolds and Kamphaus (2003) also include a conormed measure of working and short-term memory, but do not recommend including it in the calculation of the IQ indexes derived from the RIAS, but nevertheless provide the necessary statistical information and normative tables to do so for those who prefer to include this construct in the measurement of intelligence.

Reliability Evidence

Although he still finds value in profile analysis, Sattler (2001) states that it is problematic at the subtest level because the individual subtests on an intelligence test do not measure unique cognitive processes. Additionally, he argues that the subtests are not as reliable as the IQs or indexes. Several researchers have studied the stability of subtest scores and indexes on intelligence tests.

Livingston, Jennings, Reynolds, and Gray (2003) examined the test–retest stability of subtest profile scores on the WISC-R. Using a referred sample and mean length of test–retest of three years, Livingston et al. calculated the stability of individual subtest scores, IQs, and ipsatized scores. The reliability coefficients of the individual subtest scores ranged from .53 to .76 and the reliability of the IQs ranged from .48 to .92. In contrast, the reliability of the ipsatized scores ranged from .29 to .58, indicating that these scores are relatively unstable. The authors found that profile scores became more stable when the profile included IQs or indexes. This study has implications in practice, by showing that the interpretation of indexes is a more reliable practice than that of interpreting subtest score profiles.

McDermott, Fantuzzo, and Glutting (1990) also discourage the use of profile analysis by psychologists. They disagree with Wechsler's statement that the Wechsler scales (the WISC-R in particular) can be both measures of global capacity and specific abilities. McDermott and colleagues warn against the use of ipsative comparisons with the Wechsler scales by providing statistical evidence that ipsatization removes common variance in all scores. The resulting profile has less predictive efficiency and less score stability than the conventional subtest scores. An additional problem with profile analysis, as described by McDermott and colleagues, is that it is impossible to compare ipsatized scores across individuals because each is altered by a different amount (the individual's personal average). Essentially, a profile is unique to each individual client, and comparisons across clients based upon profiles cannot be made. Finally, they conclude that ipsatized scores should not direct treatment decisions because they must sum to zero. If one area of weakness is identified through ipsative comparison, and that specific area is improved, it must come at the expense of an area of strength to continue to sum to zero. Therefore, while attempting to improve a client's functioning in one cognitive area, the clinician is worsening functioning in another, as measured by intelligence tests.

Watkins and Canivez (2004) examined the temporal stability of WISC-III subtest scores. School psychologists twice tested 579 children with the WISC-III as part of the special education eligibility process and IQs, composites, and ipsative scores were compared for each child across testing. Results indicated that IQs were stable across testing, as well as classification of exceptional student status. However, the temporal stability of subtest-level strengths and weaknesses was at chance level. Children were tested with differing test–retest intervals (0.5–6 years) and when interval length was examined, the results remained insignificant. The authors state that examiners will find interpretable cognitive strengths and weaknesses for most children because of the number of possible subtest combinations. An average of six or seven interpretable cognitive strengths and weaknesses was found for each student in the present study. The authors of this study argue against interpreting subtest profiles and using ipsative comparisons to make academic recommendations because of the frequency with which significant profiles occur and the relative instability of the profile itself.

The predictive ability of profile analysis has also been scrutinized. Watkins and Glutting (2000) conducted a study in which they tested the ability of profile analysis to predict reading and math achievement scores. School psychologists typically use profile analysis to form diagnostic impressions and make academic recommendations, but Watkins and Glutting argue that in order to make academic decisions based on the profile, it must actually predict reading and math achievement.

There are three components of a profile that are important to analyze: elevation, scatter, and shape. Elevation refers to the individual mean score across subtests. Scatter is essentially the standard deviation of the subtest scores. Shape is the location of the ups and downs across the profile (i.e., higher and lower scores on individual subtests). The current study examines the profiles of Weschler Intelligence Scale for Children-Third Edition (WISC-III) subtest scores among exceptional and nonexceptional students and their scores on an achievement measure (Weschler Individual Achievement Test [WIAT] for the nonexceptional sample and Woodcock–Johnson-Revised [WJ-R] Achievement for the exceptional sample) to determine if the profile is predictive of achievement. The results indicate that elevation is predictive of WIAT reading and math scores, explaining 52% and 56% of the variance, respectively. For the WJ-R, elevation information explains 13% and 37% of the variance. Scatter information is only significant in the area of predicting WJ-R math, by explaining 1% of additional variance. Shape information is significant in all four areas, explaining between 5 and 8% of additional variance.

Results of this study indicate that cognitive profiles have some use in predicting academic achievement, but the majority of the evidence supports the case that predictive capabilities derive from the elevation of the profile, that is, mostly general intelligence with greater emphasis from crystallized intelligence and some additional contribution from fluid intelligence. One can assume that most individuals with higher overall IQs are likely to have higher overall achievement scores as well, so the elevation evidence is not surprising.

Some (e.g., Siegel, 1989) have argued that intelligence is unrelated to some important academic outcomes, most importantly, learning to read. Siegel's (1989) assertion that intelligence is unrelated to acquisition of reading is refuted not only by common sense and years of experience with children in various learning environments but more importantly by virtually hundreds if not thousands of research studies on the relationship between intelligence and achievement (e. g., see Jensen, 1998; Kamphaus, in press; Reynolds, 2008; Sattler, 2001) as well as specific work aimed directly at testing such an hypothesis (Fuchs & Fuchs, 2006; Fuchs & Young, 2006). This claim is used to support arguments for dropping assessment of intelligence or other cognitive abilities as traditionally conceived from the evaluation and diagnosis of learning disabilities (see Reynolds, 2008, for a discussion and review). With the exception of tests directly of the academic area of interest (e.g., tests of reading and its subskills), intelligence test scores remain some of the best predictors of academic as well as vocational attainment and success available to us today. As Schmidt and Hunter (2004, p. 162) tell us based on a series of empirical studies "... [g] predicts both occupational level attained and performance within one's chosen occupation and does so better than any other ability, trait, or disposition and better than job experience. The sizes of these relationships with GMA [general mental ability] are also larger than most found in psychological research."

Base Rate Evidence

One would expect that the profiles of gifted students would vary from the profile of learning disabled students, but research has proven that assumption incorrect. McDermott et al. (1990) find flaws in many studies of profile analysis that attempt to identify profiles unique to diagnostic groups. They point out that groups that have the same or similar diagnoses may not be homogeneous categories, and, therefore, any resulting profile for the group may not be reflective of the whole group. The authors further argue that one cannot use ipsative comparisons to both form diagnostic groups and find profiles that define them.

Additionally, they state that the measurement error for subtests varies with age, and that it is erroneous to pool samples across ages, which researchers to that point had done. Next, the authors caution against hypothesis testing of subtest profiles because they are not simple linear relationships as are subtest scores and cannot be measured in the same way. Finally, the authors point out that a researcher cannot claim to have discovered a unique profile without comparing it to a null hypothesis (a commonplace profile in a population of average children). The authors praised the well-validated studies of core profiles, which enable researchers to determine the uniqueness of profiles.

Fiorello, Hale, McGrath, Ryan, and Quinn (2002) conducted a study in which they used the regression commonality analysis to find the proportion of variance in FSIQ scores that was predicted by unique contributions of variables, as opposed to common or shared variance of variables. Scores from 873 children from the WISC-III–WIAT linking standardization sample data were examined. An additional 47 children from an LD sample and 51 from an ADHD sample were added to the overall sample. The profiles of each child were examined and the sample was divided into variable (n = 707) or flat (n = 166) profile groups based on variability in index scores on the WISC-III. The criterion for the variable group was 1 or more index score that was statistically significant from the others. Unique and shared variance estimates of FSIQ were calculated for each participant and compared across groups.

Results showed that the FSIQ variance in the flat profile group was 89% shared. The authors stated that interpreting the FSIQ as a general measure of ability for this group was acceptable based upon the proportion of shared variance. The amount of variance that resulted from the combination of the four index scores (g) was 64%. For the variable profile group, 36% of the variance was shared, 61% was unique, and g accounted for 2%. The authors suggested that an interpretation of FSIQ alone for this group would not provide an accurate reflection of ability and should be avoided. Similarly, the LD and ADHD groups had g accounting for variance only 3% and 2%, respectively, and unique variance 58% and 47%, respectively. The authors of this study argue against interpretation of FSIQ only for the majority of the sample (variable, LD, and ADHD groups, which make up 80% of the sample), and argue that profile analysis is needed to ensure that FSIQ accurately reflects one's ability.

SCIENTIFIC SUPPORT FOR *G*

In direct contrast, the scientific support for a single general intelligence construct has been consistent across the decades. In addition, hundreds of scientific investigations have shown that measures of g have been found to be significantly correlated with a vast array of important life outcomes including academic achievement, military training assignments, job performance, income, unlawfulness, SES of origin, achieved SES, and assortative mating (Lubinski, 2004; Schmidt & Hunter, 2004). Twin studies in particular have provided strong support for the existence of a general intelligence factor.

Johnson, Bouchard, Krueger, McGue, and Gottesman (2004) have suggested that if there is, in fact, one true measure of intelligence, g, then an individual's score for g across cognitive assessment batteries should be the same. In other words, g should not vary, on an individual basis, by test administered. To test their hypothesis, Johnson et al. used pre-existing data from the Minnesota Study of Twins Reared Apart (Bouchard et al., 1990). A total of 436 individuals (multiples themselves, spouses of multiples, and other family members) were evaluated with three cognitive ability tests, as well as a multitude of other psychological and physical examinations.

The three cognitive ability tests administered were the Comprehensive Ability Battery (CAB; Hakstian & Bennet, 1977), the Hawaii Battery, including Raven's Progressive Matrices (HB; Kuse, 1977), and the Wechsler Adult Intelligence Scale (WAIS; Weschler, 1955). In order to reduce redundancy, only those subtests that measured different constructs in different ways were administered to the participants. Also, some tests from the Educational Testing Service were added to the HB to provide a more thorough evaluation of abilities. The result of these modifications was that 14 tests were administered as part of the CAB, 17 from the HB, and 7 from the WAIS. No two subtests directly overlapped in terms of task completed.

Factor analysis was then performed to determine the number of distinct factors that comprised each test battery. The authors determined that a 6-factor solution was best for the CAB, and they named the factors Numerical Reasoning, Figural Reasoning, Perceptual Reasoning, Fluency, Memory, and Verbal. A 5-factor solution was also found to be the best fit for the HB, with the factors being Logical Reasoning, Spatial, Fluency, Visual Memory, and Patterns. The WAIS was found to consist of 3 factors: Verbal Comprehension, Freedom from Distraction, and Perceptual Organization. Correlations among the g factors on the three batteries ranged from .99 to 1.00, supporting the authors' hypothesis that tests will not vary in their measurement of g, as g is an underlying element of general intelligence.

Watkins (2006) outlined the use of the Schmid and Leiman (1957) orthogonalization procedure to determine the amount of variance explained by the FSIQ and four first-order factor scores of the WISC-IV. Results of this statistical manipulation showed that the FSIQ factor accounted for 38.3% of the total variance and 71.3% of the common variance. In addition, the FSIQ factor explained more variance within each of the 10 subtests than did any other factor score. Each subtest had considerable unique variance, which, combined with the influence of the FSIQ factor, explained more variance than did any of the first-order factors. The author concluded that general intelligence (FSIQ) accounted for the majority of the variance in the WISC-IV and should be favored over the first-order factors when making recommendations.

DiStefano and Dombrowski (2006) used exploratory and confirmatory factor analysis to determine the number of factors best measured by the Stanford Binet-Fifth Edition (SB-V). The manual of the SB-V only reports confirmatory factor analysis, with the reason being that the SB-V is a revision of a previous test (SB-IV) and a theoretical model of factors was already in place. The authors of the study argued that with the substantial revisions of this edition may come a new factor model of best fit.

The authors conducted separate analyses for each of the five age groups used in the norming sample of the SB-V and computed correlations between the 20 half-scales of the measure. Confirmatory factor analysis was also conducted by age group, and tested a series of four models: unidimensional (g), 2-factor (verbal, nonverbal), 5-factor (based on the CHC theory), and a 4-factor model (Knowledge, Abstract Visual Reasoning, Quantitative Reasoning, and Memory) based on the results of the EFA and previous editions of the SB.

Results of the exploratory factor analysis indicate that the unidimensional model (g) accounted for 46% of the variance across age groups and had the highest factor loadings. Additionally, the younger age groups (2–5 years and 6–10 years) showed evidence for the 2-factor model measuring verbal versus nonverbal intelligence. The other models were unsupported by individual age groups and the norming set as a whole. Results of the confirmatory factor analysis revealed similar findings, suggesting that the unidimensional model was the best overall model regardless of age group. The 5-factor model had the best fit indices for the youngest age group (2–5 years); however, it added little to the unidimensional model because of nonparsimony. For the remaining four age groups, the unidimensional model was the best fit. Only the 1- and 2-factor models could be estimated for the older groups because of the high correlation (.89–.98) between factors. In sum, regardless of age group and type of factor analysis used, the unidimensional model was the most representative of intelligence as measured by the SB-V.

Profile analysis is a common practice among practitioners (Pfeiffer et al., 2000), yet it is highly disputed by researchers (McDermott et al., 1990; Livingston et al., 2003; Watkins & Canivez, 2004; also see Chapter 1 of Reynolds & Kamphaus, 2003, for additional review). Research has shown the results of profile analysis to be unstable and unreliable and most researchers advise against using profile analysis in practice. In addition to the reliability problems with profile analysis, there is a base rate problem. Profiles have not been shown to differ between diagnostic groups (McDermott et al., 1990; Fiorello et al., 2002), making interpretations regarding deviance or psychopathology untenable.

Factor analytic studies have shown consistently that intelligence tests measure fewer factors than they purport to measure (DiStefano & Dombrowski, 2006; Frazier & Youngstrom, 2007; Johnson et al., 2004; Watkins, 2000) and interpretation of the overall intelligence score (g) is the most valid interpretation to be made.

Often, clinicians attempt to determine whether examinees have very specific strengths or weaknesses in cognitive abilities from an ipsative review of subtest scores on an intelligence battery. A clinician might conclude based upon such an analysis that an examinee has a weakness in oral expression or visual perception or in the ability to break visual elements into their component parts, or some other very narrow cognitive skill. The evidence is that intelligence tests cannot provide such information reliably and that such interpretations most likely lack validity when based upon this approach. This does not mean it is not desirable to assess such narrow skills nor that they are unimportant. It does lead us to the recommendation that when information about such narrow-band cognitive skills is desired, clinicians should use tests designed specifically to assess the skill of interest (e.g., Hammill, Pearson, & Voress, 1997; Reynolds, 2002, 2007; Reynolds & Voress, 2007; Reynolds, Voress, & Pearson, 2008; Wallace & Hammill, 2002).

Based on the preponderance of evidence we recommend avoiding the interpretation of intelligence tests at the level of subtest profiles, and instead interpreting only composite (part or index) and general intelligence scores that have long-term support in the scientific literature. In the special case of evaluating individuals with developmental disabilities, the interpretation of the overall composite or general intelligence test score is going to be most useful and efficient. Given that individuals with disabilities often have impairments in multiple domains of functioning, we think that the clinician's time is better spent identifying an individual's developmental needs and problems in the domains of importance for that individual's adaptation, rather than parsing cognitive strengths and weaknesses that are not well supported by science. We attempt to demonstrate this approach in the following case example.

CASE STUDY

Background Information

Darren is a 9-year-old boy who is in third grade at a public school for students with learning difficulties. He is an only child who lives with this father and stepmother. According to his father, his birth mother is deceased. Darren's mother is reported to have experienced significant health problems during pregnancy. When his mother was pregnant with Darren, she developed cancer for which she received radiation therapy. Darren was born at 28 weeks gestation via Caesarean section because of his and his mother's distress. Weighing 3 pounds at birth, he was incubated for 3 months and remained in the hospital for 5 months. He received oxygen for his first year of life. Darren was delayed in reaching developmental milestones. He began crawling at 10 months and walking at 2 years. He mastered toilet training at 5 years. He spoke his first word at 2 years of age and began speaking in sentences at the age of 5. In addition, Darren has fine motor skills deficits such as difficulty using scissors and gripping a pencil.

Darren has also suffered significant hearing loss, which was recently corrected surgically. According to teacher reports, Darren still has difficulty understanding speech in a classroom setting where there are interfering sounds. At the time of the evaluation, Darren was described as being in good physical health and was not receiving any medication.

Academic History

Darren's academic delays were noted in preschool. His teacher observed that he was unable to work at the academic level of his peers and was therefore grouped with younger children for instruction. Upon entering kindergarten Darren was not able to identify all of the colors, letters, and single-digit numbers that are typical for that age group. He was evaluated for special education in kindergarten and deemed eligible for special education with a diagnosis of mild mental retardation. He received services until his transfer to a special needs school in third grade. Darren's current teachers note that he can recognize and name letters of the alphabet (he cannot say them in order), and that he can count to 20 by himself.

Previous Psychological Testing

The results of psychological evaluation a few months prior to this one indicated that Darren's measured intelligence was in the significantly below average range (standard score of 63 on the Kaufman Brief Intelligence Test, second edition). He also scored significantly below the average range on academic achievement and readiness measures, with standard scores in the 60s in the areas of reading, spelling, and mathematics (as measured by the Wide Range Achievement Test, third edition). As a result of this evaluation, Darren was diagnosed with a mild intellectual delay.

Psychosocial History

At the ages of six and seven, Darren would get easily frustrated and angry with his parents. His mood and attitude have improved and his parents say that he is now often happy and content. Darren also is described as having strong spatial skills. Both Darren's parents and his teachers report attention and hyperactivity as areas of difficulty. He is described as having a short attention span, being easily distracted, and often jumping from one play activity to another. He is described as "very active" by his parents who say that he is always on the go, as though he is being driven by a motor. Darren talks excessively and interrupts others' conversations. He also moves about while engaged in normally stationary tasks (e.g., watching TV and playing video games). Finally, Darren's parents report some impulsive behaviors (i.e., touching others) and disorganization. He has few friends as other children seem put off by his impulsive behavior and social inappropriateness.

General Behavioral Observations

Darren was happy and in good spirits throughout the testing and rapport was easily established. He appeared healthy and was dressed appropriately for age and setting. During the evaluation, he displayed several socially immature behaviors such as hiding under the table to grab the examiner's legs and taking test materials from the examiner. Darren did not appear to have any difficulty hearing test instructions.

Darren was active and impulsive during testing. When distracted, however, he was easily redirected to the task at hand. His response style was impulsive, lacked forethought, and gave little indication of concern or awareness of potential negative consequences. In addition, Darren did not check his answers for correctness and often made mistakes without appearing to know it.

Evaluation Procedures

Behavior Assessment System for Children – Second edition (BASC-2; Reynolds & Kamphaus, 2004)

Parent Rating Scales – Child Form (PRS-C; Reynolds & Kamphaus, 2004)

Teacher Rating Scales – Child Form (TRS-C; Reynolds & Kamphaus, 2004)

Reynolds Intellectual Assessment Scales (RIAS; Reynolds & Kamphaus, 2003)

Vineland – II Adaptive Behavior Scales – Survey Interview Form (Vineland – II; Sparrow, Cicchetti, & Balla, 2006)

Wechsler Intelligence Scale for Children – Fourth Edition (WISC-IV; Weschler, 2003)

Woodcock-Johnson Tests of Academic Achievement – Third Edition (WJ-III Achievement (Woodcock, McGrew, & Mather, 2001)

Test Results and Interpretation

Wechsler Intelligence Scale for Children – Fourth Edition (WISC-IV)

The WISC-IV is an individually administered clinical instrument for assessing the intellectual ability of children aged 6 years through 16 years, 11 months. The child's performance on 10 subtests is summarized in an overall intelligence score called the Full Scale IQ (FSIQ). The WISC-IV also yields index scores for Verbal Comprehension (VCI), Perceptual Reasoning (PRI), Working Memory (WMI), and Processing Speed (PSI). Index scores have a mean score of 100 with a standard deviation of 15. Scores between 90 and 110 are considered to be within the Average range. Darren's WISC-IV index scores appear below.

Index	Standard Score	95% Confidence Interval	Percentile Rank
Verbal Comprehension	59	55–68	0.3
Perceptual Reasoning	55	51–66	0.1
Working Memory	56	52–67	0.2
Processing Speed	83	76–94	13
Full Scale IQ	54	50–60	0.1

Each index score is comprised of various subtests. WISC-IV subtest scores have a mean of 10, a standard deviation of 3, and can range from 1 to 19. Scores falling between 8 and 12 are considered average. WISC-IV subtest scores appear below.

Verbal Comprehension	Scaled Score	Percentile Rank
Similarities	1	.13
Vocabulary	2	.38
Comprehension	6	9
Perceptual Reasoning		
Block Design	2	.38
Picture Concepts	3	1
Matrix Reasoning	3	1
Working Memory		
Digit Span	1	.13
Letter–Number Sequencing	4	2.3
Processing Speed		
Coding	7	16
Symbol Search	7	16

Darren's Full Scale composite score on the WISC-IV provides an over-all estimate of cognitive development and includes all subtests. Darren earned a Full Scale score on the WISC-IV of 54 (0.1 percentile), which places his performance in the significantly below average range of cognitive development. There is a 95% probability that Darren's WISC-IV true Full Scale IQ falls between 50 and 60.

The Verbal Comprehension Index of the WISC-IV measures verbal expression and verbal reasoning abilities with subtests that require a client to define words, answer factual and common sense questions, and identify similarities between concepts. Darren scored in the significantly below average range on this index with a standard score of 59 (0.3 percentile).

The Perceptual Reasoning Index of the WISC-IV measures nonverbal reasoning and the ability to solve novel puzzles presented in a nonverbal format. This index includes activities such as forming designs with blocks, selecting pictures that share a common characteristic, and identifying a missing portion of an incomplete matrix. Darren's ability on this index fell within the significantly below average range with a standard score of 55 (0.1 percentile).

The Working Memory Index of the WISC-IV measures attention, concentration, and one's ability to hold and mentally manipulate verbal information. Activities include repeating numbers and letters in sequences. Darren's score on this index fell within the significantly below average range with a standard score of 56 (0.2 percentile).

The Processing Speed Index of the WISC-IV measures written clerical speed. Activities include searching for the presence or absence of a symbol and copying symbols paired with geometric shapes. Darren's score on this index fell within the below average range with a standard score of 83 (13th percentile). As this score is clearly higher than the others, this area represents an area of relative significant strength for Darren, suggesting that simply and highly structured copying and spatial tasks are easier for him. This scale represents one of the more common areas of strength on the WISC-IV for children with significantly below average intellectual skills as it has the lowest correlation of the various WISC-IV indexes with overall intelligence or *g*.

Reynolds Intellectual Assessment Scales (RIAS)

The RIAS is another individually administered intelligence test. Subtest scores are combined into a number of composite scores dependent upon the subtests given. The RIAS yields Indexes that are standard scores with a mean of 100 and a standard deviation of 15. Darren's RIAS composite Indexes appear below.

Composites	Standard Score	95% Confidence Interval	Percentile Rank
Composite Intelligence Index (CIX)	62	59–69	1
Subtests			
Verbal Intelligence Index (VIX)	61	57–70	<1
Nonverbal Intelligence Index (NIX)	65	61–73	1
Composite Memory Index (CMX)	79	74–86	8

Darren scored in the significantly below average range on this measure, with a CIX score of 62 (<0.1 percentile). Although somewhat higher than his scores on the WISC-IV, the RIAS results still document the presence of significant cognitive impairment. The RIAS results confirm WISC-IV results and background information suggesting that Darren finds rote tasks and some spatial tasks relatively easier to perform.

Adaptive Behavior

Vineland Adaptive Behavior Scales, Second Edition (Vineland-II)

The *Vineland Adaptive Behavior Scales, Second Edition* (Vineland-2) was administered to determine Darren's current level of adaptive skill development. The Vineland provides a measure of a child's skills in three domains: Communication (skills involved in receptive and expressive language acquisition); Daily Living Skills (skills involved in self-care, home and community living); and Socialization (skills needed for relating to others, playing, and coping with the environment). The three domain scales are combined into an Adaptive Behavior Composite. Domain and composite scores are presented as Standard Scores with a mean of 100 and a standard deviation of 15. Subdomain scores are presented as *v*-Scale scores with a mean of 15 and a standard deviation of 3.

Domain	Standard Score	Percentile Rank	Adaptive Level
Communication	67	1	Low
Daily Living Skills	74	4	Moderately Low
Socialization	76	5	Moderately Low
Adaptive Behavior Composite	71	3	Moderately Low

Subdomain	Scaled Score	Adaptive Level
Receptive Language	9	Low
Expressive Language	10	Moderately Low
Written Language	8	Low
Personal Living Skills	11	Moderately Low
Domestic Living Skills	13	Adequate
Community Living Skills	8	Low
Interpersonal Relationships	12	Moderately Low
Play and Leisure Time	10	Moderately Low
Coping Skills	10	Moderately Low

Darren's overall score, as measured by the Adaptive Behavior Composite, fell in the below average range with a standard score of 71 (3rd percentile). The Communication domain consists of the subdomains of Receptive, Expressive, and Written Communication, and assesses one's ability to understand and express verbal and written language. Darren scored significantly below average on this domain with a standard score of 67 (1st percentile). The Daily Living Domain is a measure of an individual's ability to perform daily tasks, such as age-appropriate self-care, community awareness and safety, and household chores. Darren's score on this domain fell in the below average range with a standard score of 74 (4th percentile). It is noteworthy that Darren's parents report that he has good skills in the areas of housekeeping, kitchen activities, and safety at home, but he does not know the names and values of coins and bills.

The Socialization Domain measures one's skill in the area of social interaction. Darren scored in the below average range on this domain with a standard score of 76 (5th percentile). These results indicate that Darren regularly spends time with friends and engages in small talk, but has difficulty maintaining comfortable distances between self and others.

Academic Achievement

Woodcock–Johnson Tests of Academic Achievement–Third Edition (WJ-III Achievement)

The WJ-III Achievement is an individually administered achievement test containing various subtests. The subtest scores are combined into a number of composite scores dependent upon the subtests given. Some composites could not be calculated in Darren's case because he failed to successfully complete training items on several subtests. The WJ-III Achievement yields standard scores with a mean of 100 and a standard deviation of 15. Darren's composite and subtest scores appear below.

The Basic Reading Skills Composite includes Letter–Word Identifica-

Composites	Standard Score	Confidence Intervals	Percentile Rank
Broad Math	59	54–65	0.3
Basic Reading Skills	41	34–47	<0.1
Math Calculation Skills	49	40–58	<0.1
Academic Skills	47	43–52	<0.1
Academic Applications	50	43–56	<0.1
Subtests			
Letter–Word Identification	46	41–51	<0.1
Calculation	49	39–60	<0.1
Math Fluency	51	38–65	<0.1
Spelling	46	37–54	<0.1
Passage Comprehension	34	22–46	<0.1
Applied Problems	69	63–75	2
Writing Samples	46	27–64	<0.1
Word Attack	40	27–52	<0.1

tion and Word Attack assessing a child's ability to pronounce both real and nonsense words correctly. Darren's score on this composite fell in the significantly below average range with a standard score of 41 (<0.1 percentile).

The Math Calculation composite of the WJ-III includes Calculation and Applied Problems, and measures one's abilities to compute mathematics problems and interpret simple word problems. Darren scored in the significantly below average range with a standard score of 49 (<0.1 percentile) on this composite. The Broad Mathematics composite includes Calculation, Math Fluency, and Applied Problems. Darren's score on this composite also fell in the significantly below average range with a standard score of 59 (0.3 percentile).

The written language composites were not calculated because Darren was not administered the Writing Fluency subtest (due to lack of skill in that area). On the Spelling subtest, Darren was able to print several capital letters and one lowercase letter, but did not write any words correctly. On the Writing Samples subtest, he correctly wrote his name and the word "cat" only.

Social/Emotional Adjustment

Behavior Assessment System for Children–Second Edition (BASC-2)

The *Behavior Assessment System for Children-2-Parent Rating Scales* (BASC-2-PRS) and *Teacher Rating Scales* (BASC-2-TRS) are questionnaires completed by parents and teachers in order to assess behavior, emotional and learning problems, as well as social competence. The BASC-2 forms yield T-Scores with a mean of 50 and a standard deviation of 10. Scores above 70 are considered to be indicative of significant difficulty. Scores above 60 are considered "at risk;" that is, that they are not of immediate concern but may develop into problems in the future. On the Adaptive Scales, scores below 30 are considered significantly low and scores below 40 are considered "at risk."

BASC-2 Rating Scales for Four Informants

Parent and Teacher Rating Scales	T-scores			
Clinical Scales	Father	Mother	Teacher 1	Teacher 2
Hyperactivity	74**	83**	64*	83**
Aggression	66*	71**	46	63*
Conduct Problems	70**	65*	42	66*
Anxiety	54	47	45	48
Depression	51	60*	42	42
Somatization	53	67*	43	47
Atypicality	62*	70**	50	53
Withdrawal	44	51	47	41
Attention Problems	61*	69*	68*	62*
Learning Problems	N/A	N/A	70**	70*
Adaptive Scales				
Adaptability	46	41	58	52
Social Skills	52	37*	49	51
Leadership	49	38*	42	51
Study Skills	N/A	N/A	34*	36*
Activities of Daily Living	34*	31*	N/A	N/A
Functional Communication	37*	26**	32*	34*
Composites				
Externalizing Problems	72**	76**	51	72**
Internalizing Problems	53	60*	42	45
School Problems	N/A	N/A	71**	67*
Behavioral Symptoms Index	62*	72**	54	59
Adaptive Skills	43	32*	42	44

*= At Risk; ** = Clinically Significant; N/A = Not Assessed

Parent Ratings

The Externalizing Problems composite score includes scores from the Clinical Scales of Atypicality, Withdrawal, Hyperactivity, Aggression, and Conduct Problems. Both parents endorsed items resulting in clinically significant elevations on the Hyperactivity, Aggression, Conduct Problems, and Atypicality scales. Darren was described as argumentative, purposefully annoying others, and disobedient. His parents also described him as overactive, frequently impulsive, and as having a tendency to interrupt others in conversation. The elevation on the Atypicality scale was the result of reports that he acts strangely and confused at times.

The Internalizing Composite consists of the Clinical Scales of Depression, Anxiety, and Somatization. Darren's mother reported "At Risk" levels of Depression and Somatization, indicating that he is upset easily, changes moods often, and frequently has headaches.

Also included on the rating scale is a composite representing adaptive behaviors. This composite reflects the scales of Adaptability, Social Skills, Leadership, Activities of Daily Living, and Functional Communication. Darren's parents described him as having inadequate telephone skills and not responding appropriately to questions. In addition, Darren was described as struggling to complete daily routines independently and assist around the house.

Teacher Ratings

Darren's teachers noted concerns with externalizing behavior and school problems. Specifically, they said that Darren sometimes hits others and often annoys others purposefully. In addition, Darren was described as failing to ask permission to use others' possessions, is frequently overactive, and is impulsive. Finally, both teachers indicated that Darren struggles with academics and usually has trouble keeping up in class.

A review of the Content Scales from the BASC-2 PRS and TRS scales obtained on Darren confirmed significant problems overall with behavioral control, with his greatest elevation occurring on the Executive Functioning scale. Although he has conduct problems as seen in the parent and teacher ratings, these are not particularly targeted as getting his way with others as his Bullying content scale was elevated barely into the at-risk range (T = 61), suggesting his problems with conduct and related domains is more related to his impulsivity and general difficulties with self-regulation.

Summary

Darren is a 9-year-old, third-grade male who was referred because his parents were interested in learning about his developmental status. Darren currently attends a special program for children with learning difficulties. He has been diagnosed as mild mental retardation previously.

The results of the current evaluation reveal that Darren's overall cognitive and academic abilities are in the significantly below average range, consistent with his history of cognitive developmental delay. He does perform slightly better on rote cognitive tasks that do not require complex decision making.

Darren's adaptive behavior was also found to be impaired and consistent with the prior diagnosis of mild mental retardation. Hence, the results of this evaluation indicate that Darren still meets formal diagnostic criteria for Mild Mental Retardation (Code 317) as delineated in the *Diagnostic and Statistical Manual of Mental Disorders, Fourth Edition* (*DSM–IV–TR*).

Darren's teachers and parents indicate that he suffers from inattention and hyperactivity. Specifically, he is described as struggling with sustaining attention, disorganization, distractibility, following instructions, and listening. Additionally, he displays high levels of impulsivity, hyperactivity, and consistently interrupts others. Darren displays these symptoms at home and at school and to a degree that is in excess of what would be expected given his cognitive level. Results from behavior rating scales and the parent interview indicate that Darren meets formal diagnostic criteria for Attention-Deficit/Hyperactivity Disorder, Combined Type (Code 314.01) as delineated in the *DSM–IV–TR*.

Recommendations

Darren needs to improve his phonics and sight vocabulary for early literacy skills, but also his functional reading skills. He also needs to learn to recognize common, everyday written signs and symbols such as road signs and frequented businesses (e.g., fast-food, grocery stores, clothing stores).

In order to further his academic progress Darren's parents are encouraged to make use of "teachable moments" at home and in the community. Teachable moments can include counting out the silverware when setting the table and identifying the colors of fruits and vegetables at the grocery store.

Parent Child Interaction Therapy (PCIT; Herschell, Calzada, Eyberg, & McNeil, 2002) is recommended for Darren's family to improve Darren's inattentive, hyperactive, and impulsive behaviors at home. PCIT teaches parents how to interact with their children in such a way to elicit more positive behavior. More information about PCIT can be found at www.pcit.org.

Visual activity schedules are instruction cards with pictures and words describing the steps one should take in order to complete a daily routine. They will be useful in helping Darren to independently complete daily living tasks. For example, the "evening routine" card could include pictures of pajamas, a toothbrush, a washcloth, a book, and a bed. Each picture has a word or two describing the action and the pictures are ordered according to the desired sequence. Darren can have a card for daily routines at home and at school.

Darren's parents are encouraged to consult Darren's pediatrician to determine if psychiatric evaluation or medication would be appropriate to treat his symptoms of ADHD.

Case Conceptualization.

Darren's case describes many principles of intellectual assessment for children with developmental disabilities. First, the assessment of general intelligence summarizes well the cognitive impairment possessed by Darren. He does have some areas where he performs in the below average range but he lags the general population in all cognitive and academic areas. Essentially, norm-referenced conclusions are prioritized over profile-based conclusions in this case or, said another way, his level of performance in all areas is more important for understanding his current cognitive developmental status versus the shape of his strength and weaknesses profile.

In fact, Darren's scores are consistent with the known structure of intellectual abilities making his relative strength observed on rote recall and clerical speed tasks less important to interpret for diagnostic purposes. This "strength" is consistent with the research of Carroll (1993) and others, which demonstrates that this ability is less correlated with important life outcomes due to its poor measurement of general intelligence. Second, this case is consistent with the research on children with mild mental retardation in that it reflects the higher rate of comorbidity of psychiatric disorders for children and adults with significant cognitive impairment (Kamphaus, in press. In this case the symptoms of ADHD are both normatively and developmentally very inappropriate thus warranting the diagnosis and associated treatments.

Third, as Doll discovered in the 1930s, intelligence tests are inadequate for describing the full range of skills and deficits for individuals with developmental disabilities. For intervention or treatment design purposes in particular, the intelligence test results provide less guidance than the academic achievement, adaptive behavior, and behavior rating scale results.

REFERENCES

Binet, A. (1905). New methods for the diagnosis of the intellectual level of subnormals. *L'Annee psychologique, 12,* 191–244.

Bouchard, T. J., Lykken, D. T., McGue, M., Segal, N. L. & Tellegen, A. (1990). Sources of human psychological differences: The Minnesota study of twins reared apart. *Science, 250,* 223–228.

Carroll, J. B. (1993). *Human cognitive abilities: A survey of factor analytic studies.* New York: Cambridge University Press.

DiStefano, C., & Dombrowski, S.C. (2006). Investigating the theoretical structure of the Stanford-Binet-fifth edition. *Journal of Psychoeducational Assessment, 24,* 123–136.

Doll, E.A. (1935). The Vineland Social Maturity Scale: Manual of directions. *The Training School Bulletin, 22,* 1–3.

Doll, E.A. (1953). *The measurement of social competence.* Minneapolis, MN: Educational Test Bureau.

Fiorello, C. A., Hale, J. B., McGrath, M., Ryan, K., & Quinn, S. (2002). IQ interpretation for children with flat and variable test profiles. *Learning and Individual Differences, 13,* 115–125.

Frazier, T. W., & Youngstrom, E. A. (2007). Historical increase in the number of factors measured by commercial tests of cognitive ability: Are we overfactoring? *Intelligence, 35,* 169–182.

Fuchs, D., & Fuchs, L. S. (2006). What the inclusion movement and responsiveness-to-intervention say about high-incidence disabilities. Keynote for the Inaugural International Conference of the University of Hong Kong's Center for Advancement in Special Education. Hong Kong.

Fuchs, D.. & Young, C. (2006). On the irrelevance of intelligence in predicting responsiveness to reading instruction. *Exceptional Children, 73,* 8–30.

Gustafsson, J. E. (1999). Measuring and understanding *g*: Experimental and correlational approaches. In P. L. Ackerman, P. C. Kyllonon, & R. D. Edwards (Eds.), *Learning and individual differences: Process, trait and content determinants* (pp. 275–289). Washington, DC: American Psychological Association.

Hakstian, A. R. & Bennet, R. W. (1977). Validity studies using the Comprehension Ability Battery (CAB): 1. Academic achievement criteria. *Educational and Psychological Measurement, 37,* 425–437.

Hammill, D., Pearson, N., & Voress, J. (1997). *Developmental test of visual perception* (2nd ed.). Austin, TX: Pro-Ed.

Herschell, A., Calzada, E., Eyberg, S. M., & McNeil, C. B. (2002). Parent–child interaction therapy: New directions in research. *Cognitive and Behavioral Practice, 9,* 9–16.

Jensen, A. R. (1998). *The g factor: The science of mental ability.* Westport, CN: Praeger.

Johnson, W., Bouchard, T. J., Jr., Krueger, R. F., McGue, M., & Gottesman, I. I. (2004). Just one *g*: Consistent results from three test batteries. *Intelligence, 32,* 95–107.

Kamphaus, R. W. (in press). *Clinical assessment of child and adolescent intelligence.* New York: Springer.

Kaufman, A. S. (1994). *Intelligent testing with the WISC–III.* New York: Wiley.

Kuse, A. R. (1977). Familial resemblances for cognitive abilities estimated from 2 test batteries in Hawaii. Unpublished dissertation from the University of Colorado at Boulder.

Kyllonen, P. C. (1996). Is working memory capacity Spearman's g? In I. Dennis & P. Tapsfield (Eds.), *Human abilities: Their nature and measurement* (pp. 49–75). Mahwah, NJ: Erlbaum.

Livingston, R. B, Jennings, E., Reynolds, C. R., & Gray, R. M. (2003). Multivariate analyses of the profile stability of intelligence tests: High for IQs, low to very low for subtest analyses. *Archives of Clinical Neuropsychology, 18,* 487–507.

Lubinski, D. (2004). Introduction to the special section on cognitive abilities: 100 years after Spearman's (1904) "'General intelligence,' objectively determined and measured." *Journal of Personality and Social Psychology, 86,* 96–111.

McDermott, P. A., Fantuzzo, J. W., & Glutting, J.J. (1990). Just say no to subtest analysis: A critique on Wechsler theory and practice. *Journal of Psychoeducational Assessment, 8,* 290–302.

McGrew, K.S. (2005). The Cattell–Horn–Carroll theory of cognitive abilities: Past, present, and future. In D. P. Flanagan & P. L. Harrison (Eds.), *Contemporary intellectual assessment: Theories, tests, and issues* (pp. 136–182). New York: Guilford Press.

Pfeiffer, S. I., Reddy, L. A., Kletzel, J. E., Schmelzer, E. R., & Boyer, L. M. (2000). The practitioner's view of IQ testing and profile analysis. *School Psychology Quarterly, 15,* 376–385.

Reynolds, C. R. (2008). RTI, neuroscience, and sense: Chaos in the diagnosis and treatment of learning disabilities. In E. Fletcher-Janzen & C. R. Reynolds (Eds.), *Neuropsychological perspectives on learning disabilities in the era of RTI* (pp. 14–27). New York: John Wiley & Sons.

Reynolds, C. R. (2007). *Koppitz-2: The Koppitz developmental scoring system for the Bender-gestalt test revised and expanded.* Austin, TX: Pro-Ed.

Reynolds, C. R. (2002). *Comprehensive trail-making test.* Austin, TX: Pro-Ed.

Reynolds, C. R., & Kamphaus, R. W. (2003). *Reynolds Intellectual Assessment Scales (RIAS).* Odessa, FL: PAR.

Reynolds, C. R., & Kamphaus, R. W. (2004). *Manual: Behavior Assessment System for Children-Second edition.* Circle Pines: MN: American Guidance Service.

Reynolds, C. R., & Voress, J. (2007). *Test of memory and learning* (2nd ed.). Austin, TX: Pro-Ed.

Reynolds, C. R., Voress, J., & Pearson, N. (2008). *Developmental test of auditory perception.* Austin, TX: Pro-Ed.

Sattler, J. M. (2001). *Assessment of children: Cognitive applications* (4th ed.). La Mesa, CA: Author.

Schmid, J. & Leiman, J.M. (1957) The development of hierarchical factor solutions, *Psychometrika 22,* 53–61

Schmidt, F. L. & Hunter, J. (2004). General mental ability in the world of work: Occupational attainment and job performance. *Journal of Personality and Social Psychology*. 2004, *86* 162–173.

Siegel, L. S. (1989). IQ is irrelevant to the definition of learning disabilities. *Journal of Learning Disabilities, 22*, 469–478.

Sparrow, S. S., Cicchetti, D. V. & Balla, D. A. (2006). Vineland Adaptive Behavior Scales, Second Edition – Survey Interview Form. Pearson Education, Inc. Spearman, C. (1927). *The abilities of man*. New York: Macmillan.

Wallace, G. & Hammill, D. (2002). *Comprehensive receptive and expressive vocabulary test* (2nd ed.). Austin, TX: Pro-Ed.

Watkins, M. W. (2006). Orthogonal higher order structure of the Wechsler Intelligence Scale for Children–fourth edition. *Psychological Assessment, 18*, 123–125.

Watkins, M. W., & Canivez, G. L. (2004). Temporal stability of WISC–III subtest composite: Strengths and weaknesses. *Psychological Assessment, 16*, 133–138.

Watkins, M. W., & Glutting, J. J. (2000). Incremental validity of WISC–III profile elevation, scatter, and shape information for predicting reading and math achievement. *Psychological Assessment, 12*, 402–408.

Wechsler, D. (1955). *Manual for the Wechsler Adult Intelligence Scale*. New York: Psychological Corporation.

Wechsler, D. (2003). *Wechsler, Manual for the Wechsler Intelligence Scale for Children— Fourth edition*. San Antonio, TX: Psychological Corporation.

Woodcock, R. W. McGrew, K. S., & Mather, N. (2001). *Woodcock–Johnson III Tests of Achievement*. Itasca, IL: Riverside.

5

Rating Scale Systems for Assessing Psychopathology: The Achenbach System of Empirically Based Assessment (ASEBA) and the Behavior Assessment System for Children-2 (BASC-2)

LESLIE A. RESCORLA

INTRODUCTION

Over the past three decades, standardized rating forms obtained from multiple informants have become increasingly common in both clinical and school settings for assessing children's behavioral and emotional problems. Two widely used systems that assess a broad range of problems from the perspectives of parents, teachers, and children themselves are the Achenbach System of Empirically Based Assessment (ASEBA; Achenbach & Rescorla, 2001) and the Behavior Assessment System for Children (BASC, BASC-2; Reynolds & Kamphaus, 1992; 2004). This chapter first presents the history of the ASEBA and the BASC and then summarizes the similarities between the two systems. The main focus of the chapter is a review of the important differences between the ASEBA and the BASC-2. The chapter closes with conclusions and implications.

LESLIE A. RESCORLA • Department of Psychology, Bryn Mawr College, 101 N. Merion Avenue, Bryn Mawr, PA, 19010.

J.L. Matson et al. (eds.), *Assessing Childhood Psychopathology and Developmental Disabilities*, DOI: 10.1007/978-0-387-09528-8,
© Springer Science+Business Media, LLC 2009

HISTORY OF THE ASEBA AND THE BASC

ASEBA

The ASEBA originated with efforts to identify syndromes of co-occurring problems reported for disturbed children at a time when the American Psychiatric Association's (1952) *Diagnostic and Statistical Manual–First Edition* (*DSM–I*) provided only two diagnoses for children (Achenbach, 2006; Achenbach & Rescorla, 2004). In the initial research, behavioral and emotional problems were scored from a large sample of child psychiatric records (Achenbach, 1966). Factor analyses revealed several patterns of co-occurring problems or syndromes (e.g., Aggressive Behavior, Somatic Complaints) that were not identified in *DSM–I*, plus two broadband factors that Achenbach (1966) designated as Internalizing and Externalizing.

The next step was development of the *Child Behavior Checklist* (CBCL), a rating form completed by parents. Items were created and tested through nine pilot editions from 1970 through 1976. In 1978, Achenbach and Edelbrock published CBCL findings based on data obtained for 2,300 4- to 16-year-old children on their intake into 42 mental health services. Factor analysis of these parents' ratings yielded many of the same syndromes identified by Achenbach (1966), as well as the broadband Internalizing and Externalizing scales. The 1978 CBCL also included scales designed to measure competencies. The problem and competence scales were then normed on 1,300 randomly selected nonreferred children whose parents completed the CBCL in a home interview survey. Research findings for this sample, as well as for a matched clinical sample, were published in 1981 (Achenbach & Edelbrock, 1981).

In 1983, Achenbach and Edelbrock published the first detailed manual for the CBCL. To obtain information from teachers and adolescents, Achenbach and Edelbrock (1986; 1987) developed the *Teacher's Report Form* (TRF) and the *Youth Self-Report* for ages 11 to 18 (YSR) Many syndromes derived by factor analysis for the TRF and YSR paralleled those derived for the CBCL. At around this same time, Achenbach (1986) published the *Direct Observation Form* (DOF), designed to assess problems and on-task behavior in settings such as classrooms.

In 1991, Achenbach published revised manuals for the CBCL, TRF, and YSR (Achenbach, 1991a; b; c). New factor analyses identified patterns of co-occurring problems that were common across the CBCL, TRF, and YSR, as well as across gender and age groups. A set of eight syndromes identified for all three types of informants, many of which had been found in the previous factor analyses, was normed using data from a new national sample.

A CBCL for ages 2 to 3 was published in 1992 (Achenbach, 1992), followed by the *Caregiver-Teacher Report Form* (C-TRF; Achenbach, 1997). The *Semistructured Clinical Interview for Children and Adolescents* (SCICA; McConaughy & Achenbach, 1994) was developed for assessing children's self-reports and behavior during interviews. Additionally, the *Young Adult Self-Report* (YASR) and the *Young Adult Behavior Checklist* (YABCL) were published in 1997 for ages 18 to age 30 (Achenbach, 1997).

In 2001, Achenbach and Rescorla published revisions of the CBCL and TRF (normed by gender for ages 6 to 11 and 12 to 18) and the YSR (normed by gender for ages 11 to 18). For this revision, six problem items were changed on the CBCL/6-18 and YSR and three items were changed on the TRF. Data from a new general population sample and from a new clinical sample were obtained. Both exploratory factor analyses (EFA) and confirmatory factor analyses (CFA) were used to identify a common set of eight syndromes across the three forms: *Anxious/Depressed, Withdrawn/Depressed, Somatic Complaints, Social Problems, Thought Problems, Attention Problems, Rule-Breaking Behavior,* and *Aggressive Behavior.* Additionally, a new set of *DSM-Oriented Scales* was added based on expert ratings regarding the consistency of ASEBA items with particular diagnostic categories in the *Diagnostic and Statistical Manual – Fourth Edition* (*DSM-IV;* American Psychiatric Association, 1994). These were designated as *Affective Problems, Anxiety Problems, Somatic Problems, Attention Deficit/Hyperactivity Problems, Oppositional Defiant Problems,* and *Conduct Problems.*

Achenbach and Rescorla (2000) published revised editions of the ASEBA preschool forms, McConaughy and Achenbach (2001) published a revised SCICA (to span ages 6 to 18), and Achenbach and Rescorla (2003) published revised versions of the forms for young adults (to span ages 18 to 59). Forms for ages 60 to 90+ were also published (Achenbach, Newhouse, & Rescorla, 2004). The *Test Observation Form* was published in 2004 (TOF; McConaughy, & Achenbach, 2004).

In 2007, four additional scales were published for scoring the CBCL/6-18, TRF, and YSR based on configurations of existing items that had been tested by various researchers (Achenbach & Rescorla, 2007a): *Positive Qualities* on the YSR, *Obsessive-Compulsive Problems* and *Post-Traumatic Stress Problems* on all three forms, and *Sluggish Cognitive Tempo* on the CBCL/6-18 and TRF. Also, in 2007, Multicultural Scoring Options were added to the ASEBA scoring software, Assessment Data Manager (ADM) for Ages 6 to 18, for scoring the CBCL, TRF, and YSR according to different sets of norms based on data from many countries.

BASC

Reynolds and Kamphaus (1992) reported that development of the BASC occurred over about six years. Lists of problems and positive behaviors solicited from 20 teachers and 500 students were transformed into rating scale items and added to the many items already created by the authors based on their review of other behavioral checklists, consultations with professionals, and professional experience. Two phases of item tryouts were followed by final item selection and "scale definition." Covariance structure analysis (CSA), a form of CFA, was used iteratively to refine the scale structure based on a "starting model" created by assigning items to scales.

The 1992 BASC was comprised of a Parent Rating Scale (PRS), a Teacher Rating Scale (TRS), a Self-Report of Personality (SRP), a Structured Developmental History form (SDH), and a Student Observation System (SOS). According to its authors, the BASC assessed "positive (adaptive) as well as negative (clinical) dimensions." A key goal of the BASC was to facilitate differential diagnosis among *DSM* psychiatric categories as well as among special education categories. The 1992 BASC was normed on large samples obtained through 116 school sites in 26 states and three Canadian cities, with *N*s ranging from 2,401 for the TRS to 9,861 for the SRP. Norms for children being served in clinical or school settings for behavioral or emotional problems were also provided in the 1992 BASC, based on *N*s of 401 for the PRS, 411 for the SRP, and 693 for the TRS. Several validation studies were conducted for the 1992 BASC, including seven involving 1991 versions of the ASEBA forms.

In 2004, numerous modifications were embodied in the BASC-2 (Reynolds & Kamphaus, 2004). Items that had less than optimal reliabilities were replaced with new items, and items were adjusted to increase consistency between the TRS and the PRS and across different age levels. The BASC-2 TRS and PRS have forms for ages 2 to 5, 6 to 11, and 12 to 21. The BASC-2 SRP has forms for ages 8 to 11, 12 to 21, and 18 to 25 (the latter for young adults in postsecondary school education). When the BASC was revised, the most changes were made to the SRP, in order to address concerns about reliability, form length, score distributions, and response format (Reynolds & Kamphaus, 2004).

CSA was used to determine which items needed to be eliminated and to obtain factor loadings for each BASC-2 scale. The BASC-2 added some new adaptive scales on the PRS and TRS, and some new problem scales on the SRP. Additionally, seven content scales, comprised of existing items plus some new items, were added to the TRS and PRS and four content scales were added to the SRP. Two sets of norms were obtained: General norms, derived from a general population sample recruited through schools and child care centers, and Clinical norms, derived from a clinical sample recruited through clinics, hospitals, and special education programs.

Similarities Between the ASEBA and the BASC-2

Both the ASEBA and the BASC-2 assess a broad spectrum of problems as well as positive functioning in children and adolescents from the perspectives of parents, teachers, and children themselves. In both systems, items from a given scale (e.g., Attention Problems) are dispersed among items from other scales. Both systems employ Likert scales for rating problems (except for some SRP items), and forms can be either hand- or computer-scored. Development of both systems involved sophisticated factor analytic techniques. Both systems display scores for individual items, narrowband scales, and broadband scales (e.g., Internalizing and Externalizing, Total Problems/Behavioral Symptoms Index). Additionally, both systems highlight "critical items" (e.g., setting fires, thinking about suicide) that are cause for concern, and both generate narrative reports of findings for ratings by each informant. Both systems also report strong test–retest reliability, with ASEBA *r*s ranging from .83 for the YSR to .89 for the CBCL/6-18 and BASC-2 *r*s ranging from .76 to .84 for the PRS, .79 to .88 for the TRS, and .73 to .83 for the SRP.

Both the ASEBA and the BASC-2 provide percentiles and *T* scores by age and gender based on large normative general population samples. Both systems also demarcate cutpoints for two levels of risk (ASEBA: *Clinical* and *Borderline* ranges; BASC: *Clinically Significant* and *At-Risk* ranges). Both the ASEBA and the BASC-2 provide scores for children enrolled in special education programs or attending mental health facilities and both systems have many points of contact with *DSM-IV* diagnoses. Furthermore, both systems have an instrument for recording direct observations of children in naturalistic settings such as classrooms.

Despite these important similarities between the ASEBA and the BASC-2, the systems differ in many important ways. The next sections focus on the following major differences between the ASEBA and the BASC-2 for ages 6 to 18: (a) arrangement and rating of items; (b) approach to assessing adaptive competencies; (c) method of constructing problem scales; (d) selection of cutpoints; (e) validation procedures; (f) number and variety of scales; (g) approach to handling possible informant "bias;" (h) procedures for cross-informant comparisons; (i) procedures for obtaining a general population sample; (j) choice of norm groups; (k) research base; and (l) multicultural applications.

DIFFERENCES IN ARRANGEMENT AND RATING OF ITEMS

ASEBA: Arrangement of Items

The ASEBA places items assessing positive characteristics and behavioral/emotional problems in separate sections of the form. On the CBCL and TRF, positive functioning is assessed in a competence/adaptive functioning portion of the checklist, as well as by the open-ended item, "Please describe the best things about your child/this pupil." The 120 problem items on the CBCL/6-18 and TRF tap a wide variety of behavioral and emotional difficulties (e.g., *8. Can't concentrate, can't pay attention for long; 50. Too fearful or anxious*), with no items assessing positive qualities or neutral behaviors.

The YSR also contains a separate section tapping competence, similar to that on the CBCL. In addition, the 2001 edition of the YSR contains 14 items tapping positive qualities that are dispersed among the 105 problem items. The original YSR (Achenbach & Edelbrock, 1987) contained 16 positive qualities items, but two were replaced with new problem items when the YSR was revised in 2001. The positive qualities items tap characteristics considered to be socially desirable (e.g., *I like to help others; I like to be fair to others*). They were included on the YSR to enable adolescents to endorse positive characteristics and to replace items from the CBCL and TRF that were not appropriate to ask adolescents. These 14 items are now scored on a separate Positive Qualities scale, based on research using the YSR in 24 countries suggesting the clinical utility of this scale (Achenbach & Rescorla, 2007a; b).

BASC-2: Arrangement of Items

As on the original BASC, BASC-2 items tapping positive characteristics and those tapping problems are mixed together. For example, of the 139 items on the TRS for ages 12–21, 39 describe positive characteristics (three items are on Attention Problems and two on Withdrawal, with reverse scoring). Conversely, two of the five scales tapping positive characteristics—Adaptability and Functional Communication—each contain two reverse-scored problem items. A similar mix of positive items and negative items is found on each BASC-2 form at each age level. Reverse-scored items often state the opposite of another item on the same scale (e.g., *I am liked by others* vs. *I feel that nobody likes me; Makes friends easily* vs. *Has trouble making new friends*).

ASEBA: Rating of Items

The ASEBA uses a 3-level Likert scale for rating items: *0 = Not True (as far as you know); 1 = Somewhat or Sometimes True;* and *2 = Very True or Often True.* Achenbach, Howell, Quay, and Conners (1991) compared CBCL findings for 3-level versus 4-level item ratings. The 3-level ratings were obtained by Achenbach and Edelbrock (1981) for 1,300 nonreferred children and 1,300 clinically referred children. The 4-level ratings were obtained by Achenbach et al. (1991) for 2,600 nonreferred children and 2,600 referred children. These comparisons revealed that parents of non-referred children using the 4-level scale tended to avoid the lowest rating (*Never or not at all true*), whereas parents of referred children tended to avoid the highest rating (*Very often or very much*). Scores for referred children were 2.9 times higher than those for nonreferred children using 3-level ratings (Achenbach & Edelbrock, 1981), but only 2.2 times higher using 4-level ratings (Achenbach et al., 1991), due to "differential compression" of scores toward the middle with 4-level ratings.

BASC-2: Rating of Items

The BASC-2 uses a 4-level Likert scale for rating items: *0 = Never, 1 = Sometimes, 2 = Often, 3 = Almost Always,* except for some dichotomous (*True/False*) SRP items. Reynolds and Kamphaus (1992) explained that they selected a "multipoint" rather than a "dichotomous" scale because it attains "an adequate level of reliability" using fewer items and because a 4-level scale "does not overwhelm raters with too many choices." However, they did not report any specific tests of the 4-level version versus other versions, such as a 3-level version. They did note, however, that to increase "readability and comprehensibility" for children, the 1992 SRP utilized a dichotomous scale. Reynolds and Kamphaus (2004) retained the 4-level scale for the BASC-2 PRS and the TRS, arguing that it "can improve measurement at the extremes of the behavior dimension being measured because *Never* and *Almost always* are extreme ratings" (p. 94). However, they decided to use both dichotomous and 4-level items for the SRP, based on piloting both the previous *True/False* format and their standard 4-level format.

DIFFERENCES IN APPROACH TO ASSESSING ADAPTIVE COMPETENCIES

ASEBA

Achenbach and Edelbrock (1983) piloted various approaches to assessing competencies in the CBCL. They rejected the approach of using bipolar items (e.g., *Kind to animals* vs. *Cruel to animals*) because both characteristics could be true of the same child (i.e., a boy might be nice to his dog most of the time but occasionally be cruel to it), and because they found that parents tended to avoid both poles in favor of the middle. They also rejected using items tapping age-appropriate skills (e.g., crossing the street independently), because such items did not discriminate well between children referred for help with behavioral/emotional problems and nonreferred children. Using items for rating positive qualities (e.g., *Has a good sense of humor*) was also rejected, because parents of clinically referred children endorsed most of these items almost as much as parents of nonreferred children.

After rejecting these three alternative approaches, Achenbach and Edelbrock (1983) settled on an approach to assessing competencies that involves reporting on the positive activities that children actually engage in, as well as on relations with others and functioning in school. For the CBCL/6-18 and YSR, competencies are scored on scales designated as *Activities* (participation and skill in sports, nonsports recreational activities, jobs, and chores); *Social* (participation in group activities such as clubs, teams, and groups plus relationships with friends, peers, siblings, and parents); *School* (performance in academic subjects, plus yes-or-no reports of remedial services, grade retention, and other school problems); and *Total Competence* (sum of scores on these three scales) (Achenbach & Rescorla, 2001). The TRF has two adaptive functioning scales: *Academic Performance* (performance in academic subjects) and *Total Adaptive* (sum of ratings of how hard the student is working, how appropriately the student is behaving, how much the student is learning, and how happy the student is).

BASC-2

The BASC-2 features numerous items assessing positive characteristics (e.g., *Is a "good sport; Says "please" and "thank you;" Is usually chosen as a leader*). On the TRS and PRS for ages 6 to 18, scales designated as *Adaptability, Social Skills, Leadership, Study Skills*, and *Functional Communication* are summed to yield an *Adaptive Composite*. Items comprising these scales vary somewhat across the teacher and parent versions of the forms and across age levels, but there are many common items. The SRP also has many items tapping positive qualities, including *I enjoy meeting others; My parents are proud of me*; and *I am dependable*. These items are scored on scales designated as *Relations with Parents, Interpersonal Relations, Self-Esteem*, and *Self-Reliance*, which are summed to yield a *Personal Adjustment Composite*.

DIFFERENCES IN METHOD OF CONSTRUCTING
PROBLEM SCALES

ASEBA

Since the 1960s, factor analysis has been used to derive ASEBA problem syndromes from the "bottom-up." The 2001 CBCL/6-18 syndromes were derived using EFA, principal components analysis (PCA), and CFA (Achenbach & Rescorla, 2001). The sample used to derive the 2001 syndromes included children recruited through the U.S. National Survey of Children, Youth, and Adults (Achenbach & Rescorla, 2001), children from general population samples in Australia and England, and children from outpatient and inpatient mental health services in the United States. To be included in the factor analytic sample, children had to have CBCL Total Problems scores at or above the median Total Problems score obtained by children of the same gender and age in the National Survey sample. This was to ensure that enough problems were reported to permit detection of clinically important syndromes. Ns were 4,994 for the CBCL/6-18, 4,437 for the TRF, and 2,551 for the YSR.

Ten separate EFAs were performed (i.e., by gender for ages 6 to 11 and 12 to 18 for the CBCL/6-18 and TRF and by gender for ages 11 to 18 for the YSR). These ten EFAs yielded eight factors that were similar across forms and age/gender groups. Items that had significant ($p < .01$) loadings of ≥ 20 on versions of a factor found in at least five of the ten analyses were identified. If items met these criteria for more than one factor, they were assigned to the factor with the highest mean loading across the various age/gender/form combinations. Thus, no cross-loading items were allowed in the 2001 revision of the ASEBA syndromes. All items loading on any factor were then included in analyses to test correlated 8-factor models for each gender/age group on the CBCL/6-18 and YSR. For the TRF, better fit was obtained with a correlated 7-factor model plus a hierarchical model for Attention Problems (i.e., a general Attention Problems factor plus specific *Inattention* and *Hyperactivity-Impulsivity* factors) (Achenbach & Rescorla, 2001; Dumenci, McConaughy, & Achenbach, 2004).

After the multifactor models were supported in the foregoing analyses, the models with both genders and all ages combined were tested separately for each form using CFA. The Root Mean Square Error of Approximation (RMSEA) was .06 for the 8-factor CBCL/6-18 model, .05 for the 8-factor YSR model, and .07 for the 7-factor TRF model, all below the threshold of .08 for "acceptable" fit according to Browne and Cudek (1993). The eight 2001 syndromes (Anxious/Depressed, Withdrawn/Depressed, Somatic Complaints, Social Problems, Thought Problems, Attention Problems, Rule-Breaking Behavior, and Aggressive Behavior) were essentially the same as those derived in 1991 using different data and PCA only, but two syndrome names were changed slightly (Withdrawn became Withdrawn/Depressed and Delinquent Behavior became Rule-Breaking Behavior).

Thus, the ASEBA scores the same eight syndromes for the CBCL/6-18, TRF, and YSR. Although many of the same items comprise these syndromes across the three forms, there are some differences among the items comprising particular syndrome scales on the different forms. Most notably, the TRF Attention Problems syndrome includes 26 items, whereas the CBCL/6-18 version includes 10 items and the YSR version includes 9 items.

Second-order factor analyses of the correlations between the eight 2001 syndromes for the CBCL/6-18, TRF, and YSR yielded a broadband Internalizing group of syndromes (Anxious/Depressed, Withdrawn/Depressed, and Somatic Complaints) and a broadband Externalizing group of syndromes (Rule-Breaking Behavior and Aggressive Behavior), which was exactly the same pattern found for the 1991 versions of the syndromes. The Social Problems, Thought Problems, and Attention Problems syndromes did not load as strongly on either the Internalizing or Externalizing factors as the other syndromes did and are therefore not scored on either broadband scale, as was also true in the 1991 versions.

The 2001 editions of the CBCL/6-18, TRF, and YSR are also scored on *DSM*-oriented scales, which were developed to facilitate cross-walks between ASEBA data and *DSM-IV* diagnoses. The *DSM*-oriented scales were constructed from the "top down" by having international panels of expert psychiatrists and psychologists from 16 countries identify ASEBA problem items that they judged to be very consistent with particular *DSM-IV* categories (Achenbach & Rescorla, 2001). Items that were identified by a substantial majority of experts as being very consistent with a *DSM-IV* category were used to construct Affective Problems, Anxiety Problems, Somatic Problems, Attention Deficit/Hyperactivity Problems, Oppositional Defiant Problems, and Conduct Problems scales, plus *Inattention and Hyperactivity-Impulsivity* subscales scored from the TRF. The *DSM*-oriented scales were normed on the same samples as the empirically based syndrome scales.

Some empirically based syndromes are quite similar to a *DSM*-oriented scale with a similar name (e.g., Attention Problems and Attention Deficit/Hyperactivity Problems). However, in other cases, a single empirically based syndrome combines items that the *DSM-IV* separates into different diagnostic categories (e.g., the Anxious/Depressed syndrome vs. Affective Problems and Anxiety Problems). In still other cases, two empirically based syndromes differentiate between kinds of problems that the *DSM-IV* combines in a single diagnostic category (e.g., Rule-Breaking Behavior and Aggressive Behavior syndromes vs. Conduct Problems). Rather than manipulating the empirically based syndromes to reflect *DSM-IV* categories, the ASEBA developed a parallel set of scales constructed explicitly to reflect *DSM-IV* diagnostic constructs.

Table 5.1 summarizes the Cronbach's (1951) alpha coefficients for empirically based syndromes, *DSM*-oriented scales, and Internalizing, Externalizing, and Total Problems scales on the CBCL/6-18, TRF, and YSR. Table 5.1 also displays alphas for the four new scales introduced in 2007. Alphas on the three broadband scales (Internalizing, Externalizing, and Total Problems) were >.90 for all three forms. Mean alphas across syndromes and *DSM*-oriented scales were .84 (CBCL), .87 (TRF), and .80 (YSR). Mean alphas for CBCL and YSR competence scales were .70 and .67, but the alpha for TRF Total Adaptive was .90.

Table 5.1. Internal Consistency Alpha Coefficients for
CBCL/6-18, TRF, and YSR Scales

Scale	CBCL	TRF	YSR
Broadband Scales			
Total Problems	.97	.97	.95
Internalizing	.90	.90	.90
Externalizing	.94	.95	.90
Syndromes			
Anxious/Depressed	.84	.86	.84
Withdrawn/Depressed	.80	.81	.71
Somatic Complaints	.78	.72	.80
Social Problems	.82	.82	.74
Thought Problems	.78	.72	.78
Attention Problems	.86	.95	.79
Inattention Subscale		.93	
Hyperactivity/Impulsivity Subscale		.93	
Rule-Breaking Behavior	.85	.95	.81
Aggressive Behavior	.94	.95	.86
DSM-Oriented Scales			
Affective Problems	.82	.76	.81
Anxiety Problems	.72	.73	.67
Somatic Problems	.75	.80	.75
Attention Deficit Hyperactivity	.84	.94	.77
Inattention Subscale		.94	
Hyperactive Impulsive Subscale		.90	
Oppositional Defiant Problems	.86	.90	.70
Conduct Problems	.91	.83	.90
Problem Scales mean alpha	**.84**	**.87**	**.80**
Competence/Adaptive Scales			
Total Competence	.79		.75
Activities	.69		.72
Social	.68		.55
School	.63		
Total Adaptive		.90	
Competence Scales mean alpha	**.70**	**.90**	**.67**
2007 Scales			
Obsessive-Compulsive Problems	.55	.58	.65
Posttraumatic Stress Problems	.74	.74	.75
Sluggish Cognitive Tempo	.53	.76	
Positive Qualities			.75

BASC-2

The BASC took a very different approach to construction of problem scales (Reynolds & Kamphaus, 1992). Collections of items were written to conform to an initial set of constructs chosen by the authors. Although factor analyses were performed, items were moved or deleted from factors to improve consistency of items across age levels and forms, to ensure sufficient items for each factor, and to be consistent with the authors' clinical judgment about the hypothesized factors. For example, "'Says "I want to die" or "I wish I were dead"'" was retained on the Depression scale despite low loadings because of its "clear relevance" (p. 72). Also, some scales were separated even though they appeared to form a single factor (e.g., Depression and Withdrawal; Hyperactivity and Attention Problems; p. 80).

The same approach of conceptualizing a priori scales and then refining them through statistical analysis and the authors' judgments was used for the BASC-2. As reported by Reynolds and Kamphaus (2004, p. 55), the a priori scales were "designed to sample the symptomatology associated with popular diagnostic nosologies," namely the *DSM-IV* and the special education categories of the Individuals with Disabilities Education Act (IDEA; 1997).

The factor structure of the original BASC was used as the starting model for the BASC-2. CSAs were then carried out on each scale. After each CSA, the Modification Indexes (MIs) were examined to see if model fit would be improved by moving or deleting items. Items with the highest loadings on their assigned scale were generally retained, but "items considered to be critical indicators of the construct being measured were kept even if their statistical properties were not strong" (p. 96). Items were "added or dropped from each scale" until no further gains could be obtained in reliability or scale coverage. After each scale was finalized, CSAs were performed for each form using the whole set of scales and their constituent items. Each item was placed on only one scale but scales were allowed to intercorrelate. Inspection of MIs at this stage led to dropping a few items (<10%) due to low loadings on their assigned scale or comparable loadings on two scales. No RMSEAs are reported in the BASC-2 manual for these analyses, making it impossible to judge the fit of the model whereby items were assigned to factors.

Once all the scales were finalized, CSAs were performed testing various versions of the entire BASC-2 model (i.e., items assigned to factors and factors assigned to composites). These versions differed in the broadband scales or composites to which some factors were assigned (e.g., Adaptability assigned to Internalizing vs. Adaptive Skills). As Reynolds and Kamphaus explain (p. 145), "This process was repeated until all substantial improvements to fit were explored." For the final model of each form, the RMSEAs reported for each BASC-2 form were as follows: PRS = .16 (p. 177); TRS = .16–.17 (p. 145); SRP = .11–.12 (p. 209). Although Reynolds and Kamphaus (2004) describe the model fit as "only moderate," these RMSEA values are far above the .08 threshold for "acceptable" fit according to Browne and Cudek (1993).

As on the ASEBA forms, some BASC-2 scales did not end up on a broadband scale. Thus, the Atypicality and Withdrawal scales are not part of the Internalizing, Externalizing, or School Problems scales. Whereas ASEBA Total Problems score is calculated by summing all problem items on a form, the Behavioral Symptoms Index on the BASC-2 is calculated by summing scores from only the following six of the ten problem scales: Hyperactivity, Aggression, Depression, Attention Problems, Atypicality, and Withdrawal.

Table 5.2 displays the Cronbach alpha coefficients for all scales on the PRS and the TRS for the General norm group, with mean alphas calculated from the alphas provided for four age groups in the BASC-2 manual. Alphas for composite scales were all ≥.90. Mean alphas for PRS and TRS problem

Table 5.2. Internal Consistency Alpha
Coefficients for BASC-2 PRS and TRS Scales

Scale	PRS	TRS
Composites		
Behavioral Symptoms Index	.95	.97
Intrrernalizing Problems	.90	.90
Externalizing Problems	.93	.97
Adaptive Skills	.95	.97
Clinical Scales		
Hyperactivity	.83	.94
Aggression	.86	.92
Conduct Problems	.86	.92
Anxiety	.83	.81
Depression	.87	.85
Somatization	.83	.82
Atypicality	.82	.84
Withdrawal	.80	.83
Attention Problems	.87	.94
Learning Problems		.87
Problem Scales mean alpha	**.87**	**.90**
Adaptive Scales		
Adaptability	.82	.87
Social Skills	.87	.92
Leadership	.84	.87
Activities of Daily Living	.74	
Functional Communication	.86	.89
Study Skills		.91
Adaptive Scales mean alpha	**.83**	**.89**
Content Scales		
Anger Control	.73	.82
Bullying	.83	.91
Developmental Social Disorders	.82	.89
Negative Emotionality	.74	.77
Emotional Self-Control	.80	.81
Executive Functioning	.82	.86
Resiliency	.83	.87

Note: each entry represents mean alpha across ages 6–18, calculated
from the BASC-2 Manual entries for age groups separately

scales were .87 and .90, whereas mean adaptive scale alphas were .83 and
.89. On the SRP, mean alphas were .82 for problem scales and .80 for adaptive scales. These high alphas for BASC-2 scales are to be expected given that
items were shifted following each CSA until no better fit could be achieved.

DIFFERENCES IN SELECTION OF CUTPOINTS

ASEBA

The ASEBA demarcates $T = 70$ (>97th percentile) as the Clinical range
cutpoint and $T = 65$ (>93rd percentile) as the Borderline range cutpoint

for syndromes and *DSM*-oriented scales. The downward adjustment from the 1991 Borderline cutpoint of $T = 67$ was designed to identify slightly more children as at risk. The ASEBA cutpoint on the Internalizing, Externalizing, and Total Problems broadband scales is $T = 64$ (>90th percentile) for the Clinical range and $T = 60$ (>84th percentile) for the Borderline range. ASEBA broadband scales include a larger number of items and hence reflect more generalized and diverse aspects of functioning than each narrowband scale. Therefore, cutpoints are less conservative. Cutpoints for the adaptive/competence scales are reversed, as low scores indicate poor functioning (<3rd percentile and <7th percentile for Clinical and Borderline ranges for narrowband scales and <10th percentile and < 16th percentile for Total Competence/Adaptive).

BASC-2

The *BASC*-2 uses $T = 70$ (>97th percentile) as the Clinically Significant cutpoint and $T = 60$ (>84th percentile) as the At-Risk cutpoint for narrowband problem scores. Because the 84th percentile cutpoint for the BASC-2 At -Risk range is lower than the 93rd percentile cutpoint for the ASEBA Borderline range, the BASC-2 tends to identify a larger percentage of children as At-Risk on its narrowband scales than are identified in the Borderline range on the ASEBA. For composite scores (e.g., Behavioral Symptoms Index, Internalizing, etc.), the 84th percentile BASC-2 At-Risk cutpoint is similar to the 84th percentile ASEBA Borderline cutpoint, whereas the 97th percentile BASC-2 Clinically Significant cutpoint is higher than the 90th percentile ASEBA Borderline cutpoint. Thus, more children are likely to be identified as in the Clinical range on ASEBA broadband syndromes than in the Clinically Significant range on BASC-2 broadband syndromes. As on the ASEBA, cutpoints for the BASC-2 adaptive scales are the reverse of those for problem scales.

DIFFERENCES IN VALIDATION PROCEDURES

Both the ASEBA and the BASC-2 manuals report correlations between their scales and scales from other behavior rating forms, such as the Conners Rating Scales (Conners, 1997). Each manual also reports correlations between comparable scales on parallel ASEBA/BASC-2 instruments. Table 5.3 displays the *r*s reported between the CBCL and PRS and between the TRF and the TRS for scales with comparable names and constituent items. Comparisons between the YSR and the SRP are not included in this table, because they have fewer counterpart scales. As shown in Table 5.3, the *r*s were comparable in the two studies and across informants (mean *r*s of .69 to .73). Of the 60 *r*s calculated, only two fell below Cohen's (1988) benchmark for large effects of .50, and 26 of the 60 *r*s were >.60. Thus, these pairs of ASEBA and BASC-2 scales appear to measure quite similar constructs, indicating strong reciprocal convergent validity.

Table 5.3. Correlations Between Comparable Scales for the CBCL/PRS and the TRF/TRS

Scale Pairs	ASEBA manual	BASC-2 manual
Total Problems & Behavioral Symptoms Index	.89 (P), .85 (T)	.83 (P), .76 (T)
Internalizing	.83 (P), .75 (T)	.75 (P), .74 (T)
Externalizing	.88 (P), .74 (T)	.78 (P), .76 (T)
Syndromes/Scales		
Anxious/Depressed & Anxiety	.54 (P), .54 (T)	.71 (P), .68 (T)
Anxious/Depressed & Depression	.60 (P), .56 (T)	.64 (P), .51 (T)
Withdrawn/Depressed & Withdrawal	.58 (P), .62 (T)	.67 (P), .73 (T)
Somatic Complaints & Somatization	.80 (P), .79 (T)	.63 (P), .68 (T)
Attention Problems & Attention Problems	.82 (P), .80 (T)	.73 (P), .64 (T)
Aggressive Behavior & Aggressive Behavior	.72 (P), .85 (T)	.75 (P), .69 (T)
DSM-Oriented Scales/Scales		
Affective Problems & Depression	.77 (P), .48 (T)	.61 (P), .81 (T)
Anxiety Problems & Anxiety	.55 (P), .46 (T)	.76 (P), .59 (T),
Somatic Problems & Somatization	.80 (P), .78 (T)	.63 (P), .63 (T)
Attention Deficit Hyperactivity & Hyperactivity	.70 (P), .81 (T)	.55 (P), .70 (T)
Attention Deficit Hyperactivity & Attention Problems	.75 (P), .67 (T)	.66 (P), .65 (T)
Conduct Problems & Conduct Problems	.79 (P), .84 (T)	.70 (P), .77 (T)
Mean *r*	.73 (P), .70 (T)	.69 (P), .69 (T)

ASEBA

Since 1983, the ASEBA has been validated by testing the ability of its problem and competence scales to discriminate between nonreferred children and children referred for mental health or special education services. Children comprising the nonreferred sample are drawn from the normative sample so as to match the referred sample on age, sex, and socioeconomic status (SES), which is essential because clinical samples are not demographically representative of the general population. Strong ability to discriminate between nonreferred and referred children has been demonstrated for ASEBA forms since their inception (e.g., Achenbach & Edelbrock, 1983). For the 2001 ASEBA, referred versus nonreferred comparisons were based on samples of $N = 3,210$ for the CBCL/6-18, $N = 3,086$ for the TRF, and $N = 1,938$ for the YSR.

As displayed in the 2001 ASEBA manual, problem T score means were consistently higher and competence/adaptive T score means were consistently lower for referred than for nonreferred children. The discriminative validity of the competence and problem scales was tested using multiple regressions, with referral status, SES, ethnicity, and age as predictors. Referral status accounted for 36% of the variance for CBCL/6-18 Total Competence, 28% for YSR Total Competence, and 29% for TRF Total Adaptive, all large ESs based on Cohen's (1988) benchmarks (small = 2–13%, medium = 13–26%, large >26%). For the 17 problem scales of the CBCL, five ESs were ≥30% (for *DSM*-oriented Conduct Problems, Total Problems, Externalizing, Aggressive Behavior, and Attention Problems), and the smallest ES 9% (DSM-oriented Somatic Problems). On the TRF, 19 of the 21 referral status ESs were ≥10%, with the largest ESs for Total Problems (26%) and Attention problems (22%). Referral status ESs were generally smaller on the YSR, ranging from 5% for DSM-oriented Anxiety Problems to 17% for Externalizing.

Additionally, all competence/adaptive functioning items and all problem items discriminated significantly (p < .01) between referred and nonreferred children on at least one form and generally on all forms where the item appeared (Achenbach & Rescorla, 2001). The item that discriminated best between referred and nonreferred samples was *103. Unhappy, sad, and depressed*, with referral status ESs of 29% on the CBCL, 15% on the TRF, and 14% on the YSR. The extremely strong discriminative power for this item has been found in many samples, both in the United States and in the Netherlands (Achenbach & Rescorla, 2001).

Within each age/gender group, age effects did not exceed chance expectations. On competence/adaptive functioning scales, the largest ES for SES was 6% on the TRF Academic Performance scale. SES ESs were significant but even smaller (≤2%) for 5 of 17 CBCL/6-18 problem scales and for 15 of 21 TRF problem scales. No SES ESs were significant for the YSR. With SES controlled, no ESs for ethnicity exceeded chance expectations on the CBC/6-18 or YSR, but a few small ESs (<2%) for ethnicity were significant on the TRF, with white students obtaining higher scores than African American students on adaptive functioning items. The small but significant SES differences on ASEBA scales underscore the importance of matching referred and nonreferred groups on SES when testing validity.

ASEBA scales have also been validated via categorical analysis. Children in the same matched referred and nonreferred samples were classified with respect to whether their scores on each ASEBA scale were in the deviant range (Borderline and Clinical ranges combined) versus the normal range. This classification was used as a "risk factor" to predict referred versus nonreferred status, with the outcome expressed as an odds ratio (OR). As displayed in Table 5.4, children who scored in the deviant range on CBCL Total Problems were 14 times more likely to be in the referred group than children who scored in the normal range. It is noteworthy that the OR was higher for Externalizing than for Internalizing on the CBCL (12 vs. 8) and that ORs were highest for the CBCL, lowest for the YSR, and intermediate for the TRF.

BASC-2

The Clinical samples for the BASC-2, which were larger than those for the original BASC (N = 577 to 799 for ages 6 to 11 and N = 789 to 950 for adolescents), included children with learning disability (LD), ADHD, speech/language impairment, mental retardation, emotional behavioral/ disturbance, hearing impairment, pervasive developmental disorder, and other impairments (orthopedic, visual, etc.), as defined by special education disability categories of the IDEA (1997). As noted by Reynolds and Kamphaus (2004), the Clinical sample was not representative of the U.S. general population, due to higher concentrations of boys and children from African American and Hispanic families (p. 125). It is most likely that the Clinical sample was also of lower SES, given the racial/ethnic differences, but this was not reported in the BASC-2 manual.

Table 5.4. Odds Ratios (ORs) for Predicting Referral
Status from Deviant Scores on ASEBA Scales

Scale	CBCL	TRF	YSR
Broadband Scales			
Total Problems	14	9	5
Internalizing	8	5	4
Externalizing	12	7	4
Syndromes			
Anxious/Depressed	9	5	5
Withdrawn/Depressed	10	4	4
Somatic Complaints	6	2	4
Social Problems	11	6	4
Thought Problems	12	6	4
Attention Problems	12	7	5
Inattention Subscale		5	
Hyperactivity/Impulsivity Subscale		5	
Rule-Breaking Behavior	12	6	4
Aggressive Behavior	16	9	6
DSM-Oriented Scales			
Affective Problems	13	6	6
Anxiety Problems	8	6	3
Somatic Problems	4	2	4
Attention Deficit Hyperactivity	10	6	5
Inattention Subscale		6	
Hyperactive Impulsive Subscale		5	
Oppositional Defiant Problems	13	7	4
Conduct Problems	17	8	6
Competence/Adaptive Scales			
Total Competence	15		9
Activities	8		10
Social	10		6
School	15		
Academic Performance		8	
Total Adaptive		9	

Note. N = 3,210 for CBCL, 1,938, and 3,086 TRF equally divided between
referred and nonreferred children matched on age, gender, SES, and race/
ethnicity.

The BASC-2 manual contains many tables and graphs depicting T
scores for the Clinical samples based on norms for the General sample.
T scores are also presented for 10 clinical subgroups (e.g., ADHD, learning disability, bipolar disorder, depression, speech-language impairment,
etc.). For the PRS, Ns for these clinical subgroups ranged from 2 (depression for ages 6 to 11) to 293 (ADHD for adolescents), with Ns < 40 for seven
of the 20 subgroups. For the TRS, Ns for these clinical subgroups ranged
from 7 (bipolar disorder for ages 6 to 11) to 275 (LD for adolescents), with
Ns < 40 for nine of 19 subgroups. For the SRP, Ns for clinical subgroups
ranged from 8 (bipolar disorder for adolescents) to 292 (ADHD for adolescents), with Ns < 40 for nine of 19 subgroups.

Children in the Clinical sample generally had lower scores on adaptive scales and higher scores on problem scales than children in the General sample, but no adjustments were made for demographic differences between the two samples. Mean scores in the two groups appeared to differ by .1 to .8 of a SD across scales and forms. No statistical tests of BASC-2 scores for the General versus the Clinical samples that would demonstrate discriminative validity are reported in the manual. Mean *T* scores are also provided for the different clinical subgroups at each age level, but *N*s for many of the clinical subgroups are too small to provide representative samples.

DIFFERENCES IN NUMBER AND VARIETY OF SCALES

ASEBA

The same eight empirically based syndromes, three broadband scales (Internalizing, Externalizing, and Total Problems), and six *DSM*-oriented scales are scored on the CBCL/6-18, TRF, and YSR. In addition, empirically based and *DSM*-oriented Inattentive and Hyperactive-Impulsive subscales are scored for the TRF. As described earlier, four new scales were added in 2007. The YSR Positive Qualities was already described, but the new Obsessive-Compulsive Problems (OCP), Posttraumatic Stress Problems (PTSP), and Sluggish Cognitive Tempo (SCT) scales are described next.

Using 11 CBCL items reflecting symptoms of obsessive-compulsive disorder (OCD), Nelson, Hanna, Hudziak, Botteron, Heath, and Todd (2001) conducted PFA with three demographically matched groups (children diagnosed with OCD, clinically referred without OCD, and nonreferred children from the 1991 CBCL national normative sample, total *N* = 218). Eight of the 11 items had large loadings (.49 to .70) on the first principal factor (e.g., *9. Can't get his/her mind off certain thoughts; obsessions (describe)*; *31. Fears he/she might think or do something bad*; *32. Feels he/she has to be perfect*; *66. Repeats certain acts over and over; compulsions (describe)*.

This 8-item OCP scale yielded high sensitivity, specificity, positive predictive value, and negative predictive value for discriminating between the OCD group and the other groups. Similar findings were reported by Geller et al. (2006) using the same three-group design with another sample. In samples of thousands of Dutch and American 7- to 12-year-old twins, Hudziak et al. (2004) found that genetic factors accounted for about 55% of the variance in scores on the 8-item OCP scale, whereas nonshared environmental factors accounted for about 45%.

Wolfe, Gentile, and Wolfe (1989) identified 20 CBCL items corresponding to diagnostic criteria for posttraumatic stress disorder (PTSD). Parents of two groups of sexually abused Canadian children endorsed these items much more frequently than parents in the CBCL normative sample (Wolfe & Birt, 1997; Wolfe et al., 1989). The 20 CBCL items identified by Wolfe et al. (1989) were further analyzed by Ruggerio and McLeer (2000) in U.S. samples of sexually abused children, children who were receiving outpatient psychiatric services, and children recruited from schools. Significant *r*s were found with the number of posttraumatic stress symptoms reported during diagnostic interviews or significant discrimination was obtained between abused children who did or did not meet criteria for PTSD for 14 items (e.g., *9. Can't get his/her mind off certain thoughts; obsessions (describe)*; *31. Fears he/she might think or do something bad*; *47. Nightmares*; *50. Too fearful or anxious*; *52. Feels too guilty*; *69. Secretive, keeps things to self*). Therefore, these 14 items were chosen to comprise the ASEBA PTSP scale. Wolfe and Birt (2006) found that this scale discriminated well between sexually abused and nonabused community children, but not between sexually abused children and nonsexually abused children in the care of child protection agencies when effects of SES, physical abuse, and neglect were controlled.

Using factor analysis of various problem items, Lahey et al. (1988) obtained a factor comprising sluggishness, drowsiness, and daydreaming that they labeled "Sluggish Tempo." Subsequent research has shown that what is now called Sluggish Cognitive Tempo (SCT) problems are associated with the Inattentive type of ADHD. Based on TRF ratings of 2,744 mostly Hispanic students, Carlson and Mann (2002) identified five TRF items for measuring SCT: *13. Confused or seems to be in a fog*; *17. Daydreams or gets lost in his/her thoughts*; *60. Apathetic or unmotivated*; *80. Stares blankly*; and *102. Underactive, slow moving, or lacks energy*. Students rated by teachers as ADHD Inattentive type who also had high scores on the TRF SCT items differed significantly on several other TRF scales from ADHD Inattentive type children with low scores on SCT.

In a study of 6- to 11-year-olds attending elementary schools in San Juan, Puerto Rico, Bauermeister et al. (2005) compared three groups: Combined ADHD, Inattentive type ADHD, and non-ADHD. SCT was measured with the five TRF items identified by Carlson and Mann (2002) and the four counterparts of these items on the CBCL (which lacks TRF item *60. Apathetic or unmotivated* is omitted). The ADHD Inattentive children scored significantly higher than both the ADHD Combined group and the non-ADHD group on the SCT scale.

BASC-2

The BASC-2 features 10 new content scales developed using a "rational and empirical approach" to supplement interpretation of the PRS, TRS, and SRP (Reynolds & Kamphaus, 2004). The content scales are scored from the same item pools as the BASC-2 primary scales. Only the ASSIST Plus software program for the BASC-2 (vs. the more basic scoring program) includes the utility to generate scores for content scales.

The seven PRS and TRS content scales include: *Anger Control*, which measures the tendency to become angry and to lack self-control of emotion; *Bullying*, which measures the tendency to be cruel and threatening; *Developmental Social Disorders*, which measures the tendency to show deficits in social skills, communication, interests, and activities; *Negative Emotionality*, which measures the tendency to react in an overly negative way to changes in routine; *Emotional Self-Control*, which measures the ability to regulate affect in response to environmental events; *Executive Functioning*, which measures the ability to plan, anticipate, inhibit, and maintain goal-directed activity; and *Resiliency*, which measures the ability to access internal and external support systems to relieve stress and overcome difficulties. Anger Control plus three additional content scales are provided for the SRP: *Ego Strength*, which measures emotional competence, self-awareness, self-acceptance, and self-identity; *Mania*, which measures the tendency toward extended periods of arousal, activity, and alertness; and *Test Anxiety*, which measures the tendency to worry about taking tests.

Reynolds and Kamphaus (2004) first decided what clinically relevant areas of content should be captured by the new scales and then determined if additional BASC-2 items were needed for these scales. The item composition of each scale was refined by examining *r*s among items. Content scale alpha reliabilities for genders combined for ages 6 to 18 in the General norms sample ranged from .70 to .85 on the PRS, from .74 to .92 on the TRS, and from .67 to .87 on the SRP. The BASC-2 manual does not present any research findings validating the new content scales against other scales measuring the same constructs or using relevant clinical groups.

DIFFERENCES IN APPROACH TO HANDLING POSSIBLE INFORMANT "BIAS"

ASEBA

According to Achenbach and Rescorla (2001), informants' ratings may be affected by many factors, including motivation, carefulness, candor, past experience, values, and goals. Even when each informant is motivated to respond as honestly and conscientiously as possible, their ratings are likely to differ because each informant interacts with the child in a different context or in a different way. For this reason, the ASEBA underscores the importance of systematically comparing reports from multiple informants to identify both agreements and disagreements.

As long as an informant does not leave more than eight problem items unscored, the ASEBA form is considered "valid" from the point of view of computing scores. If an informant rates problems much lower than other informants, this may suggest that the informant is denying problems, unaware of problems, or trying to minimize problems. Conversely, if an informant rates problems much higher than other informants, this may suggest that the informant is trying to exaggerate problems or has a very low threshold for what constitutes a problem. However, discrepant scores may also be clinically meaningful and important. For example, if a father's CBCL indicates many more problems for an adolescent than the mother's CBCL, three TRFs, and the YSR, then it may be that the adolescent's interactions with the father are much more troubled than his interactions with other adults. Similarly, one teacher's ratings may be much lower than ratings by several other teachers because the target child has a particularly good relationship with that teacher or a special affinity in that teacher's class.

In addition to believing that informant differences are best examined through cross-informant comparisons, the authors of the ASEBA chose not to include validity scales because research has raised questions about their value. For example, Peidmont, McCrae, Riemann, and Angleitner (2000) found higher correlations between scores on two personality inventories, higher correlations with observer reports, and comparable differentiation of "aberrant" and "normal" personality for participants whose scores were flagged as "less valid" versus "valid" on validity scales.

BASC-2

Unlike the ASEBA, both the BASC and the BASC-2 contain a variety of validity scales to deal with possible informant "bias." The BASC-2 PRS, TRS, and SRP each include an *F Index*, a *Consistency Index* (CI), and a *Response Pattern Index* (RPI); the SRP also includes a *Lie Index* and a *V Index*. The only one of these fives scales for which the BASC-2 manual provides validation data is the CI.

The *F* ("fake bad") index, designed to flag informants who may be "excessively negative," is a scale of 20 items (15 on the SRP) that were endorsed by <3% of respondents. It is scored by summing the problem items on the scale rated as *Almost always* plus the positive items rated as *Never.* Caution cutpoints are set at the 95th to 98th percentile across forms and age groups, whereas the *Extreme caution* cutpoints are at about the 99th percentile across forms and age groups. The CI, designed to identify random responding, is comprised of 20 pairs of contradictory items. High CI scores indicate that an informant has responded inconsistently to items measuring essentially the same content. To test validity of the CI, a series of random datasets were computer generated. Using CI index scores in the *Caution* or *Extreme Caution* range, about 66% of the cases with computer-generated random responses were identified. The RPI, designed to identify forms on which the "respondent was inattentive to the item content," is the sum of the number of times a response differs from the response to the previous item. Caution-High and Caution-Low ranges were set at the .5th percentile and the 99.5th percentiles, approximately.

The SRP L index is obtained by summing the number of times the child responded *True* or *Almost Always* to an unrealistically positive item plus the number of times the child responded *False* or *Never* to a mildly negative statement endorsed by most children. *Caution* cutpoints are at about the 9th and 5th percentiles for children and adolescents, respectively, whereas *Extreme Caution* cutpoints are at the 1st percentile for both age groups. Finally, the SRP also has a V Index, designed to flag forms on which the child or adolescent endorsed nonsensical items.

DIFFERENCES IN PROCEDURES FOR CROSS-INFORMANT COMPARISONS

ASEBA

Because informants typically have different perspectives on a child's problems, the ASEBA considers systematic cross-informant comparisons to be essential for comprehensive assessment. Meta-analyses of many studies of various assessment instruments have yielded a mean correlation of .60 between reports of children's problems by pairs of informants who play similar roles in relation to children, including pairs of parents, teachers, mental health workers, and observers (Achenbach, McConaughy, & Howell, 1987). The mean correlation was .28 between reports by informants who play different roles in relation to children, such as parents versus teachers versus mental health workers. Between children's self-reports and reports by adults, the mean correlation was .22. Although all these correlations were statistically significant, their modest magnitude indicates that no one informant can substitute for all others.

The ASEBA software provides three ways to quickly compare data obtained from different informants. First, the ASEBA software prints Q correlations between each pair of informants' ratings for problem items, as well as the 25th percentile, mean, and 75th percentile Q correlations found in large reference samples for similar informant pairs. Second, the ASEBA software prints a bar graph for each of the 17 problem scales common to the CBCL/6-18, TRF, and YSR scale showing the T scores obtained from ratings by up to eight informants. The bar graphs enable the clinician to quickly identify how children and adolescents function in different contexts and how they are perceived by different informants. Third, the software prints side-by-side comparisons of the 0–1–2 ratings obtained from each informant on each problem item of each scale, enabling the clinician to quickly identify items that are endorsed by all, some, or no informants.

BASC-2

The original BASC did not provide cross-informant scoring options. It was therefore necessary for users to visually compare profiles or tables of scores printed for different informants. However, the BASC-2 scoring program prints a "Multi-Rater T Score Profile" which superimposes on a single graph the profile obtained from each parent and teacher respondent (up to a maximum for five raters). Because the scales for the SRP are different, this output does not allow simultaneous display of PRS, TRS, and SRP profiles. When profiles are displayed for more than three informants, the overlapping graphs are somewhat difficult to decipher, making the table under the figure listing the T scores and percentiles for each informant on each scale especially useful. The multi-informant utility also provides correlations between pairs of raters and indicates which differences between informants are significant at $p < .05$.

DIFFERENCES IN PROCEDURES FOR OBTAINING A GENERAL POPULATION SAMPLE

ASEBA

The general population sample used to norm the 2001 ASEBA was recruited in 1999 and 2000 using multistage national probability sampling, which ensures that all individuals in the target population have similar probabilities of being selected. First, Listing Areas of about 150 households were randomly selected in 100 sites that were collectively representative of the 48 contiguous states with respect to region, ethnicity,

SES, and urbanicity. Eligible participants were then identified by interviewers who went door-to-door to all households in a listing area to determine the age, gender, and eligibility of residents. From the residents thus
identified, a stratified random sampling procedure was used to select
candidates for the survey.

Once eligible participants had been selected, a trained interviewer
then contacted the candidate interviewees. A parent was initially administered the CBCL/6-18. With parental consent, TRFs were sent to teachers
and the YSR was administered to 11- to 18-year-olds. Parent interviewees
were also asked whether their child had received mental health, substance abuse, or special education services in the preceding 12 months.
To create nonclinical normative samples (called "healthy samples" in epidemiology), ASEBA forms for children who had received services in the
preceding 12 months were excluded from the samples used to norm the
ASEBA scales.

The ASEBA manual reports *completion rates,* namely the percentage of parents, teachers, and youths invited to participate who actually completed the CBCL/6-18, TRF, or YSR (Achenbach & Rescorla,
2001). High completion rates are very important because they help
guard against selection biases. Without knowing the completion rate, it
is impossible to evaluate how representative a sample is. For ages 6 to
18, 93% of the selected parents completed the CBCL/6-18. YSRs were
completed by 96% of the 11- to 18-year-olds whose parents completed
the CBCL/6-18. After 14% of the CBCL sample and 15% of the YSR
sample had been excluded because they had received services in the
past year, the *N*s for the final normative samples were 1,753 for the
CBCL and 1,057 for the YSR.

The completion rate was lower for the TRF than for the CBCL and
YSR, possibly owing to the need to mail TRFs to teachers. Completed
TRFs were received for 72% of the children whose parents gave consent for the TRF (*N* = 1,128). Of this group, 152 children (14%) were
excluded from the normative sample because they had received services in the past year. Because the resulting *N* = 976 would have been
somewhat small, the feasibility of including TRF data from the 1989
TRF national normative sample (completion rate = 76%) was tested
statistically. When mean scores on adaptive functioning and problems
were compared for 1989 and 1999, no differences exceeded chance
expectations ($p < .01$). Consequently, 1,343 TRFs from the 1989 sample were added to the 976 from the 1999–2000 sample, yielding a
normative sample of 2,319. The CBCL, TRF, and YSR samples all cor-
responded very well with U.S. Census parameters. The samples comprised 44% boys for the CBCL/6-18, 48% boys for the TRF, and 52%
boys for the YSR. Across forms, SES based on parents' occupations
was 32–38% upper class, 46–53% middle class, and 16% lower class.
For the CBCL/6-18 and YSR, ethnicity was 60% white, 20% African
American. 8–9% Latino, and 11–12% mixed or other; for the TRF, ethnicity was 72% white, 14% African American, and 7% in each of the
other two categories.

BASC-2

A total of 375 sites in 40 states were used to collect the General sample and Clinical sample. Rather than using probability-based sampling of households, the BASC-2 recruited its general population sample through schools. Site coordinators were hired to recruit teachers for participation in the project. Once a teacher consented to participate, parents of all the children in that class received a background information form and a consent form. Teachers typically completed forms for no more than four children in a class, but PRS forms were initially sent to all parents who consented and SRP forms were initially administered to all children whose parents consented. As the data collection proceeded from 2002 to 2004, PRS and SRP forms were only obtained from participants needed to fill certain demographic cells, as defined by age, gender, SES, ethnicity, and region. The data collection continued until the targets for all cells had been reached.

This approach to sampling is sometimes referred to as poststratification. That is, once the data have been collected, participants are selected from all those providing data so as to match U.S. census parameters. Because poststratification was used, the BASC-2 General normative sample had exactly even numbers of children in each age/gender group (e.g., 600 children age 6 to 7, 50% of whom were boys) and closely matched U.S. Census parameters. Across all ages and forms, 60–66% of the sample was white, 15–20% of the sample was African American, and 16–20% was Hispanic. SES was measured by mother's education level, with the breakdown 14–16% < 11th grade, 31–34% high school graduates, 29–32% some post-high school education, and 22–24% four or more years of college.

The BASC-2 manual does not provide any information on completion rates. It is therefore impossible to know how representative the sample was of the participating school classes. Furthermore, no data are provided on how many teachers invited to participate declined, how many parents invited to give consent declined, how many parents who gave consent actually completed forms, or how many children whose parents provided consent completed the SRP.

DIFFERENCES IN CHOICE OF NORM GROUPS

ASEBA

As noted previously, ASEBA norms are based on the scores obtained by children from the general population sample who had not received mental health, substance abuse, or special education services in the past year. For the CBCL and TRF, separate norms are provided by gender for ages 6 to 11 and 12 to 18. YSR norms for ages 11 to 18 are provided by gender. Age differences within the broad age groups are not sufficient to warrant norms for narrower age bands. The rationale for the ASEBA norms is that the most appropriate and useful comparison group for a given child's scores consists of a large sample of "healthy" children of the same gender and age group in a national probability sample.

BASC-2

BASC-2 General norms and Clinical norms are available for both genders combined and for each gender separately. The age ranges for all norm sets are 6 to 7, 8 to 11, 12 to 14, and 15 to 18. Although the General norm group was recruited through general education classrooms, 17.4 to 23.3% of the children had been classified through their schools as having learning, behavioral, developmental, or other problems qualifying them for special education services (p. 121). Thus, unlike the ASEBA, the BASC-2 General norm group is not restricted to "healthy" children. In addition to providing norms for the full Clinical sample, the BASC-2 provides norms separately for LD (N = 471) and ADHD (N = 483) subgroups at both the child and adolescent levels.

Reynolds and Kamphaus (2004) state that the "General combined-sex norms will be the preferred norms, and they are recommended for general use" (p. 13). Their explanation is that the combined norms reflect the fact that boys typically obtain higher scores for certain scales (e.g., Aggression), whereas girls typically obtain higher scores for other scales (e.g., Social Skills). The combined norms indicate how commonly a score was obtained by children of the same age regardless of gender, whereas the gender-specific norms indicate how commonly a score was obtained by children of the same age and gender. The combined norms have the tendency to make a child's score more deviant on a scale typical for that child's gender but less deviant on a scale atypical for that child's gender. For example, on the TRS Aggression scale, the combined norms yield $T = 70$ for a raw score of 12, which is more deviant than a boy would score using male norms ($T = 66$) but less deviant than a girls would score using female norms ($T = 77$).

DIFFERENCES IN RESEARCH BASE

ASEBA

Over the past three decades, many empirical studies using ASEBA forms have been published. The *Bibliography of Published Studies Using ASEBA Instruments* (Bérubé & Achenbach, 2008) lists references for over 6,500 publications from 67 cultures by over 8,000 authors. References are listed according to some 450 topics (e.g., ADHD, Learning Disability, Conduct Disorder, Anxiety, Depression, Drug Studies, Outcomes, and Substance Abuse).

Numerous studies have reported significant associations between ASEBA scales and psychiatric diagnoses (e.g., Edelbrock & Costello, 1988; Kasius, Ferdinand, van den Berg, & Verhulst, 1997). In an outpatient clinic sample, CBCL/6-18 empirically based problem scales correlated from .49 to .80 (mean r = .62; N = 65) with scores on a checklist of *DSM-IV* criteria (Hudziak, 1998) and correlated from .27 to .53 (mean point biserial r = .39; N = 134) with *DSM-IV* diagnoses recorded in the children's clinic records (Achenbach & Rescorla, 2001).

ASEBA scales have also been widely used in cluster analytic and latent class analytic studies. Using cluster analysis of CBCL syndrome profiles, Edelbrock and Achenbach (1980) identified and replicated six profile types for boys and seven for girls. Compared to children with other profile types, children with the "Hyperactive" profile type had significantly lower scores on the CBCL School scale and children with the "Aggressive-Cruel" profile type had significantly lower scores on the CBCL Social scale. More recent studies have used latent class analysis with sets of ASEBA items. For example, Hudziak, Wadsworth, Heath, and Achenbach (1999) compared assignment to one of four latent classes derived from the CBCL Attention Problems scale for children in demographically matched referred and nonreferred samples ($N = 2,100$ per sample). In the nonreferred sample, 84% to 90% fell into the "none" or "mild" classes, whereas in the referred sample 74% to 83% fell into the "moderate" or "severe" classes.

A rapidly growing research area involves use of ASEBA scales as phenotypic markers in genetic studies. For example, the Aggressive Behavior syndrome has yielded high heritability estimates in many studies (e.g., 53% to 75% in Eley, Lichtenstein, & Stevenson, J. (1999)) and has significant associations with serotonergic activity (Hanna, Yuwiler, & Coates, 1995), dopamine-beta-hydroxylase (DBH) levels (Gabel, Stadler, Bjorn, Shindledecker, & Bowden, 1993), and testosterone (Scerbo & Kolko, 1994). In 1,481 Dutch twin pairs examined from ages 3 to 12 (Bartels et al., 2004), heritability for Internalizing scores decreased with age, whereas heritability for Externalizing changed less with age and was somewhat greater for boys than girls at most ages. In 2,192 Dutch twin pairs, heritability for Attention Problems was very high for all age/gender groups (70% to 74%) and accounted for most of the variance in longitudinal stability (Rietveld, Hudziak, Bartels, Beijsterveldt, & Boomsma, 2004).

ASEBA scales have been used extensively in longitudinal research. For example, parallel studies of representative samples of thousands of American and Dutch children have yielded large correlations between syndrome scores obtained at intervals of six years (Achenbach, Howell, McConaughy, & Stanger, 1995; Verhulst & van der Ende, 1992). Child and adolescent ASEBA scores also predicted adult substance abuse, trouble with the law, suicidal behavior, and referral for mental health services (Achenbach, Howell, McConaughy, & Stanger, 1998; Ferdinand & Verhulst, 1995). A Dutch longitudinal study that spanned 14 years showed that childhood scores on the Anxious/Depressed, Thought Problems, and Delinquent Behavior (Rule-Breaking Behavior) syndrome scales were exceptionally good predictors of adult problems, including *DSM-IV* diagnoses (Hofstra, van der Ende, & Verhulst, 2002).

BASC-2

In part because the BASC was first published only in 1992, fewer research studies have been published than for the ASEBA. At the time of publication of the BASC-2, the original BASC had been used in some 125 studies (Reynolds & Kamphaus, 2004; p. 10). Fewer than 50 published empirical articles are listed in the BASC/BASC-2 Research Bibliography (http://ags.pearsonassessments.com/psych/bib.asp), with most of the references being dissertation abstracts, conference presentations, reviews of the BASC, or overview chapters on child assessment measures. Reynolds and Kamphaus (2002) provide useful summaries of numerous research studies using the BASC.

Several studies have used the BASC with children diagnosed with ADHD. For example, Manning and Miller (2001) reported that children with ADHD had significantly higher scores than control children on numerous PRS and TRS scales, although their scores on many scales fell below the At-Risk cutpoint. Using a sample of 301 children identified through a large school sample, Ostrander, Weinfurt, Yarnold, and August (1998) found that the PRS was more efficient than the CBCL at differentiating children with and without ADHD and for identifying the ADHD-Combined subtype, whereas the CBCL was more efficient in identifying ADHD-Inattentive students. Doyle, Ostrander, Skare, Crosby, and August (1997) and Vaughn, Riccio, Hynd, and Hall (1997) found that the BASC and the CBCL were roughly equivalent in identifying Combined type ADHD, but Vaughn et al. found that the BASC was better at identifying Inattentive type ADHD. Sullivan and Riccio (2006) reported data for an 18-item BASC scale they described as tapping frontal lobe/executive functioning (FLEC). Children with ADHD and children with other diagnoses had higher FLEC scores than controls, but the ADHD and non-ADHD groups did not differ from each other.

Cluster analytic studies of scales on the TRS (Kamphaus, Huberty, DiStefano, & Petolsky, 1997) and PRS (Kamphaus et al., 1999) have yielded seven and nine clusters, respectively. As noted by Kamphaus et al. (1999), many of the clusters resembled those found using the CBCL (e.g., children with good adjustment, children with primarily internalizing problems, children with high levels of problems across most scales, children with attention problems, and so forth). DiStefano, Kamphaus, Horne, and Winsor (2003) replicated the seven TRS clusters in two independent samples of children.

Several studies have examined BASC scores in children with medical problems, such as survivors of childhood leukemia. For example, Shelby, Nagle, Barnett-Queen, Quattlebaum, and Wuori (1998) reported that childhood survivors did not differ on the PRS from the normative sample, whereas adolescent survivors had significantly higher BASC scores (e.g., 38% scored in the At-Risk range on the Behavioral Symptoms Index).

DIFFERENCES IN MULTICULTURAL APPLICATIONS

ASEBA

ASEBA instruments have been translated into over 85 foreign languages. Users can order Spanish versions of the CBCL/6-18, TRF, and YSR, and other translations are available by contacting ASEBA (www.ASEBA. org). More than 1,800 cross-culturally relevant ASEBA studies have been published from over 67 countries (Bérubé & Achenbach, 2008). Some of this research is summarized in *Multicultural Understanding of Child and Adolescent Psychopathology: Implications for Mental Health Assessment* (Achenbach & Rescorla, 2007b).

Many early cross-cultural studies reported rigorous statistical comparisons of ASEBA item and scale scores in large epidemiological samples for another culture vis-à-vis the United States (e.g., Lambert, Lyubansky, & Achenbach, 1998). Crijnen, Achenbach, and Verhulst (1997) pioneered a new approach to multicultural research when they compared 12 cultures on CBCL Total Problems, Externalizing, and Internalizing scores. Later studies compared CBCL syndrome scores in the same 12 cultures (Crijnen, Achenbach, & Verhulst, 1999) and YSR scores in seven cultures (Verhulst et al., 2003).

More recently, Rescorla et al. (2007a,b,c) analyzed scale scores, item scores, and age and gender differences on CBCLs from 31 societies ($N = 55,508$), TRFs from 21 societies ($N = 30,957$), and YSRs from 24 societies ($N = 27,206$). Effects of society were significant for most problem scales, but ESs were generally <10%. There was much greater variation in scores within societies than between societies. Furthermore, many societies differing in geographical region, ethnicity, religion, and political/ economic system had very similar scores, and most societies had mean scores close to the overall mean for all societies. Correlations between all pairs of societies for mean item scores indicated a great degree of consistency across societies with respect to which items tended to receive high, medium, and low ratings. There was also great consistency across societies in some striking patterns of gender differences. For example, boys obtained significantly higher Attention Problems scores than girls on the TRF and CBCL in almost every society, but not in any society on the YSR.

In a parallel set of studies using the same datasets, Ivanova et al. (2007a,b,c) tested the ASEBA syndrome model in each society using CFA. RMSEAs within the range for acceptable to good fit were obtained for every society for every form. In addition, most items loaded significantly on their predicted factors for most societies. Thus, the empirically based syndrome model derived from data collected in the United States, Britain, and Australia showed good fit to data collected using ASEBA forms in societies as different as Iran, Germany, Ethiopia, Iceland, Japan, Poland, the Netherlands, China, Turkey, and Italy.

With publication of ADM with Multicultural Options (Achenbach & Rescorla, 2007a), ASEBA users can choose to have a child's profile displayed in relation to norms from low-scoring, intermediate-scoring, or high-scoring societies. For example, ASEBA scale scores for an immigrant child can be displayed in relation to one set of norms that includes the child's home culture and in relation to a different set of norms that includes the host culture where the child resides.

BASC-2

A few published studies have reported BASC scores for children from other societies. For example, when Zhou, Peverly, Xin, Huang, and Wang (2003) compared SRP scores for Chinese American adolescents in New York City (N = 106), Mainland Chinese students (N = 120), and European American students (N = 131), they found that Chinese American students had the most negative attitudes toward school, teachers, and their own learning. Jung and Stinnett (2005), who compared BASC SRP and PRS scores for 120 Korean, Korean American, and Caucasian American children ages 8 to 11, reported that Korean children had higher Internalizing scores than American children and that Korean American children had more adjustment difficulties. Cho, Hudley, and Back (2003), who used the SRP with 51 Korean American adolescents, reported elevated social and emotional distress relative to norms.

Chapter 16 of the BASC-2 manual describes the development of the Spanish versions of the forms and presents tables regarding the Spanish-form samples, alphas, and correlations among scales. Although the manual does not report any empirical studies using the Spanish versions, McCloskey, Hess, and D'Amato (2003) compared PRS scores for 55 Hispanic children with scores from the normative sample. Some differences in associations were found for four scales on the Behavioral Symptom Index as well as for the Adaptive Composite.

CONCLUSIONS AND IMPLICATIONS

The ASEBA and the BASC-2 both provide comprehensive systems for assessing behavioral and emotional problems and positive functioning in children and adolescents from the perspectives of parents, teacher, and children themselves. Both systems report scores for items, narrowband scales, and broadband scales. Furthermore, both systems report good test–retest reliability and were normed on large samples demographically representative of the U.S. population. Both systems also report scores for clinical samples.

Despite the many similarities between the ASEBA and the BASC-2, they also differ in the following ways. (a) The ASEBA separates problem items and adaptive/competence items and uses a 3-level problem rating scale, whereas the BASC-2 mixes these two kinds of items and uses a 4-level scale; (b) the ASEBA assesses competence in the areas of activities, social relationships, and school functioning, whereas the BASC-2 has more adaptive scales and uses descriptors of positive behaviors; (c) ASEBA syndrome scales were derived by factor analysis and *DSM*-oriented scales were constructed using expert judgment, whereas BASC-2 scales were constructed based on a combination of author judgment and statistical refining; (d) because some cutpoints differ between the ASEBA and the BASC, the BASC-2 is likely to identify more children as At-Risk on narrowband scales than the ASEBA identifies as Borderline, whereas the ASEBA is likely to identify more children in the Clinical range on broadband scales than the BASC-2 identifies as Clinically Significant; (e) the ASEBA manual reports extensive validation procedures involving differentiation of referred from nonreferred children, whereas the BASC-2 presents scores for both General and Clinical groups but does not report any statistical tests of these differences; (f) the ASEBA has 17 problem scales common to all forms, plus four new scales on some forms, whereas the BASC-2 has few scales common to the PRS/TRS and the SRP and has 10 new content scales; (g) the ASEBA addresses possible informant bias using cross-informant comparisons, whereas the BASC-2 employs several validity scales, only one of which is itself validated; (h) the ASEBA yields cross-informant bar graphs for up to eight informants on the 17 scales common to all three forms, tables of ratings by all informants on all items, and correlations between all pairs of raters, whereas the BASC-2 yields overlapping profiles for up to five informants on the PRS and SRP, tables with scores for all informants, and correlations between pairs of informants; (i) the ASEBA recruited its normative sample using probability sampling and reported completion rates that are very high for the CBCL and YSR and moderate for the TRF, whereas the BASC-2 recruited its General sample through schools, used poststratification, and reported no completion rates; (j) ASEBA norms are based on a "healthy" sample and separated by gender and age group, whereas BASC-2 norms for both General and Clinical samples are provided with genders pooled and genders separated; (k) More than 6,500 research studies report use of ASEBA forms, whereas fewer than 50 studies report use of BASC and BASC-2 forms; and (l) more than 1,800 studies report ASEBA findings from other cultures, allowing development of multicultural scoring norms, whereas only a few international studies have been published using the BASC.

Awareness of these differences is important for trainers in clinical and school psychology as well as for experts in test construction and psychometrics. However, the many differences between the ASEBA and the BASC-2 may vary in their importance depending on the needs and preferences of different users. For example, the ASEBA's strong research base, empirical derivation of syndromes, probability sampling with high completion rates, and extensive validation may be particularly important features for some users. Conversely, the BASC-2's mix of problem and positive items, approach to measuring adaptive functioning, validity scales, and content scales may be particularly attractive features for other users. Practitioners who assess children and adolescents should consider which differences are most relevant to their needs as they decide on which of the two systems is best for their professional use.

REFERENCES

Achenbach, T. M. (1966). The classification of children's psychiatric symptoms: A factor-analytic study. *Psychological Monographs, 80,* (*No. 615*).

Achenbach, T. M. (1986). *The direct observation form of the child behavior checklist* (rev. ed.). Burlington, VT: University of Vermont, Department of Psychiatry.

Achenbach, T. M. (1991a). *Manual for the Child Behavior Checklist/4-18 and 1991 Profile.* Burlington, VT: University of Vermont, Department of Psychiatry.

Achenbach, T. M. (1991b). *Manual for the Teacher's Report Form and 1991 Profile.* Burlington, VT: University of Vermont, Department of Psychiatry.

Achenbach, T. M. (1991c). *Manual for the Youth Self-Report and 1991 Profile.* Burlington, VT: University of Vermont, Department of Psychiatry.

Achenbach, T. M. (1992). *Manual for the Child Behavior Checklist/2-3 and 1992 Profile.* Burlington, VT: University of Vermont, Department of Psychiatry.

Achenbach, T. M. (1997). *Guide for Caregiver-Teacher Report Form for Ages 2–5.* Burlington, VT: University of Vermont, Department of Psychiatry.

Achenbach, T. M. (1997). *Manual for the Young Adult Self-Report and Young Adult Behavior Checklist.* Burlington, VT: University of Vermont, Department of Psychiatry.

Achenbach, T.M. (2006) Applications of the Achenbach System of Empirically Based Assessment (ASEBA) to children, adolescents, and their parents. In S. R. Smith & L. Handler (Eds.), *The clinical assessment of children and adolescents: A practitioners' guide.* Mahwah, NJ: Erlbaum (pp. 329–346).

Achenbach, T. M., & Edelbrock, C. (1981). Behavioral problems and competencies reported by parents of normal and disturbed children aged four to sixteen. *Monographs of the Society for Research in Child Development, 46* (1, Serial No. 188).

Achenbach, T. M., & Edelbrock C. (1983). *Manual for the Child Behavior Checklist/4-18 and Revised Child Behavior Profile.* Burlington, VT: University of Vermont, Department of Psychiatry.

Achenbach, T. M., & Edelbrock, C. (1986). *Manual for the Teacher's Report Form and Teacher Version of the Child Behavior Profile.* Burlington, VT: University of Vermont, Department of Psychiatry.

Achenbach, T. M., & Edelbrock, C. (1987). *Manual for the Youth Self-Report and Profile.* Burlington, VT: University of Vermont, Department of Psychiatry.

Achenbach, T. M., Howell, C. T., McConaughy, S. H., & Stanger, C. (1995). Six-year predictors of problems in a national sample: III. Transitions to young adult syndromes. *Journal of the American Academy of Child and Adolescent Psychiatry, 34,* 658–669.

Achenbach, T. M., Howell, C. T., McConaughy, S. H., & Stanger, C. (1998). Six-year predictors of problems in a national sample: IV. Young adult signs of disturbance. *Journal of the American Academy of Child and Adolescent Psychiatry, 37,* 718–727.

Achenbach, T. M., Howell, C. T., Quay, H. C., & Conners, C. K. (1991) National survey of problems and competencies among 4- to 16-year olds. *Monographs of the Society for Research in Child Development. Serial No.* 225, 56, 3.

Achenbach, T. M., McConaughy, S. H., & Howell, C. T. (1987). Child/adolescent behavioral and emotional problems: Implications of cross-informant correlations for situational specificity. *Psychological Bulletin, 101,* 213–232.

Achenbach, T. M., Newhouse, P. A., & Rescorla, L. A. (2004). *Manual for the ASEBA Older Adult Forms & Profiles.* Burlington, VT: University of Vermont, Research Center for Children, Youth, and Families.

Achenbach, T. M., & Rescorla, L. A. (2000). *Manual for the ASEBA Preschool Forms & Profiles.* Burlington, VT: University of Vermont, Department of Psychiatry.

Achenbach, T. M., & Rescorla, L. A. (2001). *Manual for the ASEBA School-Age Forms & Profiles.* Burlington, VT: University of Vermont, Research Center for Children, Youth, and Families.

Achenbach, T. M., & Rescorla, L. A. (2003). *Manual for the ASEBA Adult Forms & Profiles.* Burlington, VT: University of Vermont, Research Center for Children, Youth, and Families.

Achenbach, T. M., & Rescorla, L. A. (2004). The Achenbach System of Empirically Based Assessment (ASEBA) for ages 1.5 to 18 years. In M. E. Maruish (Ed.), *The use of psychological testing for treatment planning and outcomes assessment* (3rd ed). Mahwah, NJ: Erlbaum (pp. 179–213).

Achenbach, T. M., & Rescorla, L. A. (2007a). *Multicultural supplement for the manual for the ASEBA School-Age Forms and Profiles.* Burlington, VT: University of Vermont, Research Center for Children, Youth, and Families.

Achenbach, T. M., & Rescorla, L. A. (2007b). Multicultural understanding of child and adolescent psychopathology: Implications for mental health assessment. New York: Guilford.

American Psychiatric Association. (1952;1994). *Diagnostic and statistical manual of mental disorders* (1st ed., 4th ed.). Washington, DC: American Psychiatric Association.

Bartels, M., van den Oord, E. J. C. G., Hudziak, J. J., Rietveld, M. J. H., van Beijsterveldt, C. E. M., & Boomsma, D. I. (2004). Genetic and environmental mechanisms underlying stability and change in problem behaviors at ages 3, 7, 10, and 12. *Developmental Psychology, 40,* 852–867

Bauermeister, J. J., Matos, M., Reina, G., Salas, C. C., Martínez, J. V., Cumba, E., et al. (2005). Comparison of the DSM-IV combined and inattentive types of ADHD in a school-based sample of Latino/Hispanic children. *Journal of Child Psychology and Psychiatry, 46,* 166–179.

Bérubé, R. L., & Achenbach, T. M. (2008). *Bibliography of published studies using the Achenbach System of Empirically Based Assessment (ASEBA): 2008 edition.* Burlington, VT: University of Vermont, Research Center for Children, Youth, & Families.

Browne, N. W., & Cudeck, R. (1993). Alternative ways of assessing model fit. In K. A. Bollen & J. S. Long (Eds.), *Testing structural equation models* (pp. 136–162). Newbury Park, CA: Sage.

Carlson, C. L., & Mann, M. (2002). Sluggish cognitive tempo predicts a different pattern of impairment in the attention deficit hyperactivity disorder, predominantly inattentive type. *Journal of Clinical Child and Adolescent Psychology, 31,* 123–129.

Cho, S. J., Hudley, C., & Back, H. J. (2003). Cultural influences on ratings of self-perceived social, emotional, and academic adjustment for Korean American adolescents. *Assessment for Effective Intervention, 29,* 3–14.

Cohen, J. (1988). *Statistical power analysis for the behavioral sciences* (2nd ed.). New York: Academic Press.

Conners, C. K. (1997). *Conners' Parent Rating Scale-Revised.* North Tonawanda, NY: Multi-Health Systems.

Crijnen, A. A. M., Achenbach, T. M., & Verhulst, F. C. (1997). Comparisons of problems reported by parents of children in 12 cultures: Total Problems, Externalizing, and Internal-izing. *Journal of the American Academy of Child and Adolescent Psychiatry, 36,* 1269–1277.

Crijnen, A. A. M., Achenbach, T. M., & Verhulst, F. C. (1999). Comparisons of problems reported by parents of children in twelve cultures: The CBCL/4-18 syndrome constructs. *American Journal of Psychiatry, 156,* 569–574.

Cronbach, L. J. (1951). Coefficient alpha and the internal structure of tests. *Psychometrika, 16,* 297–334.

DiStefano, C., Kamphaus, R. W., Horne, A. M., & Winsor, A. P. (2003). Behavioral adjustment in the U.S. elementary school: Cross-validation of a person-oriented typology of risk. *Journal of Psychoeducational Assessment, 21,* 338–357.

Doyle, A., Ostrander, R., Skare, S., Crosby, R. D., & August, G. (1997). Convergent and criterion-related validity of the Behavior Assessment System for Children-Parent Rating Scales. *Journal of Clinical Child Psychology, 26,* 276–284.

Dumenci, L., McConaughy, S. H., & Achenbach, T. M. (2004). A hierarchical three-factor model of inattention-hyperactivity-impulsivity derived from the attention problems syndrome of the Teacher's Report Form. *School Psychology Review, 33,* 287–301.

Edelbrock, C., & Achenbach, T. M. (1980). A typology of Child Behavior Profile patterns: Distribution and correlates for disturbed children aged 6–16. *Journal of Abnormal Child Psychology, 8,* 441–470.

Edelbrock, C., & Costello, A. J. (1988). Convergence between statistically derived behavior problem syndromes and child psychiatric diagnoses. *Journal of Abnormal Child Psychology, 16,* 219–231.

Eley, T. C., Lichtenstein, P., & Stevenson, J. (1999). Sex differences in the etiology of aggressive and nonaggressive antisocial behavior: Results from two twin studies. *Child Development, 70,* 155–168.

Ferdinand, R. F., & Verhulst, F. C. (1995). Psychopathology in Dutch young adults: Enduring or changeable? *Social Psychiatry and Psychiatric Epidemiology, 30,* 60–64.

Gabel, S., Stadler, J., Bjorn, J., Shindledecker, R., & Bowden, C. (1993). Dopamine-beta-hydroxylase in behaviorally disturbed youth. Relationship between teacher and parent ratings. *Biological Psychiatry, 34,* 434–442.

Geller, D. A., Doyle, R., Shaw, D., Mullin, B., Coffey, B., Petty, C., et al. (2006). A quick and reliable screening measure for OCD in youth: reliability and validity of the obsessive compulsive scale of the Child Behavior Checklist. *Comprehensive Psychiatry, 47,* 234–240.

Hanna, G. L., Yuwiler, A., & Coates, J. K. (1995). Whole blood serotonin and disruptive behaviors in juvenile obsessive-compulsive disorder. *Journal of the American Academy of Child and Adolescent Psychiatry, 34,* 28–35.

Hofstra, M. B.,van der Ende, J., & Verhulst, F. C. (2001). Adolescents' self-reported problems as predictors of psychopathology in adulthood: 10-year follow-up study. *British Journal of Psychiatry, 179*, 203–209.

Hofstra, M. B., van der Ende, J., & Verhulst, F. C. (2002). Child and adolescent problems predict DSM-IV disorders in adulthood: A 14-year follow-up of a Dutch epidemiological sample. *Journal of the American Academy of Child and Adolescent Psychiatry, 41*, 182–189.

Hudziak, J. J. (1998). *DSM-IV Checklist for Childhood Disorders.* Burlington, VT: Univertsity of Vermont, Research Center for Children, Youth and Families.

Hudziak, J. J., van Beijsterveldt, C. E. M., Althoff, R. R., Stanger, C., Rettew, D. C., Nelson, E. C., et al. (2004). Genetic and environmental contributions to the Child Behavior Checklist obsessive-compulsive scale: A cross-cultural twin study. *Archives of General Psychiatry, 61*, 608–616.

Hudziak, J. J., Wadsworth, M. E., Heath, A. C., & Achenbach, T. M., (1999). Latent class analysis of Child Behavior checklist Attention Problems. *Journal of the American Academy of Child and Adolescent Psychiatry, 38*, 985–991.

Individuals with Disabilities Education Act (IDEA), 1997, 20 USC et seq. (Fed Reg 64, 1999).

Ivanova, M. Y., Achenbach, T. M., Dumenci, L., Rescorla, L. A., Almqvist, F., Bilenberg, N., et al. (2007a). *Testing the 8-syndrome structure of the CBCL in 30 societies. Journal of Child and Adolescent Clinical Psychology, 36*, 405–417.

Ivanova, M. Y., Achenbach, T. M., Rescorla, L. A., Dumenci, L., Almqvist, F., Bathiche, et al. (2007b). *The generalizability of Teacher's Report Form syndromes in 20 societies. School Psychology Review, 36*, 468–483.

Ivanova, M. Y., Achenbach, T. M., Rescorla, L. A., Dumenci, L., Almqvist, F., Bilenberg, N., et al. (2007c). *The generalizability of the Youth Self-Report syndrome structure in 23 societies. Journal of Consulting and Clinical Psychology, 75*, 729–738.

Jung, W. S., & Stinnett, T. A. (2005). Comparing judgments of social, behavioral, emotional, and school adjustment functioning for Korean, Korean American, and Caucasian American children. *School Psychology International 26*, 317–329.

Kamphaus, R. W., Huberty, C. J., Distefano, C., & Petoskey, M. D. (1997). A typology of teacher-rated child behavior for a national U.S. sample. *Journal of Abnormal Child Psychology, 25*, 453–463.

Kamphaus, R. W., Petoskey, M. D., Cody, A. H., Rowe, E. W., Huberty, C. J., & Reynolds, C. R. (1999). A typology of parent-rated child behavior for a national U.S. sample. *Journal of Child Psychology and Psychiatry and Allied Disciplines, 40*, 1–10.

Kasius, M. C., Ferdinand, R. F., van den Berg, H., & Verhulst, F. C. (1997). Associations between different diagnostic approaches for child and adolescent psychopathology. *Journal of Child Psychology and Psychiatry, 38*, 625–632.

Lahey, B. B., Pelham, W. E., Schaughency, E. A., Atkins, M. S., Murphy, H. A., Hynd, G. W., et al. (1988). Dimensions and types of attention deficit disorder. *Journal of the American Academy of Child and Adolescent Psychiatry, 27*, 330–335.

Lambert, M. C., Lyubansky, M., & Achenbach, T. M. (1998). Behavioral and emotional problems among adolescents of Jamaica and the United States: Parent, teacher, and self-reports for ages 12 to 18. *Journal of Emotional and Behavioral Disorders, 6*, 180–187.

Manning, S. C, & Miller, D. C. (2001). Identifying ADHD subtypes using the Parent and Teacher Rating Scales of the Behavior Assessment Scale for Children. *Journal of Attention Disorders, 5*, 41–51.

McCloskey, D. M., Hess, R. S., & D'Amato, R. C. (2003). Evaluating the utility of the Spanish version of the Behavioral Assessment System for Children-Parent Report System. *Journal of Psychoeducational Assessmemt, 21*, 325–357.

McConaughy, S. H., & Achenbach, T. M. (1994). *Manual for the Semistructured Clinical Interview for Children and Adolescents.* Burlington, VT: University of Vermont, Research Center for Children, Youth, and Families.

McConaughy, S. H., & Achenbach, T. M. (2001) *Manual for the Semistructured Clinical Interview for Children and Adolescents* (2nd ed.). Burlington, VT: University of Vermont, Research Center for Children, Youth, and Families.

McConaughy, S. H., & Achenbach, T. M. (2004). *Manual for the Test Observation Form for Ages 2–18.* Burlington, VT: University of Vermont, Research Center for Children, Youth, and Families.

Nelson, E. C., Hanna, G. L., Hudziak, J. J., Botteron, K. N., Heath, A. C., & Todd, R. D. (2001). Obsessive-compulsive scale of the Child Behavior Checklist: Specificity, sensitivity, and predictive power. *Pediatrics, 108,* E14.

Ostrander, R., Weinfurt, K. P., Yarnold, P. R., & August, G. J. (1998). Diagnosing attention deficit disorders with the Behavior Assessment System for Children and the Child Behavior Checklist: Test and construct validity analyses using optimal discriminant classification trees. *Journal of Consulting and Clinical Psychology, 66,* 660–672.

Piedmont, R. L., McCrae, R. R., Riemann, R., & Angleitner, A. (2000). On the invalidity of validity scales: Evidence from self-report and observer rating in volunteer samples. *Journal of Personality and Social Psychology, 78,* 582– 593.

Rescorla, L. A, Achenbach, T. M., Ivanova, M. Y, Dumenci, L., Almqvist, F., Bilenberg, N., et al. (2007a). *Problems reported by parents of children ages 6 to 16 in 31 cultures* (in review).

Rescorla, L. A., Achenbach, T. M., Ginzburg, S., Ivanova, M. Y., Dumenci, L., Almqvist, F., et al. (2007b, in press). Problems reported by teachers of children ages 6 to 15 in 21 countries. *School Psychology Review.*

Rescorla, L. A, Achenbach, T. M., Ivanova, M. Y., Dumenci, L., Almqvist, F., Bilenberg, N., et al. (2007c, in press). Problems reported by adolescents ages 11 to 16 in 22 countries. *Journal of Consulting and Clinical Psychology.*

Reynolds, C. R., & Kamphaus, R. W. (1992). *Behavior Assessment System for Children.* Circle Pines, MN: American Guidance Service.

Reynolds, C. R., & Kamphaus, R. W. (2002). The clinician's guide to the Behavior Assessment System for Children. New York: Guilford.

Reynolds, C. R., & Kamphaus, R. W. (2004). *Behavior Assessment System for Children – 2.* Circle Pines, MN: American Guidance Service.

Rietveld, M. J. H., Hudziak, J. J., Bartels, M., Van Beijsterveldt, C. E. M., & Boomsma, D. I. (2004). Heritability of attention problems in children: Longitudinal results from a study of twins, age 3 to 12. *Journal of Child Psychology and Psychiatry, 45,* 577–588.

Ruggiero, K. J., & McLeer, S. V. (2000). PTSD scale of the Child Behavior Checklist: Concurrent and discriminant validity with non-clinic-referred sexually abused children. *Journal of Traumatic Stress, 13,* 287–299.

Scerbo, A. S., & Kolko, D. (1994). Salivary testosterone and cortisol in disruptive children: Relationship to aggressive, hyperactive, and internalizing behaviors. *Journal of the American Academy of Child and Adolescent Psychiatry, 33,* 1174–1184.

Shelby, M. D., Nagle, R. J., Barnett-Queen, L. L., Quattlebaum, P. D., & Wuori, D. F. (1998). Parental reports of psychosocial adjustment and social competence in childhood survivors of acute lymphocytic leukemia. *Children's Health Care, 27,* 113–129.

Sullivan, J. R., & Riccio, C. A. (2006). An empirical analysis of the BASC Frontal Lobe/Executive Control scale with a clinical sample. *Archives of Clinical Neuropsychology, 21,* 495–501.

Vaughn, M. L., Riccio, C. A., Hynd, G. W., & Hall, J. (1997). Diagnosing ADHD (predominantly inattentive and combined type sybtypes): Discriminant validity of the Behavior Assessment for Children and the Achenbach Parent and Teacher Rating Scales. *Journal of Clinical Child Psychology, 26,* 349–357.

Verhulst, F. C., Achenbach, T. M., van der Ende, J., Erol, N., Lambert, M. C., Leung, P. W. L., Silva, M. A., Zilber, N., & Zubrick, S. R. (2003). Comparisons of problems reported by youths from seven countries. *American Journal of Psychiatry 160,* 1479–1485.

Verhulst, F. C., & van der Ende, J. (1992). Six-year stability of parent-reported problem behavior in an epidemiological sample. *Journal of Abnormal Child Psychology, 20,* 595–610.

Wolfe, V. V., & Birt, J. H. (1997). Child sexual abuse. In E. Mash and L. Terdal (Eds.), *Assessment of childhood disorders* (3rd ed., pp. 569–623). New York: Guilford.

Wolfe, V. V., & Birt, J. H. (2006). The Children's Peritraumatic Experiences Questionnaire: A measure to assess DSM-IV PTSD criterion A2 (unpublished manuscript).

Wolfe, V. V., Gentile, C., & Wolfe, D. A. (1989). The impact of sexual abuse on children: A PTSD formulation. *Behavior Therapy, 20,* 215–228.

Zhou, Z., Peverly, S. T., Xin, T, Huang, A. S., & Wang, W. (2003). School adjustment of first generation Chinese-American adolescents. *Psychology in the Schools, 40,* 71–84.

6

Neuropsychological Disorders of Children

WM. DREW GOUVIER, AUDREY BAUMEISTER, and KOLA IJAOLA

There is one fundamental axiom that governs the practice of neuropsychological assessment of children. That is that they are not little adults. Every aspect of the evaluation process must be changed to adapt to this fact. A special set of adapted techniques must be used to get background history and clarify the referral question; different strategies are needed to build rapport and maintain cooperation throughout the evaluation; the interpretation of assessment results is modulated by principles of dynamic localization (Vygotsky, 1960) and neuroplasticity (Stein, Brailowsky, & Will, 1995), and the reporting and communication of results is invariably a multiparty process quite different from a typical doctor–patient consultation (Ryan, Hammond, & Beers, 1998).

There are a variety of reasons why a child might be referred to a neuropsychologist for an assessment. These include examining the impact of congenital neurodevelopmental disorders, determining the effects of acquired injuries and tracking their recovery, or simply to better understand current learning and behavior issues and to understand how to best remediate them or mitigate their deleterious influences (Baron, 2004). This is particularly true for children who are experiencing academic problems in school or behavioral problems due to ADHD, learning disorders, or other conditions that place them neuropsychologically at risk. Neuropsychological assessments are requested by parents, teachers, counselors, and medical professionals when a child is noted to be developmentally off track in terms of cognitive, sensory, or motor development, and typically include but go beyond the normal rating scale assessment by others for social and behavioral problems, and the more comprehensive individually administered psychoeducational evaluation conducted for circumscribed academic problems.

WM. DREW GOUVIER, AUDREY BAUMEISTER, and KOLA IJAOLA • Department of Psychology, Louisiana State University, Baton Rouge, LA 70803.

J.L. Matson et al. (eds.), *Assessing Childhood Psychopathology and Developmental Disabilities*, DOI: 10.1007/978-0-387-09528-8,
© Springer Science+Business Media, LLC 2009

It should be clear, therefore, that not all problems assessed by a neuropsychologist are necessarily neurological in nature. For example, in the conduct of a psychoeducational examination, it is incumbent on the psychologist to establish which of several possible reasons account for the question of why Johnny can't read? Possible answers include poor schooling, poor general health, specific health conditions such as strabismus or nystagmus, poor attentional abilities, focal learning disability, low intellect, poor memory, low motivation or apathy, comorbid psychiatric problems, or even effortful motivation to appear impaired. Any of these vectors could result in the behavioral presentation of impaired reading, even though many have nothing to do with the neurological pathways involved in reading per se.

There are numerous journals and scholarly textbooks that address the field of pediatric neuropsychology, and it is a field far too broad to be represented in any single chapter. The reader is referred to several excellent recent texts that provide a more thorough introduction and review of the field than is possible here. These include Rourke, van der Vlugt, and Rourke's (2002) *Practice of Child Clinical Neuropsychology: An Introduction*, Baron's (2004) *Neuropsychological Evaluation of the Child*, and the edited volumes by Segalowitz and Rapin (2003) entitled *Handbook of Neuropsychology (2nd ed.). Volume 8: Child Neuropsychology, Parts I and II*. Also noteworthy are the edited volumes by Farmer, Warschausky, and Donders (2006) *Treating Neurodevelopmental Disorders: Clinical Research and Practice* and Hunter and Donders (2007) *Pediatric Neuropsychological Intervention*, and the lifespan developmental perspective offered in Goldstein and Reynolds' (2005) edited *Handbook of Neurodevelopmental and Genetic Disorders in Adults*. Given the immensity of the field, the present chapter limits its focus to identifying and reviewing some of the more common sources of neuropsychological dysfunction in children.

DEVELOPMENTAL NEUROPSYCHOLOGICAL DISORDERS

Speech and Language

Language impairment has been cited as one of the most frequent reasons for outpatient neuropsychological evaluation of children (Baron, 2004). Language is a broad construct referring to the communication of meaningful symbols (Benson & Ardila, 1996) whereas speech is a more limited subset involving the mechanical aspect of oral communication (Baron, 2004). Analysis of language behavior can provide a window for establishing the presence of a variety of psychological disorders. When considering the autistic spectrum, for example, a child with comprehension deficits, language formulation deficits, but relatively intact single-word production may fit the profile of childhood autism, whereas the presence and utilization of the prosodic component of speech along with pragmatic language may be more indicative of a child with Asperger's syndrome.

It is noteworthy that the *DSM-IV-TR* (APA, 2000) lists only two types of formal developmental language disorders. There is the expressive language disorder and the mixed receptive/expressive language disorder. Following the logic of the computer programmer's dictum "garbage in, garbage out" there is no stand-alone receptive language disorder. Thus, the appearance of an isolated receptive language problem in a child mandates a search for an acquired rather than developmental etiology.

The speech and language portion of a neuropsychological evaluation typically includes assessment of the following: conversational fluency, phonological processing, generative fluency, comprehension, repetition, naming, reading, writing, spelling, calculation, and oral motor praxis. The following may be evaluated through general conversation: fluency and fluidity of word usage, articulation and clarity, rate, rhythm, intonation, grammar, syntax, level of vocabulary, length or utterance, and comprehension. Paraphasia (production of unintended syllables, words, or phrases during the effort to speak) is rarely observed in childhood, whereas impaired word finding (dysnomia), dyscalculia, and impaired written formation is more common among children. Shyness, stranger anxiety, and elective mutism must be ruled out as possible confounds (Baron, 2004).

In brain injured children, aphasia may be prominent in acute stages, but typically resolves into a subtle deficit, whereas visuospatial functions appear more vulnerable to lasting deficit (Marsh & Whitehead, 2005). The relatively quicker recovery of acquired language deficits in children is taken as evidence supporting the notion of greater cerebral plasticity at early ages. Flight of function to the nonaffected hemisphere is often seen in children under age 5, who after receiving focal left hemispheric injury, demonstrate organized language development in homotopic areas of the injury-free right cerebral hemisphere (Baron, 2004).

ADHD and Learning Disabilities

As ADHD is often comorbid with LD, numerous attempts have been made to differentiate between children with ADHD versus LD based on their academic, social, and neuropsychological profiles (Hynd, Lorys, Semrud-Clikeman, Nieves, Huettner, & Lahey, 1991). Van der Meere, van Baal, and Sergeant (1989) used a continuous performance test (CPT) and found that children with LD had lower abilities in the memory search and decision processes aspects (e.g., is that a signal or not?), whereas children with hyperactivity showed poorer motor-decision abilities (e.g., do I respond to this or not?). In a longitudinal CPT study of omission and commission error rates, Kupietz (1990) compared LD and ADHD children and found no initial differences in the number of correct detections and commission errors, but with increasing age, the LD group improved more than the ADHD group, and that children with comorbid ADHD and LD are much more affected by distracters than children with either ADHD or LD only.

In the area of ADHD specifically, Barkley (1997) offered a broad reinterpretation of the core deficits seen in children with ADHD combined type. He proposed that these children suffered a deficit in generalized executive functioning more so than simple deficits in attentional or inhibitory abilities. A developmental model of executive functioning, offered by Anderson (2002), describes this aspect of cognitive processing as involving four discrete but interrelated domains. Attentional control, cognitive flexibility, goal setting, and information processing are thought to operate in a coordinated manner to enable "executive control" of behavior to be exercised and regulated. According to this formulation, the developmental maturation of these domains proceeds along a predictable path, with attentional control emerging in infancy and maturing quickly thereafter, whereas cognitive flexibility, goal setting, and information processing skills begin their critical period of development between ages 7 and 9, and reach maturity by 12 years of age. Only after these components are in place and relatively developed can "executive control" abilities be observed, beginning with the start of adolescence and not completing their development until full myelination of the prefrontal areas is completed in the early 20s.

Despite the elegance and plausibility of Barkley's theory, research aimed at its support has been lacking. In a recent study of 43 seven- to eleven-year-old children with ADHD combined or inattentive types, executive functioning profiles were not significantly related to symptoms of their ADHD, but only to comorbid symptoms of depression and autism symptomology (Jonsdottir, Bouma, Sergeant, & Scherder, 2006). Teacher ratings of inattention were not correlated with executive functioning profiles either, but were robustly predicted by the children's language skill. Another study offered similar findings (Geurts, Verte, Roeyers, & Sergeant, 2005). Using groups of 16 boys with no ADHD, ADHD inattentive type, and ADHD combined type, carefully matched for age, IQ, and the presence of oppositional defiant and conduct disorders, no differences between the two ADHD groups were observed on any of the five executive functioning domains under study, and significant between-group differences were noted only between the control children and the ADHD combined group on measures related to inhibition but not on the other four domains of executive functioning.

The topic of executive functioning has received attention in the area of learning disabilities as well. In a study comparing 42 children with dyslexia and 42 nondyslexic children, Reiter, Tucha, and Lange (2005) describe a number of deficits in the children with dyslexia that were far more than simple reading problems. For example, these children showed "obvious differences" in their working memory capacity, their inhibitory capabilities were impaired on demanding, but not simple go–no go tasks, and they showed significant impairment in both verbal and figural fluency functions. Although concept formation skills were equivalent between the groups, actual problem-solving skills (initiating a response to the concepts) were poorer among the children with dyslexia.

A number of authors have proposed that the core deficit in developmental dyslexia results from phonological impairments, that is, difficulties processing the sound structure of language (Peterson, McGrath, Smith, & Pennington, 2007), and this suggestion has received considerable support in the literature. For example, the posterior areas of the reading network have been observed to show a lack of activation in functional neuroimaging (fMRI) during word and pseudoword reading conditions in persons with familial dyslexia, and this activation deficit persists whether the family members have learned to compensate for their deficit or not (Brambati et al., 2006). Anatomic research from this same group has shown corresponding regional reductions in the volume of grey matter in the posterior reading network areas among other persons with familial dyslexia (Brambati et al., 2004).

Several classification schemes have been offered to expand on the 3 Rs set of learning disorders outlined in the *DSM-IV*. In addition to the traditional reading disorder, mathematics disorder, and disorder of written expression, Rourke and his colleagues have spent decades developing an alternative scheme that offers a potential to account for the verbal and performance discrepancies often seen in the profiles of children referred for evaluation due to academic or behavioral problems (Rourke et al., 2002; Drummond, Ahmad, & Rourke, 2005). He suggests that the pie can be sliced into Basic Phonological Processing Deficits (BPPD) and Nonverbal Learning Disabilities (NLD). Classification rules that were generated, tested, and well validated on children between 9 and 15 have been developed, and now extended for use with younger children in the 7- to 8-year-old range (Drummond et al., 2005). Such rules can be useful for helping to determine whether a comprehensive neuropsychological evaluation is warranted, and might be useful in guiding future research into the relatively less studied phenomena of NLDs.

In another massive effort, D'Amato, Dean, and Rhodes (1998) sought to subtype children's learning disabilities empirically. Using a sample of 1,144 school-age children with learning disabilities, all of whom had completed extensive neuropsychological, intellectual, and academic evaluation, a cluster analysis was performed to identify coherent groupings among the children. Four interpretable clusters were identified, which the authors labeled as (1) Verbal-Sequential-Arithmetic, (2) Motor Speed and Cognitive Flexibility Deficits, (3) Mixed Language-Perceptual Deficits, and (4) No Deficit Subtype. They describe these subtypes as showing unique profiles, and also each having distinct differences in their developmental etiology. This approach, although showing clear empirical promise, failed to generate much interest in formulating a new approach to classifying the learning disabilities.

In keeping with recent trends toward support-based rather than deficit-based models of disability, D'Amato and colleagues have recently taken another stab at reformulating our way of viewing the area of learning disorders (D'Amato, Crepeau-Hobson, Huang, & Geill, 2005). This recent paper contends that children with learning disabilities are better served when their evaluation and educational intervention are conceptualized within an ecological perspective rather than a deficit-based one. Taken this way, instead of considering the problem as residing within the child, better results and more favorable outcomes will occur when the problem is analyzed with the child viewed as just one part of a learning environment in an educational system that possesses (and lacks) certain resources.

Viewed from this ecological neuropsychology perspective, a strength-based analysis that considers the child and the resources available within his or her educational environment as part of an interconnected and reciprocally influenced system, can be conducted. One thing is clear, however. No matter how far the pendulum swings to a "response to treatment" model rather than a deficit-focused model, the more thoroughly our health care and educational professionals understand the organism that lies between the stimulus and response, between the blackboard and the test paper, the better equipped those people will be to act as effective agents of change in the child's life (Silver et al., 2006).

Regarding verbal memory, children with ADHD have shown deficits on memory tasks requiring organized, deliberate rehearsal strategies, whereas LD children have shown a more general verbal deficit (Douglas and Benezra, 1990). In contrast Robins (1992) found no neuropsychological differences on tasks requiring verbal memory, verbal learning to trials, or sustained attention between ADHD and LD children. However, behavioral symptoms did differentiate between the groups; children with ADHD showed more impulsive behavior, impaired accuracy on timed tasks, aggression, and poor ability to work independently in the classroom.

Korkman and Pesonen (1994) devised a study using the Neuropsychological Assessment of Children (NEPSY). They tested 60 eight-year-old children to compare deficits among children who met criteria for ADHD ($N = 21$), LD ($N = 12$), or comorbid ADHD and LD ($N = 27$). The examiners used the 19 NEPSY subtests which focus on attention, learning, language, sensory–motor, visual–spatial, and memory functions. Reading and spelling abilities were also assessed. Children with ADHD demonstrated deficiencies in phonological awareness, verbal memory (digit) span, storytelling, and verbal IQ. Children with comorbid ADHD and LD showed more pervasive attention problems and greater visual–motor problems. All three groups showed impairment in visual–motor precision and name retrieval.

Although these impairments were shared, it was suggested that different mechanisms underlie these impairments. Linguistic impairment was believed to be the cause of name retrieval deficits in the LD group, and would also contribute to their noted reading and spelling problems. Attention problems and poor active memorization were blamed for name-retrieval deficiencies in the ADHD group, which were interpreted as unrelated to specific reading and spelling problems. The comorbid group showed a double dose of disability, with features of both core problems present in their profiles. These findings validated earlier studies that found impaired control and inhibition of impulses to be the main symptom of ADHD, whereas phonological and linguistic deficiencies were prevalent among those with LD (Boliek & Obrzut, 1997).

Hypotheses regarding neurological dysfunction associated with ADHD have implicated various areas of the brain from the brain stem to the frontal lobes, but little evidence points to any specific causal area (Reynolds & Fletcher-Janzen, 1997). Other hypotheses have implicated neurochemical dysfunction as a cause of ADHD. Both norepinephrine and dopamine have been implicated in the pathophysiology of ADHD (Calis, Grothe, & Elia, 1990). At this time many controversies remain on the subject, although with rapid advances in psychopharmacological treatment and increasingly sensitive psychometrics, the underlying neurological aspects of ADHD may soon be clarified (Reynolds & Fletcher-Janzen, 1997).

Several studies have found ADHD to be related to thyroid abnormalities. Evidence has shown that between 46 and 70% of children who have a generalized resistance to thyroid hormone (GRTH) also meet diagnostic criteria for ADHD (Hauser et al., 1993; Refetoff, Weiss, & Usala, 1993). The pathophysiologic relationship between GRTH and ADHD is not fully understood but it has been shown that those with comorbid GRTH and ADHD are afflicted with altered brain glucose uptake (Hauser, Zametkin, Vitiello, Martinex, Mixson, & Weintraub, 1992). It has also been theorized that the brain's exposure to high levels of thyroid hormone may result in ADHD, which is reasonable given that thyroid hormone is known to have powerful stimulant properties.

Relatively few neuroimaging studies have been conducted with children, although many of these have focused on the neuroanatomical correlates of ADHD. In a group of pure ADHD Hyperactive Type children, cerebral blood flow (rCBF) neuroimaging techniques were used and significant hypoperfusion in the right striatum of the caudate nucleus was identified. When methylphenidate was administered to these children, a significant increase in perfusion occurred in the right and left stratum, but more so in the left striatum (Lou, Henriksen, Bruhn, Bomer, & Neilsen, 1989). Others have found a smaller left caudate nucleus in ADHD children when compared to normal children (Hynd et al., 1993; Lou et al., 1989). This may result in a right-sided bias in choline acetyltransferase and dopamine, which has been associated with increased motor activity (Hynd et al., 1993).

The corpus callosum has also been a structure of interest as it plays a role in interhemispheric coordination and regulation (Lassonde, 1986). An early MRI study found the genu (anterior aspect of the corpus callosum) was significantly smaller in children with ADHD than normal controls (Hynd et al., 1991). This is particularly significant, as this is the structure that connects homologus areas of the premotor, orbitofrontal, and prefrontal regions of the brain. Hynd et al. note that the smaller genu in children with ADHD correlates with frontal lobe deficits in motor regulation, persistence, and inhibition. Several studies have found children with ADHD to demonstrate behavior similar to adults with frontal lobe damage (Gualtieri & Hicks, 1985).

Shue and Douglas (1992) administered a test battery to children with ADHD and normal controls, which included measures of motor control as well as complex problem-solving skills. These tests had previously shown sensitivity to frontal lobe damage. Children with ADHD had significantly more difficulty than controls across tasks and their patterns of performance were similar to patients with frontal lobe damage. Children with ADHD were not able to inhibit motor responses as well as normal controls. Performance deficits shown by the ADHD children did not reflect generalized cognitive impairment, but impairment specific to those with frontal lobe dysfunction.

INTELLECTUAL DISABILITY AND AUTISM SPECTRUM DISORDERS

New techniques in neuroscience research are being applied more and more frequently in trying to enhance our understanding of these severely disabling childhood problems (Temple, 2002). Disorders classified along the Autism Spectrum (previously known as Pervasive Developmental Disorders) are described as impairment in social reciprocity, communication, and cognition (Cook & Leventhal, 1992). Whereas children with intellectual disability (previously known as mental retardation) tend to show delayed development across a broad range of functions, autistic children often show relatively higher scores on visual–spatial tests and rote memory, while showing poorly developed verbal comprehension (Dawson & Castelloe, 1995). Children with autism demonstrate high rates of retardation (70%), epilepsy (25%), attentional deficits, and aggressive and impulsive disorders (Cook & Leventhal, 1992). They have also been described as sharing behavioral similarities with children with Tourette's syndrome (Comings, 1990) as well as comorbid sleep disturbances and mood disorders (APA, 1994).

Older analytic theories cited parent–child relationships as the causal factor in the development of autism, and later behavioral theories suggested the abnormal behaviors seen among persons with autism were learned, however, neurodevelopmental theories have now come to the forefront. There are numerous research reports suggesting a role of EEG abnormalities (APA, 1994), hippocampal abnormalities (Minshew & Goldstein, 1993), ventricular enlargement (Bigler, 1988; Hauser, Delong, & Rosman, 1975), cortical atrophy (Bigler, 1989), right–left asymmetry abnormalities (Prior & Bradshaw, 1979), reticular activating system dysfunctions (Rimland, 1964), and limbic system, brain stem, and cerebellar abnormalities (Courchesne, 1989, 1997). Evidence has shown that autistic children do not show typical patterns of hemispheric specialization and dominance (Escalante-Mead, Minshew, & Sweeney, 2003), and also that autistic children are chronically overaroused, with such arousal adversely affecting information processing abilities (Teeter & Semrud-Clikeman, 1997). Children with autism have demonstrated lower levels of executive control and frontal lobe function (Bishop, 1993). Such results have been evidenced through high error count on the Wisconsin Card Sorting Task as well as inefficient completion of the Tower of Hanoi (Ozonoff, Pennington, & Rogers, 1990).

Among individuals with intellectual disabilities, differences can be identified among various subgroups. For example, among persons with Down's syndrome, a unique profile of cognitive abilities emerges during development, with performance in visuospatial abilities often better developed than verbal/linguistic abilities. Further deficiencies in motor development (e.g., greater clumsiness) are observed in this group than in similarly affected persons with etiologies other than Down's syndrome (Vicari, 2006). One other group does share a propensity to show pronounced motor problems along with occasional intellectual disabilities. Among girls with Turner's syndrome, decreased motor speed is frequently observed, and a careful analysis of this phenomenon has shown it to be a problem of muscle initiation and not one of motor planning (Nijhuis-Van der Sanden, Eling, Van Asseldonk, & Van Galen, 2004). Curiously, even among persons with Turner's syndrome who are of normal intelligence, spatial disorientation is commonly seen, and these individuals often show poor performance on nonverbal and visuomotor tests and mathematics tests, even though their verbal scores are often average or higher (Berkow & Fletcher, 1992). But even in persons with intellectual disability, not all cognitive functions are impaired. Singh et al. (2005) offer data from a group of 20 children with mild mental retardation that shows their capacity for facial recognition and interpretation of facial expressions are quite similar to those of children in the general population.

Although spastic cerebral palsy (SCP) is often regarded as a circumscribed motor system problem, neuropsychological analysis of children shows otherwise. Many of the executive functions described above involve motor planning, inhibition, and the capacity to choose optimal paths toward goals, an activity that typically involves direct action upon some persons or entities within the child's environment. White and Christ (2005) used this reasoning to hypothesize that SCP would not disrupt the associative aspects of learning and memory, but would interfere with the executive aspects such as the imposition of efficient learning strategies, strategic processing, and effective inhibition of irrelevant responses. Their predictions were confirmed; controlling for general verbal ability, their children with SCP and normal controls performed comparably on measures of initial learning and retention over time, suggesting intact medial temporal brain processing in both groups. But the children with SCP showed impairment in benefiting from repeated trials (learning strategy) and in inhibiting inappropriate intrusive responses, especially among the younger children in the SCP group. These findings suggest a developmental delay in the maturation of the prefrontally mediated executive aspects of learning and memory.

Prenatal Substance Exposure

Studies have shown that over 100,000 babies are born each year with exposure to cocaine and/or other drugs (Chasnoff, Landress, & Barrett, 1990). Cocaine is both water and liposoluble and passes easily through the placenta (Woods, Plessinger, & Clark, 1987). The fetus may actually be exposed to the drug for a longer period of time than adults because of the quicker excretion time in the drug-abusing host than in the resident fetus (Singer, Garber, & Kliegman, 1991). Cocaine also causes vasoconstriction in the uterus, resulting in reduced blood and oxygen flow into the fetus (Woods, et al., 1987). Newborn children vary in their expression and severity of cocaine exposure symptoms. Koren (1993) suggests that differences in frequency of use and individual metabolic abilities account for such variation. Maternal cocaine use has been associated with spontaneous abortions, premature placental detachment, and meconium-stained amniotic fluid (Frank et al., 1988).

Given these untoward effects, it is not surprising that higher rates of prematurity have also been found among these children (MacGregor, Keith, Bachicha, & Chasnoff, 1989), and these abnormalities may also be linked to the early neurodevelopmental delays shown by these children (Oro & Dixon, 1987). Smaller head size and slower brain growth have also been demonstrated in these children (Coles, Platzman, Smith, James, & Falek, 1991; Eisen et al., 1991). Neurological abnormalities found among neonates exposed to cocaine prenatally include cerebral infarcts, as well as EEG and brainstem auditory evoked response (BAER) abnormalities (Chasnoff, Griffith, MacGregor, Dirkes, & Burns, 1989; Dixon & Bejar, 1989).

Studies have shown that children exposed to cocaine in utero can display subtle language delays as well as diminished development of problem-solving skills (Hawley, Halle, Drasin, & Thomas, 1995). When purely cocaine exposed infants are compared to alcohol or marijuana-only exposed infants, no differences were found in global scores on the Bayley Intelligence Scale-Fourth Edition or the Stanford Binet Intelligence Scale-Fourth Edition at age 3, although a difference was found between prenatal drug exposed groups and nonexposed groups (Griffith, Azuma, & Chasnoff, 1994). Receptive language impairments have been found among children of mothers involved in drug rehab programs (Malakoff, Mayes, & Schottenfeld, 1994). Sensory and behavioral deficits have also been found (Chasnoff et al., 1989; Coles et al., 1991; Neuspiel et al., 1991). Limited research is available regarding long-term effects of prenatal drug exposure, although given the subtle language deficits and problem solving difficulties found, it is possible that these may develop into later difficulties in executive functioning and language processing (Teeter & Semrud-Clikeman, 1997).

Perhaps even more teratogenic than cocaine is the influence of maternal alcohol abuse (Riley et al., 2003). Fetal alcohol syndrome (FAS) is caused by prenatal exposure to alcohol and is evidenced by growth deficiency, facial anomalies, and sympathetic nervous system dysfunction (Streissguth, 1994). Children with FAS typically exhibit delayed development, overactivity, motor clumsiness, attention deficits, learning problems, cognitive retardation, and seizure disorders. FAS is estimated to occur in 1 to 3 per 1,000 live births (National Institute on Alcohol Abuse and Alcoholism, 1990), although rates have been reported to be much higher on Native American reservations (May, Hymbaugh, Aase, & Samet, 1983) and in Russia (Mattson, Riley, Matveeva, & Marintcheva, 2003).

Severity of FAS has been related to how much alcohol is consumed, the period of gestation during which the mother drank, how frequently she drank, and age of mother (Overholser, 1990; Russell et al., 1991). Streissguth, Sampson, and Barr (1989) found that children exposed to alcohol before birth demonstrated cognitive delays, memory and attention deficits, motor difficulties, organizational and problem-solving difficulties, as well as social and adaptive behavior problems. Anatomical studies of the brains of children diagnosed with FAS have shown decreases in total brain size, especially in the cerebrum and cerebellum, along with smaller basal ganglia and diminished volume, or occasional agenesis, of the corpus callosum (Mattson et al., 1994). Only 28% of samples show normal head size (Streissguth, Randels, & Smith 1991). Newborns of alcoholic mothers have shown delay in their response to the environment and typically have low birth weight (Day, 1992; Greene et al., 1991). A long-term outcome study of children with FAS found that the majority of children showed borderline or mild intellectual disability and that their IQs remained low and stable over time (Steinhausen, Willms, & Spohr, 1994).

In a study of adaptive behavior skills, Streissguth, Clarren, and Jones (1985) found that daily living skills, although below expectations for given age, were often an area of strength for FAS children, whereas socialization skills were most deficient. Areas that were particularly difficult for children included acting without considering consequences, taking initiative, inability to read social cues, and inability to establish social relationships. Psychopathology appears to create great difficulty in adolescence and adulthood for persons with FAS patients (Dorris, 1989). Problems with disinhibition and executive control, characteristic of the prefrontal problems noted in other groups with cognitive disabilities are present among persons with FAS, but one cannot chalk all of the social and behavioral deficits of these persons to neuropsychological dysfunction. Very few groups come from a more troubled or dysfunctional family environment (Teeter & Semrud-Clikeman, 1997). Regarding psychosocial factors Streissguth, Aase, Clarren, Randels, LaDue, and Smith (1991) found that 69% of biological mothers of FAS children were deceased at a 5- to 12-year follow-up, and 33% of FAS children are given up for adoption or abandoned at the hospital. Indeed, FAS children experience tumultuous home environments.

Academic problems abound in these children as well. In a study of adolescents with FAS, Streissguth, Randels, and Smith (1991) found that arithmetic and word attack skills were most impaired. Regarding school placement, 6% were in regular education with no support, 28% were in self-contained special education classrooms, 15% were not in school or were working, and 9% were in sheltered workshops. Regarding language skills, FAS children have not been found to be especially deficient, as once again, language development seems to often proceed more normally, even at the expense of delayed development in other key areas (Greene et al., 1990).

ACQUIRED NEUROPSYCHOLOGICAL DISORDERS

Abuse and Neglect

Neuropsychological techniques have also been used to differentiate among children from another class of children who are multiply at risk for dysfunction. The role of potential maternal prenatal alcohol or drug consumption was not controlled in this study, however, the report of Nolin and Ethier, (2007) is enlightening all the same. Using a neuropsychological battery that measured motor functions, attention, memory and learning, visuomotor integration, language, intelligence, and frontal/executive functions, these authors reported that discriminant analysis could successfully use the neuropsychological profiles to accurately distinguish between children who suffered neglect with physical abuse, children who were neglected but not physically abused, and normal control children, all of whom were matched for age, gender, and annual family income.

Relative to the control children, the children who were merely neglected showed relative deficiencies in auditory attention and visuomotor integration, and those who were neglected and physically abused showed these deficits and more; problem solving, abstraction, and planning were all impaired in this more seriously maltreated group. This finding suggests a dose–response curve in which neuropsychological functioning appears to be sensitive to the severity of horrific childhood experiences.

Acquired Brain Injuries

Kraus (1995) reported that approximately 180 per 100,000 children under age 15 experience Traumatic Brain Injury (TBI). Lescohier and DiScala (1993) found that among hospital-treated cases, approximately 75% are mild and 135 are severe. For children under age 5, there is a similar level of risk across genders. Risk rises for boys through childhood and adolescence (Kraus, 1995). Regarding cause of injury, younger children are more frequently injured in falls and abuse, whereas older children and adolescents are more likely injured in collisions, sports activities, and other types of violence (Warschausky, Kewman, Bradley, & Dixon, 2003). Severe TBI typically leads to increased intracranial pressure. This increased pressure results in diminished cerebral blood flow which can cause ischemic and hypoxic injury (Warschausky, Kewman, & Selim, 1996).

The assessment of the severity of TBI typically includes examination of the depth of coma, differentiation between the damage due to diffuse versus focal injuries, level of elevated intracranial pressure, length of post-traumatic amnesia, presence or absence of hypoxic insult, and pupillary reactivity. The Glasgow Coma Scale (GCS: Teasdale & Jennett, 1974) is used to assess the depth of coma using specific ratings of eye opening and movement as well as verbal and motoric responses. Neuroimaging typically involves a CT scan and less frequently an MRI. Several instruments are available to assess posttraumatic amnesia (where the patient's ability to consolidate and retain new memories is impaired). One such test is the Children's Orientation and Amnesia Test (COAT: Ewing-Cobbs, Levin, Fletcher, Minerm, & Eisenberg, 1990) which includes a brief set of questions that may be administered on a daily basis.

As a child undergoes recovery, behavioral symptoms, such as high levels of agitation may occur. The Rancho Los Amigos Scale (Hagen, Malkmus, & Durham, 1979) provides an ordinal description of levels of cognitive and behavioral recovery ranging from coma to purposeful/appropriate functioning. One prevalent finding in pediatric TBI patients is slowed processing speed. The WISC-III processing speed index has demonstrated the highest sensitivity among the WISC- III index scores, showing strong correlation with severity of injury measured by depth and length and depth of coma. On the other hand, digit span tasks are not sensitive to TBI (Warschausky et al., 1996), and should not be mistaken as a measure or even a screener for memory functions.

Executive dysfunction is also common among TBI patients and has been differentially associated with severity of injury, brain lesion volume size, and location of the primary lesions (Levin et al., 1997). Severity of injury has also been associated with magnitude of memory impairment on the California Verbal Learning Test-Children's Version (Delis, Kramer, Kaplan, & Ober, 1994). Regarding academic achievement difficulties, no evidence exists of a specific learning disability pattern following TBI, however, moderate to severe injury is associated with a decline in general adaptive functioning, therefore assessment of adaptive behavior is critical for individuals sustaining these more severe injuries (Max, Koele, Lindgren, et al., 1998).

In a recent study of children with mild developmental learning disabilities who then sustained head trauma, Wood and Rutherford (2006) report that there were only minimal between-groups differences between the LD group and non-LD but head-injured comparison group. These were on two measures of complex speeded information processing, the Trails B and the Digit Symbol subtest from the Wechsler scales. Much more pronounced were the neurobehavioral problems evident among the LD group. These participants reported greater adjustment problems with higher levels of anxiety and depression, mood swings, and more frequent instances of impulsive aggression. This finding reflects the same process of a double dose of disability described in earlier sections, and probably represents support for the neuronal reserve theory of recovery from brain damage (Stein, Brailowsky, & Will, 1995).

There is some disagreement about whether there is a generalized impairment in cognitive skills resulting from early head injury, or whether the deficits are more circumscribed. In support to the former, is the report of Levine and colleagues (Levine, Kraus, Alexander, Suriyakham, & Huttenlocher, 2005) who describe a group of 15 children who sustained TBI before age 7. IQ testing was conducted on each child at age 7, and repeated several years later. They report that post-7 IQ scores were significantly lower than pre-7 IQ scores, and this effect was present whether the lesion size was large or small. In fact, those with largest lesions showed the lowest pre-7 IQ scores, whereas those with the smallest lesions had the highest pre-7 IQ scores but showed the greater IQ decline over time. Perhaps this is because they had more to lose following their initial injury, but these findings show dramatically that the cognitive outcome of TBI in children, even those producing relatively small lesions, changes over time.

On the other hand Marsh and Whitehead (2005) report that among children who sustain skull fracture during infancy, when tested five years later against the performance of matched controls, the only deficit they showed was in memory for faces and in the domain of visual attention. Their performance equaled that of the controls in language skills, sensory motor abilities, visuomotor and visuospatial functions, grades, and parent/teacher reports.

Nonetheless, there is a substantial body of research that supports the presence of persisting memory deficits following childhood TBI (Lowther & Mayfield, 2004; Alexander & Mayfield, 2005), and it is probably true that enduring deficits in inhibitory control persist as well (Levin, Hanton, Zhang, Swank, & Hunter, 2004). Nothing is simple, however, and as in the Nolan and Ethier (2007) study of abused and neglected children, the contribution of the family environment within which the child is raised cannot be dismissed as having some causative or moderating role.

For example, Goldstrohm and Arffa (2005) examined the premorbid, neurocognitive, behavioral, and familial functioning of 33 preschoolers who sustained mild to moderate TBI, compared to 34 matched controls. Despite the matching procedures, substantial premorbid differences emerged, with the TBI children having higher rates of premorbid behavior difficulties, lower cognitive functioning, poorer preacademic skills, and greater reported situational issues and life stressors among the parents than the control children and their families. It causes one to speculate about whether these differences represent risk factors that resulted in the children's injuries in the first place, by mechanisms such as being too harried or rushed to worry about seatbelts or tricycle helmets and the like.

Some evidence has shown that early in recovery, nonverbal functions such as visuoperceptual and visuoconstructive skills are more severely impaired than verbal functions. Donders (1997) found a strong association between severity of injury and the WISC- III perceptual organization index. Although verbal intellect and vocabulary are relatively spared early in recovery, discourse cohesion and capacity to draw inferences have shown impairment following injury. Such impairments may in turn have adverse effects on social interactions (Lezak, 1978a).

TBI can lead to numerous psychological, behavioral, and social changes. Those with TBI compared with controls have shown higher levels of affective instability, aggression, rage, inattention, impaired social judgment, and apathy (Brown, Chadwick, Shaffer, Rutter, & Traub, 1981; Taylor, Yeates, Wade, Drotar, Klein, and Stancin, 1999). Additionally, among children with severe injuries, up to 25% of children show depressive symptomatology and receive their first psychiatric diagnoses post injury (Kirkwood et al., 2000; Max, Koele, Smith, et al., 1998). Personality changes have been demonstrated in TBI at levels as high as 40% (Max et al., 2000), and are often regarded as more disabling than any of the acquired neurocognitive changes that may persist (Lewinsohn & Graf, 1973; Lezak, 1978b).

TBI may also result in the development of posttraumatic seizures; however this occurs only in about 2% of the population (McLean, Kaitz, Kennan, Dabney, Cawley, & Alexander, 1995). This incidence of seizures goes up dramatically when there is a fracture to the skull, however, and even greater still when it is a depressed fracture. New onset of seizure disorders become the rule rather than the exception when the insult involves any sort of compound depressed fracture or gunshot wound (Hauser & Hesdorffer, 1990; Lezak, Howieson, & Loring 2004).

Epilepsy

Seizure disorders are a common concomitant with many of the developmental and medical disorders of childhood. Epileptic disorders can be idiopathic or acquired, but given that the peak lifetime prevalence of epilepsy occurs between 10 and 50 years of age, it is merely the authors' choice to discuss epilepsy under the section of acquired disorders. This is reasonable, but not fair, because even among epilepsy syndromes that emerge later in life, most do not have a clearly identifiable etiology, although numerous risk factors are known to accrue over time (Hauser & Hesdorffer, 1990).

Our understanding of seizure disorders is evolving as more sophisticated neuroscience research on the topic is completed. As with many other neuropsychiatric disorders that were initially conceptualized as either present or absent, the evolving concept of the epilepsy spectrum disorder has been gaining ground among many professionals as well (Hines, Kubu, Roberts, & Varney, 1995). Rather than regarding epilepsy as a disease that is simply present or absent, spectrum theorists assert that there are subclinical variants of epilepsy that exist without stereotypic spells, but that do involve paroxysmal affective, psychosensory, and cognitive symptoms.

Because of the on again–off again phenomenology of these symptoms, such as memory gaps, episodic irritability, jamais vu and déjà vu, auditory or visual illusions, abrupt mood shifts, abnormal somatic sensations, intrusive thoughts, and parasomnias to name a few, this condition has often been considered some form of a cycling mood disorder such as a bipolar or cythlothymic variant, and treated with mood stabilizing medications (Varney, Garvey, Campbell, Cook, & Roberts, 1993). It is more than a mere coincidence that these same medications, when used in neurological settings are classified as anticonvulsants, and there is little doubt that the etiology of these conditions lies at the borderland between psychiatry and neurology (Varney, Hines, Bailey, & Roberts, 1992). But more on this follows later.

The child with epilepsy is three times more likely to experience cognitive problems than children with other neurological pathologies for at least three different reasons: the effect of the epilepsy itself contributing to brain dysfunction, any associated deficit due to the structural or functional lesion responsible for the epileptic focus, and the neurodepressant side effects of antiepileptic medications (Campo-Castello, 2006).

Generally speaking, children with epilepsy show diminished reaction times and reduced capacity for speeded information processing, along with impairments in the domains of attention, language, and memory, but different specific epilepsy syndromes differentially have an impact on the neuropsychological and intellectual performance profiles of the affected children, with a direct relationship between measures of the severity of the epilepsy (based on age of onset, duration of active epilepsy, seizure frequency, the number of episodes of status epilepticus, and the use of polypharmacotherapy), and the resultant profile of intellectual and neuro-cognitive deficits (Nolan et al., 2003).

Among the children most likely to receive psychiatric rather than neurologic diagnoses, are the ones with temporal lobe epilepsy. Although these children typically have normal IQs, they are likely to show deficits relative to matched controls on measures of attention, complex speeded information processing, complex problem-solving, and a broad range of verbal learning and memory problems (Guimareaes et al., 2007).

Even among children with subclinical paroxysmal discharges, expected patterns of lateralization can be observed, with relatively superior visuospatial functioning among those whose primary discharge focus was in the left hemisphere, and relatively superior planning and executive functioning among those whose primary focus was in the right hemisphere (Carvajal-Molina Iglesias-Dorado, Morgade-Fonte, Martin-Plasencia, & Perez-Abalo, 2003). One procedure useful for evaluating hemispheric differences in persons with epilepsy spectrum disorders is the dichotic listening procedure, in which the typical right ear advantage phenomenon is directly affected by the hemispheric side of the primary focus of abnormal electrical activity (Roberts, Varney, Paulsen, & Richardson, 1990). This procedure has proven useful in working with children with formal epilepsy diagnoses as well, and can be used to help distinguish between the primary and secondary (mirror) focus in cases of generalized seizures when the testing is administered during the relatively quiet interictal intervals (Korkman, Granström, & Berg, 2004).

Specific Medical Conditions

Tumors

Numerous other conditions can lead to the development of seizures as a corollary symptom of the condition and not as the primary disorder itself. Most notable among these are brain tumors, which have a peak lifetime prevalence of diagnosis in children between the ages of three and nine years (Carpentieri & Mulhern, 1993). Although few studies have investigated the psychosocial effects of CNS tumors (Mulhern, Hancock, Fairclough, & Kun, 1992) between 1,200 and 1,500 new cases are diagnosed each year (Kun, 1992).

Risk factors for the development of brain tumors include genetic factors such as neurofibromatosis and tuberous sclerosis, family history of epilepsy and stroke, as well as immunosuppression prior to organ transplant (Cohen & Duffner, 1994). Treatments typically involve whole-brain radiation, chemotherapy, and/or surgical interventions, and with such treatments, 50 to 60% of children are cancer-free after five years (Carpentieri & Mulhern, 1993). The highest survival rates occur in children with an astrocytoma in the cerebellum, and the lowest survival rates are among those with a brain stem glioma (Duffner et al., 1986).

The most commonly diagnosed tumor type is the astrocytoma (Cohen & Duffner, 1994). In children under age two, the most common types are the medulloblastoma (in the medulla portion of the brain stem), low-grade astrocytomas, and ependymomas (which arise from the lining of the ventricles and spinal cord or ependyma). In children ages five to nine, the most common types of tumors include the low- and high-grade astrocytomas, cerebellar astrocytomas, and medulloblastomas (Cohen & Duffner, 1993).

Prompt and accurate diagnosis of brain tumors is crucial for successful survival (Price, Goetz, & Lovell, 1992). Studies have shown that brain tumors cause behavioral, personality, academic, intellectual, and neuropsychological deficits in children (Mulhern, Kovnar, Kun, Crisco, & Williams, 1988). Depending on the type, size, and location of the tumor, as well as the presence or absence of hydrocephalus and/or increased intracranial pressure, different manifestations occur (Price et al., 1992). Nausea, headaches, visual deficits, lateralized sensory or motor impairments, vomiting, or seizures may precede the tumor, and presence of such symptoms warrants referral to a child neurologist who may recommend CT, MRI, or other neurological scans (Teeter & Semrud-Clikeman, 1997). Neurological signs may not always appear early, as low-grade (less malignant) tumors tend to have a slow gradual effect on displacement and compression of neural tissue (Carpentieri & Mulhern, 1993).

Regarding cognitive effects of cancer treatment, it has been found that children diagnosed under the age of seven show a mean loss of 27 IQ points across the first two years (Radcliff et al., 1992). Older children do not demonstrate such a decrease. Moore, Copeland, Reid, and Levy (1992) found that children receiving cranial radiotherapy in addition to chemotherapy presented with more compromised neuropsychological functioning than those with chemotherapy without radiation or those who received no form of CNS treatment. Other predictors of neuropsychological functioning include pre- and postoperative mental status, need for shunt, extent of tumor, and postoperative infections (Packer, Meadows, Rourke, Goldwein and D'Angio, 1987).

The readers are cautioned by Butler and Haser (2006) that the trends toward increasing survival and decreasing morbidity among children with cancer render these older data suspect, and the older studies from 1995 and earlier probably overestimate the morbidity of cancer and its successful treatment, and underestimate the survival rates of treatment itself. Support for this position can be seen in a recent paper on outcomes in children successfully treated for leukemia via chemotherapy or combined chemotherapy plus radiation (Reddick et al., 2006).

The treated children, compared to their siblings as controls, showed statistically significant deficits in nearly every domain of neuropsychological performance, however, only in the domain of attention was a clinically significant effect size of one standard deviation obtained. The degree of impairment was directly correlated with anatomic measures of white matter volume, and this anatomic measure was significantly diminished among those children who received irradiation therapy in addition to their chemotherapy.

The strongest links between declines in intelligence and cranial radiation among children have been found among measures of verbal fluency, visual attention, memory skills, and the Picture Arrangement and Block Design subtests of the WISC (Garcia-Perez, Sierransesumaga, Narbona-Garcia, Calvo-Manuel, & Aguierre-Vantallo, 1994). Such declines varied with level of radiation dose, even when controlling for the direct effects of the tumor. Other studies have replicated these results (Moore, Ater, & Copeland 1992; Morrow, O'Conner, Whitman, & Accardo, 1989; Riva, Milani, Pantaleoni, Ballerini, & Giorgi, 1991; Teeter & Semrud-Clikeman, 1997).

Regarding specific brain structures, Dennis et al. (1991) found that among children and adolescents with brain tumors with specific damage to the putamen and/or globus pallidus, deficits in all memory skills were found. Dennis et al. theorized that the putamen and globus pallidus may serve as a "final common pathway" for memory functions. Packer et al. (1987) found that survivors of medulloblastomas of the posterior fossa held IQs and reading abilities in the average range, but demonstrated deficits in mathematics. Significant memory deficits were also found in 73% of their sample, in addition to delayed motor speed, dexterity, and visuomotor skills.

Sickle Cell Disease

This disturbance of the red blood cells is unique among persons of native African descent. It typically does not become disabling until early adulthood, and then usually only in those individuals homozygous for the trait. This later disability is usually due to compounding influence of the progressive worsening of their chronic anemia, coupled with the accumulation of untoward vascular events such as pulmonary emboli, occlusion of vessels supplying vital areas, renal failure, and intercurrent infections (Berkow & Fletcher, 1992).

Pediatric sickle cell disease is not without consequence. In fact, children with sickle cell disease are at increased risk for acquired deficits in intellectual functioning, attention and executive functioning, memory, language, visuomotor abilities, and academic achievement (Berkelhammer et al., 2007). The etiology of these deficits appears to be due to the children's increased risk of cerebral infarction (stroke), and these often occur without externally seen or internally perceived symptoms, a phenomenon known as silent infarction. Their impact on performance depends on the brain regions that are affected. When the infarcts are in the region of the frontal lobes, affected children show performance patterns of behavioral disinhibition also seen in children with frontal TBI, and are not observed in children with sickle cell disease who do not have cerebral infarctions (Christ, Moinuddin, McKinstry, DeBaun, & White, 2007).

Neuropsychological deficits accrue and worsen as the disease progresses through a series of frank and/or silent infarcts, eventually affecting a broad range of functions including attention and concentration, executive functioning, visuomotor speed, and coordination (Kral, Brown, & Hynd, 2001).

Meningitis

The meninges are a layer of tissue that surrounds the spinal cord and the brain. This layer protects the brain from infection, cushions it from injury, and serves as a barrier to foreign objects. Meningitis results when the meninges (particularly the arachnoid and pia mater layers) become inflamed or infected. The infection may be related to sinusitis, ear infections, and other abscesses. Infection may also be acquired by neonates in the birth canal (Teeter & Semrud-Clikeman, 1997). The most common form, bacterial meningitis, affects nearly 40,000 people per year in the United States (Green & George, 1979). Among children, the most frequently involved are those between ages one and five (Taylor, Schatschneider, & Reich, 1992). Hemophilus (Hib) meningitis has been related to significant developmental disability (Jadavji, Biggar, Gold, & Prober, 1986; Klein, Feigin, & McCracken, 1986), and occurs among 30 to 70 per 100,000 children (Snyder, 1994). The highest incidence rates have been found among the Navajo and Alaskan Yupik Eskimo ethnic groups (Coulehan et al., 1976; Fraser, 1982).

Young children afflicted with meningitis tend to present with fever, low appetite, nausea, irritability, jaundice, respiratory problems, and a bulging fontanel (Snyder, 1994). Older children tend to present a fever, headache, generalized seizure activity, nausea, vomiting, a stiff neck, and depressed consciousness. Visual field defects, facial palsy, ataxia, paralysis, and seizure activity, all demonstrative of cranial nerve deficits, may also occur. Additionally, CT scans may show hydrocephalus, edema, or cortical atrophy (Taylor et al., 1992).

For diagnosis, a sample of cerebrospinal fluid (CSF) is taken. If meningitis is present, the CSF is generally cloudy and pressure is elevated. For treatment, usually high doses of antibiotics, often ampicillin, are given for ten days. Fluids are closely monitored and CT, MRI, and EEG scans are ordered as needed (Schaad et al., 1990).

The effects of meningitis depend on age of onset, length of time prior to diagnosis, nature of infectious agent, severity of infection, and treatment used (Weil, 1985). Neonatal patients experience the highest risk for mortality due to meningitis. Children experiencing coma and subdural infections experience the most severe neurological and neuropsychological deficits (Lindberg, Rosenhall, Nylen, & Ringner, 1977). Children experiencing seizures prior to meningitis onset experience the poorest cognitive result posttreatment (Emmett, Jeffrey, Chandler, & Dugdale, 1980; Klein et al., 1986). Sell (1983) examined the long-term effects of meningitis in children and found that 50% of patients showed significant cognitive and physical difficulty, language deficits, hearing problems, cognitive and motor delays, and most frequently, visual impairments. Given the neuropsychological deficits that may arise, comprehensive neuropsychological batteries are recommended in addition to repeated hearing and vision screenings (Teeter & Semrud-Clikeman, 1997).

Encephalitis

Encephalitis is a general inflammatory state of the brain, and is often associated with inflammation of the meninges. Encephalitis occurs in 1,400 to 4,300 individuals per year in the United States (Ho & Hirsch, 1985). The disease is typically caused by viruses and can occur perinatally or postnatally. For most cases, the direct cause cannot be identified; however, Herpes simplex and insect bites are known culprits (Adler & Toor, 1984). Acute and chronic forms have been reported, where acute forms are evidenced within days or weeks of infection, and chronic forms can take months to become symptomatic. Diagnosis typically involves examination of CSF for viral agents, as well as CT scans and EEG analysis.

Encephalitis symptoms include fever, headache, vomiting, loss of energy, lassitude, irritability, and depressive symptoms. Increased confusion and disorientation are seen as the disease progresses. Paralyses or muscle weakness, gait problems, and speech problems have also been documented (Hynd & Willis, 1988). Mental retardation, irritability and lability, seizure disorder, hypertonia, and cranial nerve involvement can occur in more severe cases (Ho & Hirsch, 1985). Treatment for encephalitis typically involves antiviral agents if a viral cause has been verified. If no virus has been identified, treatment involves antibiotics and monitoring of the disease process.

Cardiac, Circulatory, and Pulmonary Problems

Children who survive surgical treatment of congenital heart defects typically develop normal memory and intellectual functioning and no abnormal psychiatric or behavioral functioning, but show weaknesses in language and motor development. It is not clear whether attentional and executive functioning are affected; some studies show an effect and others do not, but none show a protective or enhancement effect of heart surgery on these functions, so there probably is an effect that is inconsistently observed (Miatton, De Wolf, Francois, Thiery, & Vingerhoets, 2006).

Children with migraine headaches may be referred for neuropsychological evaluation, but a recent study showed relatively normal neurocognitive profiles among pediatric migraineurs, with deficits only on a measure of simple visual reaction time. The degree of this deficit was significantly correlated with increased frequency of headache attack and reduced interictal interval. No differences were observed between children whose migraines were preceded by an aura versus those without aura, and both types showed a profile of internalizing problems in the Child Behavior Checklist (Riva et al., 2006).

Among children with sleep-related breathing disorders, deficits in visual attention and executive functioning have been observed, as well as deficits in phonological awareness, a skill crucial to the development of proficient reading. It is not clear whether these findings reflect neurocognitive dysfunction secondary to hypoxia or due to sleep fragmentation, but there is evidence to support a role of the latter in the negative correlation between neurocognitive abilities and daytime arousal level. (O'Brien et al., 2004). Certainly hypoxic exposure can have an impact, however. Among children who survive severe burn injuries, the neuropsychological and emotional outcomes of those who sustain hypoxic episodes in the course of their injuries are much poorer than the outcomes of children who suffer equivalent burn injuries without hypoxic injuries (Rosenberg et al., 2005).

Psychiatric Disorders

Nowhere on the borderland between psychiatric disorders and neurologic disorders is the atmosphere more murky than when investigating the neuropsychological profiles of children with psychiatric disorders. Although there may appear to be a clear border between the two domains when viewed from a great distance, the closer one looks, the blurrier and grayer the differences become. For example, in a voxel-based morphometric study of the brains of children with obsessive compulsive disorder (OCD) compared to a matched group of healthy children, clear and reliable structural differences emerged in terms of decreased cingulate area and frontal gray matter, and decreased bilateral frontal white matter densities. These regions have been extensively related to action monitoring and error signal processing, and this study's authors (Carmona et al., 2007) go so far as to suggest that these structural brain abnormalities represent the primary cause of deficit in cases of childhood OCD. Children with symptoms of both anxiety and depression have been studied and found to have deficiencies in sequencing, alternation, and problem-solving compared to their healthy peers (Emerson, Mollison, & Harrison, 2005). Children with depression alone have been shown to have problems comprehending the prosodic and nonverbal emotional aspects of speech (Emerson, Harrison, & Everhart, 1999), and also show corresponding asymmetry in the grip strength portion of the psychomotor examination (Emerson, Harrison, Everhart, & Williamson, 2001).

As we move further along the spectrum of depression severity, numerous studies have identified substantial neuropsychological deficits in youngsters with bipolar disorder. With matching controls for ADHD, age and gender, bipolar disorder produced large effect sizes, with affected participants showing significant deficits in sustained attention, working memory, and processing speed, and deficits of a moderate effect size on measures of interference control, abstract problem-solving, and verbal learning (Doyle et al., 2005). Another recent study has shown that children with bipolar disorder demonstrate deficits in attentional set shifting and visuospatial memory (Dickstein et al., 2004). The clinical and neuropsychological characteristics of child and adolescent bipolar disorders have recently been reviewed, and the reader is referred to Kyte, Carlson, and Goodyear (2006) for this excellent review that offers a comparison of the similarities and differences between childhood, adolescent, and adult onset bipolar disorders and mania syndromes.

A similar comparison between adolescent onset and adult onset schizophrenia examined the neuropsychological profiles and subsequent cognitive development of cohorts of early onset versus young adult onset persons with schizophrenia and matched healthy adolescents and young adults. Quite simply, the earlier the onset of schizophrenic symptoms, the greater were the resultant deficits in working memory, language, and motor functioning. (White, Ho, Ward, O'Leary, & Andreasen, 2006). This provides a plausible neuropsychological account of why prognosis in persons with schizophrenia is inversely related to age of onset.

Even persons with problems more typical of the personality disorders of Axis II have not escaped neuropsychological scrutiny. In a study of 325 school-age boys who were classified by cluster analysis into one of four groups: controls, childhood limited antisocial traits, adolescent limited antisocial traits, and life-course persistent antisocial traits, any participants who exhibited antisocial traits during childhood (childhood-limited and life-course groupings) showed persisting impairment on measures of visuospatial and memory functioning. (Raine et al., 2005). These deficits were robust despite controlling statistically for abuse, psychosocial adversity, head injury, and hyperactivity. To paraphrase the words of neuroscientist Joseph LeDoux, "no matter where you feel it or what it is, if it's happening to you, it's happening in your brain" (LeDoux, personal communication, October, 2007, Baton Rouge, LA).

ASSESSMENT PROCEDURES IN PEDIATRIC NEUROPSYCHOLOGY

The following is a good example of preliminary assessment for a child adapted largely from Ryan et al., 1998. Baron (2004) suggests an approach that involves preliminary screening of the child along a number of dimensions of behavior, and then a more focused examination to follow up on deficit areas identified in the preliminary exam. This is best conducted using a flexible approach to testing, although most of these same domains can be more thoroughly covered in the initial stage by using a comprehensive battery such as the Halstead Neuropsychological Test Battery for Children from 9 to 14 years old (Reitan & Davison, 1974), the Reitan Indiana

Neuropsychological Test Battery for Children (Reitan, 1974) or the Luria Nebraska Neuropsychological Battery for Children (Golden, 1981, 1997). In either approach, the important challenge is to ensure adequate coverage of the listed domains, with representative screening measures suggested for each, as per Ryan et al., 1998 and others.

ATTENTION: WISC-III Digit Span, Continuous Performance Testing, Seashore Rhythm
Test d2 Test of Attention
MOTOR SPEED/EYE HAND COORDINATION/FINE MOTOR DEXTERITY: Finger
Oscillation Test, Grooved Pegboard, Purdue Pegboard
PSYCHOMOTOR EFFICIENCY/SPEEDED INFORMATION PROCESSING: WISC-III
Coding
LEARNING AND MEMORY: Wide Range Assessment of Memory and Learning, Test of Memory and Learning, California Verbal Learning Test Childrens'Version, Rey-Osterreith Complex Figure (immediate and delayed memory trials)
VISUOCONSTRUCTIONAL SKILLS: WISC-III Block Design, WISC-III Object
Assembly, Rey-Osterreith Complex Figure (copy trial); Clock Drawing Test
EXECUTIVE FUNCTIONS/MENTAL FLEXIBILITY: Trail Making Test, WISC-III
Mazes, Tactual Performance Test
HYPOTHESIS TESTING/REASONING: Wisconsin Card Sorting Test, Children's
Category Test
ACADEMIC ACHEIVEMENT: Wide Range Achievement Test; Wechsler Individual
Achievement Test
GENERAL INTELLIGENCE: Reynolds Intellectual Assessment Scales; Short Form
WISC-III (Information, Comprehension, Picture Completion, Block Design), Test of Nonverbal Intelligence-III
LANGUAGE COMPREHENSION AND EXPRESSION: Aphasia Screening Test, Token Test, Peabody Picture Vocabulary Test, Controlled Word Association Test

The reader is referred to Spreen and Strauss (1998), Lezak et al. (2004), and Strauss, Sherman, and Spreen (2006) for comprehensive references detailing the administration, normative referencing, and informed commentary on each of the above-mentioned measures. It is at the point of completing the screening battery that the assessment process becomes truly interesting, for the real detective work, involving the formulation and testing of hypotheses about the nature of the underlying dysfunction, begins in earnest. This process involves using and adapting additional measures in an attempt to tease out the reason why certain tests are failed, and to identify what specific supports or props might be used to allow a deficient skill to be expressed and developed. This creative use of evaluation procedures has direct relevance to the development of recommendations for teachers and other professionals who work to support the success of these children in educational and other community settings.

SUMMARY AND CONCLUSIONS

Neuropsychological testing offers clinical practitioners an exquisitely sensitive window into the functioning of the brain. As the reader completes this review, he or she might be impressed, not just with the sensitivity of neuropsychological testing, but also with its lack of specificity. Fortunately for all of us and our patients, the early years of neuropsychology, where neurosurgeons sought our opinion about where in the brain to cut, are behind us now, and the role of neuropsychology has evolved to become more of a discipline that focuses on the identification of strengths and weaknesses for the purposes of planning more effective treatments and making disability determinations to help guide the appropriate granting of accommodations in the educational or workplace settings.

Frontal lobe and executive functioning problems appear in nearly every section of this chapter. These brain regions and the corresponding functions dependent on the integrity of those regions are vulnerable for a number of reasons. They are among the last to mature and myelinate developmentally, and thus, their successful development is at least in part dependent on the successful development of all other structures and functions that emerge along the developmental course beforehand. They are also positioned most precariously within the cranial vault. No region is more vulnerable to acceleration/ deceleration insults than the diagonal axis that cuts through the anterior frontal and anterior temporal lobes, regardless of where the acceleration/deceleration forces are applied, and the underside of these structures, rich with connections to the limbic system, are ripe for contusion whenever the brain is jostled about on the cribiform plate.

Whenever a patient has trouble getting together the resources to do something, such as saying what needs to be done, planning how to do it, deciding what to do next, or bringing the task to completion, the problem is likely in the frontal–prefrontal executive functions system. When the problem appears to be more a lack of comprehension or understanding, the first place to look is at the posterior half of the brain and perceptual recognition and language comprehension systems that are dependent on posterior brain integrity.

REFERENCES

Adler, S. P., & Toor, S. (1984). Central nervous system infections. In J. M. Pellock & E. C. Meyer (Eds.), *Neurologic emergencies in infancy and childhood* (pp. 237–256). New York: Harper& Row.

Alexander, A. I., & Mayfield, J. (2005). Latent factor structure of the test of memory and learning in a pediatric traumatic brain injured sample: Support for a general memory construct. *Archives of Clinical Neuropsychology, 20,* 587–598.

American Psychiatric Association. (1994). *Diagnostic and Statistical Manual of Mental Disorders* (4th ed.). Washington, DC: Author.

American Psychiatric Association. (2000). *Diagnostic and Statistical Manual of Mental Disorders* (4th ed., with text revision). Washington, DC: Author.

Anderson, P. (2002). Assessment and development of executive function (EF) during childhood. *Child Neuropsychology, 8*, 71–82.

Barkley, R. A. (1997). Behavioral inhibition, sustained attention, and executive functions: Constructing a unifying theory of ADHD. *Psychological Bulletin, 121*, 65–94.

Baron, I. S. (2004). *Neuropsychological evaluation of the child.* New York: Oxford University Press.

Benson, D. F., & Ardila, A. (1996). *Aphasia: A clinical perspective.* New York: Oxford University Press.

Berkelhammer, L. D., Williamson, A. L., Sanford, S. D., Dirksen, C. L., Sharp, W. G., Margulies, A. S., & Prengler, R. A. (2007). Neurocognitive sequelae of pediatric sickle cell disease: A review of the literature. *Child Neuropsychology, 13*, 120–131.

Berkow, R., & Fletcher, M. B. (Eds.) (1992) *The Merck manual* (16th ed.). Rahway, NJ: Merck Labs.

Bigler, E. (1988) Good outcomes associated with cerebral reconstitution in hydrocephalus. *Journal of Child Neurology, 3*, 297–298.

Bigler, E.. (1989). On the neuropsychology of suicide. *Journal of Learning Disabilities, 22*(3), 180–185).

Bishop, D. V. M. (1993). Annotation: Autism, executive functions and theory of mind: A neuropsychological perspective. *Journal of Child Psychology and Psychiatry, 34*, 279–293.

Boliek, C. A., & Obrzut, J. E. (1997). Neuropsychological aspects of Attention Deficit/Hyperactivity Disorder. In C. R. Reynolds & E. Fletcher-Janzen (Eds.), *Handbook of clinical child neuropsychology* (2nd ed., pp. 619–633). New York: Plenum.

Boucher, J. & Warrington, E. K. (1976). Memory deficits in early infantile autism: Some similarities to the amnesic syndrome. *British Journal of Psychology, 67*, 73–87.

Brambati, S. M., Termine, C., Ruffino, M., Danna, M., Lanzi, G., Stella, G., Cappa, S. F., & Perani, D. (2006). Neuropsychological deficits and neural dysfunction in familial dyslexia. *Brain Research, 1113*, 174–185.

Brambati, S. M., Termine, C., Ruffino, M., Stella, G., Fazio, F., Cappa, S. F., & Perain, D. (2004) Regional reductions of gray matter volume in familial dyslexia. *Neurology, 63*, 742–745.

Brown, G., Chadwick, O., Shaffer, D., Rutter, M., & Traub, M. (1981). A prospective study of children with head injuries: III. Psychiatric sequelae. *Psychological Medicine,11*, 63–78.

Butler, R. W., & Haser, J. K. (2006). Neurocognitive effects of treatment for childhood cancer. *Mental Retardation and Developmental Disabilities Research Reviews, 12*, 184–191.

Calis, K. A., Grothe, D. R., & Elia, J. (1990). Attention-deficit hyperactivity disorder. *Clinical Pharmacy, 9*, 632–642.

Campo-Castello, J. (2006). Neuropsychology de la epilepsia: que factores estan implicados? *Revista De Neurologia, 43*, 59–70.

Carmona, S., Bassas, N., Rovira, M., Gispert, J. D., Soliva, J. C., Prado, M., Thomas, J., Bublena, A., & Vilarroya, O. (2007). Pediatric OCD structural brain deficits in conflict monitoring circuits: A voxel-based morphometry study. *Neuroscience Letters, 421*, 218–223.

Carpentieri, S. C., & Mulhern, R. K. (1993). Patterns of memory dysfunction among children surviving temporal lobe tumors. *Archives of Clinical Neuropsychology, 8*, 345–357.

Carvajal-Molina F., Iglesias-Dorado, J., Morgade-Fonte, R. M., Martin-Plasencia, P., & Perez-Abalo, M. C. (2003). Neuropsychological study of 8 to 15-year-old children with lateralized sub-clinical paroxysmal discharges and poor academic achievement. *Revista de Neurologia, 36*, 212.

Chasnoff, I. J., Griffith, D., MacGregor, S., Dirkes, K., & Burns, K. (1989). Temporal patterns of cocaine use in pregnancy. *Journal of the American Medical Association, 261*, 1741–1744.

Chasnoff, I. J., Landress, H., & Barrett, M. (1990). The prevalence of illicit drug or alcohol use during pregnancy and discrepancies in mandatory reporting in Pinellas County, Florida. *New England Journal of Medicine, 322,* 1202–1206.

Christ S. E., Moinuddin, A., McKinstry, R. C., DeBaun, M., & White, D. A. (2007). Inhibitory control in children with frontal infarcts related to sickle cell disease. *Child Neuropsychology, 13,* 132–141.

Cohen, M. E., & Duffner, P. K. (1994). Tumors of the brain and spinal cord including leukemic involvement. In K. Swaiman (Ed.), *Pediatric neurology.* St. Louis, MO: Mosby.

Coles, C. D., Platzman, K., Smith, I., James, M., & Falek, A. (1991). Effects of cocaine, alcohol, and other drugs used in pregnancy on neonatal growth and neurobehavioral status. *Neurotoxicology and Teratology, 13,* 1–11.

Comings, D. E. (1990). *Tourette syndrome and human behavior.* Durante, CA; Hope Press.

Cook, E. H., & Leventhal, B. L. (1992). Neuropsychiatric disorders of childhood and adolescence. In S. C. Yudofsky & R. E. Hales (Eds.), *The American Psychiatric Press textbook of neuropsychiatry* (2nd ed., pp. 639–662). Washington, DC: American Psychiatric Press.

Coulehan, J., Michaels, R., Williams, K. L. D., North, Q., Welty, T., & Rogers, K. (1976). Bacterial meningitis in Navajo Indians. *Public Health Reports, 91,* 464–468.

Courchesne, E. (1989). Neuroanatomical systems involved in autism: The implications of cerebellar abnormalities. In G. Dawson (Ed.). *Autism: Nature, diagnosis, and treatment* (pp. 120–143). New York: Guildford Press.

Courchesne, E. (1997). Brainstem, cerebellar, and limbic neuroanatomical abnormalities in autism. *Current Opinions in Neurobiology, 7,* 269–278.

D'Amato, R. C., Crepeau-Hobson, F., Huang, L. V., & Geill, M. (2005). Ecological neuropsychology: An alternative to the deficit model for conceptualizing and serving students with learning disabilities. *Neuropsychology Review, 15,* 97–103.

D'Amato, R. C., Dean, R. S., & Rhodes, R. L. (1998). Subtyping children's learning disabilities with neuropsychological, intellectual, and achievement measures. *International Journal of Neuroscience, 96,* 107–125.

Dawson, G. & Castelloe, P. (1995). Autism. In C. E. Walker & M. C. Roberts (Eds.). *Handbook of clinical child psychology.* New York: Plenum Press.

Day, N. L. (1992). The effects of prenatal exposure to alcohol. *Alcohol Health and Research World, 16,* 238–244.

Delis, D. C., Kramer, J. H., Kaplan, E., & Ober, B. A. (1994). *California Verbal Learning Test-Children's Version.* San Antonio, TX: Psychological Corporation.

Dennis, M., Spiegler, B. J., Hoffman, H. J., Hendrick, E. B., Humphreys, R. P., & Becker, L. E. (1991). Brain tumors in children and adolescents-I. Effects on working, associative, and serial-order memory of IQ, age at tumor onset, and age of tumor. *Neuropsychologia, 29,* 813–827.

Dickstein, D. P., Treland, J. E., Snow, J., McClure, E. B., Mehta, M. S., Towbin, K. E., Pine, D. S., & Leibenluft, E. (2004). Neuropsychological performance in pediatric bipolar disorder. *Biological Psychiatry, 55,* 32–39.

Dixon, S., & Bejar, R. (1989). Echoencephalogoraphic findings in neonates associated with maternal cocaine and methamphetamine use: Incidence and correlates. *Journal of Pediatrics, 117,* 770–778.

Donders, J. (1997). Sensitivity of the WISC-III to injury severity in children with traumatic head injury. *Assessment, 4,* 107–109.

Dorris, M. (1989). *The broken cord.* New York: Harper & Row.

Douglas, V. I., & Benezra, E. (1990). Supra-span verbal memory in attention deficit disorder with hyperactivity normal and reading-disabled boys. *Journal of Abnormal Child Psychology, 18,* 617–638.

Doyle, A. E., Wilens, T. E., Kwon, A., Seidman, L. J., Faraone, S. V., Fried, R., Swezey A., Snyder, L., & Biderman, J. (2005). Neuropsychological functioning in youth with bipolar disorder. *Biological Psychiatry, 58,* 540–548.

Drummond, C. R., Ahmad, S. A., & Rourke, B. P. (2005). Rules for the classification of younger children with nonverbal learning disabilities and basic phonological processing disabilities. *Archives of Clinical Neuropsychology, 20,* 171–182.

Duffner, P. K., Cohen, M E., Horowitz, M., et al. (1986). Postoperative chemotherapy and delayed irradiation in children less than 36 months of age with malignant brain tumors. *Annals of Neurology, 20,* 424–430.

Eisen, L., Field, T., Bandstra, E., et al. (1991). Perinatal cocaine effects on neonatal stress behavior and performance on the Brazelton Scale. *Pediatrics, 88,* 477–480.

Emerson, C. S., Harrison, D. W., & Everhart, D. E. (1999). Investigation of receptive affective prosodic ability in school age boys with and without depression. *Neuropsychiatry, Neuropsychology, and Behavioral Neurology, 12,* 102–109.

Emerson, C. S., Harrison, D. W., Everhart, D. E., & Williamson, J. B. (2001). Grip strengthasymmetry in depressed boys. *Neuropsychiatry, Neuropsychology, and Behavioral Neurology, 14,* 130–134.

Emerson, C. S., Mollet, G. A., & Harrison, D. W. (2005). Anxious-depression in boys: An evaluation of executive functioning. *Archives of Clinical Neuropscyhology, 20,* 539–546.

Emmett, M., Jeffrey, H., Chandler, D., & Dugdale, A. (1980). Sequelae of *Hemophilus influenzae* meningitis. *Australian Paediatric Journal, 16,* 90–93.

Escalante-Mead, P. R., Minshew, N. J., & Sweeney, J. A. (2003). Abnormal brain lateralization in high-functioning autism. *Journal of Autism and Developmental Disorders, 33,* 539–543.

Ewing-Cobbs, L., Levin, H. S., Fletcher, J. M., Minerm, M. E., & Eisenberg, H. M. (1990). The Children's Orientation and Amnesia Test: Relationship to severity of acute head injury and to recovery of memory. *Neurosurgery, 27,* 683–691.

Farmer, J. E., Warschausky, S. A., & Donders, J. (Eds.) (2006).*Treating neurodevelopmental disabilities: Clinical research and practice.* New York: Guilford Press.

Frank, D. A., Zuckerman, B. S., Amaro, H., et al. (1988). Cocaine use during pregnancy: Prevalence and correlates. *Pediatrics, 82,* 888–895.

Fraser, D. (1982). *Haemophilus influenzae* in the community and the home. In S. H. Sell & P. F. Wright (Eds.), *Haemophilus influenzae: Epidemiology, immunology, and prevention of disease* (pp. 11–24). New York: Elsevier Biomedical.

Garcia-Perez, A., Sierransesumaga, L., Narbona-Garcia, L., Calvo-Manuel, F., & Aguierre-Ventalló, M. (1994). Neuropsychological evaluation of children with intracranial tumors: Impact of treatment modalities. *Medical and Pediatric Oncology, 23,* 116–123.

Geurts, H. M., Verte, S., Oosterlaan, J., Roeyers, H., & Sergeant, J. A. (2005). ADHD subtypes: Do they differ in their executive functioning profile? *Archives of Clinical Neuropsychology, 20,* 457–477.

Golden, C.J. (1981) The Luria Nebraska Children's Battery: Theory and initial formulation. In G. Hynd & S. Obrzut (Eds.) *Neuropsychological assessment of the school aged child: Issues and procedures.* New York: Grune & Stratton.

Golden, C. J., (1997) The Nebraska Neuropsychological Children's Battery. In C. R. Reynolds & E. Fletcher-Janzen (Eds.), *Handbook of clinical child neuropsychology.* New York: Plenum.

Goldstein, S., & Reynolds, C. R. (Eds.). (2005). *Handbook of neurodevelopmental and genetic disorders in adults.* New York: Guilford Press.

Goldstrohm, S. L., & Arffa S. (2005). Preschool children with mild to moderate traumatic brain injury: An exploration of immediate and post-acute morbidity. *Archives of Clinical Neuropsychology, 20,* 675–695.

Green, S. H., & George, R. H. (1979). Bacterial meningitis. In F. C. Rose (Ed.), *Pediatric neurology* (pp. 569–581). Oxford: Blackwell Scientific.

Greene, T. H., Ernhart, C. B., Ager, J., Sokol, R. J., et al. (1991). Prenatal alcohol exposure and cognitive development in the preschool years. *Neurotoxicology and Teratology, 13,* 57–68.

Greene, T. H., Ernhart, C. B., Martier, S., Sokol, R. et al. (1990). Prenatal alcohol exposure and language development. *Alcoholism: Clinical and Experimental Research, 14,* 937–945.

Griffith, D. Azuma, S. D., & Chasnoff, I. J. (1994). Three-year outcome of children exposed prenatally to drugs. *Journal of the American Academy of Child and Adolescent Psychiatry, 33,* 20–27.

Gualtieri, C. T., & Hicks, R. E. (1985). Neuropharmacology of methylphenidate and a neural substrate for childhood hyperactivity. *Psychiatric Clinics of North America, 8,* 975–892.

Guimareaes, C. A., Li, L. M., Rzezak, P., Fuentes, D., Franzon, R. C., Montenegro, M. A., Cendes, F., Thome-Souza, S., Valente, K., & Guerreiro, M. M. (2007). Temporal lobe epilepsy in childhood: Comprehensive neuropsychological assessment. *Journal of Child Neurology, 22,* 836–840.

Hagen, C., Malkmus, D., & Durham, P. (1979). *Levels of cognitive functioning.* In *Rehabilitation of the head injured adult: Comprehensive physical management.* Downey, CA: Professional Staff Association of Rancho Los Amigos Hospital, Inc.

Hauser, P., Zametkin, A. J., Martinez, P., Vitiello, B., Matochik, J., Mixson, A., & Weintraub, B. (1993). Attention deficit hyperactivity disorder in people with generalized resistance to thyroid hormone. *New England Journal of Medicine, 328,* 997–1001.

Hauser, P., Zametkin, A. J., Vitiello, B., Martinex, P., Mixson, A. J., & Weintraub, B. D. (1992). Attention deficit hyperactivity disorder in 18 kindreds with generalized resistance to thyroid hormone [Abstract]. *Clinical Research, 40,* 388A..

Hauser, S. L., Delong, G. R., & Rosman, N. P. (1975). Pneumographic findings in the infantile autism syndrome: A correlation with temporal lobe disease. *Brain, 98,* 677–688.

Hauser, W. A., & Hesdorffer, D. C. (1990). *Epilepsy: Frequency, causes, and consequences.* New York: Demos

Hawley, T. L., Halle, T. G., Drasin, R. E., & Thomas, N. G. (1995). Children of addicted mothers: Effects of the "crack epidemic" on the caregiving environment and the development of preschoolers. *American Journal of Orthopsychiatry, 65,* 364–378.

Hines, M. E., Kubu, C. S., Roberts, R. J., & Varney, N. R. (1995). Characteristics and mechanisms of epilepsy spectrum disorder: An explanatory model. *Applied Neuropsychology,2,* 1–6.

Ho, D. D., & Hirsch, M. S. (1985). Acute viral encephalitis. *Medical Clinics of North America, 69,* 415–429.

Hunter, S., & Donders, J. (Eds.) (2007). *Pediatric neuropsychological intervention.* New York: Cambridge University Press.

Hynd, G. W., Hern, K. L., Novey, E. S., Eliopulos, D., Marshall, R., Gonzalez, J. J., & Voeller, K. K. (1993). Attention deficit-hyperactivity disorder and asymmetry of the caudate nucleus. *Journal of Child Neurology, 8,* 339–347.

Hynd, G. W., Lorys, A. R., Semrud-Clikeman, M., Nieves, N., Huettner, M., & Lahey, B. (1991). Attention deficit disorder without hyperactivity (ADD/WO): A distinctive behavioral and neurocognitive syndrome. *Journal of Child Neurology,* 6(Suppl.), S37–S41.

Hynd, G. W., Semrud-Clikeman, M., Lorys, A. R., Novey, E. S., Eliopulos, D., & Lyytinen, H. (1991). Corpus callosum morphology in attention deficit- hyperactivity disorder: Morphometric analysis of MRI. *Journal of Learning Disabilities, 24,* 141–146.

Hynd, G. W., & Willis, W. G. (1988). *Pediatric neuropsychology.* Orlando, FL: Grune & Stratton.

Jadavji, T., Biggar, W., Gold, R., & Prober, C. (1986). Sequelae of acute bacterial meningitis in children treated for seven days. *Pediatrics, 78,* 21–25.

Jonsdottir, S., Bouma, A., Sergeant, J. A., & Scherder, E. J. (2006). Relationships between neuropsychological measures of executive function and behavioral measures of ADHD symptoms and comorbid behavior. *Archives of Clinical Neuropscyhology, 21,* 383–394.

Kirkwood, M., Janusz, J., Yeates, K. O., Taylor, H. G., Wade, S. L., Stancin, T., & Drotar, D. (2000). Prevalence and correlates of depressive symptoms following traumatic brain injuries in children. *Child Neuropsychology, 6*(3), 195–208.

Klein, J., Feigin, R., & McCracken, G. J. (1986). Report of the task force on diagnosis and management of meningitis. *Pediatrics, 78,* 959–982.

Koren, G. (1993). Cocaine and the human fetus: The concept of teratophilia. *Neurotoxicology and Teratology, 15,* 301–304.

Korkman, M., Granström, M. L., & Berg, S. (2004). Dichotic listening in children with focal epilepsy: Effects of structural brain abnormality and seizure characteristics. *Journal of Clinical and Experimental Neuropsychology, 26,* 83.94.

Korkman, M., & Pesonen, A. E. (1994). A comparison of neuropsychological test profiles of children with attention deficit-hyperactivity disorder and/or learning disorder. *Journal of Learning Disabilities, 27,* 383–392.

Kral, M. C., Brown, R. T., & Hynd, G. W. (2001). Neuropsychological aspects of pediatric sickle cell disease. *Neuropsychology Review, 11,* 170–196.

Kraus, J. F. (1995). Epidemiological features of brain injury in children: Occurrence, children at risk, causes and manner of injury, severity and outcomes. In S. H. Broman & M. E. Michel (Eds.), *Traumatic head injury in children* (pp. 22–39). New York: Oxford University Press.

Kun, L. E. (1992). Brain tumors in children. In A. Perez & W. Brady (Eds.), *Principles and practices of pediatric oncology* (pp. 1417–1441). Philadelphia: Lippincott.

Kupietz, S. S. (1990). Sustained attention in normal and in reading-disabled youngsters with and without ADHD. *Journal of Abnormal Child Psychology, 18*, 357–372.

Kyte, Z. A., Carlson, G. A., & Goodyer, I. M. (2006). Clinical and neuropsychological characteristics of child and adolescent bipolar disorder. *Psychological Medicine, 36*, 1197–1211.

Lassonde, M. (1986). The facilitory influence of the corpus callosum on interhemispheric processing. In F. Lepore, M. Ptito, & H. Jasper (Eds.), *Two hemispheres-one brain* (pp. 385–401). New York: Liss.

Lescohier, I., & DiScala, C. (1993). Blunt trauma in children: Causes and outcomes of head versus intracranial injury. *Pediatrics, 91*, 721–725.

Levin, H. S., Hanten, G., Zhang, L., Swank, P. R., & Hunter, J. (2004). Selective impairment of inhibition after TBI in children. *Journal of Clinical and Experimental Neuropscyhology, 26*, 589–597.

Levin, H. S., Song, J., Scheibel, R. S., Fletcher, J. M., Harward, H., Lilly, M., & Goldstein, F. (1997). Concept formation and problem-solving following closed head injury in children. *Journal of the International Neurological Society, 3*, 598– 607.

Levine, S. C., Kraus, R., Alexander, E., Suriyakham, L. W., & Huttenlocher, P. R. (2005). IQ decline following early unilateral brain injury: A longitudinal study. *Brain and Cognition, 59*, 114–123.

Lewinsohn, P., & Graf, M. (1973). A follow-up study of persons referred for vocational rehabilitation who have suffered brain injury. *Journal of Community Psychology, 1*, 57–62.

Lezak, M. (1978a). Subtle sequelae of brain damage: Perplexity, distractibility, and fatigue. *American Journal of Physical Medicine, 57*, 9–15.

Lezak, M. (1978b). Living with the characterologically altered brain injured patient. *Journal of Clinical Psychiatry, 39*, 592–598.

Lezak, M., Howieson, D. B., & Loring, D. W. (2004) *Neuropsychological assessment* (4th ed.), New York: Oxford University Press.

Lindberg, J., Rosenhall, U., Nylen, O., & Ringner, A. (1977). Long-term outcome of Hemophilus *influenzae meningitis* related to antibiotic treatment. *Pediatrics, 60*, 1–6.

Lou, H. C., Henriksen, L., Bruhn, P., Borner, H., & Neilson, J. B. (1989). Striatal dysfunction in attention deficit and hyperkinetic disorder. *Archives of Neurology, 46*, 48–52.

Lowther, J. L., & Mayfield, J. (2004). Memory functioning in children with traumatic brain injuries: a TOMAL validity study. *Archives of Clinical Neuropsychology, 19*, 105–118.

Luria, A.R. (1973) *The working brain: An introduction to neuropsychology*, New York: Basic Books.

MacGregor, S., Keith, L., Bachicha, J., & Chasnoff, I. J. (1989). Cocaine use during pregnancy: Correlation between prenatal care and perinatal outcome. *Obstetrics and Gynecology, 74*, 882–885.

Malakoff, M. E., Mayes, L. C., & Schottenfeld, R. S. (1994). Language abilities of preschool-age children living with cocaine-using mothers. *American Journal of Addictions, 3*, 346–354.

Marsh, N., & Whitehead, G. (2005). Skull fracture during infancy: A five-year follow-up. *Journal of Clinical and Experimental Neuropsychology, 27*, 352–366.

Mattson, S. N., Riley, E. P., Jernigan, T. L., Garcia, A., et al. (1994). A decrease in the size of the basal ganglia following prenatal alcohol exposure: A preliminary report. *Neurotoxicology and Teratology, 16*, 283–289.

Mattson, S. N., Riley, E. P., Matveeva, A., & Marintcheva, G. (2003) Fetal alcohol syndrome in Moscow, Russia: Neuropsychology test performance. Described in E. P. Riley, S. N. Mattson, T. K. Li, S. W. Jacobson, C. D. Coles, P. W. Kodituwakku, C. M. Adnams, & M. I. Korkman (2003). Neurobehavioral consequences of prenatal alcohol exposure: An international perspective. *Alcoholism-Clinical and Experimental Research, 27,* 362–373.

Max, J. E., Koele, S., Castillo, C. C., Lindgren, S. D., Arndt, S., Bokura, H., et al. (2000). Personality change disorder in children and adolescents following TBI. *Jounral of the International Neuropsychological Society, 6*(3), 279–289.

Max, J. E., Koele, S., Lindgren, S. D., Robin, D. A., Smith, W. L., Sato, Y., & Arndt, S. (1998). Adaptive functioning following TBI and orthopedic injury: A controlled study. *Archives of Physical Medicine and Rehabilitation, 79,* 893–899.

Max, J. E., Koele, S. L., Smith, W. L., Sato, Y., Lindgren, S. D., Robin, D. A., & Arndt, S. (1998). Psychiatric disorders in children and adolescents after severe TBI: A controlled study. *Journal of the American Academy of Child and Adolescent Psychiatry, 37*(8), 832–840.

May, P. A., Hymbaugh, K. J., Aase, J. M., & Samet, J. M. (1983). Epidemiology of fetal alcohol syndrome among American Indians of the Southwest. *Social Biology, 30,* 374–387.

McLean, D. E., Kaitz, E. S., Kennan, C. J., Dabney, K., Cawley, M. F., & Alexander, M. A. (1995). Medical and surgical complications of pediatric brain injury. *Journal of Head Trauma Rehabilitation, 10,* 1–12.

Miatton, M., De Wolf, D., Francois, K., Thiery, E., & Vingerhoets, G. (2006). Neurocognitive consequences of surgically corrected congenital heart defects: A review. *Neuropsychology Review, 16,* 65–68.

Minshew, N. J., & Goldstein, G. (1993). Is autism an amnesic disorder? Evidence from the California Verbal Learning Test. *Neuropsychology, 7,* 206–219.

Moore, B. D., Ater, J. L., & Copeland, D. R. (1992). Improved neuropsychological functioning in children with brain tumors diagnosed during infancy and treated without cranial irradiation. *Journal of Child Neurology, 7,* 281–290.

Moore, B. D., Copeland, D. R., Reid, H., & Levy, B. (1992). Neurophysiological basis of cognitive deficits in long-term survivors of childhood cancer. *Archives of Neurology, 49,* 809–817.

Morrow, J., O'Conner, D., Whitman, B., & Accardo, P. (1989). CNS irradiation and memory deficit. *Developmental Medicine and Child Neurology, 31,* 690–691.

Mulhern, R. K., Hancock, J., Fairclough, D., & Kun, L. E. (1992). Neuropsychological status of children treated for brain tumors: A critical review and integration. *Medical and Pediatric Oncology, 20,* 181–192

Mulhern, R. K., Kovnar, E. H., Kun, L. E., Crisco, J. J., & Williams, J. M. (1988). Psychologic and neurologic function following treatment for childhood temporal lobe astrocytoma. *Journal of Child Neurology, 7,* 1660–1666.

National Institute on Alcohol Abuse and Alcoholism. (1990). *Seventh special report to the U.S. Congress on Alcohol and Health,* DHHS Pub. No. (ADM) 90–1656. Washington, DC: U.S. Government Printing Office.

Neuspiel, D. R., Hamel, S. C., Hochberg, E., Green, J., & Campbell, D. (1991). Maternal cocaine use and infant behavior. *Neurotoxicology and Teratology, 13,* 229–233.

Nijhuis-Van der Sanden, M. W., Eling, P. A., Van Asseldonk, E. H., & Van Galen, G. P. (2004). Decreased movement speed in girls with Turner syndrome: A problem in motor planning or muscle initiation? *Journal of Clinical and Experimental Neuropsychology, 26,* 795–618.

Nolan, M. A., Redoblado, M. A., Lah, S., Sabaz, M., Lawson, J. A., Cunningham, A. M., Bleasel, A. F., & Bye, A. M. (2003). Intelligence in childhood epilepsy syndromes. *Epilepsy Research, 53,* 139–150.

Nolin, P., & Ethier, L. (2007). Using neuropsychological profiles to classify neglected children with or without physical abuse. (2007). *Child Abuse and Neglect, 31,* 631–643.

O'Brien, L. M., Mervis, C. B., Holbrook, C. R., Bruner, J. L., Smith, N. H., McNally, N., McClimment, M. C., & Gozal, D. (2004). Neurobehavioral correlates of sleep-disordered breathing in children. *Journal of Sleep Research, 13,* 165–172.

Oro, A. S., & Dixon, S. D. (1987). Perinatal cocaine and methamphetamine exposure: Maternal and neonatal correlates. *Journal of Pediatrics, 111,* 571–578.

Overholser, J. C. (1990). Fetal alcohol syndrome: A review of the disorder. *Journal of Contemporary Psychotherapy, 20,* 163–176.

Ozonoff, S., Pennington, S. F., & Rogers, S. J. (1990). Are there emotion perception deficits in young autistic children? *Journal of Child Psychology and Psychiatry and Allied Disciplines, 31*, 343–361.

Packer, R. K., Meadows, A. T., Rourke, L. B., Goldwein, J. L., & D'Angio, G. (1987). Long-term sequelae of cancer treatment on the central nervous system in childhood. *Medical and Pediatric Oncology, 15*, 241–253.

Peterson, R. L., McGrath, L. M., Smith, S. D., & Pennington, B. F. (2007). Neuropsychology and genetics of speech, language, and literacy disorders. *Pediatric Clinics of North America, 54*, 543–561.

Price, T. P., Goetz, K. L., & Lovell, M. R. (1992). Neuropsychiatric aspects of brain tumors. In S. C. Yudofsky & R. E. Hales (Eds.), *The American Psychiatric Press textbook of neuropsychiatry* (2nd ed., pp. 473–498). Washington, DC: American Psychiatric Press.

Prior, M. R., & Bradshaw, J. L. (1979). Hemispheric functioning in autistic children. *Cortex, 15*, 73–81.

Radcliff, J., Packer, R. J., Atkins, T. E., Bunin, G. R., Schut, J., Goldwein, J. W., & Sulton, L. N. (1992). Three-and four-year cognitive outcome in children with non-cortical brain tumors treated with whole-brain radiotherapy. *Annals of Neurology, 32*, 551–554.

Raine, A., Moffitt, T. E., Caspi, A., Loeber, R., Stouthamer-Loeber, M., & Lynam, D. (2005). Neurocognitive impairments in boys on the life-course persistent antisocial path. *Journal of Abnormal Psychology, 114*, 38–49.

Reddick, W. E., Shan, Z. Y., Glass, J. O., Helton, S., Xiong, X. P., Wu, S. J., Banner, M. J., Howard, S. C., Christensen, R., Khan, R. B., Pui, C. H., & Mulhern, R. K. (2006). Smaller white-matter volumes are associated with larger deficits in attention and learning among long-term survivors of acute lymphoblastic leukemia. *Cancer, 106*, 941–949.

Refetoff, S., Weiss, R. E., & Usala, S. J. (1993). The syndromes of resistance to thyroid hormone. *Endocrine Review, 14*, 348–399.

Reitan, R. M. Psychological effects of cerebral lesions in children of early school age. In R. M. Reitan & L. A. Davison. (1974) *Clinical neuropsychology: Current status and applications.* Washington, DC: Winston and Sons

Reitan, R. M., & Davison, L. A. (1974) *Clinical neuropsychology: Current status and applications.* Washington, D.C.: Winston and Sons.

Reiter, A., Tucha, O., & Lange, K. W. (2005). Executive functions in children with dyslexia. *Dyslexia, 11*, 116–131.

Reynolds, C. R., & Fletcher-Janzen, E. (Eds.) (1997), Handbook *of clinical child neuropsychology* (2nd ed.). New York: Plenum

Riley, E. P., Mattson, S. N., Li, T. K., Jacobson, S. W., Coles, C. D., Kodituwakku, P. W., Adnams, C. M., & Korkman, M. I. (2003). Neurobehavioral consequences of prenatal alcohol exposure: An international perspective. *Alcoholism- Clinical and Experimental Research, 27*, 362–373.

Rimland, B. (1964). *Infantile autism.* New York: Appleton-Century-Crofts.

Riva, D., Aggio, F., Vago, C., Nichelli, F., Andreucci, E., Paruta, N., D'Arrigo, S., Pantaeoni, C., & Bulgheroni, S. (2006). Cognitive and behavioural effects of migraine in childhood and adolescence. *Cephalalgia, 26*, 596–603.

Riva, D., Milani, N., Pantaleoni, C., Ballerini, E., & Giorgi, C. (1991). Combined treatment modality for medulloblastoma in childhood: Effects on neuropsychological functioning. *Neuropediatrics, 22*, 36–42.

Roberts, R. J., Varney, N. R., Paulsen, J. S., & Richardson E. D. (1990). Dichotic listening and complex partial seizures. *Journal of Clinical and Experimental Neuropsychology, 12*, 448–458.

Robins, P. M. (1992). A comparison of behavioral and attentional functioning in children diagnosed as hyperactive or learning-disabled. *Journal of Abnormal Child Psychology, 20*, 65–82.

Rosenberg, M., Robertson, C., Murphy, K. D., Rosenberg, L., Micak, R., Robert, R. S., Herndon, D. N., & Meyer, W. J. (2005). Neuropsychological outcomes of pediatric burn patients who sustained hypoxic episodes. *Burns, 31*, 883–889.

Rourke, B., Van der Vlugt, H., & Rourke, S. (2002) *The practice of child clinical neuropsychology: An introduction.* Lisse, The Netherlands: Swets & Zeitlinger.

Russell, M., Czarnecki, D. M., Cowan, R., McPherson, E., et al. (1991). Measures of maternal alcohol use as predictors of development in early childhood. *Alcoholism: Clinical and Experimental Research, 15,* 991–1000.

Ryan, C. M., Hammond, K., & Beers, S. (1998) General assessment issues for a pediatric population. In P. J. Snyder & P. D. Nussbaum (Eds.) *Clinical neuropsychology: A pocket handbook for assessment.* Washington, DC: American Psychological Association.

Schaad, U., Suter, S., Gianella-Borradori, A., Pfenninger, J., Auckenthaler, R., Bernath, O., Cheseaux, J. J., & Wedgewood, J. (1990). A comparison of ceftriaxone and cefuroxime for treatment of bacterial meningitis in children. *New England Journal of Medicine, 322,* 141–147.

Segalowitz, S. J., & Rapin, I. (Eds.), (2003). *Volume 8. Child neuropsychology. Parts I and II.* in F. Boller & J. Grafman, (Eds.) *Handbook of neuropsychology* (2nd ed.). Amsterdam: Elsevier.

Sell, S. H. (1983). Long term sequelae of bacterial meningitis in children. *Pediatric Infectious Disease, 2,* 90–93.

Shue, K. L., & Douglas, V. I. (1992). Attention deficit hyperactivity disorder and the frontal lobe syndrome. *Brain and Cognition, 20,* 104–124.

Silver, C. H., Blackburn, L. B., Sharon, A., Barth, J. T., Bush, S. S., Koffler, S. P., Pliskin, N. H., Reynolds, C. R., Ruff, R. M., Troster, A. I., Moser, R. S., & Elliott, R. W. (2006). The importance of neuropsychological assessment for the evaluation of childhood learning disorders: NAN policy and planning committee. *Archives of Clinical Neuropsychology, 21,* 741–744.

Singer, L. T., Garber, R., & Kliegman, R. (1991). Neurobehavioral sequelae of fetal cocaine exposure. *The Journal of Pediatrics, 119,* 667–672.

Singh, N. N., Oswald, D. P., Lancioni, G. E., Ellis, C. R., Sage, M., & Ferris, J. R. (2005). The neuropsychology of facial identity and facial expression in children with mental retardation. *Research in Developmental Disabilities, 26,* 33–40.

Snyder, R. D. (1994). Bacterial meningitis of infants and children. In K. Swaiman (Ed.), *Principles of neurology* (pp. 611–642). St. Louis, MO: Mosby.

Spreen, O., & Strauss, E. (1998). A compendium of neuropsychological tests: Administration, Norms, and Commentary (2nd ed.). New York: Oxford University Press.

Stein, D. G., Brailowsky, S., & Will, B. (1995). *Brain repair.* New York: Oxford University Press.

Steinhausen, H. C., Willms, J., & Spohr, H. L. (1994). Correlates of psychopathology and intelligence in children with fetal alcohol syndrome. *Journal of Child Psychology and Psychiatry and Allied Disciplines, 35,* 323–331.

Strauss, E., Sherman, E., & Strauss, O. A compendium of neuropsychological tests: Administration, norms, and commentary (3rd ed.). New York: Oxford University Press.

Streissguth, A. P. (1994). A long-term perspective of FAS. *Alcohol Health and Research World, 18,* 74–81.

Streissguth, A. P., Aase, J. M., Clarren, S. K., Randels, S. P., LaDue, R. A., & Smith, D. F. (1991). Fetal alcohol syndrome in adolescents and adults. *Journal of the American Medical Association, 265,* 1961–1967.

Streissguth, A. P., Clarren, S. K., & Jones, K. L. (1985). Natural history of the fetal alcohol syndrome: A ten-year follow-up of eleven patients. *Lancet, 2,* 85–91.

Streissguth, A. P., Randels, S. P., & Smith, D. F. (1991). A test-retest study of intelligence in patients with fetal alcohol syndrome: Implications for care. *Journal of the American Academy of Child and Adolescent Psychiatry, 30,* 584–587.

Streissguth, A. P., Sampson, P. D., & Barr, H. M. (1989). Neurobehavioral dose-response effects of prenatal alcohol exposure in humans from infancy to adulthood. Conference of the Behavioral Teratology Society, the National Institute on Drug Abuse, and the New York Academy of Sciences: Prenatal abuse of licit and illicit drugs. *Annals of the New York Academy of Sciences, 562,* 145–158.

Taylor, H. G., Schatschneider, C., & Reich, D. (1992). Sequelae of Haemophilus influenzae meningitis: Implications for the study of brain disease and development. In M. G. Tramontana and S. Hooper (Eds.), Advances in child Neuropsychology: Vol. I (pp.109–137). New York: Springer-Verlag.

Taylor, H. G., Yeates, K. O., Wade, S. L., Drotar, D., Klein, S. K., & Stancin, T. (1999). Influences on first-year recovery from TBI in children. *Neuropsychology, 13*(1), 76–89.

Teasdale, G., & Jennett, G. (1974). Assessment of coma and impaired consciousness. *Lancet, 2,* 81.

Teeter, P. A., & Semrud-Clikeman, M. (1997). *Child neuropsychology: Assessment and interventions for neurodevelopmental disorders.* Needham Heights, MA: Allyn & Bacon.

Temple, E. (2002). The developmental cognitive neuroscience approach to the study of developmental disorders. *Behavioral and Brain Sciences, 25,* 771.

Van der Meere, J., van Baal, M., & Sergeant, J. (1989). The additive factor method: A differential diagnostic tool in hyperactivity and learning disability. *Journal of Abnormal Child Psychology, 17,* 409–422.

Varney, N. R., Garvey, M., Campbell, D., Cook, B., & Roberts, R. J. (1993). Identification of treatment resistant depressives who respond favorably to carbamazepine. *Annals of Clinical Psychiatry, 5,* 117–222.

Varney, N. R., Hines, M. E., Bailey, C., & Roberts, R. J. (1992). Neuropsychiatric correlates of theta bursts in patients with closed head injury. *Brain Injury, 6*(6), 499–508.

Vicari, S. (2006). Motor development and neuropsychological patterns in persons with Downs syndrome. *Behavior Genetics, 36,* 355–364.

Vygotsky, L. S. (1960). *Development of higher mental functions.* Moscow, Russia: Academy of Pedagogy. (Russian). Cited in Luria, A. R. (1973) *The working brain: An introduction to neuropsychology,* New York: Basic Books.

Warschausky, S., Kewman, D. G., Bradley, A., & Dixon, P. (2003). Pediatric neurological conditions: Brain and spinal cord injury and muscular dystrophy. In M. C. Roberts (Ed.), *Handbook of pediatric psychology* (3rd ed., pp. 375–391). New York: Guilford Press.

Warschausky, S., Kewman, D., & Selim, A. (1996). Attentional performance of children with traumatic brain injury: A quantitative and qualitative analysis of digit span. *Archives of Clinical Neuropsychology, 11*(2), 147–153.

Weil, M. L. (1985). Infections of the nervous system. In J. H. Menkes (Ed.), *Textbook of child neurology* (3rd ed., pp. 316–431). Philadelphia: Lea & Febiger.

White, D. A., & Christ, S. E. (2005). Executive control of learning and memory in children with bilateral spastic cerebral palsy. *Journal of the International Neuropsychological Society, 11,* 920–924.

White, T., Ho, B. C., Ward, J., O'Leary, D., & Andreasen, N. (2006). Neuropsychological performance in first-episode adolescents with schizophrenia: A comparison with first-episode adults and adolescent control subjects. *Biological Psychiatry, 60,* 463–471.

Wood, R. L., & Rutherford, N. A. (2006). The impact of mild developmental learning difficulties on neuropsychological recovery from head trauma. *Brain Injury, 20,* 477–484.

Woods, J. R., Plessinger, M. A., & Clark, K. E. (1987). Effects of cocaine on uterine blood flow and fetal oxygenation. *Journal of the American Medical Association, 257,* 957–961.

PART III

Assesment of Specific Psychopathologies

7

Assessment of Conduct Problems

NICOLE R. POWELL, JOHN E. LOCHMAN, MELISSA F. JACKSON, LAURA YOUNG, and ANNA YAROS

The completion of this chapter has been supported by grants to the second author from the National Institute on Drug Abuse (DA 08453; DA 16135), the Centers for Disease Control and Prevention (R49/CCR 418569), and the Office of Juvenile Justice and Delinquency Prevention (2006-JL-FX-0232). Correspondence about this paper can be directed to: John E. Lochman, Ph.D., Department of Psychology, Box 870348, The University of Alabama, Tuscaloosa, AL 35487.

ASSESSMENT OF CONDUCT DISORDERS

Conduct Disorder is one of the most common reasons for referral of a child or adolescent for psychological or psychiatric treatment (Nelson, Finch, & Hart, 2006). The prevalence and the nature of Conduct Disorder and other disruptive behavior problems exact a high cost to identified children and their families, as well as to the educational system, the community, and society at large. As a result, the need for services for children displaying serious behavior problems is clear, and a thorough comprehensive assessment is a critical first step in making an accurate diagnosis and identifying key factors that serve to maintain or exacerbate symptoms. In this chapter, we define Conduct Disorder and related behavior problems, provide information on associated factors, and describe relevant issues in the assessment of these problems in children and adolescents.

NICOLE R. POWELL, JOHN E. LOCHMAN, MELISSA F. JACKSON, LAURA YOUNG, and ANNA YAROS • Department of Psychology, University of Alabama, Tuscaloosa, AL.

J.L. Matson et al. (eds.), *Assessing Childhood Psychopathology and Developmental Disabilities*, DOI: 10.1007/978-0-387-09528-8,
© Springer Science+Business Media, LLC 2009

Conduct Disorder and Related Problems

Conduct disorders, aggression, and delinquency are all terms that refer to antisocial behaviors that indicate an inability or failure of an individual to conform to his or her societal norms, authority figures, or respect the rights of others (Frick, 1998; Lochman, 2000). These behaviors can range from chronic annoying of others and argumentativeness with adults to stealing, vandalism, and physical harm to others. Although these behaviors cover a broad spectrum of problems, they are highly correlated, with few children showing one type of behavior in the absence of others (Frick et al., 1993). This relatedness of behaviors is considered to be indicative of a single psychological dimension, generally referred to as antisocial behaviors or conduct problems.

Antisocial behaviors of children and adolescents have long been a major concern of society, in part because of the enormous public costs. The costs of a life of crime include government expenditures for criminal justice investigation, arrest, adjudication, and incarceration; as well as costs to victims, such as medical costs, time missed from work, the value of stolen property as well as loss of life, and costs that accrue to the criminal and his or her family, such as lost wages (Foster, Jones, & Conduct Problems Prevention Research Group [CPPRG], 2005). The social cost of adolescent delinquency exceeds $70,000 over a seven-year period (Foster et al., 2005). As a result, society has given increased attention to juvenile correction facilities, early intervention programs such as Fast Track developed by the CPPRG (2004a), and evidence-based intervention programs that have been found to produce reductions in delinquency and serious conduct problem behavior (Chamberlain & Reid, 1998; Henggeler, Melton, & Smith, 1992; Lochman & Wells, 2004). Aggressive and disruptive behaviors are among the most enduring dysfunctions in children, and if left untreated, frequently result in high personal and emotional cost to the child, the family, and to society in general. As a direct result, much research has investigated the causes, treatment, and prevention of conduct problems.

As a clinical syndrome with a broad list of symptoms, it is logical to expect much heterogeneity within the group that falls under the umbrella term of conduct problems. In addition to heterogeneity in the type of conduct problems manifested, children with conduct problems also can differ in the causal factors involved, the developmental course of the problems, the response to treatment, and the interaction between any of these.

There is strong agreement that children with conduct problems are a very heterogeneous group, however, there is significantly less consensus about the most appropriate method of classifying conduct problems into meaningful subtypes. One of the most widely used and accepted classifications of disruptive behavior disorders is in the fourth edition of the *Diagnostic and Statistical Manual of Mental Disorders (DSM-IV;* American Psychiatric Association [APA], 1994). The criteria employ a two-dimensional approach with an explicit symptom list for making a diagnosis. This system divides conduct problems into two syndromes: Conduct Disorder (CD) and Oppositional Defiant Disorder (ODD).

CD encompasses symptoms that fall into one of four classes of behavioral problems consisting of: aggressive conduct that threatens physical harm to other people or animals (bullies, threatens, or intimidates others;

often initiates physical fights; uses a weapon), nonaggressive conduct that causes property loss or damage (fire setting; property destruction), deceitfulness and theft (stealing; breaking into someone's house or car), and serious violations of rules (truancy from school; running away from home). The diagnosis of CD is made if the child or adolescent has displayed at least 3 of the 15 symptoms during the past twelve months.

The *DSM-IV* also distinguishes between children who begin showing conduct problems in early childhood from those who begin showing conduct problems closer to adolescence. If any symptoms are present prior to age 10, with the child meeting criteria for CD, he or she is classified as Childhood-Onset Type. However, if criteria are met for CD and no symptoms are present prior to age 10, the child is classified Adolescent-Onset Type. CD children with childhood-onset are more likely to display the aggressive component of the disorder, are more likely to drop out of school, and are more likely to persist in their conduct problems over time (Nelson et al., 2006).

Although childhood-onset conduct problems tend to reflect aggressive behavior, adolescent-onset conduct problems tend to reflect more delinquent behavior such as vandalism and theft (Zoccolillo, 1993). This distinction between Childhood-Onset and Adolescent-Onset CD is consistent with Moffitt's (1993) identification of youth with life-course persistent antisocial behavior, in contrast to other delinquent youth who have adolescent-limited antisocial behavior. Youths with life-course persistent antisocial behavior are at early risk because of combined biological and family factors. Conversely, children classified as Adolescent-Onset type typically display disruptive behaviors, particularly in the company of peers, but do not usually exhibit severe behavior problems or continued conduct problems into adulthood.

Conceptually there seems to be an important relationship between CD and ODD. ODD is defined as a recurrent pattern of negativistic, defiant, disobedient, and hostile behavior toward authority figures. ODD behaviors are usually apparent in the preschool years, and have been linked to problematic temperaments in infancy and childhood. Research indicates that CD is a developmentally advanced form of ODD, and that there are similar correlates for both ODD and CD. Both children with ODD and children with CD come from lower socioeconomic status (Frick et al., 1992; Keenan, Loeber, Zhang, Stouthamer-Loeber, & Van Kammen, 1995), are more likely to have a parent with a history of Antisocial Personality Disorder (APD; Faraone, Biederman, Kenean, & Tsuang, 1991; Frick, et al., 1992), and to have parents who use ineffective discipline practices (Frick et al., 1993).

Undoubtedly, the frequency with which children or adolescents manifest clinically significant and impairing levels of conduct problems is greatly determined by the definition used for such conduct when surveying populations. The *DSM-IV* notes a prevalence ranging between 2 and 16% for ODD (APA, 1994). For CD, rates of 6–16% for males and 2–9% for females have been cited (APA, 1994). Sex ratios in research studies have been approximately 3–4:1(males to females) for both ODD and CD. Both disorders, therefore, occur more commonly in males than in females, but ratios vary widely as a function of both the age of the child and the definition of the disorder (APA, 1994; Hinshaw & Anderson, 1996). The higher rate for boys is associated primarily with childhood-onset; the male to female ratio evens out in adolescence. Characteristic symptom patterns tend to differ as well. Males with CD are especially likely to develop substance abuse problems and APD in adulthood (Nelson et al., 2006)

Children who meet criteria for ODD or CD are likely to meet criteria for other disorders as well. This co-existence of more than one disorder is referred to as comorbidity. Comorbidity with ODD and CD is the rule rather than the exception, especially with regard to Attention-Deficit/Hyperactivity Disorder (ADHD). In clinic samples of children with CD, 75–90% had co-occurring ADHD (Abikoff & Klein, 1992). Comorbidity with ADHD seems to affect the manifestation and course of conduct disorders. The presence of ADHD in CD/ODD children produces more severe, chronic, and aggressive conduct problems and increased peer rejection (Abikoff & Klein, 1992). CD and ODD can also be comorbid with anxiety (60–75% of clinic-referred CD children) and depression (15–31% of CD children; Hinshaw, Lahey & Hart, 1993). For these comorbid children, affect regulation difficulties may lead to co-occurring problems with children's expression of anger, anxiety, and depression.

Researchers are beginning to identify psychological features in some antisocial youth that are linked to subsequent psychopathy (Barry, Frick, DeShazo, McCoy, Ellis, & Loney, 2000). These youth who have psychopathic features display manipulation, impulsivity, and remorseless patterns of interpersonal behavior, are usually referred to as "callous/unemotional," and are considered to be conceptually different from youth diagnosed with CD who do not have these features (Hart & Hare, 1997). Low levels of fearfulness have been associated with higher levels of the callous and unemotional traits in delinquent adolescents (Pardini, Lochman, & Frick, 2003).

One of the most distressing qualities of conduct disorders is the enduring stability of these disorders over the course of childhood and adolescence and even potentially into adulthood. Aggression may be one of the most enduring forms of psychopathology in children (Frick, 1998). Longitudinal research has indicated that CD is often a precursor of APD in adulthood (Myers, Burket, & Otto, 1993). It is estimated that 80% of youth who have severe antisocial behavior are likely to have future psychiatric disorders (Kazdin, 2004), and approximately half of children with CD will develop significant APD symptomatology. Two factors that predict the development of APD are the number of CD symptoms the child exhibits and early age of onset of symptoms (APA, 1994). In addition, ODD and CD children who show pervasive symptoms in a variety of settings (e.g., home, school, community) are at risk for a wide range of negative outcomes in adolescence including, truancy, substance use, early teenage parenthood, and delinquency (Lochman & Wayland, 1994).

Contributing Factors

Empirical research has identified numerous factors associated with the development and maintenance of aggressive and disruptive behaviors. These contributing factors can be conceptualized within a contextual social-cognitive model (Lochman & Wells, 2002), which describes how certain family and community characteristics influence conduct problems directly, as well as indirectly through their impact on mediating processes. The contextual social-cognitive model posits that stressors within the family and neighborhood can adversely affect children's behavior; in addition, these stressors affect parenting practices, influencing child psychological and social processes and, in turn, resulting in behavioral consequences such as aggression, delinquency, and substance abuse.

For clarity of presentation, contributing factors encompassed in the contextual social-cognitive model of child conduct problems are presented in two categories: contextual factors and child-level factors. Although several of these factors are malleable and represent clear targets for assessment and intervention, others are less susceptible to change. Nonetheless, it is useful to assess for each of these factors as part of a thorough case conceptualization that can guide treatment planning and goals.

Contextual Factors

Family Factors

Disruptive behavior problems in children have been associated with family characteristics such as low SES and poverty, low levels of maternal education, and teenage parenthood (Keenan et al., 1995; McLeod & Shanahan, 1996; Nagin & Tremblay, 2001). Parents who experience mental health issues such as depression (e.g., Barry, Dunlap, Cotton, Lochman, & Wells, 2005), substance abuse (e.g., Loeber, Green, Keenan, & Lahey, 1995), and APD (e.g., Lahey et al., 1995) are more likely to have a child with disruptive behavior problems. Conduct problems are also more common in children whose families experience stressful life events (e.g., Barry et al., 2005), marital discord (e.g., Erath, Bierman, & CPPRG, 2006), and multiple changes in family composition (Ackerman, Brown, D'Eramo, & Izard, 2002). This set of risk factors can lead to less effective parenting practices and, as a result, increased child behavior problems.

Parenting Factors

The relation between parenting practices and child behavior problems is reciprocal and ongoing; poor parenting can exacerbate child behavior problems, and on the other hand, negative, oppositional child behaviors can elicit ineffective reactions from parents (e.g., Fite, Colder, Lochman, & Wells, 2006). Specific parenting practices that are associated with child behavior problems include punitive discipline practices, spanking, physical aggression, inconsistency, low levels of warmth and involvement, and poor monitoring (e.g., Haapasalo & Tremblay, 1994; Stormshak, Bierman, McMahon, Lengua, & CPPRG, 2000).

Peer Factors

Similar to the reciprocal relation between parenting practices and child conduct problems, peer relations and child behavior also affect each other in a bidirectional manner (CPPRG, 2004b). Aggressive children are at increased risk of peer rejection (Cillessen, Van IJzendoorn, Van Lieshout, & Hartup, 1992), and aggressive children who are rejected by their peers demonstrate increasing conduct problems over time (e.g., Coie, Lochman, Terry, & Hyman, 1992). Children and adolescents who are rejected by peers in general are more likely to associate with a deviant peer group, leading to modeling, reinforcement, and increased opportunity for antisocial behaviors (Dishion, Andrews, & Crosby, 1995).

Community Factors

The broader environmental context also has an effect on child behavior prolems, and certain neighborhood and school characteristics are associated with increased conduct problems in children. With regard to neighborhood factors, high levels of community violence can lead directly to increased child conduct problems and can influence children's beliefs about the acceptability of aggression (Guerra, Huesmann, & Spindler, 2003). Neighborhood problems can also exacerbate child behavior problems through their negative effect on parenting practices (Pinderhughes, Nix, Foster, Jones, & CPPRG, 2001). Other neighborhood risk factors for conduct problems include high levels of residential instability, poverty, and elevated unemployment rates (see Leventhal & Brooks-Gunn, 2000 for a review).

In the school setting, children who are exposed to high levels of peer aggression tend to increase their own aggressive behavior (Barth, Dunlap, Dane, Lochman, & Wells, 2004). Over the course of several grades, children who spend more time in classrooms characterized by high rates of aggression exhibit more aggressive behavior than peers who have less exposure to classroom aggression (Thomas, Bierman, & CPPRG, 2006). Children's attitudes about school can also affect their behavior, and those who are poorly bonded to their schools are also at risk for increased behavior problems and substance abuse (Maddox & Prinz, 2003).

Child-Level Factors

Social-Cognitive Factors

Children and adolescents who exhibit conduct problems have been shown to demonstrate characteristic deficits in their cognitive processing of interpersonal situations. The social-information processing model presented by Crick and Dodge (1994) provides a useful framework to describe the difficulties exhibited by disruptive children. This model encompasses six steps, and, as a group, aggressive children have been shown to have problems at each of these; however, individual aggressive children generally exhibit deficits at only a few steps (Orobio de Castro, Veerman, Koops, Bosch, & Monshouwer, 2002).

The steps of the social-information processing model include: (1) encoding of relevant cues, (2) interpretation of cues, (3) identification of social goals, (4) response formulation, (5) selection of a response, and (6) behavioral enactment. In the first step, disruptive children tend to selectively recall aggressive, rather than neutral, cues related to an event, to display a pronounced recency effect in their recall of cues, and to recall fewer relevant cues overall (Crick & Dodge, 1994). In the second step, disruptive children tend to ascribe hostile intent to others' actions in neutral or ambiguous situations (i.e., hostile attribution bias; Orobio de Castro et al., 2002), but underestimate their own aggressive behavior (Lochman, 1987; Lochman & Dodge, 1998).

When identifying their social goals in an interpersonal interaction, the third step of processing, disruptive children are more likely to pursue goals of retaliation and dominance over social affiliation and constructive problem-solving goals (Erdley & Asher, 1996). In the fourth step of processing, response formulation, disruptive children display deficiencies in both the quantity and the quality of solutions they generate (Lochman, Meyer, Rabiner, & White, 1991). Although most disruptive children are able to formulate an adequate number of possible social problem-solving solutions, the most seriously aggressive youth produce fewer options (Lochman & Dodge, 1994). Qualitatively, solutions to interpersonal problems generated by disruptive children tend to be less developmentally advanced and less effective in preserving relationships. For example, disruptive children tend to identify more direct-action and help-seeking solutions, and fewer solutions involving verbal assertion and compromise (Larson & Lochman, 2002).

In the fifth step of processing, selection of a response, individuals must identify and evaluate the consequences of each possible solution, then use this information to select the response that is most consistent with an identified goal. Aggressive and disruptive children tend to view aggression as a useful and acceptable solution that will help them to achieve their goals, and may be more likely to select an aggressive response to an interpersonal problem (Larson & Lochman, 2002). Behavioral enactment, the final processing step, may present a challenge for disruptive children who are more likely to have difficulties in carrying out prosocial behaviors (Dodge, Pettit, McClaskey, & Brown, 1986).

In the assessment of conduct problems, an awareness of these potential social-cognitive deficiencies is important in identifying the specific processes that may influence and maintain disruptive behaviors in a given child, which has useful implications for treatment. For example, a child who displays a strong hostile attribution bias can be helped to view frustrating situations in a more productive way through perspective-taking exercises, whereas a child who displays an overreliance on direct-action or help-seeking responses to interpersonal conflict can be coached in the use of verbal assertion and compromise.

Self Regulation and Self Control

Strong, unregulated emotional arousal and impulsivity have been associated with disruptive behavior problems in children (Larson & Lochman, 2002). Compared with nonaggressive children, children with disruptive behaviors have been shown to display more intense reactions on physiological indicators in response to provocation and frustration (van Goozen, Matthys, Cohen-Kettenis, Gispen-de Wied, Wiegant, & van

Engeland, 1998; Williams, Lochman, Phillips, & Barry, 2003). Under conditions of emotional arousal, aggressive children tend to problem-solve in an automatic, reactive manner, generating less competent, direct-action solutions than when they are calm and able to use more deliberate problem-solving strategies (Rabiner, Lenhart, & Lochman, 1990). Increases in physiological arousal may also lead to more pronounced cognitive distortions (Williams et al., 2003). In the absence of adequate self-regulatory and self-control skills, disruptive children may quickly become overaroused in conflictual situations, leading to problematic cognitive processes and behaviors.

ASSESSMENT OF BEHAVIOR

Rating Scales

The assessment of behavior via rating scales allows for a standardized means of obtaining information regarding the child's symptoms and behaviors. These ratings can be used to compare the child's symptom levels across time, as well as to compare her symptom level to that of other children her age. The accuracy of reports obtained through rating scales depends on the scales' reliability and validity, as well as the reporter's ability to rate the child openly, honestly, and adequately. Amidst the various scales used to assess for conduct disorders, there are opportunities to obtain self-, teacher-, and parent-reports of behaviors. Although many scales only utilize one informant, the Achenbach rating forms, Conners' rating forms, and the Behavior Assessment System for Children represent three sets of assessment instruments that include parent, teacher, and self-report versions.

Within the set of Achenbach measures, the Child Behavior Checklist (CBCL; Achenbach, 1991a) is a parent-report measure, the Teacher's Report Form (TRF; Achenbach, 1991b) relies on teacher-report, and the Youth Self Report (YSR; Achenbach, 1991c) is a self-report measure. Each of these measures assesses externalizing and internalizing problems in children and adolescents. The CBCL is a 120-item measure, scored on a 3-point scale, with nine subscales intended for ages 4 to 18 years. The TRF also contains 120 items scored on a 3-point scale, but it has only eight subscales (it does not include the sex problems subscale) and is intended for ages 6 to 18 years. Both the CBCL and TRF take approximately 10 to 15 minutes to complete. They also both produce an externalizing score (the sum of the delinquent behavior and aggressive behavior subscales), an internalizing score, and a total problem score. The YSR, which can be completed in approximately 30 minutes, contains 119 items scored on a 3-point scale and is intended for ages 11 to 18 years. It contains nine scales that include social problems, attention problems, delinquent behavior, and aggressive behavior. The internal consistency of the various measures range from .56 to .92 for the CBCL, .63 to .96 for the TRF, and .59 to .90 for the YSR. All three scales are thought to have satisfactory validity. Whereas the Achenbach set of measures allows for a cross-informant assessment, some of the scales have rather low reliability. This measure should be viewed as a broad-based screening measure.

The Behavior Assessment System for Children-Second Edition (BASC-2; Reynolds & Kamphaus, 2005) includes the BASC-2 Parent Rating Scale (BASC-2 PRS), Teacher Rating Scale (BASC-2 TRS), and Self-Report of Personality (BASC-2 SRP). Each measure is intended to assess psychological functioning in children and adolescents, including adaptive and problem behaviors.

The BASC-2 PRS can be completed in about 20 minutes, consists of 134 to 160 items, is scored on a 4-point scale, and is intended for ages 2 to 21 years. From these items, 14 subscales (including aggression and conduct problems subscales) and four composite scores (including an externalizing problems composite, adaptive skills composite, and behavioral symptoms index) are created.

The BASC-2 TRS contains 109 to 148 items scored on a 4-point scale, is intended for ages 4 to 18 years, and is typically completed within 30 minutes. The BASC-2 TRS contains 15 subscales (including aggression and conduct problem subscales) and five composite scores (including an externalizing problems composite, adaptive skills composite, and behavioral symptoms index).

The BASC-2 SRP has 139 to 176 items, with some items scored on a 4-point scale and some using a true–false scoring method. This self-report measure is intended for ages 8 to 21 years, and it takes about 30 minutes to complete. The BASC-2 SRP contains 16 subscales (including hyperactivity, interpersonal relations, school adjustment, and social stress subscales) and five composite scores (including inattention/hyperactivity, personal adjustment, and school problems composite scores).

The internal consistency of the BASC-2 measures ranges from .80 to .95 for the BASC-2 PRS, .62 to .95 for the BASC-2 TRS, and .78 to .94 for the BASC-2 SRP. This set of BASC measures also allows for cross-informant assessment, and is particularly strong at evaluating externalizing problems.

The Conners' Rating Scales-Revised (CRS-R; Conners, 1997) have a primary emphasis on externalizing problems. Within this set of instruments are the Conners' Parent Rating Scale–Revised (CPRS-R), the Conners' Teacher Rating Scale-Revised (CTRS-R), and the Conners–Wells' Adolescent Self-Report Scale (CASS). Each measure has a short and long form version.

The CPRS-R has a 27-item short version with four subscales (including oppositional and hyperactivity scales) and an 80-item long version with ten subscales (including those listed in the short form plus such scales as the social problems subscale). Both versions use a 4-point rating scale and are intended for use with children aged 3 to 17 years. The short version takes approximately 5 to 10 minutes to complete, and the long version will typically take 15 to 20 minutes. The CTRS-R includes a 28-item short form with four subscales and a 59-item long form with nine subscales. The short and long form versions of the CTRS-R are similar to the CPRS-R in terms of subscales and length of administration.

The CASS is designed for ages 12 to 17 years, has both a 27-item short form with five subscales and an 87-item long form with eight subscales, and utilizes a 4-point rating scale.

Both forms have conduct problems, anger control problems, and hyperactive-impulsive subscales. The internal consistency of the Conners' scales ranges from .73 to .96 for the CPRS-R and CTRS-R and from .75 to .92 for the CASS. The measures have satisfactory to good convergent and discriminant validity. The CRS-R scales in general are quite useful for evaluating externalizing problems. However, although the CASS may be useful in determining general distress, its focus is limited to social and emotional problems.

Parent Informant Scales

In addition to the sets of measures described above, the Devereux Scales of Mental Disorders and the Personality Inventory for Children-Second Edition are parent-report measures useful for assessing conduct disorders. The Devereux Scales of Mental Disorders (DSMD; Naglieri, LeBuffe, & Pfeiffer, 1994) can be used with children ages 5 to 18 years, and consist of 110 (adolescent version) or 111 (child version) items that can be completed in 15 minutes and are scored on a 5-point scale. Both the child and adolescent versions create externalizing, internalizing, and critical pathology composite scores. Additionally, they both contain six subscales, which include conduct and attention subscales for children, and conduct and delinquency subscales for adolescents. Although the DSMD has limited validity, its internal consistency ranges from .70 to .99.

The Personality Inventory for Children-Second Edition (PIC-2; Wirt, Lachar, Seat, & Broen, 2001) is a 275-item true–false measure of behavioral, emotional, cognitive, and interpersonal adjustment in children and adolescents ages 5 to 19 years old that takes approximately 40 minutes to complete. The PIC-2 consists of 21 adjustment subscales and nine adjustment scales, including a delinquency scale. The adjustment scale's internal consistency ranges from .75 to. 91 and its convergent and discriminant validity are satisfactory. The PIC-2 covers a range of problems and provides validity scales.

Teacher Informant Scales

The Devereux Scales of Mental Disorders (DSMD) utilize the same exact measure for the parent- and teacher-informant versions. As such, see the above discussion of the DSMD for details regarding the teacher-informant version of this measure. Among teachers, the DSMD has internal consistency ranging from .76 to .98.

The Revised Behavior Problem Checklist (RBPC; Quay & Peterson, 1996) is an 89-item measure intended for ages 5 to 18 years that takes approximately 15 to 20 minutes to complete. The RBPC focuses primarily on externalizing problems, with six subscales including conduct disorder, socialized aggression, and attention problems–immaturity. Items are rated on a 3-point scale. Internal consistency ranges from .68 to .95 and validity is satisfactory.

The Student Behavior Survey (SBS; Lachar, Wingenfeld, Kline, & Gruber, 2000) contains 102 items, is meant for ages 5 to 18 years, and contains three sections with 14 total subscales. The adjustment problems and disruptive behavior sections include such subscales as verbal aggression, physical aggression, behavior problems, oppositional defiant, and conduct problems. All subscales are scored on a 4-point scale, except for the performance subscale which uses a 5-point scale. The internal consistency of the SBS ranges from .86 to .95, and its convergent and discriminant validity are satisfactory. Although its validity is satisfactory, the SBS should be used cautiously, as some of its scales demonstrate low test–retest reliability (ranging from .29 to .94).

Self-Report Scales

The Personality Inventory for Youth (PIY; Lachar & Gruber, 1995a,b) is a companion measure to the parent-reported PIC-2. The PIY contains 270 true–false items, takes 30 to 60 minutes to complete, and is intended for youth aged 10 to 18 years. Among its nine scales are an impulsivity and distractibility scale, delinquency scale, and social skills deficits scale. These nine scales are broken down further into 24 subscales which include impulsivity, antisocial behavior, dyscontrol, noncompliance, and conflict with peers. Its internal consistency ranges from .71 to .90, and it has satisfactory validity.

The Minnesota Multiphasic Personality Inventory-Adolescent (MMPI-A; Butcher et al., 1992) can provide useful information on adolescent psychopathology. It is designed for adolescents ages 14 to 18 years old, contains 478 true–false items, takes 60 to 90 minutes to complete, and has 10 basic scales, 7 validity scales, and 15 content scales. The basic scales include a psychopathic deviate scale, and the content scales include an anger scale and conduct problems scale. The internal consistency is low to moderate, ranging from .40 to .89, as is the validity. MMPI-A can only be used with a limited age range, and some items may be difficult for younger adolescents to understand. It may provide useful information on psychopathology, however, users should be aware of the MMPI-A's low reliability and validity and be sure to consult the manuals for interpretation purposes.

The Adolescent Psychopathology Scale (APS; Reynolds, 1998a,b) and Adolescent Psychopathology Scale-Short Form (APS-SF; Reynolds, 2000) assess externalizing and internalizing disorders in children and adolescents ages 12 to 19 years. The APS has 346 items, takes 45 to 60 minutes to complete, measures the 25 *DSM–IV–TR* disorders as well as various social and emotional problems, and contains 40 scales (including Conduct Disorder, Oppositional Defiant Disorder, Anger, Aggression, Interpersonal Problem, and Emotional Lability scales). The APS-SF has 115 items, takes 15 to 20 minutes to complete, assesses 12 central components of social and emotional functioning, and has 14 subscales (including Conduct Disorder, Oppositional Defiant Disorder, Anger/Violence Proneness, and Interpersonal Problems subscales). Both the APS and APS-SF have variable rating scales throughout their subscales. The internal consistency ranges from .69 to .95 for the APS and .80 to .91 for the APS-SF, and both scales have good validity. Both of these scales provide strong assessments of critical components of adolescent psychopathology.

Interview Measures

Another way of obtaining information regarding a child's presenting problems is through a clinical assessment interview. These interviews can take on various forms. They may be an unstructured interview in which the interviewee is encouraged to describe concerns with some guidance from the interviewer. This form of interview allows the interviewer to structure the time as desired and to follow up on statements made by the interviewee. The semi-structured interview provides guidelines for the interview, but still allows for the examiner to rephrase as needed, follow leads, and have more liberty when interpreting results.

The Hare Psychopathy Checklist: Youth Version (PCL:YV; Forth, Kosson, & Hare, 2003) is an example of a semi-structured interview that assists with the assessment of psychopathology in adolescents. It is intended for ages 12 to 18 years and takes approximately 90 to 120 minutes to complete the interview section and 60 minutes to complete the collateral review 20-item rating scale. The PCL:YV measures interpersonal, affective, behavioral, and emotional features related to psychopathy.

Another semi-structured interview is the Child Assessment Schedule (CAS; Hodges, Kline, Stern, Cytryn, & McKnew, 1982). This interview includes a parent and child version and is intended for use in assessing children ages 7 to 16 years. Responses are scored on a 3-point scale. This interview contains 11 content scales addressing overall functioning and psychopathology, including measurements of mood and behavior, acting out, and social relationships. The CAS has adequate reliability and validity.

Structured interviews are highly structured with set protocols for the progression through the interview. These stringent guidelines are used to increase reliability and validity of the interviews and decrease interviewer bias and clinical inference. These interviews require some specialized training.

The Child and Adolescent Psychiatric Assessment (CAPA; Angold et al., 1995) is a structured interview with versions for children ages 9 to 18 years and their parents. It is divided into 15 domains, including a disruptive behavior disorders domain which includes assessment of symptoms related to ODD, CD, Delinquency, and ADHD. The interview can be completed in approximately 90 minutes and allows a detailed examination of symptom ratings.

The Diagnostic Interview Schedule for Children Version IV (DISC-IV; Shaffer, Fisher, Lucas, Dulcan, & Schwab-Stone, 2000) is a structured interview that assesses current and lifetime childhood disorders. The parent-informant version is intended for children ages 6 to 17 years, and the youth-informant version is intended for children ages 9 to 17 years. This interview is composed of 358 standard questions and 1,341 optional probes. It is divided into six diagnostic sections, including a section for disruptive behavior disorders. The administration time varies on level of symptom endorsement and may range between 70 minutes and 120 minutes. This measure has high reliability and validity. However, it is often thought to have an overly rigid structure.

The Diagnostic Interview for Children and Adolescents-Revised (DICA-R) was created in 1998 to classify *DSM–III–R* categories of disorders and represents a revised version of the DICA (Herjanic & Reich, 1982). There are child and parent versions of the DICA-R, intended for ages 6 to 17 years. The interview elicits yes or no responses and takes approximately 60 minutes to administer. The sections of the DICA-R cover several mental disorders including conduct disorders.

ASSESSMENT OF ASSOCIATED FEATURES—CHILDREN AND ADOLESCENTS

Measures of Peer Relations

Sociometrics

Children with conduct disorders often have impairments in social functioning that play out in their relationships with peers. Several types of assessments exist for evaluating how children with conduct disorders get along with their peers. The first type, peer-referenced assessments, involves the child's peers in the evaluative process. This usually takes the form of sociometric peer nominations, which measure social acceptance or social status at school (Coie, Dodge, & Coppotelli, 1982). Children are asked to rank their peers, often in a class at school, on items such as "like most," and "like least." Using this type of assessment, children who have CD are often identified as disliked by their peers.

Although this is the only widely used peer-referenced assessment technique, it can be used to ask a variety of types of questions about children. Using a similar nomination method, clinicians can also ask peers about various other impressions of a child. Other questions that have been employed in sociometric instruments include items about other forms of social status such as power and popularity (Vaillancourt & Hymel, 2006). Other questions can ask peers about impressions of child characteristics and behaviors, such as attractiveness and aggressiveness (Coie et al., 1982). Reliability data suggest that these types of questions about social status and child behaviors (α = .76 to .91) may have more internal consistency than the classic "like most/like least" questions (α = .65; Coie et al., 1982; Vaillancourt & Hymel, 2006). The drawback of using such an assessment is the level of effort required to get information on one child for clinical purposes.

Social Skills Measures

Measures of social skills are easier to collect than sociometrics, but less informative about a child's real-life peer relationships. The connection often observed between rejection by peers and conduct disorders may, in some cases, be linked to deficits in social skills. Several measures evaluate social skills in children with CD. Some omnibus measures of child behavior include items that relate directly to social behavior.

As described above, the BASC-2 (Reynolds & Kamphaus, 2005) contains a variety of questions pertaining to primary features of conduct disorders, but also includes scales measuring social skills. Similarly, the CBCL, the TRF, and the YSR (Achenbach, 1991a,b,c) include questions pertaining to children's social skills, which make up the "Social Problems" subscale. Some of these ask teachers, parents, and children to rate the extent to which the child "Acts too young for his/her age" and "Gets teased a lot."

Measures developed entirely to evaluate children's social skills are also a good option for determining skill levels and deficits in children with conduct disorders. The Social Skills Rating Scales (SSRS; Gresham & Elliot, 1990) is one such social skills measure that includes checklists for the teacher, parent, and child. It is a good measure of social skills, while also containing scales of problem behaviors and academic competence. The internal consistency of the SSRS is $\alpha = .83$ indicating that it has adequate reliability, although interrater reliability across parent, teacher, and child report forms is generally poor ($r = .03$ to .29; Disperna & Volpe, 2005).

The Social Behavior Assessment Inventory (SBAI) is another measure of social skills, but only as they occur in one setting. It asks teachers to report on children's social behavior in a variety of school-related contexts. Psychometrics of this test indicate good reliability and validity (Kelley, Reitman, & Noell, 2003). Finally, the Home and Community Social Behavior Scale (HCSBS; Merrell & Calderella, 2002) and the School Social Behavior Scale (SSBS; Merrell, 2002) make up the Social Behavior Scales (SBS). The two components of the SBS differ primarily in the settings where they are administered and both include Social Competence and Antisocial Behavior subscales. Internal consistency of the SBS is excellent, with alpha coefficients as high as .98.

MEASURES OF SOCIAL COGNITION

As indicated in previous sections of this chapter, aggression and related behaviors in conduct disorders are associated with elements of social cognition. Several instruments have been developed to measure the stages of social-information processing, but few show strong reliability and validity across extensive utilization.

Attending to social cues is a first step of processing information in interpersonal situations. A test of attention to social cues is the Recall Task developed by Milich and Dodge (1984). The test presents children with a series of neutral, positive, and hostile statements intermixed. The child then reports what he or she can recall. In aggressive children, responses often tend toward the recall of the hostile statements and the addition of hostile rephrasing of the neutral and positive statements.

Tests of children's processes during the interpretation step in the social information processing model often rely on measures of hostile attribution bias. One measure of hostile attribution bias is Dodge et al.'s (1986) measure using vignettes to assess how children interpret ambiguous cues. Children report whether they interpret the antagonist in the vignettes as doing things accidentally or with hostility. Subsequent adaptation of the measure has yielded a collection of vignettes that have alpha coefficients above .70 and that reliably distinguish aggressive from nonaggressive children (Lochman & Dodge, 1994). Leff and colleagues (2006) have also developed a cartoon-based hostile attribution measure designed expressly for African American girls. The measure showed strong internal consistency (α = .76) and test–retest reliability (r = .79 to .82) in an African American sample of urban girls aged 9 to 10 years.

The goal-setting step of social cognition can be measured using the Child Social Goal Measure (Lochman, Wayland, & White, 1993). The scale uses vignettes of parent–child and child–peer conflict to assess what children hope to gain from their attempt to resolve the conflict. Choices reflect goals of avoidance, dominance, revenge, and affiliation.

The stage of the social information processing model involved in response access and response decision is supported by a robust group of measures of child problem-solving. To test children's access to various responses, clinicians can use the Means-Ends Problem-Solving Procedure (MEPS; Spivack, Shure, & Platt, 1985). The measure presents the child with a story that includes a problem and its resolution and asks the child to develop the solution that led to the resolution. Reliability (α = .80 to .84) and validity of this measure support its utility in assessment of children with CD.

Measures of response decision typically rely on self-report of how a problem was solved. The Problem Solving Inventory (PSI; Heppner, 1988), although developed for adults, can also be used with adolescents (Baker & Roberts, 1989). Scales of the PSI measure Problem-Solving Confidence, Personal Control, and Approach-Avoidance Style. Additionally, strong internal consistency (α = .72 to .85) and test–retest correlations (r = .83 to .89) make it a good choice for a clinician wanting to quickly measure problem solving abilities. The Problem-Solving Measure for Conflict (PSM-C; Lochman & Dodge, 1994) uses vignettes missing their middle parts in the same way that the MEPS does. Responses are coded for problem-solving strategy used (e.g., Verbal Assertion, Direct Action, Help Seeking). This measure exhibits interrater reliability kappas above .66 and is able to discriminate between aggressive and nonaggressive children. An important use of measures of social cognition in children with conduct disorder is to gain qualitative information about symptoms in social situations; however, measures of social cognition are unlikely to be useful in making diagnoses because most lack norms and cutoff scores.

Record Review

School Records

Beyond teacher and parent reports of children's behavior, records from schools and courts provide insight into how children with conduct disorders are functioning in their environment. School records often provide data about disruptive behaviors that contribute to an accurate diagnosis of conduct disorders. School records take various forms and differ widely across different schools. Some of the most informative records are children's grades, attendance records, and discipline records.

Because children with conduct disorders often struggle to succeed in school, grades are an important indicator of the child's functioning. However, grades are affected not just by academic competence, but also by a variety of behavioral factors. Many children with conduct disorders fall behind in coursework because they are sent out of the class and/or suspended due to disruptive behavior. As such, poor grades are not always valid measures of ability in children who have conduct disorders.

Attendance records give clinicians data about truancy that may be hard to gather based on self-report or parent-report assessments. Behaviorally disordered youth and their parents may be reluctant to admit truant behaviors to clinicians, and, furthermore, children and adolescents with conduct disorders may be truant without the knowledge of their parents. Attendance issues brought to light by school records also suggest that possible deviant behaviors might occur during truant times, when monitoring is absent.

Discipline records provide information on symptoms of conduct disorders, such as aggression, vandalism, and deception. These records can help a clinician pinpoint behaviors that occur at school, as well as evaluate institutional responses to these behaviors. By understanding what type of discipline has been tried at school, and under what conditions, an evaluator can make informed treatment recommendations to pass on to the child's parents and school.

Court Records

Public records of arrests, charges, and convictions of crimes verify the existence of actions consistent with conduct disorders and help researchers track recidivism of children with juvenile records. For the clinician, court records can offer detailed information of an incident that might not otherwise be available or easy to recall. Similarly, a child's juvenile justice records provide clues to the severity and frequency of antisocial behavior. Still, it is important to note that court records do not provide information about behaviors and practices for which a child has yet to be caught.

ASSESSMENT OF ASSOCIATED FEATURES—CAREGIVERS

Although the diagnostic criteria for ODD and CD are based on features presented by the child, the assessment of associated caregiver variables is useful in determining treatment goals and caregiver features that may exacerbate and/or contribute to the child's symptoms. The assessment of caregiver features should be theoretically driven and should utilize multiple assessment methods and multiple informants whenever possible (McMahon & Metzler, 1998). Parenting skills, familial and environmental stress, and caregiver mental health conditions are the three areas that need to be considered as a part of a comprehensive assessment. Given the personal nature of the caregiver variables being investigated and the potential for misunderstandings about the purpose of such questions, this portion of the assessment must be handled with great care and sensitivity.

Prior to delving into the following areas, it is recommended that clinicians give informants an explanation about the importance and relevance of these factors in the assessment of the child's behavior problems.

Parenting Skills

As summarized above, certain parenting practices are associated with child behavior problems and may play a causal, maintenance, and/or exacerbating role in children's disruptive behaviors (Hinshaw & Lee, 2003). As such, it is important that assessment of parenting behaviors (e.g., discipline practices, supervision, and monitoring) and the parent–child relationship be included in a comprehensive evaluation for conduct problems. Parenting skills should be evaluated through multiple informants utilizing multiple methods such as structured and/or unstructured observations, the clinical interview, and measures specific to evaluating parenting behaviors.

Observing the interactions of the caregiver and child throughout the evaluation is vital and should be considered a part of the assessment battery. Structured observation techniques may also be useful, although they can be time-consuming and may involve more complex techniques (i.e., including a "blind" rater). Structured observation techniques may include teaching activities (e.g., asking the parent to teach the child a new math concept) and/or family play activities. Although observations are considered to be the most complex and time-consuming techniques to assess parenting skills, research has demonstrated that observations are more sensitive than other methods and are more consistent (Zaslow et al., 2006).

The clinical interview should include questions related to parenting style. One way this can be evaluated is by asking the caregiver to describe situations that resulted in the child being disciplined. Specifically, the caregiver might be asked about the context of the situation, the specific incident, why this incident was a problem for the parent, how the parent handled the situation, how the child reacted, and how the situation was resolved. This method allows the evaluator to determine whether the caregiver's expectations are developmentally appropriate and whether the discipline techniques being used are appropriate and effective.

Familial and Environmental Stress

Familial and environmental stress have been shown to be associated with behavior disorders in children (Haapasalo & Tremblay, 1994; Schachar & Tannock, 1995). Stressors should be evaluated through multiple informants utilizing the clinical interview and standardized measures. The clinical interview with the caregivers might include questions to gather information related to daily hassles, marital problems, financial problems, and child-related stressors (e.g., absent from work due to school conferences). Two specific measures have been used frequently to measure caregiver stress: the Parenting Stress Index, Third Edition (Abidin, 1997) and the Daily Life Experience Checklist (DLE, Stone & Neale, 1982).

The Parenting Stress Index has been used to assess child and caregiver characteristics that place a family at risk for dysfunctional interactions. The DLE is a checklist that includes daily stressors, yielding a rich source of information on parents' current life stressors. These measures used together as part of a "familial and environmental stress" assessment battery may yield important information relevant to assessment and treatment.

Caregiver Mental Health

Children whose caregivers have severe psychopathology are at an increased risk of experiencing caregiver–child interactional difficulties, poor monitoring, and other maladaptive caregiver behaviors (Hinshaw & Lee, 2003). As noted above, depression, substance abuse, and antisocial behavior patterns in caregivers have been shown to be related to child behavior problems (Hinshaw & Lee, 2003; Murray, Sinclair, Cooper, Ducournau, & Turner, 1999). A comprehensive evaluation of caregiver mental health would include a clinical interview with questions related to family criminal and arrest history; family mental health history; a broadband measure of caregiver functioning; disorder-specific measures to further assess scales that came out clinically significant on the broadband measure; and a follow-up interview to determine the severity of the caregiver's pathology, in the cases where significant mental health issues do arise.

SUMMARY

In this chapter, we have provided an overview of conduct problems and relevant contributing factors, and have presented a number of techniques and instruments for use in the evaluation of conduct disorders. Serious behavior problems in children and adolescents may present in any number of ways and, for youth with conduct disorders, the clinical picture tends to be complex. Due to the multifaceted nature of these problems and their contributing factors, thorough comprehensive assessment is critical for accuracy in diagnosis and in identifying targets for intervention. Specifically, features of the family, school, and community environments, peer relationships, and child social-cognitive functioning should be considered in addition to the referred child's behavioral functioning.

It is important to note that children's strengths should not be overlooked in such assessments; positive qualities are areas to capitalize on in clinical work with disruptive youth, and may represent valuable sources of motivation for behavior change (as in the case of an athletically gifted adolescent motivated to remain in school to play on a basketball team). Therefore, any evaluation involving conduct problems should also include an assessment of personal strengths and positive interests. As the first step in clinical work with children with conduct problems, comprehensive assessment can provide an invaluable guide to case conceptualization, treatment planning, and intervention.

REFERENCES

Abidin, R. (1997). Parenting stress index: A measure of the parent-child system. In C. P. Zalaquet & R. J. Wood (Eds.), *Evaluating stress: A book of resources*. Lanham, MD: Scarecrow Education.

Abikoff, H., & Klein, G. (1992). Attention-deficit hyperactivity and conduct disorder: Co-morbidity and implications for treatment. *Journal of Consulting and Clinical Psychology, 60,* 881–892.

Achenbach, T. M. (1991a). Manual for the Child Behavior Checklist and 1991 Profile. Burlington, VT: University Associates in Psychiatry.

Achenbach, T. M. (1991b). *Manual for the Teacher's Report Form and 1991 Profile.* Burlington, VT: University Associates in Psychiatry.

Achenbach, T. M. (1991c). *Manual for the Youth Self-Report and 1991 Profile.* Burlington, VT: University Associates in Psychiatry.

Ackerman, B. P., Brown, E. D., D'Eramo, K. S., & Izard, C. E. (2002). Maternal relationship instability and the school behavior of children from disadvantaged families. *Developmental Psychology, 38,* 694–704.

American Psychiatric Association. (1994). *The Diagnostic and Statistical Manual of Mental Disorders* (4th ed.). Washington, DC: Author.

Angold, A., Prendergast, M., Cox, A., Harrington, R., Simonoff, E., & Rutter, M. (1995). The Child and Adolescent Psychiatric Assessment (CAPA). *Psychological Medicine, 25,* 739–753.

Baker, S. B., & Roberts, D. M. (1989) The factor structure of the problem-solving inventory: Measuring perceptions of personal problem solving. *Measurement & Evaluation in Counseling & Development, 21,* 157–164.

Barry, C. T., Frick, P. J., DeShazo, T. M., McCoy, M., Ellis, M. E., & Loney, B. R. (2000). The importance of callous-unemotional traits for extending the concept of psychopathy to children. *Journal of Abnormal Psychology, 109,* 335–340.

Barry, T. D., Dunlap, S. T., Cotton, S. J., Lochman, J. E., & Wells, K. C. (2005). The influence of maternal stress and distress on disruptive behavior problems in children. *Journal of the American Academy of Child and Adolescent Psychiatry, 44,* 265–273.

Barth, J. M., Dunlap, S. T., Dane, H., Lochman, J. E., & Wells, K. C. (2004). Classroom environment influences on aggression, peer relations, and academic focus. *Journal of School Psychology, 42,* 115–133.

Butcher, J. N., Williams, C. L., Graham, J. R., Archer, R. P., Tellegen, A., Ben-Porath, Y. S., & Kaemmer, B. (1992). *MMPI-A (Minnesota Multiphasic Personality Inventory-Adolescent): Manual for administration, scoring, and interpretation.* Minneapolis: University of Minnesota Press.

Chamberlain, P., & Reid, J. B. (1998). Comparison of two community alternatives to incarceration for chronic juvenile offenders. *Journal of Consulting and Clinical Psychology, 66,* 624–633.

Cillessen, A. H., Van IJzendoorn, H. W., Van Lieshout, C. F., & Hartup, W. W. (1992). Heterogeneity among peer-rejected boys: Subtypes and stabilities. *Child Development, 63,* 893–905.

Coie, J. D., Dodge, K. A., & Coppotelli, H. (1982) Dimensions and types of social status: A cross-age perspective. *Developmental Psychology, 18,* 557–570.

Coie, J. D., Lochman, J. E., Terry, R., & Hyman, C. (1992). Predicting early adolescent disorder from childhood aggression and peer rejection. *Journal of Consulting and Clinical Psychology, 60,* 783–792.

Conduct Problems Prevention Research Group (2004a). The effects of the Fast Track program on serious problem outcomes at the end of elementary school. *Journal of Clinical Child and Adolescent Psychology, 33,* 650–661.

Conduct Problems Prevention Research Group (2004b). The Fast Track experiment: Translating the developmental model into a prevention design. In J. B. Kupersmidt & K. A. Dodge (Eds.), *Children's peer relations: From development to intervention* (pp.181–208). Washington, DC: American Psychological Association.

Conners, C. K. (1997). *Conners' Rating Scales-Revised: Technical manual.* North Tonawanda, NY: Multi-Health Systems.

Crick, N. R., & Dodge, K. A. (1994). A review and reformulation of social information-processing mechanisms in children's social adjustment. *Psychological Bulletin, 115,* 74–101.

Dishion, T. J., Andrews, D. W., & Crosby, L. (1995). Antisocial boys and their friends in early adolescence: Relationship characteristics, quality, and interactional process. *Child Development, 66,* 139–151.

Disperna, J. C. & Volpe, R. J. (2005) Self-report on the Social Skills Rating System: Analysis of reliability and validity for an elementary sample. *Psychology in the Schools, 42,* 345–354.

Dodge, K. A., Pettit, G. S., McClaskey, C. L., & Brown, M. M. (1986). Social competence in children. *Monographs of the Society for Research in Child Development, 51,* 1–85.

Erath, S. A., Bierman, K. L., & Conduct Problems Prevention Research Group. (2006) Aggressive marital conflict, maternal harsh punishment, and child aggressive-disruptive behavior: Evidence for direct and indirect relations. *Journal of Family Psychology, 20,* 217–226.

Erdley, C. A., & Asher, S. R. (1996). Children's social goals and self-efficacy perceptions as influences on their responses to ambiguous provocation. *Child Development, 67,* 1329–1344.

Faraone, S. V., Biederman, J., Keenan, K., & Tsuang, M. T. (1991). Separation of *DSM–III* attention deficit disorder and conduct disorder: Evidence from a family genetic study of American child psychiatry patients. *Psychological Medicine, 21,* 109–121.

Fite, P. J., Colder, C. R., Lochman, J. E., & Wells, K. C. (2006). The mutual influence of parenting and boys' externalizing behavior problems. *Journal of Applied Developmental Psychology, 27,* 151–164.

Forth, A. E., Kosson, D. S., & Hare, R. D. (2003). *The Psychopathy Checklist: Youth Version.* Toronto, ON: Multi-Health Systems.

Foster, E. M., Jones, D., & Conduct Problems Prevention Research Group (2005). The high costs of aggression: Public expenditures resulting from Conduct Disorder. *American Journal of Public Health, 95,* 1767–1772.

Frick, P. J. (1998). *Conduct disorders and severe antisocial behavior.* New York: Plenum.

Frick, P. J., Lahey, B. B., Loeber, R., Stouthamer-Loeber, M., Christ, M. A., & Hanson, K. (1992). Familial risk factors to oppositional defiant disorder and conduct disorder: Parental psychopathology and maternal parenting. *Journal of Consulting and Clinical Psychology, 60,* 49–55.

Frick, P. J., Lahey, B. B., Loeber, R., Tannenbaum, L. E., Van Horn, Y., Christ, M. A., Hart, E. A., & Hanson, K. (1993). Oppositional defiant disorder and conduct disorder: A meta-analytic review of factor analyses and cross-validation in a clinic sample. *Clinical Psychology Review, 13,* 319–340.

Gresham, F. M., & Elliot, S. N. (1990) *The Social Skills Rating System.* Circle Pines, MN: American Guidance Service.

Guerra, N. G., Huesmann, L. R., & Spindler, A. (2003). Community violence exposure, social cognition, and aggression among urban elementary school children. *Child Development, 74,* 1561–1576.

Haapasalo, J., & Tremblay, R. E. (1994). Physically aggressive boys from ages 6 to 12: Family background, parenting behavior, and prediction of delinquency. *Journal of Consulting and Clinical Psychology, 62,* 1044–1052.

Hart R. D., & Hare R. D. (1997). Psychopathy: Assessment and association with criminal conduct. In D. M. Stoff, J. Breiling, & J. D. Maser (Eds): *Handbook of antisocial behavior* (pp. 22–35). New York: Wiley.

Henggler, S. W., Melton, G. B., & Smith, L. A. (1992). Family preservation using multisystemic therapy: An effective alternative to incarcerating serious juvenile offenders. *Journal of Consulting and Clinical Psychology, 60,* 953–961.

Heppner, P. P. (1988). *The problem-solving inventory.* Palo Alto, CA: Consulting Psychologist Press.

Herjanic, B., & Reich, W. (1982). Development of a structured psychiatric interview for children: Agreement between child and parent on individual symptoms. *Journal of Abnormal Child Psychology, 10,* 307–324.

Hinshaw, S. P., & Anderson, C. A. (1996). Conduct and oppositional defiant disorders. In E. J. Mash & R. A. Barkley (Eds.), *Child psychopathology* (pp. 113–152). NewYork: Guilford Press.

Hinshaw, S. P., Lahey, B. B., & Hart, E. L. (1993). Issues of taxonomy and co-morbidity in the development of conduct disorder. *Development and Psychopathology, 5*, 31–50.

Hinshaw, S. P., & Lee, S. S. (2003). Conduct and oppositional defiant disorders. In E. J. Mash & R. A. Barkley (Eds.), *Child psychopathology* (2nd ed). New York: Guilford Press.

Hodges, K., Kline, J., Stern, L., Cytryn, L., & McKnew, D. (1982). The development of a child assessment interview for research and clinical use. *Journal of Abnormal Child Psychology, 10(2)*, 173–189.

Kazdin, A. E. (2004). Psychotherapy with children. In M. J. Lambert (Ed.), *Bergin and Garfield's handbook of psychotherapy and behavior change* (5th ed., pp. 543–589). New York: Wiley.

Keenan, K., Loeber, R., Zhang, Q., Stouthamer-Loeber, M., & Van Kammen, W. B. (1995). The influence of deviant peers on the development of boys' disruptive and delinquent behavior: A temporal analysis. *Development and Psychopathology, 7*, 715–726.

Kelley, M. L., Reitman, D., & Noell, G. H. (2003). *Practitioner's guide to empirically based measures of school behavior.* New York: Kluwer Academic/Plenum.

Lachar, D., & Gruber, C. P. (1995a). *Personality Inventory for Youth (PIY) manual: Technical guide.* Los Angeles: Western Psychological Services.

Lachar, D., & Gruber, C. P. (1995b). *Personality Inventory for Youth (PIY) manual: Administration and interpretation guide.* Los Angeles: Western Psychological Services.

Lachar, D., Wingenfeld, S. A., Kline, R. B., & Gruber, C. P. (2000). *Student behavior survey.* Los Angeles: Western Psychological Services.

Lahey, B. B., Loeber, R., Hart, E. L., Frick, P., Applegate, B., Zhang, Q., Green, S. M., & Russo, M. F. (1995). Four-year longitudinal study of conduct disorder in boys: Patterns and predictors of persistence. *Journal of Abnormal Psychology, 104*, 83–93.

Larson, J., & Lochman, J. E. (2002). *Helping schoolchildren cope with anger: A cognitive behavioral intervention.* New York: Guilford Press.

Leff, S. S., Crick, N. R., Angelucci, J., Haye, K., Jawad, A. F., Grossman, M., et al. (2006). Social cognition in context: Validating a cartoon-based attributional measure for urban girls. *Child Development, 77*, 1351–1358.

Leventhal, T., & Brooks-Gunn, J. (2000). The neighborhoods they live in: The effects of neighborhood residence on child and adolescent outcomes. *Psychological Bulletin, 126*, 309–337.

Lochman, J. E. (1987). Self and peer perceptions and attributional biases of aggressive and nonaggressive boys in dyadic interactions. *Journal of Consulting and Clinical Psychology, 55*, 404–410.

Lochman, J. E. (2000). Conduct disorder. In W. E. Craighead & C. B. Nemeroff (Eds.), *The Corsini encyclopedia of psychology and neuroscience* (3rd edition, pp. 343–345). New York: Wiley.

Lochman, J. E., & Dodge, K. A. (1994). Social-cognitive processes of severly violent, moderately aggressive, and nonaggressive boys. *Journal of Consulting & Clinical Psychology, 62*, 366–374.

Lochman, J. E., & Dodge, K. A. (1998). Distorted perceptions in dyadic interactions of aggressive and nonaggressive boys: Effects of prior expectations, context, and boys' age. *Development & Psychopathology, 10*, 495–512.

Lochman, J. E., Meyer, B. L., Rabiner, D. L., & White, K. J. (1991). Parameters influencing social problem-solving of aggressive children. In R. Prinz (Ed.), *Advances in behavioral assessment of children and families* (Vol. 5, pp. 31–63). Greenwich, CT: JAI Press.

Lochman, J. E., & Wayland, K. K. (1994). Aggression, social acceptance, and race as predictors of negative adolescent outcomes. *Journal of the American Academy of Child and Adolescent Psychiatry, 33*, 1026–1035.

Lochman, J. E., Wayland, K. K., & White, K. J. (1993). Social goals: Relationship to adolescent adjustment and to social problem solving. *Journal of Abnormal Child Psychology, 21*, 135–151.

Lochman, J. E., & Wells, K. C. (2002). Contextual social-cognitive mediators and child outcome: A test of the theoretical model in the Coping Power Program. *Development and Psychopathology, 14,* 971–993.

Lochman, J. E., & Wells, K. C. (2004). The Coping Power program for preadolescent aggressive boys and their parents: Outcome effects at the one-year follow-up. *Journal of Consulting and Clinical Psychology, 72,* 571–578.

Loeber, R., Green, S. M., Keenan, K., & Lahey, B. B. (1995). Which boys will fare worse? Early predictors of conduct disorder in a six-year longitudinal study. *Journal of the American Academy of Child and Adolescent Psychiatry, 34,* 499–509.

Maddox, S. J. & Prinz, R. J. (2003). School bonding in children and adolescents: Conceptualization, assessment, and associated variables. *Clinical Child and Family Psychology Review, 6,* 31–49.

McLeod, J. D. & Shanahan, M. J. (1996). Trajectories of poverty and children's mental health. *Journal of Health and Social Behavior, 37,* 207–220.

McMahon, R. J., & Metzler, C. W. (1998). Selecting parenting measures for assessing family-based prevention interventions. In R. S. Ashery, E. B. Robertson, & K. L. Kumpfer (Eds), *Drug abuse prevention through family intervention.* NIDA Research Monograph 177: Rockville, MD: National Institute on Drug Abuse.

Merrell, K. W. (2002). *School Social Behavior Scales, Second Edition.* Eugene, OR: Assessment-Intervention Resources.

Merrell, K. W., & Caldarella, P. (2002). *Home and Community Social Behavior Scales.* Eugene, OR: Assessment-Intervention Resources.

Milich, R., & Dodge, K. A. (1984). Social information processing in child psychiatric populations. *Journal of Abnormal Child Psychology, 12,* 471–490.

Moffitt, T. E. (1993). Adolescence-limited and life-course persistent antisocial behavior: A developmental taxonomy. *Psychology Review, 100,* 674–701.

Murray, L., Sinclair, D., Cooper, P., Ducournau, P., & Turner, P. (1999). The socioemotional development of 5-year-old children of postnatally depressed mothers. *Journal of Child Psychology and Psychiatry, 40,* 1259–1271.

Myers, W. C., Burket, R. C., & Otto, T. A. (1993). Conduct disorder and personality disorders in hospitalized adolescents. *Journal of Clinical Psychology, 54,* 21–26.

Nagin, D. S., & Tremblay, R. E. (2001). Parental and early childhood predictors of persistent physical aggression in boys from kindergarten to high school. *Archives of General Psychiatry, 58,* 389–394.

Naglieri, J. A., LeBuffe, P. A., & Pfeiffer, S. I. (1994). *Devereux Scales of Mental Disorders.* San Antonio, TX: Psychological Corporation.

Nelson, W. M., Finch, A. J., & Hart, K. J. (2006). *Conduct Disorders: A practitioner's guide to comparative treatments.* New York: Springer.

Orobio de Castro, B., Veerman, J. W., Koops, W., Bosch, J. D., & Monshouwer, H. J. (2002). Hostile attribution of intent and aggressive behavior: A meta-analysis. *Child Development, 73,* 916–934.

Pardini, D.A., Lochman, J.E., & Frick, P.J. (2003). Callous/unemotional traits and social cognitive processes in adjudicated youth. *Journal of the American Academy of Child and Adolescent Psychiatry, 42,* 364–371.

Pinderhughes, E. E., Nix, R., Foster, E. M., Jones, D., & Conduct Problems Prevention Research Group (2001). Parenting in context: Impact of neighborhood poverty, residential stability, public services, social networks and danger on parental behaviors. *Journal of Marriage and Family, 63,* 941–953.

Quay, H. C., & Peterson, D. R. (1996). *Revised Behavior Problem Checklist, PAR Edition.* Odessa, FL: Psychological Assessment Resources.

Rabiner, D. L., Lenhart, L., & Lochman, J. E. (1990). Automatic vs. reflective social problem solving in relation to children's sociometric status. *Developmental Psychology, 26,* 1010–1026.

Reynolds, C. R., & Kamphaus, R. W. (2005). *Behavior Assessment System for Children, Second Edition (BASC-2).* Circle Pines, MN: American Guidance Service.

Reynolds, W. M. (1998a). *Adolescent Psychopathology Scale: Administration and interpretive manual.* Odessa, FL: Psychological Assessment Resources.

Reynolds, W. M. (1998b). *Adolescent Psychopathology Scale: Psychometric and technical manual.* Odessa, FL: Psychological Assessment Resources.

Reynolds, W. M. (2000). *Adolescent Psychopathology Scale-Short Form: Professional manual.* Odessa, FL: Psychological Assessment Resources.

Schachar, R., & Tannock, R. (1995). Test of four hypotheses for the comorbidity of attention-deficit hyperactivity disorder and conduct disorder. *Journal of the American Academy of Child and Adolescent Psychiatry, 34,* 639–648.

Shaffer, D., Fisher, P., Lucas, C., Dulcan, M., & Schwab-Stone, M. (2000). NIMH Diagnostic Interview Schedule for Children Version IV (NIMH DISC-IV): Description, differences from previous versions, and reliability of some common diagnoses. *Journal of the American Academy of Child and Adolescent Psychiatry, 39,* 28–38.

Spivack, G., Shure, M. B., & Platt, J. J. (1985). *Means-Ends Problem Solving (MEPS). Stimuli and scoring procedures supplement.* Unpublished document, Philadelphia: Hahnemann University, Preventive Intervention Research Center.

Stone, A. A., & Neale, J. M. (1982). Development of a methodology for assessing daily experiences. In A. Baum & J. Singer (Eds), *Advances in environmental psychology. environment and health. Volume IV.* Hillsdale, NJ: Erlbaum.

Stormshak, E. A., Bierman, K. L., McMahon, R. J., Lengua, L. J., & Conduct Problems Prevention Research Group (2000). Parenting practices and child disruptive behavior problems in early elementary school. *Journal of Clinical Child Psychology, 29,* 17–29.

Thomas, D. E., Bierman, K. L., & the Conduct Problems Prevention Research Group (2006). The impact of classroom aggression on the development of aggressive behavior problems in children. *Development and Psychopathology, 18,* 471–487.

Vaillancourt, T., & Hymel, S. (2006) Aggression and social status: The moderating roles of sex and peer-valued characteristics. *Aggressive Behavior, 32,* 396–408.

van Goozen, S. H. M., Matthys, W., Cohen-Kettenis, P. T., Gispen-de Wied, C., Wiegant, V. M., & van Engeland, H. (1998). Salivary cortisol and cardiovascular activity during stress in oppositional-defiant disorder boys and normal controls. *Biological Psychiatry, 43,* 531–539.

Williams, S. C., Lochman, J. E., Phillips, N. C., & Barry, T. D. (2003). Aggressive and nonaggressive boys' physiological and cognitive processes in response to peer provocations. *Journal of Clinical Child & Adolescent Psychology, 32,* 568–576.

Wirt, R. D., Lachar, D., Seat, P. D., & Broen, W. E., Jr. (2001). *Personality Inventory for Children – Second Edition.* Los Angeles: Western Psychological Services.

Zaslow, M. J., Weinfield, N. S., Gallagher, M., Hair, E. C., Ogawa, J. R., Egeland, B., et al. (2006). Longitudinal prediction of child outcomes from differing measures of parenting in a low-income sample. *Developmental Psychology, 42,* 27–37.

Zoccolillo, M. (1993). Gender and the development of conduct disorder. *Development and Psychopathology, 5,* 65–78.

8

Evidence-Based Assessment of Attention-Deficit/ Hyperactivity Disorder (ADHD)

PAULA SOWERBY and GAIL TRIPP

Following recognition of the need for evidence-based treatments for childhood disorders there is increasing awareness that the assessment procedures we use with children should also be evidence-based. In this chapter we briefly review what is known about attention-deficit/hyperactivity disorder (ADHD) before considering the informants, methods, and measures that can be used to conduct evidence-based assessments for children presenting with problems suggestive of ADHD. We also consider the difficulties in combining data across informants and measures and the important issue of incremental validity: that is, when does more assessment lead to better assessment and outcome? Although the focus of the chapter is the assessment of ADHD in school-aged children we briefly address the assessment of ADHD in preschoolers, adolescents, and adults. In preparing this chapter we have been guided by Mash and Hunsley's description of

PAULA SOWERBY • ADHD Research Clinic, Department of Psychology, University of Otago, Dunedin, New Zealand.
GAIL TRIPP • ADHD Research Clinic, Department of Psychology, University of Otago, Dunedin, New Zealand and Human Developmental Neurobiology Unit, Okinawa Institute of Science and Technology, Okinawa, Japan.

J.L. Matson et al. (eds.), *Assessing Childhood Psychopathology and Developmental Disabilities*, DOI: 10.1007/978-0-387-09528-8,
© Springer Science+Business Media, LLC 2009

evidence based assessment, "... assessment methods and processes that are based on empirical evidence in terms of both their reliability and validity as well as their clinical usefulness for prescribed populations and purposes" (Mash & Hunsley, 2005, p. 364).

Attention-deficit/hyperactivity disorder has been the subject of a great deal of research attention over the last three decades with many research articles and books published describing its nature, assessment, and treatment. It is not possible to do justice to this extensive literature in a single chapter. Where appropriate, throughout the chapter we refer the reader to more detailed sources. We recommend those planning to conduct evidence-based assessments with children referred for difficulties consistent with ADHD consult these sources.

BACKGROUND

Description of ADHD and Current Diagnostic Criteria

Attention-deficit/hyperactivity disorder is the diagnosis given to children, adolescents, and adults who display developmentally inappropriate levels of inattention, overactivity, and impulsivity. These symptoms cause significant impairment in the individual's functioning in both the home and school or work environments (American Psychiatric Association, APA, 2000)

The criteria set out in the fourth edition of the *Diagnostic and Statistical Manual of Mental Disorders–Text Revision* (APA, 2000) are the current standard for the diagnosis of ADHD in the United States of America and increasingly throughout the rest of the world. These criteria are reproduced in Table 8.1. The current criteria include two 9-item symptom lists; the first includes nine symptoms of inattention, and the second, six symptoms of hyperactivity and three of impulsivity.

Briefly, in order for an individual to meet *DSM–IV* criteria for a diagnosis of ADHD the following are required: (a) the individual must exhibit six or more symptoms of inattention and/or hyperactivity-impulsivity which have been present for at least six months and which are present to such a degree that they are maladaptive and inconsistent with the individual's developmental level; (b) some symptoms causing impairment appeared before seven years of age; (c) some impairment from symptoms is apparent in two or more settings (e.g., home and school/work); (d) there must be clear evidence of clinically significant impairment in social, academic, or occupational functioning, and (e) the symptoms are not better accounted for by another disorder nor do they occur exclusively during the course of Pervasive Developmental Disorder, Schizophrenia, or other Psychotic Disorder.

Three subtypes are recognized, predominantly inattentive (six or more symptoms of inattention but fewer than six symptoms of hyperactivity/impulsivity), predominantly hyperactive/impulsive (six or more symptoms of hyperactivity/impulsivity but fewer than six symptoms of inattention), and combined type (at least six symptoms of inattention and six symptoms of hyperactivity/impulsivity) (APA, 2000).

Table 8.1. *DSM–IV–TR* Diagnostic Criteria for ADHD.

A. Either (1) or (2)

    (1) Six (or more) of the following symptoms of **inattention** have persisted for at least 6 months to a degree that is maladaptive and inconsistent with developmental level:

Inattention

        (a) Often fails to give close attention to details or makes careless mistakes in school-work, work, or other activities

        (b) Often has difficulty sustaining attention in tasks or play activities

        (c) Often does not seem to listen when spoken to directly

        (d) Often does not follow through on instructions and fails to finish schoolwork, chores, or duties in the workplace (not due to oppositional behaviour or failure to understand instructions)

        (e) Often has difficulty organising tasks and activities

        (f) Often avoids, dislikes, or is reluctant to engage in tasks that require sustained mental effort (such as schoolwork or homework).

        (g) Often loses things necessary for tasks or activities (e.g. toys, school assignments, pencils, books, or tools)

        (h) Is often easily distracted by extraneous stimuli

        (i) Is often forgetful in daily activities

    (2) Six (or more) of the following symptoms of **hyperactivity-impulsivity** have persisted for at least 6 months to a degree that is maladaptive and inconsistent with developmental level

Hyperactivity

        (a) Often fidgets with hands or feet or squirms in seat

        (b) Often leaves seat in classroom or in other situations in which remaining seated is expected

        (c) Often runs about or climbs excessively in situations in which it is inappropriate (in adolescents or adults, may be limited to subjective feelings of restlessness)

        (d) Often has difficulty playing or engaging in leisure activities quietly

        (e) Is often "on the go" or often acts as if "driven by a motor"

        (f) Often talks excessively

Impulsivity

        (g) Often blurts out answers before questions have been completed

        (h) Often has difficulty awaiting turn

        (i) Often interrupts or intrudes on others (e.g., butts into conversations or games)

        B. Some hyperactive-impulsive or inattentive symptoms that caused impairment were present before age 7 years.

C. Some impairment from the symptoms is present in two or more settings (e.g., at school [or work] and at home).

D. There must be clear evidence of clinically significant impairment in social, academic, or occupational functioning.

E. The symptoms do not occur exclusively during the course of a Pervasive Developmental Disorder, Schizophrenia, or other Psychotic Disorder and are not better accounted for by another mental disorder (e.g., Mood Disorder, Anxiety Disorder, Dissociative Disorder, or a Personality Disorder)

The World Health Organization's *International Classification of Disease* tenth edition (WHO, 1992) also provides criteria for the diagnosis of Hyper-kinetic Disorder. These criteria emphasize the presence of abnormal levels of inattention and hyperactivity in the home and school settings together with the direct observation of inattention or hyperactivity. Unlike the *DSM–IV*, the ICD-10 criteria do not allow for comorbid mood, anxiety, or psychotic disorders.

Despite the differences between the *DSM–IV* and ICD-10 there appears to be substantial overlap among the groups formed by these criteria (Lahey et al., 2006; Tripp, Luk, Schaughency, & Singh, 1999). Tripp et al. (1999) found most children with hyperkinetic disorder met criteria for *DSM–IV* ADHD, whereas slightly less than half of those meeting criteria for ADHD also met criteria for hyperkinetic disorder. In the Lahey et al. (2006) study, all children who met full criteria for hyperkinetic disorder also met full *DSM–IV* criteria for ADHD, and only 26% of those with ADHD met criteria for hyperkinetic disorder. The *DSM–IV* criteria for ADHD identify a broader group of children than those identified by ICD-10 criteria. Lahey et al. (2006) report both the ICD-10 and *DSM–IV* criteria exhibit predictive validity over a six-year period.

Epidemiology of ADHD

ADHD is one of the most frequently diagnosed disorders of childhood. Published prevalence rates vary widely reflecting differences in study populations, assessment methods, diagnostic criteria, and their application. Barkley (2006) provides a detailed summary of prevalence estimates from studies from a number of countries utilizing different research methodologies. The DSM–IV Text Revision reports prevalence rates of 3–7% in school-aged children. Follow-up studies indicate as many as 80% of those diagnosed as hyperactive in childhood continue to evidence significant symptoms in adolescence (Faigel, Sznajdeerman, Tishby, Turel, & Pinus, 1995; Hechtman, 1991). Community studies in New Zealand using clinical diagnostic criteria report prevalence estimates of 2–3% in 15-year-olds (Fergusson, Horwood, & Lynskey, 1993; McGee et al., 1990). The results of a population screen of American adults indicate 2.9% meet narrowly defined criteria for ADHD (Farone & Biederman, 2005). A slightly higher rate of 4.4% was identified amongst participants in the National Comorbidity Survey Replication (Kessler et al., 2006).

Epidemiological studies investigating the different subtypes of ADHD report the Inattentive subtype is the most common, with prevalence estimates ranging between 4.5 and 9% of children in the general population. Rates of between 1.9 and 4.8% are reported for ADHD combined type, whereas only 1.7 to 3.9% of children meet criteria for ADHD predominately hyperactive-impulsive type (Brown, 2000). These subtype prevalence estimates contrast with the subtype diagnoses made in clinical samples, where ADHD Combined type is by far the most common. This discrepancy probably reflects the fact that children presenting with hyperactive-impulsive symptoms in addition to inattentive symptoms are more likely to be identified with problematic externalizing behavior symptoms (Eiraldi, Power, & Nezu, 1997).

Attention-deficit/hyperactivity disorder is more commonly identified in boys than girls. In epidemiological studies the reported ratio for boys to girls is around 3:1. This increases up to 9:1 in clinical settings (APA, 2000). In their meta-analysis of gender differences in ADHD, Gaub and Carlson (1997) reported that compared to boys, girls with ADHD were found to exhibit greater intellectual impairment, and fewer symptoms of hyperactivity and other externalizing behaviors. This finding raises questions about the validity of the *DSM–IV-TR* criteria for identifying significant ADHD symptoms in girls.

Comorbidity and Associated Difficulties

Both epidemiological and clinical studies indicate that ADHD is associated with significant comorbidity (Biederman, Newcorn, & Sprich, 1991, Biederman et al., 1998; Fergusson et al., 1993; Jensen, Martin, & Cantwell, 1997; Kadesjö & Gillberg, 2001; Steinhausen et al., 2006). As with prevalence rates for ADHD, reported rates for coexisting psychiatric disorders/problems vary as a function of study population and methodology.

Irrespective of these methodological variations, available studies indicate co-existing problems are common in ADHD, and indeed, having a diagnosis of ADHD increases the risk of having one or more additional psychiatric diagnoses (Brown, 2000). Across studies investigating comorbidity in ADHD, rates for anxiety disorders are in the range 25–35%, mood disorders 9–32%, ODD/CD 45–84% (Barkley, 2006), and as many as 25% are likely to have coexisting learning difficulties (Tannock & Brown, 2000).

In addition to experiencing high rates of comorbid diagnoses, children meeting criteria for a diagnosis of ADHD, and those with elevated levels of ADHD symptomatology, frequently experience a range of associated difficulties. These associated difficulties are often what precipitates presentation to clinical services and may include: social difficulties, emotional lability, low frustration tolerance, bossiness, an excessive need for attention from others, insistence that things be done "their way", strong reliance on routine and structure, poor self-esteem and academic under-achievement (APA, 2000).

Etiology

Despite decades of active research to identify the cause of ADHD the disorder's etiology remains unknown. The weight of available evidence indicates that the disorder has a neurobiological basis, however, no single cause has been identified (Swanson et al., 1998; Biederman, 2005; Nutt et al., 2007). Although environmental factors such as exposure to toxins, and pregnancy and birth complications (including prematurity) have been associated with the development of ADHD symptomatology, the child's psychosocial environment is not considered to be causal (Biederman, 2005). It has been suggested, however, that the ADHD phenotype, including the presence of comorbid disruptive disorders, may reflect the influence of the child's environment acting upon genetic factors (Nutt et al., 2007).

The disorder shows strong familial links being more common amongst relatives than in the general population (Biederman, Faraone, Keenan, Knee, & Tsuany, 1990, Biederman et al., 1992; Biederman, 2005; Faraone et al., 1992, 2005). A number of candidate genes have been identified, however, their individual contributions to the disorder are small and researchers suggest that ADHD symptomatology may be caused by multiple genes of small effect (Asherson, Kuntsi, & Taylor, 2005; Faraone et al., 2005; Waldman & Gizer, 2006). A recent review of the past decade of molecular genetic studies found that the dopamine D4 and D5 receptors, and the dopamine and serotonin transporters are all significantly associated with ADHD (Bobb, Castellanos, Addington, & Rapoport, 2005).

Imaging studies have shown variation in anatomical brain structures in children with ADHD involving the fronto-striato-cerebellar circuitry, namely, reduced brain volumes in frontal regions, the caudate nucleus, the splenium of the corpus callosum, and the cerebellum (Valera, Faraone, Murray, & Seidman, 2007). Imaging studies have also identified different activation patterns in children with and without ADHD. When undertaking tasks designed to assess response inhibition, children with ADHD show inefficient recruitment of frontal-striatal regions (Bush, Valera, & Seidman, 2005; Scheres, Milham, Knutson, & Castellanos, 2007). However, it is unclear what these differences in neuronal functioning reflect.

The effectiveness of a range of stimulant, and more recently, nonstimulant, drugs in the management of symptoms of ADHD suggest some dysfunction in neurotransmitter and neuromodulator systems in the brains of those with ADHD (Biederman, 2005; Chamberlain, Robbins, & Sahakian, 2007). As previously identified, many of the candidate genes associated with ADHD involve the dopamine system, and most psychotropic treatments for ADHD act on the dopamine and norepinephrine systems (Waldman & Gizer, 2006; Arnsten, 2006).

Neuropsychological studies of children and adolescents with ADHD have shown that some children with ADHD perform poorly on tasks that assess executive functioning skills, namely: response inhibition, vigilance, working memory, and planning (Willcutt, Doyle, Nigg, Faraone, & Pennington, 2005). In the past decade there has been considerable research investigating the possible role of executive functioning deficits in the development of ADHD symptomatology. A recent review of these studies, however, found a lack of universality of executive functioning deficits in children diagnosed with ADHD, and suggests that executive functioning deficits should be viewed as an associated difficulty, rather than a cause of ADHD symptoms (Willcutt et al., 2005).

The complexity of the disorder and its varied presentation suggest that there may well be multiple pathways leading to the symptoms that are defined as ADHD.

ASSESSMENT OF ADHD

Purpose of Assessment

The reason an individual presents or is referred for assessment will influence the assessment strategy. In research settings focusing on a particular disorder or group of disorders a standard predetermined assessment plan is likely to be followed, with additional assessment being conducted as appropriate when resources permit. In such settings individuals with similar presenting problems are likely to be referred or recruited. A primary goal of assessment may be diagnosis to aid the formation of homogeneous groups to address specific research questions.

In clinical practice, patient groups are likely to be more heterogeneous. In these settings initial assessment findings will guide the nature, breadth, and depth of subsequent assessment. In these settings diagnosis will also be an assessment goal, however, the focus may be on carrying out a functional analysis of the individual's presenting problems to aid in treatment planning and intervention and subsequent outcome evaluation.

Planning the Assessment

Whatever the assessment setting and purpose assessment practices should follow guidelines for evidence-based assessment. Hunsley and Mash (2007) define evidence-based assessment as that which "emphasizes the use of research and theory to inform the selection of assessment targets, the methods and measures used in assessment, and the assessment process" (p. 29). In addition to considering the reliability and validity of individual assessment instruments they emphasize the importance of the context in which the instruments are used, their appropriateness for different genders and populations, and the purposes for which they were designed (e.g., single versus multiple administrations). They also argue that issues of incremental validity, and clinical utility should be considered throughout assessment.

In planning and undertaking assessment with a child referred for an evaluation of ADHD or whose reported difficulties suggest symptoms of ADHD, the clinician or researcher should consider the essential information required (a) to make or exclude a diagnosis of ADHD, and (b) to develop and monitor an appropriate intervention plan. The assessor should remain mindful that referral information may not match closely the child's presentation. Preassessment planning should be regarded as tentative and open to change.

Diagnosis of ADHD

In order to determine if a child's behavior meets DSM–IV criteria for ADHD the clinician or researcher requires information on the number, type (inattentive, hyperactive, impulsive), and duration of DSM–IV symptoms of ADHD that are developmentally inappropriate. Information on symptom frequency and severity is useful in determining whether a child's behaviors are developmentally appropriate. The assessor must also obtain information regarding the presence and severity of impairment from current symptoms across settings, together with the age of onset of symptoms of ADHD which caused impairment in the child's functioning. Finally, the clinician or researcher must obtain sufficient background information to rule out alternative medical, sensory, psychiatric, or psychosocial explanations for the presence of symptoms of ADHD which cause impairment.

Treatment/Management of ADHD

Most clinicians would agree that children diagnosed with ADHD present to helping services, not only because of the presence of symptoms of ADHD, but because of associated difficulties which frequently co-occur with ADHD. As a consequence any assessment carried out to inform treatment planning is necessarily broader in scope than a diagnostic assessment.

In addition to the information described above, for treatment purposes the assessment should identify all presenting problems and areas of impairment, including comorbidity and associated difficulties. This information can then be used to prioritize targets for intervention. A functional behavioral analysis (FBA) should then be carried out on those presenting problems/areas of impairment targeted for intervention. This FBA may help to identify both resources to support intervention, and potential barriers to its implementation (e.g., family functioning, comorbid psychiatric problems).

Below we address the who (which informants) and how (which methods and measures) of assessment of ADHD. This is followed by a discussion of the issues surrounding combining information across informants and methods and the extent to which additional sources of information (informants and methods) contribute to better assessment (incremental validity).

From Whom Should We Seek Information?

Irrespective of the methods and measures used to collect diagnostic and background information the selection of informants should take account of the length of time they have known the child (to establish if symptoms meet minimum duration criteria) and their familiarity with the child's behavior in a given setting. Parents and teachers are seen as natural informants in the child assessments (Collet, Ohan & Myers, 2003a,b; Jensen et al., 1996, 1999). Practice guidelines for ADHD recommend the use of multiple informants in the assessment of ADHD (American Academy of Pediatrics, AAP, 2001, American Academy of Child and Adolescent Psychiatry, AACAP, 2007) and certainly DSM–IV criteria require the presence of impairment from symptoms in more than one setting. The extent to which parents and teachers contribute unique information to the assessment process is considered in the later discussion of incremental validity. Opinions differ regarding the usefulness of child informants with respect to externalizing symptoms, with children typically being seen as better able to provide information regarding their internal state (e.g., Loeber, Green, & Lahey, 1989) and less willing than adults to report their externalizing behavior (Jensen et al., 1999). Irrespective of whether the child being assessed is required to complete formal assessment measures they should participate in the assessment process.

How Should We Obtain Assessment Information?
Interviews

Clinical interviews are probably the most widely utilized form of data collection in research and clinical practice. They provide the clinician or researcher with the opportunity to collect information on presenting problems and symptoms, including the context in which these occur, their onset, frequency, severity, chronicity, and impact on functioning. The interview also provides an opportunity to collect information about the child's medical and developmental history and significant life events. In addition interviews permit the clinician to form an impression of the parents' and child's functioning (social, emotional, cognitive) and if interviewed together, the nature and quality of the parent–child interactions.

Interviews vary in the degree of imposed structure ranging from unstructured interviews which are highly flexible without a preset agenda through semi-structured interviews that provide general, but flexible, guidelines for the collection and recording of information through to highly structured interviews that specify the wording and order of questions and the manner in which the obtained information is recorded (Sattler & Mash, 1998).

Unstructured interviews have a long history in the assessment of children's behavioral and emotional difficulties. Numerous texts are available detailing their form and use with children and adults (e.g., Hughs & Baker, 1990; McConaughy, 2005; Sattler, 1998). Although such interviews allow the clinician to follow up leads and change direction as necessary, this freedom makes it difficult to establish their reliability and validity. The information collected by different interviewers or the same interviewer across cases is not standardized and the interviewer may omit important questions. There is also opportunity for the clinicians' biases to influence attention to, or interpretation of, the responses given (Sattler & Mash, 1998). Diagnoses made by clinicians using unstructured interviews are thought to be subject to a number of biases including: making a diagnosis prior to the collection of all relevant information; selective collection of information to confirm diagnoses; nonsystematic approaches to combining different types of information; and allowing familiarity with particular problems or disorders to influence decision making (McClellan & Werry, 2000).

Structured interviews were developed as a means of reducing variability in the manner in which interviews were conducted in an effort to increase the reliability of the information elicited (McClellan & Werry, 2000). Despite their structure Sattler and Mash (1998) question the extent to which structured interviews are reliable, identifying several possible sources of unreliability and variability.

Several structured and semi-structured interviews are now available for use with parents and children which are designed to elicit the information required to make specific *DSM–IV* diagnoses. Some were developed for administration by trained lay interviewers and others, typically the semi-structured interviews, require clinical training. In 2000 the *Journal of the American Academy of Child and Adolescent Psychiatry* included a series of articles on the most widely used and researched structured and semi-structured research psychiatric diagnostic interviews for assessing psychopathology in children and adolescents. This series of articles provides a useful starting point for anyone considering the use of diagnostic interviews. Six interviews are described including their target populations, requirements for administration, known psychometric properties and access details.

Three structured interviews are included: the NIMH Diagnostic Interview Schedule for Children Version IV (NIMH DISC-IV) is a highly structured diagnostic interview that can be administered by trained lay interviewers. The DISC-IV assesses over 30 psychiatric disorders which may occur in children and adolescents (Shaffer, Fisher, Lucas, Dulcan, & Schwab-Stone, 2000); the Children's Interview for Psychiatric Syndromes (ChIPS) is another highly structured interview for use by trained lay interviewers. It screens for 20 Axis I disorders and psychosocial stressors (Weller, Weller, Fristad, Rooney, & Schecter, 2000); the Child and Adolescent Psychiatric Assessment (CAPA) is an interviewer-based structured psychiatric interview which collects information on symptom onset, duration, frequency, and intensity. The interviewer is required to continue asking questions until a decision is reached regarding symptom presence (Angold & Costello, 2000).

Three semi-structured interviews are included: the Diagnostic Interview for Children and Adolescents (DICA) previously described as a structured interview can be used in semi-structured format with interviewer judgment required (Reich, 2000); the Schedule for Affective Disorders and Schizophrenia for School-Age Children (K-SADS) is a semi-structured interview requiring substantial interviewer training. It assesses current, past, and lifetime diagnostic status in children and adolescents (Ambrosini, 2000); the Interview Schedule for Children and Adolescents (ISCA), previously the Interview Schedule for Children, is a semi-structured symptom-oriented inventory designed for administration by experienced clinicians trained in the use of semi-structured interviews (Sherrill & Kovacs, 2000). As a useful supplement to this series of articles Anastopoulos and Shelton (2001) provide useful commentary on the psychometric properties together with the advantages and disadvantages of the DISC-IV, DICA-IV, and K-SADS in the comprehensive assessment of ADHD.

Although structured and semi-structured diagnostic interviews are useful for determining the presence of symptoms required for specific diagnoses they offer limited information for use in treatment planning (i.e., the nature and degree of impairment from symptoms and associated difficulties, a functional analysis of presenting problems, child and family resources, and potential barriers to intervention). This information, along with the child's developmental, educational, and medical history either needs to be collected as part of a supplementary unstructured interview or through the use of appropriate questionnaires.

Pelham and colleagues have questioned whether the resources required for the use of structured and semi-structured diagnostic interviews are better utilized in the collection of information required for treatment planning and monitoring. They suggest psychometrically sound symptom rating scales can provide the same diagnostic information more economically and efficiently (Pelham, Fabiano, & Massetti, 2005). As far as we are aware there are currently no published studies available that directly compare the accuracy of diagnoses made using rating scales and questionnaires with diagnostic interviews.

Current *DSM–IV* criteria require some impairment from symptoms in two or more settings. As children spend significant time in the school setting teachers are important participants in the assessment process. Clinicians regularly request that teachers complete broadband and narrowband rating scales for children undergoing assessment. Interviews with teachers can also provide important assessment information on children's relationships with teachers and peers, academic skills and progress, and ability to follow rules and directions. This information may be especially important for identifying impairment and targets for intervention. DuPaul and Stoner

(2003) offer useful suggestions on the type and nature of information which should be collected from teachers. To the best of our knowledge structured diagnostic interviews for teachers are not currently available.

Most structured and semi-structured interviews for *DSM–IV* provide child/adolescent versions, however, our experience is that children at the lower end of the age ranges for which these are recommended often struggle to provide meaningful answers to the questions posed. Thus clinicians and researchers planning to use such interviews should consider carefully if such practices are appropriate for a given child. Those unfamiliar with interviewing children are likely to find the texts on interviewing children referenced above helpful.

Rating Scales and Questionnaires

Another commonly used method for obtaining information for diagnosis and to establish baseline symptom levels to monitor intervention, is the use of questionnaires and rating scales. Rating scales or questionnaires used in the assessment ADHD can be divided into two categories, broadband and narrowband. Broadband scales are designed to identify a wide range of psychopathology, including hyperactivity/impulsivity, aggression, conduct problems, depression, anxiety, inattention, somatic difficulties, and in some cases, adaptive functioning. Narrowband scales are specific to ADHD, or at least to externalizing behaviors, and the actual items are often based around diagnostic symptoms. Some narrowband scales are effectively symptom lists from the DSM–IV diagnostic criteria for ADHD, which the respondent rates according to presence and severity.

When undertaking an evidence-based assessment of ADHD, the choice of rating instrument needs to take into account the reliability and validity of the rating scale, and the purpose to which it is being applied (Winters, Collett, & Myers, 2005). For example, in a situation where repeated administrations of the questionnaire are required (e.g., pre-and postintervention) issues such as test–retest reliability are of special consideration.

Where data from different respondents will be collected during the assessment, interrater reliability may be important. The validity of the measures to be used is also critical from an evidence-based perspective, and can provide important information regarding incremental validity and the clinical utility of the data collected. A scale that has a very high convergent validity score with a rating scale already used in the assessment would suggest information redundancy. Equally, a scale that shows limited discriminant validity, the ability to distinguish clinical from nonclinical groups, may be of limited clinical utility (Winters et al., 2005). The reader is referred to Pelham et al. (2005) and Collett et al. (2003a,b) for extensive reviews of the reliability and validity of rating scales/questionnaires typically used in the assessment of ADHD.

Other important considerations regarding the purpose to which a rating scale is applied concerns the ethnicity, sex, and age of the child being assessed. Many of the commonly used broadband and narrowband scales were developed and normed in the United States of America. The ethnicity of the normative samples is generally at best reflective of the ethnic make-up of the American state or states in which the norming procedures were undertaken. This said, many of these rating scales have been extensively translated and used cross-culturally, with some of these studies undertaken including sufficiently large samples to provide normative data for these additional populations. The broadband Child Behaviour Checklist rating scale (Achenbach, 1991; Achenbach & Rescorla, 2001) has been especially widely used, having been translated into 75 languages, and used in over 67 different cultures. The Achenbach System for Empirically Based Assessment (ASEBA) website provides a list of all translations and multicultural studies using the CBCL. With respect to sex and age, most broadband questionnaires provide norms specific to both gender and broad age categories.

Broadband Scales

Popular broadband scales have both teacher- and parent-respondent forms, or a single form that can be used in both school and home settings. Commonly used broadband scales that evidence good reliability and validity include: The Child Behaviour Checklist (CBCL, Achenbach & Rescorla, 2001); the Behaviour Assessment System for Children, Second Edition (BASC-2, Reynolds & Kamphaus, 2004); and the Conners' Parent and Teacher Rating Scales Revised (CRS-R, Conners, Sitarenios, Parker, & Epstein, 1998a,b). The CBCL and BASC-2 questionnaires have both recently been updated and renormed, and although the authors report reasonable reliability and validity data, there is currently little external published research regarding these updated editions. The CRS- R long form can be considered a broadband questionnaire, however, its heavy loading of ADHD-specific items means that it is often used as a narrowband ADHD-specific measure. A notable feature of the CRS-R is that care was taken to obtain norms for African Americans, which increases the clinical utility of this instrument when working with this population.

Broadband rating scales are not advised as a sole means of diagnosing ADHD (Clinical Practice Guidelines, AAP, 2001), however, these assessment guidelines, along with the recently updated guidelines of the American Academy of Child and Adolescent Psychiatry (AACAP, 2007) indicate a role for broadband questionnaires in screening for ADHD-type difficulties and level of impairment. Given the high prevalence of ADHD the AACAP guidelines recommend all children presenting in a clinical setting should be screened for symptoms of ADHD. Recent research using the Child Behaviour Checklist (CBCL, Achenbach, 1991, Achenbach & Rescorla, 2001) suggests that broadband scales such as the CBCL may be useful in identifying possible comorbid difficulties in children already diagnosed with ADHD (Biederman, Monuteaux, Kendrick, Klein, & Faraone, 2005). These questionnaires may also be useful in the differential diagnosis of ADHD and Bipolar disorder.

Narrowband Scales

Narrowband rating scales are largely based on the DSM–IV symptoms of ADHD. Popular ADHD rating scales that are both reliable and valid include the ADHD rating scale –IV: home and school versions (DuPaul, Power, Anastopoulos, & Reid, 1998), the Vanderbilt Rating Scale (Wolraich, 2003; Wolraich, Feurer, Hannah, Baumgaertel, & Pinnock, 1998; Wolraich et al., 2003), and the Attention Deficit Disorders Evaluation Scale, 3rd edition (ADDES-3, McCarney & Arthaud, 2004). From an evidence-based perspective, an advantage of the ADDES-3 is that items are rated on the basis of symptom frequency counts and allow the rater to identify when an item is not observed because it is not within the child's developmental ability (i.e., 0 = Not developmentally appropriate for age; 1 = not observed; 2 = one to several times per month; 3 = one to several times per week; 4 = one to several times per day; 5 = one to several times per hour). This feature not only increases rater reliability, but also adds to the scale's clinical utility by providing a quantifiable indication of impairment.

Other *DSM–IV* criterion-based scales such as the current version of the SNAP or Swanson, Nolan, & Pelham rating scale (Atkins, Pelham, & Licht, 1985; Swanson et al., 2001) and the Disruptive Behaviour Disorders rating scale (DBD, Pelham, Evans, Gnagy, & Greenslade, 1992; Pelham, Griener, & Gnagy, 1998) are also extensively used, although Pelham et al. (2005) and Collett et al. (2003a,b) note that there are limited normative data available for these measures, and there are also no convergent and discriminant validity data available on the DBD. An advantage of the DBD, however, is that it assesses the presence of ADHD, ODD, and CD symptomatology, which are commonly co-occuring externalizing behavior disorders.

Rating Scales to Assess Impairment

Although both broadband and narrowband rating scales provide some indication of impairment from symptoms, with the exception of the ADDES, this information is often nonspecific and of limited utility in terms of guiding intervention. Winters et al. (2005) recently reviewed rating scales designed to assess functional impairment in children. Their review includes summaries of rating scales which assess global functioning and impairment (e.g., Children's Global Assessment Scale [CGAS], Shaffer et al., 1983; Columbia Impairment Scale [CIS], Bird et al., 1993) and multidimensional scales assessing adaptive functioning and impairment.

Scales designed to assess adaptive functioning that have good reliability and validity include the Vineland Adaptive Behaviour Scales (VABS, Sparrow, Cicchetti, & Balla, 1984), the Adaptive Behaviour Assessment System–second edition (ABAS-2, Harrison & Oakland, 2003), and the Child and Adolescent Functional Assessment Scale (CAFAS, Hodges, 1994). The Vineland Adaptive Behavior Scales have been revised and renormed (VABS-2, Sparrow, Cicchetti, & Balla, 2005) and although the VABS-2 has maintained a questionnaire format for teacher-respondents; the parent/caregiver version is better described as a semi-structured interview. These multidimensional adaptive functioning scales provide specific information regarding the child's level of functioning in different behavioral and social domains (e.g., daily living skills/motor skills, communication, social skills). As it is often difficulties in these domains that lead to a child's presentation for assessment and treatment, this information is often the most pertinent in guiding intervention (Pelham et al., 2005).

A recently developed scale that may be of particular utility in the assessment of impairment in children with ADHD is the Impairment Rating Scale (IRS) developed by Fabiano et al. (2006). The IRS parent and teacher versions include items which are based upon domains of behavior known to be often impaired in ADHD, including: relationship with peers; relationship with siblings/parents/teacher; academic progress; self-esteem; influence on family functioning; and overall impairment. Fabiano et al. (2006) found the IRS to demonstrate reasonable test–retest reliability over a one-year period, for both parents and teachers, even when completed by two different teachers.

The IRS has also demonstrated good concurrent validity with the parent-completed Diagnostic Interview for Children (DISC) and teacher-completed Disruptive Behaviour Disorders (DBD) questionnaire. The teacher-completed IRS demonstrated incremental predictive validity in predicting a rating of global impairment one year later. Using cut-off scores, the IRS also accurately discriminated between children with and without ADHD. As Fabiano and colleagues note, however, this assessment measure is still very new, and requires the collection of further normative data from larger populations. They also note that the assessment of impairment in ADHD that is unique to ADHD symptoms is challenging given that all stages of a diagnosis of ADHD require evidence of impairment.

Social Skills Assessment

One of the most common difficulties associated with ADHD symptomatology is problems in social interactions. Such difficulties are likely to be identified during the interview stage of the assessment, and may be highlighted through the use of broadband questionnaires. Should further investigation of social skills be required, questionnaires such as the Social Skills Rating System (SSRS, Gresham & Elliot, 1990) and the Matson Evaluation of Social Skills with Youngsters (MESSY, Matson, Rotatori, & Helsel, 1983b) may be useful. The SSRS is described as having good reliability and validity, and was normed on a moderate-sized North American sample of school-age children (Kelley, Reitman, & Noell 2003).

The SSRS provides teacher, parent, and self-report scales designed to assess social skills, problem behaviors, and academic competencies (Kelley et al., 2003). The Social skills questions are the major focus, and include items covering the three domains of Cooperation, Assertion, and Self-Control. The SSRS comes with an Assessment-Intervention Record (AIR) which can be used to integrate information across informants, and provides a useful summary of the composite data (Kelley et al., 2003).

The MESSY consists of teacher- and self-report rating scales. Norms, reliability, and validity are all good, although it is noted that the original normative population was largely Caucasian. The items are described as being concrete, easily observable behaviors which provide good face validity (O'Callaghan & Reitman, 2003). The number of factors identified by the MESSY differs between the teacher and self-report forms.

The self-report form identifies five factors: Appropriate Social Skills, Inappropriate Assertiveness, Impulsive/Recalcitrant, Overconfident, and Jealousy/Withdrawal; whereas the teacher-report identifies only two: Appropriate Social Skills and Inappropriate Assertiveness. The MESSY is described as quick and easy to administer and score (O'Callaghan & Reitman, 2003). The specificity and high face validity of the items provide useful information regarding social skills and behavior. The MESSY has been translated into Chinese and Spanish with these translations continuing to provide good clinical utility. It has been noted, however, that the factor structure of the MESSY is not consistent across different populations and studies (Teodoro et al., 2005).

Background Information Questionnaires

Questionnaires may also be useful in collecting information regarding the child's developmental and medical history. There are numerous questionnaires available which fulfill this role, including those from the BASC-2 and Achenbach's CBCL assessment series. The questionnaires provide standardized items regarding maternal pregnancy (including adverse events during pregnancy), early development and milestones, child medical history, and family medical and psychiatric history. These questionnaires can be sent out to families prior to the parent interview, with the proviso that any difficult-to-complete items can be reviewed during the interview.

This allows parents and extended family to more readily confer regarding questions that may be difficult to recall when "on the spot". It may also reduce maternal discomfort when answering items relating to possible alcohol or drug consumption during pregnancy. Having these questionnaires completed prior to the parental interview can reduce the time required for the parental interview by up to an hour. An obvious disadvantage of using such questionnaires is that recording such complicated information requires a certain degree of literacy. There is also increased potential for data to be misplaced or lost.

Direct Observation

The information obtained through interviews and behavioral rating scales may be subject to the biases of the interviewers, interviewees, and respondents. Observational measures are seen as providing more objective information about a child's behavior and their interactions with others. A number of behavioral coding systems have been developed for use with children with ADHD and other externalizing behavior problems. These are designed for use in natural (e.g., classroom) or analogue settings to code for the presence of a range of behaviors such as negative vocalizations, off-task behavior, and motor activity. In general these coding systems demonstrate adequate reliability and validity. They are able to discriminate between children with and without ADHD, subtypes of ADHD, and are sensitive to the effects of intervention (see Pelham et al., 2005 for a brief review of the nature and psychometric properties of several such coding systems).

Although the direct observation of behavior, especially in the school setting, provides valuable information on the nature and frequency of problem behaviors, observational methods have a number of limitations which preclude or limit their use in routine clinical practice. Direct observation is time consuming and costly, raters require training, and multiple observations over time and across settings are required to ensure representative samples of behavior are obtained. Low-base rate, but significant, behaviors are difficult to observe with the time sampling procedures typically used in behavioral observation. Many behavioral observation coding systems lack extensive normative data, and the behavior observed in clinical analogue settings may not be representative of the child's usual behavior (Anastopolos & Shelton, 2001; DuPaul & Stoner, 2003; Pelham et al., 2005).

In light of these difficulties Pelham et al. (2005) suggest cost-effective measures such as having teachers track how much work a student produces may be an effective proxy measure of on-task behavior. They also describe the Individualized Target Behavior Evaluation (ITBE), an observational system using parent or teacher frequency counts as proxies for extensive observations by independent raters, in which target behaviors are operationalized and criteria for each behavior set and evaluated. The ITBE is reported to be reliable with acceptable temporal stability (Pelham et al., 2005).

In carrying out an assessment clinicians and researchers informally observe the child's behavior during interview and testing procedures. Edwards, Schulz, Chelonis, Philyaw, Gardner, and Young (2005) recently evaluated the validity and utility of such unstructured clinical observations in the assessment of ADHD. They found clinician ratings of hyperactive-impulsive and inattentive behaviors correlated significantly with parent, but not teacher, ratings of these behaviors. Clinician ratings showed higher specificity (probability that a child without ADHD will not show observable levels of ADHD behaviors in the clinic setting) than sensitivity (probability that a child diagnosed with ADHD will show observable levels of ADHD behaviors in the clinic). Clinician observations correctly classified between 23 and 44% of children identified as ADHD (by different measures) and 75 and 94% of those identified as not having ADHD. The authors concluded their findings provide limited support for the validity and utility of unstructured observations in the assessment and diagnosis of ADHD. They went on to interpret their findings as evidence that clinic observations are not a suitable substitute for assessing children's behavior in the school setting.

Functional Behavioral Analysis (FBA)

A functional behavioral analysis (FBA) of presenting problems is essential when conducting any psychiatric assessment where the goal is psychosocial intervention. An FBA evaluates the roles of antecedents and consequences in the development and maintenance of problematic behavior. That is, it assesses whether an individual's personal characteristics, or factors within the individual's environment, influence the likelihood of a particular problematic behavior occurring, and then reoccurring. An FBA can provide information that can be directly targeted in treatment planning. It may also provide differential diagnostic information by demonstrating that factors in the individual's environment, rather than internal psychopathology are primarily responsible for the onset and maintenance of a problematic behavior. Northup and Gulley (2001) review the contribution of functional analysis to the assessment of behaviors associated with ADHD.

Psychological and Laboratory Tests

Where there are concerns that lowered general cognitive ability is contributing to presentation, or is thought to be responsible for a child's symptoms, a standardized assessment of intellectual ability is indicated to establish current levels of cognitive functioning. Assessment of intellectual ability may also be indicated to establish if coexisting academic difficulties, which are common in children with ADHD, are due to comorbid learning difficulties or are secondary to the symptoms of ADHD.

When an assessment of intellectual functioning is necessary the clinician's choice of assessment instrument should take account of the measure's psychometric properties and the populations for whom norms are available. All other things being equal, the possibility of repeat assessments, administration time, clinician experience with the measure, and the experience for the child should be considered. Sattler (2001) reports that the scales designed to assess intellectual functioning with the highest reliability and validity, which are well-normed, and up to date include the Wechsler series (i.e., Wechsler Preschool and Primary Scales of Intelligence-Third Edition (WPPSI-III, Wechsler, 2002) 2–6 years; Wechsler Intelligence Scale for Children-Fourth Edition (WISC-IV, Wechsler, 2003) 6–16 years; Wechsler Adult Intelligence Scale-Third Edition (WAIS-III, Wechsler, 1997) 16 years to adult; the Stanford-Binet Intelligence Scales 2–85+ years (Roid, 2003); and the Differential Ability Scales 2 ½ years to 18 years (Elliot, 2006). Difficulties with the Stanford-Binet and DAS scales include the lack of a comparable battery of subtests across the different age ranges which can be assessed with these measures (Sattler, 2001).

Along with the intelligence tests described above, numerous standardized scales are available for the assessment of academic achievement (see Sattler, 2001 for a review). The choice of test selected will depend on a number of factors, including the age of the respondent, what area of achievement is the focus of the assessment, and which other cognitive measures have been administered.

The administration of comprehensive neuropsychological test batteries is not recommended in the routine assessment of ADHD (AACAP, 2007). Gordon, Barkley and Lovett (2006) review several neuropsychological tests that are commonly employed in the assessment of individuals with or suspected of having ADHD. These include measures assessing various aspects of executive function as well as those designed to assess symptoms of attention and impulsivity. With the possible exception of continuous performance tests (CPT), which have been extensively studied and show reasonable sensitivity and specificity, none of the tests reviewed are recommended for diagnostic use.

When reports from parents or teachers, including school reports, or performance on tests of intellectual ability suggest specific areas of cognitive deficit then the clinician may consider further neuropsychological testing to more fully describe and evaluate areas of strength and weakness with respect to treatment planning. Under these circumstances the clinician should select tests which assess the domains of interest that have appropriate standardization samples and good psychometric properties.

Nichols and Waschbusch (2004) recently reviewed evidence for the criterion validity, discriminant validity, and response to treatment of currently used laboratory measures of ADHD symptoms. They concluded, "No lab tasks can yet be recommended as valid for clinical purposes."

Medical Evaluation

As part of any assessment for ADHD, particularly with children, where there is any indication of sensory disturbance, vision and hearing tests should be undertaken. It is also important to consider whether there are any factors in the individual's daily environment that may have a direct influence on symptom presentation (e.g., anti-histamine medications; specific foods; disturbed sleep). This information should be identified through a functional behavior analysis of problem behavior. If a child has not recently been evaluated by a physician then a medical checkup should be considered to rule out any medical or physical causes for their symptom presentation. There are of course currently no medical or laboratory tests for ADHD.

Pearl, Weiss, and Stein (2001) suggest there are some medical conditions that include ADHD symptomatology as part of their presentation (i.e., neurofibromatosis, fetal alcohol syndrome, and lead poisoning), whereas other conditions are commonly comorbid, or may require differential diagnosis (e.g., Tourette's syndrome, learning disabilities, mental retardation). These authors suggest that when undertaking an assessment for possible ADHD the clinician or researcher should be particularly mindful of possible sleep disorders (especially obstructive sleep apnoea), epilepsy (especially absence-type seizures), and thyroid disorder.

Incremental Validity

Incremental validity refers to the issue of whether more information (informants and/or methods) contributes unique information to decision making and whether this information improves diagnostic accuracy or treatment planning. Although multiple informants and multiple methods are recommended in the evaluation of ADHD, Johnston and Murray (2003) note that for the empirical evidence that exists, multiple sources and types of information contribute incrementally to the child assessment process. In acknowledging the limited empirical literature dealing with incremental validity in child assessment they make a number of suggestions for determining if a given piece of evidence or information contributes incrementally to the assessment process. They suggest: the usefulness of multiple informants may vary with a child's age, as will the value of assessing different constructs (developmental and contextual issues); the extent to which additional information has incremental validity may depend on uses of the information (criterion uncertainty); the incremental validity of a given piece of information may depend on what other information is available (specificity of incremental validity). For low base rate disorders they acknowledge it may be difficult to demonstrate incremental validity.

For ADHD, the available evidence suggests the incremental validity of multiple informants is a function of informant age and the purpose to which the information is put, that is, ruling in versus ruling out a diagnosis of ADHD. Parent and teacher reports of externalizing behaviour problems show higher correlations with outcome than child-reports (Loeber, Green, Lahey, & Stouthamer-Loeber, 1991), whereas adolescent self-report does not predict adolescent behavior beyond parent-reports (Smith, Pelham, Gnagy, Molina, & Evans, 2000). Power et al. (1998) found a single informant approach was most useful in ruling out a diagnosis of ADHD, with a multi-informant approach being best for positively diagnosing the disorder. Tripp, Schaughency, and Clarke (2006) found parent- and teacher-completed rating scales contributed differently to confirmatory and differential diagnosis of ADHD providing further support for the inclusion of multiple informants in the assessment process.

The incremental validity of multiple methods in the assessment of ADHD is less well established. In preschool children with ADHD standardized ratings of disruptive behavior during testing demonstrated incremental validity in predicting impairment over and above demographic characteristics and parent and teacher reports (Willicutt, Hartung, Lahey, Loney, & Pelham, 1999). Tripp et al. (2006) interpreted the imperfect performance of parent and teacher rating scales in predicting ADHD diagnostic status as support for the need to include other assessment methodologies in the diagnosis and differential diagnosis of ADHD.

Making a Diagnosis of ADHD

Once diagnostic information has been collected from the different informants (e.g., parents, teachers, and child) using the methods described above the clinician or researcher must use this information to reach a decision regarding whether the child's behavior meets current criteria for a diagnosis of ADHD. Here the decision-maker faces two related challenges: how to combine or integrate data across informants and how to apply the DSM–IV diagnostic criteria in practice. How these tasks are carried out will influence which children ultimately receive a diagnosis of ADHD. Although the diagnosis itself may not affect how a clinician decides to treat a given child or family's difficulties it may influence access to further services and/ or the nature of those services.

Although the *DSM–IV* criteria for ADHD have been described as having the strongest evidence-base in the history of the diagnosis (Barkley, 2003), these criteria are not without problems. Reported concerns include: (a) the number of symptoms required for a diagnosis, and whether these symptom cut-off scores are appropriate across all ages; (b) the appropriateness of symptom content for the wide age range covered by the criteria; (c) insufficient information regarding what is considered developmentally inappropriate behavior for a given age; (d) whether both symptom cut-off scores and content are appropriate for girls as well as boys; (e) whether there is sufficient evidence to justify the age of onset criterion; and (f) the lack of guidance supplied by the *DSM–IV* criteria with regard to what constitutes evidence of impairment in two settings (Barkley, 2003).

In addition the *DSM–IV* does not provide clear guidance on how the criteria for ADHD should be applied in practice, including how symptom counts should be obtained across informants (Barkley & Edwards, 2006). As a consequence there is variability in the manner in which clinicians and researchers apply these criteria. In a recent study Wolraich et al. (2004) assessed the effect of different methods for combining parent and teacher reports to obtain symptom counts on the diagnosis of ADHD. This varied from combining parent- and teacher-reported symptoms to achieve a total symptom count of at least six symptoms in either dimension (lenient criteria) through to requiring a minimum of six symptoms reported by both parents and teacher (strict criteria). Their results clearly showed the method used to combine parent and teacher reports influenced ADHD prevalence. This single aspect of applying the *DSM–IV* criteria for ADHD has implications for the number of children who are diagnosed with ADHD and the issue of subtypes. In consulting the literature clinicians and researchers are advised to consider how studies of interest applied diagnostic criteria.

Reaching a decision regarding whether a given child's behavior meets criteria for a diagnosis of ADHD is a complex process even when there is agreement between informants regarding the nature and severity of a child's difficulties. In practice informant discrepancies are common in the assessment of child psychopathology (e.g., Achenbach, McConaughy, & Howell; 1987; De Los Reyes & Kazdin, 2005). Although such discrepancies may reflect problems with the reliability or validity of the different information sources, it is generally assumed that each piece of assessment data provides unique or additional information that will assist the assessment process (Johnston & Murray, 2003). As yet we lack adequate models regarding how discrepant information across informants is best integrated into the diagnostic decision-making process.

To assist clinicians and researchers with the diagnostic decision-making process Anastopoulos and Shelton (2001) devote a chapter of their book, including worked case examples, to the process of applying the *DSM–IV* diagnostic criteria for ADHD. This includes useful consideration of the order in which the assessor should address the various criteria. Those unfamiliar with applying the *DSM–IV* criteria will find this chapter very helpful, those more experienced may benefit from further consideration of how a diagnoses of ADHD is reached.

Assessment Strategies for Different Age Groups

An important consideration when assessing the reliability and validity of rating scales, questionnaires, and structured and semi-structured interviews is the age-appropriateness of the items for the population being assessed. An underlying problem in the assessment of ADHD in divergent age groups is that the DSM–IV diagnostic criteria for ADHD are strongly biased towards school-age individuals. The majority of assessment measures have been developed for school-age children, and there are obvious difficulties with using these measures with younger and older age groups.

Preschoolers

Measuring ADHD-type behaviors in preschool-age children is especially problematic given the issue of what should be considered developmentally inappropriate. As McLellan and Speltz (2003) point out, studies that have applied DSM–IV criteria to preschoolers have produced inflated levels of externalizing behavior disorders and mood disorders. They raise a concern that applying psychopathological criteria to what may be transient developmental problems could led to inappropriate treatment.

Although caution is needed in the assessment of ADHD symptoms in children under 4–5 years of age, diagnosis and treatment may sometimes be necessary for child safety or to address family and caregiver stress in response to the child's behavior.

There are limited narrowband rating scales available to assess ADHD symptomatology in children under five years of age. The ADDES-3 (McCarney & Arthaud, 2004) was normed on children aged 4 through 18 years of age. Given the facility for the respondent to indicate that a symptom is outside the child's developmental range, this measure can be used with a younger population. Caution should be exercised, however, as many of the ADHD symptoms may not be applicable (e.g., 'rushes through assignments with little or no regard for the accuracy or quality of work').

A number of broadband questionnaires have age-appropriate forms that have been normed on a younger age group; the most commonly used of these are the CBCL and the BASC-2. The Child Behaviour Checklist preschool form covers ages 18 months through to 5 years. Preschool norms are available from the original 1991 sample, with the more recent edition being normed on an additional 700 children. The BASC-2 preschool version was normed as a part of the normative population sample (aged 2–21 years). The BASC-2 preschool version shows good internal reliability, reasonable test–retest reliability, and good interrater reliability. There are limited validity data available.

The Early Childhood Inventory-4 (ECI-4, Gadow & Sprafkin, 1997; Sprafkin, Volpe, Gadow, Nolan, & Kelly, 2002) is another broadband questionnaire that assesses ADHD symptomatology, ODD, CD, Peer Conflict, Anxiety, Depression, sleep problems, elimination problems, feeding problems, and pervasive developmental disorder. The parent and teacher ECI-4 checklists were normed with reasonable sized samples, $n = 431$ and $n = 398$, respectively. The normative population was predominantly Caucasian, although there was a reasonable socioeconomic distribution. The ECI-4 reports reasonable test–retest reliability for the parent checklist for some, but not all of the indices over a three-month period.

Similarly, the predictive and concurrent validity were adequate for only the more commonly occurring disruptive behavior disorders (Kelly et al., 2003). It is suggested the ECI-4 would serve as an adequate screening tool for identifying common difficulties in preschool-aged children, but that there is insufficient support for its ability to identify less common difficulties, such as Generalised Anxiety disorder.

Adolescents

As Wasserstein (2005) and Brown (2000) point out, a key issue when assessing ADHD symptoms in adolescence is often the complexity of the presentation. These authors suggest that when ADHD is first assessed in adolescence there are likely to be more comorbid problems, such as substance abuse, antisocial behavior, mood/anxiety disorders, and learning disabilities that may disguise symptoms of ADHD. Robin (1998) argues that not only is the adolescent's presentation more complex, environmental factors, such as adversity, family structure, parental psychopathology, and parental problem-solving skills are more complex, and need to be thoroughly assessed due to their impact upon treatment effectiveness. In this age group any intervention strategies need to target not only ADHD symptoms, but also family dynamics (Robin, 1998). Care must also be taken at all stages of assessment and treatment to maintain a collaborative relationship between the clinician/assessor and the adolescent patient, to motivate the adolescent to remain engaged in treatment.

The assessment techniques for measuring ADHD symptomatology in adolescence differ little from those for assessing children. The assessor should be aware, however, that symptoms of overactivity are often not as overt as in childhood. As a consequence the role of self-report becomes more important in the assessment of the adolescent. Research suggests that although adolescents may underestimate the degree of difficulty they experience due to ADHD symptomatology and externalizing behavior, adolescent self-report is the most reliable means of obtaining information relating to internalizing symptoms and covert behaviors (e.g., Achenbach et al., 1987; Andrews, Garrison, Jackson, Addy, & McKeown, 1993; Cantwell et al., 1997). Both the BASC-2 and Achenbach series provide self-report rating scales for adolescents which report good reliability. The BASC-2 provides a Self-Report of Personality rating scale for ages 8–11 years, and 12–21 years; whereas Achenbach's CBCL series includes the Youth Report for ages 11 to 18 years.

The majority of parent- and teacher-respondent rating scales are normed on a wide age range that encompass the adolescent period. Of note, the BASC-2 provides a separate measure and norms for adolescents between 12 and 18 years of age, and the Conners' ADHD rating scales has adolescent and adult forms, which may allow for increased age-appropriateness of items.

Adults

As with adolescents, the DSM–IV diagnostic criteria for ADHD are not readily applied to adults (McGough & Barkley, 2004). Given the increasing acceptance that ADHD symptoms persist into adulthood, it is likely that diagnostic criteria in the DSM–V will include items more relevant to adult ADHD. Until this time, any assessment of possible adult ADHD needs to include a thorough assessment of differential diagnostic possibilities, and also demonstrate a clear developmental history of ADHD symptomatology. Differential diagnostic factors to consider include the obvious medical causes such as head injury, epilepsy, hyper- or hypothyroidism, and sleep disorders. Careful assessment of drug and alcohol use should also be undertaken. Differential diagnosis becomes particularly difficult in cases where personality disorders, such as Borderline Personality Disorder, have been previously diagnosed. In these situations the developmental history and a family psychiatric history are essential. Strong evidence of childhood ADHD symptoms and a diagnosis of ADHD in a first-degree relative would help form a strong case for ADHD, which may or may not be comorbid with a personality disorder.

A number of rating scales have been developed to assess ADHD in adulthood (Murphy & Adler, 2004). The Brown Attention Deficit Disorders Scales (Brown, 1996) largely focus on inattentive and executive functioning type difficulties. The Conners' Adult ADHD Rating Scale (CAARS, Conners, Erhardt, & Sparrow, 1999) includes inattention and hyperactivity/impulsivity items, and provides self-report and observer rating scales. The long form of the CAARS also includes measures of impulsivity/emotional lability and problems with self-concept.

The Wender Utah Rating Scale (WURS; Ward, Wender, & Reimherr, 1993) relies on retrospective self-report of adults to describe their childhood ADHD symptoms. Although this measure correlated highly with parent reports of childhood ADHD symptoms, it is reported to have poor discriminant validity (McCann, Scheele, Ward, & Roy-Byrne, 2000). McCann et al. (2000) found that although the WURS correctly identified 72% of patients with a diagnosis of ADHD, its ability to discriminate adults without a diagnosis was little better than chance, suggesting poor specificity.

The Adult Self Report Scale (ASRS; Adler, Kessler, & Spencer, 2004) is based around the *DSM–IV-TR* items but incorporates more adult-appropriate item examples. The ASRS also provides a six-item Adult ADHD Self-Report Scale screener (ASRS-v1.1; Adler et al., 2004) which can be obtained from the website listed in the references. Nutt et al. (2007) suggest that rating scales alone are insufficient for the diagnosis of ADHD, but may be helpful as part of a broader assessment. They recommend the use of measures to assess the presence and severity of comorbid symptoms, and general impairment rating scales.

CONCLUSIONS

In the preceding sections we have attempted to provide a framework for planning and conducting evidence-based assessments with children whose presentation is suggestive of ADHD. We have also included some details on the assessment of ADHD in other age groups. The specific form an assessment takes will be influenced by the characteristics of the child, the purpose of the assessment, and the available resources. Clinicians and researchers are reminded that evidence-based assessment involves more than the use of psychometrically sound methods and measures. The context in which these measures are used, their incremental validity, and their clinical utility must all be considered.

The empirical literature on incremental validity in the assessment of ADHD is limited. However, the available research supports recommendations to obtain information from multiple informants. Given the DSM–IV requirement of evidence of impairment from symptoms across settings, the frequently reported academic and social difficulties of children with ADHD, and the significant time children spend in the school setting, teachers are an obvious and appropriate source of information in addition to parents and the referred child.

There is also some empirical support for the use of multiple assessment methods in ADHD evaluations. A number of broadband and narrowband rating scales are available that have acceptable psychometric properties. Narrowband scales contribute to diagnostic decision making through identification of symptom presence or absence. Broadband scales provide important additional information on comorbid difficulties and impairment. They can also assist in determining the developmental appropriateness of behavior. Data collection via questionnaires and rating scales is time efficient and cost effective, however, it remains an empirical question whether symptom rating scales could or should replace the currently favored structured and semi-structured interviews for the collection of diagnostic information. There appear to be a number of psychometrically sound scales available that can be successfully used to collect information on functional impairment. Such information is important to both diagnosis and treatment planning.

Specialized assessment procedures, for example, formal behavioral observations and comprehensive neuropsychological assessment procedures, are not recommended as a routine part of assessment. Such assessment procedures should be included when their results are likely to clarify the nature and extent of a child's difficulties contributing to diagnosis and/or treatment planning. When academic difficulties are present the assessment of general intellectual ability may be appropriate to help clarify the nature of these difficulties. The use of laboratory measures to assess ADHD symptoms in clinical practice is not currently supported by the literature. If the child has not had a recent medical evaluation one should be considered to rule out the contribution of any medical conditions to symptoms.

In short the assessment of children who present with difficulties suggestive of ADHD should include informants who know the child sufficiently well to provide reliable and valid information regarding his or her behavior. The methods and measures used to collect information must be psychometrically sound and appropriate for use in the given assessment context. Information should be collected that allows for the ruling in as well as the ruling out of a diagnosis of ADHD. This includes careful consideration of alternative explanations for the presence of symptoms consistent with a diagnosis of ADHD. The clinician or researcher should consider issues of incremental validity and clinical utility remembering at the end of the assessment decisions will need to be made regarding diagnostic status and appropriate intervention.

REFERENCES

Achenbach, T. M. (1991). *Integrative guide for the 1991 CBCL/4-18, YSR, and TRF profiles.* Burlington, VT: University of Vermont, Department of Psychiatry.

Achenbach, T. M., McConaughy, S. H., & Howell, C. T. (1987). Child/adolescent behavioural and emotional problems: implications of cross-informant correlations for situational specificity. *Psychological Bulletin, 101,* 213–232.

Achenbach, T. M., & Rescorla, L. A. (2001). *Manual for ASEBA School-Age Forms & Profiles.* Burlington, VT: University of Vermont, Research Center for Children, Youth & Families. See http://www.aseba.org/index.html.

Adler, L. A., Kessler, R. C., Spencer, T. (2004). *Adult ADHD Self-Report Scale- v1.1 (ASRS-v1.1) Symptom Checklist.* New York, Available at: www.med.nyu.edu/psych/assets/adhdscreen18.pdf.

Ambrosini, P. (2000). Historical development and present status of the Schedule for Affective Disorders and Schizophrenia for School-Age Children (K-SADS). *American Academy of Child and Adolescent Psychiatry 39,* 49–58.

American Academy of Child and Adolescent Psychiatry. (2007). Practice parameters for the assessment and treatment of children and adolescents with Attention-Deficit Hyperactivity disorder. *Journal of the American Academy of Child and Adolescent Psychiatry, 46,* 894–921.

American Academy of Pediatrics. (2001). Clinical practice guideline: Treatment of the school-aged child with Attention-Deficit/Hyperactivity Disorder. *Pediatrics, 108,* 1033–1044.

American Psychiatric Association: (2000). *Diagnostic and statistical manual of mental disorder, fourth edition, text revision.* Washington, DC, American Psychiatric Association.

Anastopoulos, A. D., & Shelton, T. L. (2001). *Assessing attention-deficit/hyperactivity disorder.* New York: Kluwer Academic/Plenum.

Andrews, V. C., Garrison, C. Z., Jackson, K. L., Addy, C. L., & McKeown, R. E. (1993). Mother-adolescent agreement on the symptoms and diagnoses of adolescent depression and conduct disorders. *Journal of the American Academy of Child and Adolescent Psychiatry, 32,* 731–738.

Angold, A., & Costello, E. J. (2000). The child and adolescent psychiatric assessment (CAPA). *American Academy of Child and Adolescent Psychiatry, 39,* 39–48.

Arnsten, A. F. (2006). Stimulants: Therapeutic action in ADHD. *Neuropsychopharmacology 31*(11): 2376–2383.

Asherson, P., Kuntsi, J., & Taylor, E. (2005). Unravelling the complexity of attention-deficit hyperactivity disorder: A behavioural genomic approach. *British Journal of Psychiatry, 187,*103–105.

Atkins, M. S., Pelham, W. E., & Licht, M. (1985). A comparison of objective classroom measures and teacher ratings of attention deficit disorder. *Journal of Abnormal Child Psychology, 13,* 155–167.

Barkley, R. A. (2003). Issues in the diagnosis of attention-deficit/hyperactivity disorder in children. *Brain Development, 25,* 77–83.

Barkley, R. A. (2006). *Attention-deficit hyperactivity disorder: A handbook for diagnosis and treatment.* New York: The Guilford Press.

Barkley, R. A., & Edwards, G. (2006). Diagnostic interview, behaviour rating scales, and the medical examination. In R. A. Barkley, *Attention-deficit hyperactivity disorder: A handbook for diagnosis and treatment - third edition* (pp. 337–368). New York: Guilford Press.

Biederman, J. (2005). Attention-deficit/hyperactivity disorder: A selective overview. *Biological Psychiatry, 57* 1215–1220.

Biederman, J., Faraone, S. V., Keenan, K., Benjamin, J., Krifcher, B., Moore, C., et al. (1992). Further evidence for family-genetic risk factors in attention deficit hyperactivity disorder. Patterns of comorbidity in probands and relatives in psychiatrically and pediatrically referred samples. *Archives of General Psychiatry, 49,* 728–738.

Biederman, J., Faraone, S. V., Keenan, K., Knee, D., & Tsuany, M. T. (1990). Family genetic and psychosocial risk factors in *DSM–III* attention deficit disorder. *Journal of the American Academy of Child and Adolescent Psychiatry, 29,* 526–533.

Biederman, J., Faraone, S. V., Taylor, A., Sienna, M., Williamson, S., & Fine, C. (1998). Diagnostic continuity between child and adolescent ADHD: Findings from a longitudinal clinical sample. *Journal of the American Academy of Child and Adolescent Psychiatry, 37,* 305–313.

Biederman, J., Monuteaux, M. C., Kendrick, E., Klein, K. L., & Faraone, S. V. (2005). The CBCL as a screen for psychiatric comorbidity in paediatric patients with ADHD. *Archives of Disease in Childhood, 90,* 1010–1015.

Biederman, J., Newcorn, J., & Sprich, S. (1991). Comorbidity of attention deficit hyperactivity disorder with conduct, depressive, anxiety and other disorders. *The American Journal of Psychiatry, 148,* 564–577.

Bird, H. R., Shaffer, D., Fisher, P., Gould, M. S., Staghezza, B., Chen, J. Y. et al. (1993). The Columbia Impairment Scales (CIS): Pilot findings on a measure of global impairment for children and adolescents. *International Journal of Methods in Psychiatric Research, 3,* 167–176.

Bobb, A. J., Castellanos, F.X., Addington, A. M., & Rapoport, J.L. (2005). Molecular genetic studies of ADHD: 1991–2004. *American Journal of Medical Genetics Part B (Neuropsychiatric Genetics), 132B,* 109–125.

Brown, T. E. (1996). *Brown Attention-Deficit Disorder Scales.* San Antonio, TX: Psychological Corporation.

Brown, T. E. (2000). Emerging understandings of attention-deficit disorders and comorbitites. In T. E. Brown (Ed.),. *Attention-deficit disorders and comorbidities in children, adolescents and adults* (pp. 3–36). Washington, DC: American Psychiatric Press.

Bush, G., Valera, E. M., & Seidman, L. J. (2005). Functional neuroimaging of attention-deficit/hyperactivity disorder: A review and suggested future directions. *Biological Psychiatry, 57,* 1273–1284.

Cantwell, D. P., Lewinsohn, P. M., Rohde, P., & Seeley, J. R. (1997). Correspondence between adolescent report and parent report of psychiatric diagnostic data. *Journal of the American Academy of Child and Adolescent Psychiatry, 36,* 610–619.

Chamberlain, S. R., Robbins, T. W., & Sahakian, B. J. (2007). The neurobiology of attention-deficit/hyperactivity disorder. *Biological Psychiatry, 15,* 1317–1319.

Collett, B. R., Ohan, J. L., & Myers, K. M. (2003a). Ten-year review of rating scales, V: Scales assessing attention-deficit/hyperactivity disorder. *Journal of the American Academy of Child and Adolescent Psychiatry, 42,* 1015–1037.

Collett, B. R., Ohan, J. L., & Myers, K. M. (2003b). Ten-year review of rating scales. VI: scales assessing externalizing behaviours. *Journal of the American Academy of Child and Adolescent Psychiatry, 42,*1143–1170.

Conners, C. K., Erhardt, D., & Sparrow, M. A. (1999). *Conners Adult ADHD Rating Scales (CAARS)* New York: Multi Health Systems Inc.

Conners, C. K., Sitareniso, G., Parker, J. D., & Epstein, J. N. (1998a). Revision and restandardization of the Conners' Teacher Rating Scale (CTRS-R): Factor structure reliability, and criterion validity. *Journal of Abnormal Child Psychology, 26,* 279–291.

Conners, C. K., Sitarenios, G., Parker, J. D., & Epstein, J. N. (1998b). The revised Conners' Parent Rating Scale (CPRS-R): Factor structure, reliability, and criterion validity. *Journal of Abnormal Child Psychology, 26,* 257–268.

De Los Reyes, A., & Kazdin, A. E. (2005). Informant discrepancies in the assessment of childhood psychopathology: A critical review, theoretical framework, and recommendations for further study. *Psychological Bulletin, 131,* 483–509.

DuPaul, G. J., Power, T. J., Anastopoulos, A. D., & Reid, R. (1998). *ADHD Rating Scale IV: Checklists, norms and interpretation.* New York: Guilford Press.

DuPaul, G. J., & Stoner, G. (2003). *ADHD in the Schools: Assessment and intervention strategies - second edition.* New York: Guilford Press.

Edwards, M. C., Schulz, E. G., Chelonis, J., Philyaw, A., Gardner, E., & Young, J. (2005). Estimates of the validity and utility of unstructured clinical observations of children in the assessment of ADHD. *Clinical Pediatrics, 44,* 49–56.

Eiraldi, R. B., Power, T. J., & Nezu, C. M. (1997). Patterns of comorbidity associated with subtypes of attention-deficity hyperactivity disorder among 6- to 12-yr-old children. *Journal of the American Academy of Child and Adolescent Psychiatry, 36,* 503–514.

Elliot, C. D. (2006). *Differential Ability Scales - Second Edition (DAS–II) Adminstration and scoring manual.* San Antonio, TX: The Psychological Corporation.

Fabiano, G. A., Pelham, W. E. Jr., Waschbusch, D.A., Gnagy, E.M., Lahey, B. B., Chronis, A. M., et al. (2006). A practical measure of impairment: Psychometric properties of the Impairment Rating Scale in samples of children with attention deficit hyperactivity disorder and two school-based samples. *Journal of Clinical Child and Adolescent Psychology, 35,* 369–385.

Faigel, H. C., Sznajderman, S., Tishby, O., Turel, M., & Pinus, U. (1995). Attention deficit disorder during adolescence: A review. *Journal of Adolescent Health, 16,* 174–184.

Faraone, S. V., & Biederman, J. (2005). What is the prevalence of adult ADHD? Results of a population screen of 966 adults. *Journal of Attention Disorders, 9,* 384–391.

Faraone, S. V., Biederman, J., Chen, W. J., Krifcher, B., Keenan, K., Moore, C. et al. (1992). Segregation analysis of attention deficit hyperactivity disorder: Evidence for single gene transmission. *Psychiatric Genetics, 2,* 257–275.

Faraone, S. V., Perlis, R. H., Doyle, A. E., Smoller, J. W., Goralnick, J. J., Homgren, M. A. et al. (2005). Molecular genetics of Attention-Deficit/Hyperactivity Disorder *Biological Psychiatry, 57,* 1313–1323..

Fergusson, D. M., Horwood, L. J., & Lynskey, M. T. (1993). Prevalence and comorbidity of DSM–III–R diagnoses in a birth cohort of 15 year olds. *Journal of the American Academy of Child and Adolescent Psychiatry, 32,*1127–1141.

Gadow, K. D. & Sprafkin, J. (1997). *Early Childhood Symptom Inventory: Norms manual.* Stoney Brook, NY: Checkmate Plus.

Gaub, M., & Carlson, C. L. (1997). Gender differences in ADHD: A meta-analysis and critical review. *Journal of the American Academy of Child and Adolescent Psychiatry, 36,* 1036–1045.

Gordon, M., Barkley, R. A., & Lovett, B. J. (2006). Tests and observational measures. In R. A. Barkley (Ed.), *Attention-deficit hyperactivity disorder: A handbook for diagnosis and treatment - third edition* (pp. 369–388). New York: Guilford Press.

Gresham, F. M., & Elliot, S. N. (1990). *Social skills rating system: Manual.* Circle Pines, MN: American Guidance Systems.

Harrison, P. L., & Oakland, T. (2003). *Adaptive behaviour assessment system, 2nd edition.* San Antonio, TX: Psychological Corporation.

Hechtman, L. (1991). Resilience and vulnerability in long term outcome of attention deficit hyperactive disorder. *Canadian Journal of Psychiatry, 36,* 415–421.

Hodges, K. (1994). *The Child and Adolescent Functional Assessment Scale (CAFAS), self-training manual.* Ypsilanti: Eastern Michigan University, Department of Psychology.

Hughes, J. N., & Baker, D. B. (1990). *The clinical child interview.* New York: Guilford Press.

Hunsley, J., & Mash, E. J. (2005). Introduction to the special section on developing guidelines for the evidence-based assessment (EBA) of adult disorders. *Psychological Assessment, 17* (3), 251–255.

Hunsley, J., & Mash, E. J. (2007). Evidence-based assessment. *Annual Review of Clinical Psychology, 3,* 29–51.

Jensen, P. S., Martin, D., & Cantwell, D. P. (1997). Comorbidity in ADHD: Implications for research, practice and *DSM–IV. Journal of the American Academy of Child and Adolescent Psychiatry, 36,* 1065–1079.

Jensen, P. S., Rubio-Stipec, M., Canino, G., Bird, H. R., Dulcan, M. K., Schwab-stone, M. E., et al. (1999). Parent and child contributions to diagnosis of mental disorder: Are both informants always necessary? *Journal of the American Academy of Child and Adolescent Psychiatry, 38,* 1569–1579.

Jensen, P. S., Watanabe, H. K., Richters, J. E., Roper, M., Hibbs, E. D., Salzberg, A. D., et al. (1996). Scales, diagnoses and child psychopathology: II Comparing the CBCL and the DISC against external validators. *Journal of Abnormal Child Psychology,* *24,* 151–168).

Johnston, C., & Murray, C. (2003). Incremental validity in the psychological assessment of children and adolescents. *Psychological Assessment, 15,* 496–507.

Kadesjö, B., & Gillberg, C. (2001). The comorbidity of ADHD in the general population of Swedish school-aged children. *Journal of Child Psychology and Psychiatry, 42,* 487–492.

Kelley, M., Reitman, D., & Noell, G. H. (2003). *Practictioner's guide to empirically based measures of school behavior.* New York: Kluwer Academic/Plenum

Kessler, R. C., Adler, L., Barkley, R. A., Biederman, J., Conner, C. K., Demler, O., et al. (2006). The prevalence and correlates of adult ADHD is the United States: Results from the national comorbidity survey replication. *Evidence Based Mental Health, 9,* 716–723.

Lahey, B. B., Pelham, W. E., Chronis, A., Massetti, G., Kipp, H., Ehrhardt, A., et al. (2006). Predictive validity of ICD-10 hyperkinetic disorder relative to *DSM–IV* attention-deficit/hyperactivity disorder among younger children. *Journal of Child Psychology and Psychiatry, 47,* 472–479.

Loeber, R., Green, S., & Lahey, B. B. (1989). Mental health professionals' perception of the utility of children, mothers, and teachers as informants on childhood psychopathology. *Journal of Clinical Child Psychology, 19,* 136–143.

Loeber, R., Green, S. M., Lahey, B. B., & Stouthamer-Loeber, M. (1991). Differences and similarities between children, mothers, and teachers as informants on disruptive behaviour disorders. *Journal of Abnormal Child Psychology, 19,* 75–95.

Mash, E. J., & Hunsley, J. (2005). Special Section: Developing guidelines for the evidence-based assessment of child and adolescent disorders. *Journal of Clinical Child and Adolescent Psychology, 34,* 362–379.

Matson, J. L., Rotatori, A. F., & Helsel, W. J. (1983b). Development of a rating scale to measure social skills in children: The Matson evaluation of social skills with youngsters (MESSY). *Behaviour Research and Therapy, 21,* 335–340.

McCann, B. S., Scheele, L., Ward, N., & Roy-Byrne, P. (2000). Discriminant validity of the Wender Utach Rating Scale for Attention Deficit/Hyperactivity disorder in adults. *Journal of Neuropsychiatry and Clinical Neuroscience, 12,* 240–245.

McCarney, S. B., & Arthaud, T. J. (2004). *Attention Deficit Disorders Evaluation Scale - Third Edition (ADDES-3) Home Version Technical Manual.* Columbia MO: Hawthorne Educational Services Inc.

McClellan, J. M., & Speltz, M. L. (2003). Psychiatric diagnoses in preschool children. *Journal of the American Academy of Child and Adolescent Psychiatry, 42,* 127–128.

McClellan, J. M., & Werry, J. S. (2000). Introduction: Special section: Research psychiatric diagnostic interviews for children and adolescents. *Journal of the American Academy of Child and Adolescent Psychiatry, 39,* 19–27.

McConaughy, S. H. (2005). *Clinical interviews for children and adolescents: Assessment to intervention.* New York: Guilford Press.

McGee, R., Feehan, M., Williams, S., Partridge, F., Silva, P. A., & Kelly, J. (1990). *DSM–III* disorders in a large sample of adolescents. *Journal of the American Academy of Child and Adolescent Psychiatry, 29,* 611–619.

McGough, J. J., & Barkley, R. A. (2004). Diagnostic controversies in adult attention deficit hyperactivity disorder. *American Journal of Psychiatry, 161,* 1948–1956.

Murphy, K. R., & Adler, L. A. (2004). Assessing attention-deficit/hyperactivity disorder in adults: Focus on rating scales. *Journal of Clinical Psychiatry, 65* (Supplement 3), 12–17.

Nichols, S. L., & Waschbusch, D. A. (2004). A review of the validity of laboratory cognitive tasks used to assess symptoms of ADHD. *Child Psychiatry and Human Development, 34,* 297–315.

Northup, J., & Gulley, V. (2001). Some contributions of functional analysis to the assessment of behaviours associated with attention deficit hyperactivity disorder and the effects of stimulant medication. *School Psychology Review, 30,* 227–.238.

Nutt, D. J., Fone, K., Asherson, P., Bramble, D., Hill, P., Matthews, K., et al. (2007). Evidence-based guidelines for management of attention-deficit/hyperactivity disorder in adolescents in transition to adult services and in adults: Recommendations from the British Association for Psychopharmacology. *Journal of Psychopharmacology, 21,* 10–41.

O'Callaghan, P. M., & Reitman, D. (2003). The Matson Evaluation of Social Skills with Youngsters: Self report version, teacher report version (Review). *Practictioner's guide to empirically based measures of school behaviour.* M. Kelley, D. Reitman, & G. H. Noell. New York: Kluwer Academic/Plenum.

Pearl, P. L., Weiss, R. E., & Stein, M. A. (2001). Medical mimics: Medical and neurological conditions simulating ADHD. *Annals of the New York Academy of Sciences, 931,* 97–112.

Pelham, W. E., Evans, S. W., Gnagy, E. M., & Greenslade, K. E. (1992). Teacher ratings of *DSM–III–R* symptoms for the disruptive behaviour disorders: Prevalence, factor analyses, and conditional probabilities in a special education sample. *School Psychology Review, 21,* 285–299.

Pelham, W. E., Jr., Fabiano, G. A., & Massetti, G. M. (2005). Evidence-based assessment of attention deficit hyperactivity disorder in children and adolescents. *Journal of Clinical Child and Adolescent Psychology, 34,* 449–476.

Pelham, W. E., Griener, A., & Gnagy, E. M. (1998). *Summer treatment program manual.* Buffalo, NY: Comprehensive Treatment for Attention Deficit Hyperactivity Disorder.

Power, T. J., Andrews, T. J., Eiraldi, R. B., Doherty, B. J., Ikeda, M. J., DuPaul, G. J., et al. (1998). Evaluating attention deficit hyperactivity disorder using multiple informants: The incremental utility of combining teacher with parent reports. *Psychological Assessment, 10,* 250–260.

Reich, W. (2000). Diagnostic interview for children and adolescents (DICA). *American Academy of Child and Adolescent Psychiatry, 39,* 59–66.

Reynolds, C. R., & Kamphaus, R. W. (2004). *Behavior Assessment System for Children, Second Edition (BASC-2).* Bloomington, MN: Pearson Assessments. See: http://ags.pearsonassessments.com/

Robin, A. L. (1998). *ADHD in Adolescents: Diagnosis and Treatment.* New York: Guilford Press.

Roid, G. (2003). *Stanford-Binet Intelligence Scales, Fifth Edition.* Rolling Meadows, IL: Riverside Publishing.

Sattler, J. M. (1998). *Clinical and forensic interviewing of children and families: Guidelines for the mental health, education, pediatric, and child maltreatment fields.* San Diego: Jerome M. Sattler.

Sattler, J. M. (2001). *Assessment of children: Cognitive applications - fourth edition.* San Diego: Jerome. M. Sattler.

Sattler, J. M. & Mash, E, J. (1998). Introduction to clinical assessment interviewing. In J. M. Sattler (Ed.), *Clinical and forensic interviewing of children and families: Guidelines for the mental health, education, pediatric, and child maltreatment fields* (pp. 2–44). San Diego: Jerome M. Sattler.

Scheres, A., Milham, M. P., Knutson, B., & Castellanos, F.X. (2007). Ventral striatal hyporesponsiveness during reward anticipation in attention-deficit/hyperactivity disorder. *Biological Psychiatry, 61,* 720–724.

Shaffer, D., Gould, M. S., Brasic, J., Ambrosini, P., Fisher, P., Bird, H., et al. (1983). A children's global assessment scale (CGAS). *Archives of General Psychiatry, 40,* 1228–1231.

Shaffer, D., Fisher, P., Lucas, C. P., Dulcan, M. K., Schwab-Stone, M. E. (2000). NIMH diagnostic interview for children version IV (NIMH DISC-IV): Description, differences from previous versions, and reliability of some common diagnoses. *American Academy of Child and Adolescent Psychiatry, 39,* 28–38.

Sherrill, J. T., & Kovacs, M. (2000). Interview schedule for children and adolescents (ISCA). *Journal of the American Academy of Child and Adolescent Psychiatry, 39,* 67–75.

Smith, B. H., Pelham, W. E., Gnagy, M., Molina, B., & Evans, S. (2000). The reliability, validity, and unique contributions of self-report by adolescents receiving treatment for attention-deficit/hyperactivity disorder. *Journal of Consulting and Clinical Psychology, 68,* 489–499.

Sparrow, S. S., Cicchetti, D. V., & Balla, D. A. (1984). *Interview Edition Survey Form manual: Vineland Adpative Behaviour Scales.* Circle Pines, MN: American Guidance Service.

Sparrow, S. S., Cicchetti, D. V., & Balla, D. A. (2005). *Vineland Adaptive Behaviour Rating Scales - second edition (Vineland-II) Survey Form manual.* American Guidance Services (AGS).

Sprafkin, J., Volpe, R. J., Gadow, K. D., Nolan, E. E., & Kelly, K. (2002). A *DSM–IV*-referenced screening instrument for preschool children: The Early Childhood Inventory - 4. *Journal of the American Academy of Child and Adolescent Psychiatry, 41,* 604–612.

Steinhausen, H., Novik, T, Baldursson, G., Curatolo, P., Lorezo, M. J., Pereira, R. R., et al. (2006). Co-existing psychiatric problems in ADHD in the ADORE cohort. *European Child and Adolescent Psychiatry, 15*(Supplement 1), 1/25 – 1/29.

Swanson, J., Schuck, S., Mann, M., Carlson, C., Hartmann, K., Sergeant, J., et al. (2001). *Categorical and dimensional definitions and evaluations of symptoms of ADHD: the SNAP and SWAN rating scales.* Available at: http://www.adhd.net.

Swanson, J. M., Sergeant, J. A., Taylor, E., Sonuga-Barke, E. J. S., Jensen, P. S., & Cantwell, D. P. (1998). Attention-deficity hyperactivity disorder and hyperkinetic disorder. *The Lancet, 351,* 429–433.

Tannock, R., & Brown, T. E. (2000). Attention deficit disorders with learning disorder in children and adolescents. In T. E. Brown (Ed.), *Attention-deficit disorder and comorbidities in children, adolescents and adults* (pp. 231–296). Washington, DC: American Psychiatric Press.

Teodoro, M. L. M., Käppler, K. C., Rodrigues, J. de L., Freitas, P. M de., & Haase, V. G. (2005). The Matson Evaluation of Social Skills with Youngsters (MESSY) and its adaptation for Brazilian children and adolescents. *Interamerican Journal of Psychology, 39* (2), 239–246.

Tripp, G., Luk, S. L., Shaughency, E. A., & Singh, R. (1999). *DSM–IV* and ICD-10: A comparison of the correlates of ADHD and hyperkinetic disorder. *Journal of the American Academy of Child and Adolescent Psychiatry, 38,* 156–164.

Tripp, G., Shaughency, E. A., Clarke, B. (2006). Parent and teacher rating scales in the evaluation of attention-deficit hyperactivity disorder: Contribution to diagnosis and differential diagnosis in clinically referred children. *Journal of Developmental Behavioural Pediatrics, 27,* 209–218.

Valera, E. M., Faraone, S. V., Murray, K. E., & Seidman, L. J. (2007). Meta-analysis of structural imaging findings in attention-deficit/hyperactivity disorder. *Biological Psychiatry, 61,* 1361–1369.

Waldman, I. D., & Gizer, I. R. (2006). The genetics of attention deficit hyperactivity disorder. *Clinical Psychology Review, 26,* 396–432.

Ward, M. F., Wender, P. H., & Reimherr, F. W. (1993). The Wender Utah Rating Scale: An aid in the retrospective diagnosis of childhood attention deficit hyperactivity disorder. *American Journal of Psychiatry, 150,* 885–890.

Wasserstein, J. (2005). Diagnostic issues for adolescents and adults with ADHD. *Journal of Clinical Psychology, 61,* 535–547.

Wechsler, D. (1997). *Wechsler Adult Intelligence Scale - third edition.* San Antonio, TX: Psychological Corporation.

Wechsler, D. (2002). *Wechsler Preschool and Primary Scale of Intelligence - third edition: Administration and scoring manual.* San Antonio, TX: Psychological Corporation.

Wechsler, D. (2003). *Wechsler Intelligence Scale for Children - fourth edition: Administration and scoring manual.* San Antonio TX: Psychological Corporation.

Weller, E. B., Weller, R. A., Fristad, M. A., Rooney, M. T., & Schecter, J. (2000). Children's interview for psychiatric syndromes (ChIPS). *American Academy of Child and Adolescent Psychiatry, 39,* 76–84.

Willcutt, E. G., Doyle, A. E., Nigg, J. T., Faraone, S. V., & Pennington, B. F. (2005). Validity of the executive functioning theory of attention deficit/hyperactivity disorder: A meta-analytic review. *Biological Psychiatry, 57,* 1336–1346.

Willcutt, E. G., Hartung, C. M., Lahey, B. B., Loney, J., & Pelham, W. E. (1999). Utility of behaviour ratings by examiners during assessments of preschool children with attention-deficit/hyperactivity disorder. *Journal of Abnormal Child Psychology, 27,* 463–472.

Winters, N. C., Collett, B. R., & Myers, K. M. (2005). Ten-year review of rating scales, VII: Scales assessing functional impairment. *Journal of the American Academy of Child and Adolescent Psychiatry, 44,* 309–338.

Wolraich, M. L. (2003). *Vanderbilt ADHD Teacher Rating Scale (VADTRS) and the Vander-bilt ADHD Parent Rating Scale (VADPRS)*. Oklahoma City: University of Oklahoma Health Sciences Centre: Available online at: www.nichq.org.

Wolraich, M. L., Feurer, I. D., Hannah, J. N., Baumgaertel, A., & Pinnock, T. Y. (1998). Obtaining systematic teacher reports of disruptive behaivour disorders utilizing *DSM–IV. Journal of Abnormal Child Psychology, 26*, 141–152.

Wolraich, M. L., Lambert, E. W., Bickman, L., Simmons, T., Doffing, M. A., & Worley, K. A. (2004). Assessing the impact of parent and teacher agreement on diagnosing attention-deficit hyperactivity disorder. *Journal of Developmental and Behavioral Pediatrics, 25*, 41–47.

Wolraich, M. L., Lambert, W., Doffing, M. A., Bickman, L., Simmons, T., & Worley, K. (2003). Psychometric properties of the Vanderbilt ADHD diagnostic parent rating scale in a referred population. *Journal of Pediatric Psychology, 28*, 559–568.

World Health Organization. (1992). *International classification of diseases (tenth edition). Classification of mental and behavioural disorders.* Geneva: World Health Organisation.

9

Assessment of Mood Disorders in Children and Adolescents

C. EMILY DURBIN and SYLIA WILSON

The research literature on mood disorders in children and adolescents has grown considerably over the past 20 years, following empirical demonstrations that children and adolescents can present with classic signs of mood disorders as evinced by adults (Carlson & Cantwell, 1980), and that depressive disorders identified in adulthood often onset at a relatively young age (Kessler, Avenevoli, & Merikangas, 2001). Although developmental psychopathology research on depression has lagged behind that on externalizing disorders, considerable data regarding the phenomenology, course, and correlates of mood disorders in children and adolescents has accumulated. This literature has pointed to a number of issues and challenges related to the conceptualization and assessment of depression across the lifespan. In this chapter, we review key issues in the measurement of depression in children and adolescents as they relate to phenomenology, etiology, course, and treatment outcome.

Existing data indicate that the prevalence of frank mood disorders exhibits a strong developmental trend, with very low rates in preschool-aged children (Kashani & Carlson, 1987), increasing slightly in the elementary school age (Fleming & Offord, 1990; Cohen et al., 1993), and rising to levels similar to that among adults in adolescents (Kessler et al., 1994; Lewinsohn, Rohde, & Seeley, 1998). Therefore, researchers and clinicians working with depressed children and adolescents must keep in mind that the base rates of threshold levels of these disorders are quite low. Nonetheless, it appears that early onset mood disorders and depressive symptoms in childhood and adolescence are linked to a number of indicators of poor outcome, including later psychopathology and impairment in important

C. EMILY DURBIN and SYLIA WILSON • WCAS Psychology, 2029 Sheridan Road #1202, EV2710, Northwestern University, 633 Clark Street, Evanston, IL 60208.

J.L. Matson et al. (eds.), *Assessing Childhood Psychopathology and Developmental Disabilities*, DOI: 10.1007/978-0-387-09528-8,
© Springer Science+Business Media, LLC 2009

life domains (Harrington, Fudge, Rutter, Pickles, & Hill, 1990; Luby, Todd & Geller, 1996; Birmaher et al., 1996; Rudolph, Hammen & Burge, 1994). Therefore, depressive disorders and symptoms present an important assessment issue for clinical and research work with children and adolescents, and the assessment of childhood onset of these disorders is relevant to understanding course and outcome among adult samples.

In this chapter, we review key issues in the assessment of depressive disorders (Major Depressive Disorder (MDD) and Dysthymic Disorder (DD)) in children and adolescents with the aim of providing broad guidelines derived from the empirical literature on depression in children and adolescents, as well as developmental science regarding emotion, mood, and self-report in youngsters. We describe the best validated measures across broad categories (diagnostic interviews, questionnaires, etc.) in order to illustrate some of the important considerations and questions in the measurement of depressive disorders that are specific to children and adolescents. Finally, we detail areas in which assessment questions illuminate substantive issues in the study of depression in young populations.

GENERAL DEVELOPMENTAL CONSIDERATIONS

It is important for assessment in both research and clinical contexts that assessors are attuned to developmental norms for moods and behaviors when judging the presence and severity of particular depressive symptoms. Given the relative paucity of research on the presentation of depression in younger samples, it behooves clinicians and researchers to keep in mind the dual concerns of maximizing the information value of existing research on depression in adults when assessing depression in youngsters, and the necessity of incorporating a truly developmental perspective into the assessment of mood disorders and related phenomena in children and adolescents. We propose that best practice assessment of mood disorders should proceed from an understanding of the body of evidence related to mood disorders across the lifespan, taking into account evidence (when existing) on developmental specificity in clinical samples of children and adolescents, as well as incorporating information from basic science on mood, motivation, and self-report in children and adolescents when clinical research is lacking regarding a particular assessment issue.

TAILORING ASSESSMENT DECISIONS
TO ASSESSMENT NEEDS

Psychological assessments are conducted for a variety of purposes, and the procedures and measures selected should provide the optimal match to the goals of the assessment. Therefore, evaluation of existing assessment measures and development of new measures can only be conducted in the context of the match between an assessment need and a particular measure. Assessment may be conducted in order to derive a diagnosis consonant with a specific classification system, to evaluate factors predictive of prognosis, to measure potential treatment targets, to track treatment progress, to evaluate treatments, and to evaluate client suitability for particular interventions. It is important to note that the validity and utility of any particular assessment measure may vary across these different assessment contexts, as well as across specific populations (e.g., children vs. adolescents, different ethnic/racial groups), or the setting in which the assessment is conducted (e.g., primary medical setting vs. specialty mental health clinic). As a result, researchers and clinicians alike must consider the suitability of a particular instrument for a specific assessment purpose and setting, rather than making global judgments about the validity of a particular instrument.

Assessment for Diagnostic Purposes

Since the seminal work of Carlson and Cantwell (1980), the field now recognizes that adolescents and young children can exhibit classic symptoms of mood disorders, including MDD and DD. Moreover, existing studies indicate that the symptom presentation of these disorders tends to be quite similar in children and adolescents, compared to adults, with some minor differences in the prevalence of particular symptoms across age groups (e.g., Ryan et al., 1987). For example, somatic complaints and low self-esteem appear to decrease with age, whereas anhedonia and psychomotor retardation increase (Carlson & Kashani, 1988).

Minor efforts have been made to adjust diagnostic criteria for younger individuals, with only two such modifications instituted in the current incarnation of the Diagnostic and Statistical Manual of Mental Disorders – Fourth Edition (DSM-IV; American Psychiatric Association [APA], 1994). First, irritability may be substituted for the core depressed mood symptom among children and adolescents for both MDD and DD; unfortunately, there is no literature exploring the validity of this substitution or its impact on the rates of mood disorders in young samples (Kessler et al., 2001). Second, for DD, the total duration of the syndrome need be only one year, compared to two in adults. Therefore, in terms of the constructs assessed, diagnosis of unipolar mood disorders in children and adolescents is quite similar to that for adults.

Despite similarities in the symptom and course requirements for mood disorders across development, assessment of these conditions must take into account the ways in which each criterion may be influenced by a child's developmental stage. First, the typical symptom profile may be influenced by children's level of cognitive, social, and physical maturity. Current *DSM* criteria for MDD and DD may not all be applicable to the life context and experiences of young children in particular (Luby et al., 2002). Although very young children may exhibit negative moods (such as sadness or irritability), fatigue, and difficulty with sleep and appetite, they may be less likely to exhibit classic indicators of guilt, hopelessness, suicidality, and problems with libido (Garber & Horowitz, 2002).

Clinical research on the developmental course of these and other symptoms, as well as basic research on the development of processes underlying these systems may prove useful for articulating more developmentally sensitive guidelines for assessing depressive symptoms in children and adolescents. For example, Luby et al. (2002) recently demonstrated initial construct validity for modifications to existing *DSM–IV* criteria for MDD in preschoolers. Specifically, they found that anhedonia, as expressed by lack of pleasure in play and activities, as well as death- or suicide-related themes in play, appeared to be valid markers of mood disturbance, along with typical vegetative signs (activity, appetite, and sleep changes).

Absent such data for all developmental periods, clinicians and researchers must draw upon existing knowledge of normal development in order to probe for symptoms and impairment across domains that are relevant to younger depressed individuals, as well as to distinguish symptoms of pathology from developmentally normative expressions. For example, anhedonia may be more likely to take the form of social withdrawal and disinterest in play activities in younger children, and low self-esteem may be more salient among all adolescents regardless of mood disorder status. Thus, diagnostic assessment must attend to the developmental context, both for defining the areas of behavior and functioning in which depressive symptoms may manifest, as well as for making the distinction between normal and abnormal behavior.

Unfortunately, for many constructs relevant to depression, basic normative data are lacking. Clarifying these boundaries between normal and pathological expression is important for assessment, but also for core substantive questions regarding the nature of depression and its relationship to normal functioning (i.e., whether it is continuous with normal processes or discrete). Moreover, in addition to training interviewers in developmental context and putative developmentally specific manifestations of mood disorders, clinicians and researchers must also make decisions about who will be the source of information for diagnostic decisions. As discussed below, diagnostic interviewing may be complicated by the existence of differences across reporters in the salience and information value of their reports of children and adolescents' mood symptoms.

Assessing Comorbidity

Mood disorders in children and adolescents tend to be highly comorbid conditions, most commonly associated with anxiety disorders (Kovacs & Devlin, 1998; Angold, Costello, & Erkanli, 1999), but also with externalizing/disruptive disorders (Angold et al., 1999). Assessment of depressive disorders and comorbid problems requires careful attention to features specific to depression and those that are common across multiple disorders.

Because depressive and anxiety disorders share components of negative affectivity/distress (Clark & Watson, 1991; Lonigan, Phillips, & Hooe, 2003), distinguishing among these disorders can be challenging, particularly when assessment data consist of questionnaires or ratings scales. Many self-report questionnaires measuring depression and/or anxiety are heavily loaded with items/scales that tap the shared distress components of these disorders, relative to the unique aspects of depression. In interview assessment, careful attention to temporal parameters and course may be particularly important for distinguishing between anxiety and depression. There is some evidence that anxiety disorders may temporally precede depressive disorders in children and adolescents (Kovacs, Gatsonis, Paulauskas, & Richards, 1989; Avenevoli, Stolar, Li, Dierker, & Merikangas, 2001). This pattern of temporal ordering could represent a distinct etiological pathway wherein depression develops in response to earlier psychological problems. Such a patterning may have implications for treatment decisions.

The presence of comorbid externalizing problems is an important arena of assessment for depression. This is particularly the case for depressed children and adolescents, who appear to exhibit greater comorbid externalizing problems, particularly conduct disorder, compared to depressed adults (Avenevoli et al., 2001). Given that externalizing problems are often more salient to informants (such as parents or teachers) than are internalizing problems, assessors should keep in mind that mood disorders that co-occur with exernalizing problems may be underrecognized by others in the child's environment.

Proper diagnostic assessment of mood disorders in youngsters involves the challenge of distinguishing among mood, substance, and behavioral disorders, both for differential diagnosis and for documenting co-existing disorders that may affect treatment planning and/or be predictive of prognosis. Comorbidity among depressed children and adolescents has several important implications. First, comorbidity is important in a practical sense, as it predicts poorer treatment response, less benign course, greater overall impairment, and may potentially obscure the identification of another disorder. Second, although empirical data for treatment matching is lacking, depressed children and adolescents with comorbid conditions may be less responsive to treatments developed to target depression alone, and therefore require treatment modifications. Finally, when selecting assessment instruments for the purpose of diagnosis, researchers and clinicians must also attend carefully to the measurement properties of instruments for assessing other conditions in addition to depression (such as anxiety or externalizing problems).

Assessment for Treatment Planning and Evaluation

In addition to determining whether a child meets diagnostic criteria for MDD and DD (and therefore is suitable for empirically validated treatments for those conditions), treatment planning for depressed children and adolescents likely should also include some measures of important prognostic indicators. Unfortunately, very little is known about factors that predict responsiveness to treatment among depressed youngsters or characteristics associated with differential response to distinct interventions. Therefore, treatment planning might be limited to collecting baseline measures of symptom severity and impairment for the purpose of identifying targets for treatment and serving as a baseline measure against which to compare scores during and after treatment.

However, treatment decisions may be guided by knowledge of a depressed youngster's profile on known predictors of poorer course of the disorder. Specifically, a number of variables have been linked to poorer outcome among depressed youngsters, including comorbidity, early age of

onset, suicidality, comorbid MDD/DD, adverse family environment characteristics, depressotypic cognitions, stressful life events, and familial
loading for mood disorders (Birmaher, Arbelaez, & Brent, 2002). Thus,
clinical assessment should include some measurement of these factors in
order to identify those children whose mood episodes are likely to have a
poorer course. As the mechanisms linking these factors to outcome are not
well understood, these indicators may not be ideal candidates for treatment targets, but they may inform decisions about termination, maintenance sessions, or other aspects of clinical care.

Decisions regarding assessment for the purposes of treatment monitoring
and evaluation will necessarily be influenced by treatment goals and the
form and type of intervention conducted. However, a few general issues are
relevant. First, dimensional measures are more appropriate for the assessment
of change over time than are dichotomous measures, such as diagnoses.
Therefore, rating scales, questionnaires, or clinician severity ratings are
among the possibilities for tracking change and outcome in treatment.

Second, repeated administration of the same measure results in attenuation effects that are not specific to depression, but present across a range
of measures of psychopathology (Egger & Angold, 2004). Obviously, this
indicates that severity may appear to decrease over the course of treatment
for spurious reasons. Thus, clinicians should keep in mind that decreases
in measures of disorder severity may be inflated by this process.

Third, given that parents and children often disagree about problems
that could be the focus of treatment (Yeh & Weisz, 2001), it may be important to track changes across multiple dimensions that are relevant to both
child/adolescent clients and important family members who are actively
involved in treatment.

Finally, measuring changes in levels of depression and related phenomena may be complicated by the high stability of these constructs in
children and adolescents (e.g., Tram & Cole, 2006). To the extent that
measures of depression exhibit high stability, there will be (1) less change
evident in these measures, and (2) less remaining variance in these measures to be predicted by other measures. As a result, it may be difficult to
determine predictors of change in depression over time, particularly in
naturalistic follow-up studies.

Assessing Prognostic Indicators, Risk Factors, and Correlates of Depression

Correlates of child depression include impairment in family, social, and
academic domains, as well as neurobiological correlates, which have
important clinical and theoretical implications. From a clinical perspective,
evidence that psychosocial factors may influence the course and maintenance of depression suggests that the development of treatment plans
should incorporate not only a clinical assessment of diagnosable depression or depression symptoms, but should also include a comprehensive
evaluation of family, social, and academic factors. Assessing for increased
family conflict, family and peer relationship difficulties, and/or problems
in academic functioning can not only provide the clinician with a greater

sense of the degree of depression experienced by the child, but also informs clinical practice in terms of areas on which to focus additional treatment interventions, while illuminating existing family or social environments that may impede or facilitate treatment gains.

From a theoretical perspective, research on correlates of depression, and, in particular, investigation into the temporal nature of these correlates (i.e., whether they precede the development of depression, suggesting causal effects, or whether they develop subsequent to the development of depression, suggesting contributions to the course or maintenance of the disorder) further informs our conceptualization of depression, both in children and in adults.

Depression is associated with significant family dysfunction, including lower family support (Sheeber, Hops, Alpert, Davis, & Andrews, 1997), increased family conflict and sibling discord (Cole & McPherson, 1993; Kaslow, Deering, & Racusin, 1994; Sheeber et al., 1997), and abuse or neglect (Kashani & Carlson, 1987), as well as negative family circumstances, such as stressful life events and parental divorce or loss (Goodyer, Wright, & Altham, 1988; Hammen, Adrian, Gordon, Jaenicke, & Hiroto, 1987). Research investigating these correlates has focused both on the impact of the family environment on the development and maintenance of depression symptoms in the child, as well as the impact of the child's depressive symptomatology on the family environment. Further research regarding the transactional nature of family relationships, and, in particular and as discussed below, research utilizing multimethod, multi-informant approaches will greatly improve our understanding of the temporal and likely bidirectional effects of child depression and the family environment (e.g., Hammen, Burge, & Stansbury, 1990; Radke-Yarrow, 1998; Messer & Gross, 1995).

In addition to experiencing significant impairment within the family environment, children with depression also appear to be significantly impaired in social domains. Common social correlates of depression include difficulties in interpersonal relationships, as well as maladaptive social problem-solving, coping, and emotion regulation (Hammen & Rudolph, 2003). Research indicates that not only do children with depression perceive themselves to be less socially competent and as having poorer peer relationships and friendships (for reviews, see Gotlib & Hammen, 1992; Weisz, Rudolph, Granger, & Sweeney, 1992), they are also rated as less socially competent than children without depression by teachers (Rudolph & Clark, 2001), parents (Goodyer, Wright, & Altham, 1990; Puig-Antich et al., 1993), and independent observers (Rudolph et al., 1994). Furthermore, compared to children without depression, children with depression exhibit less prosocial and more hostile problem-focused strategies (Quiggle, Garber, Panak, & Dodge, 1992; Rudolph, Kurlakowsky, & Conley, 2001), more passive and helpless coping when faced with challenges (Ebata & Moos, 1991; Herman-Stahl & Petersen, 1999; Rudolph et al., 2001), and difficulty with emotional regulation in situations of high arousal (Zahn-Waxler, Klimes-Dougan, & Slattery, 2000).

Academic impairment also appears to be a correlate of child depression, although the literature is somewhat inconsistent, with some research suggesting that depression is associated with perceived, as opposed to actual, academic competence, and other research suggesting an association with both perceived and actual academic competence. Depressive symptoms are generally associated with poorer academic grades (Forehand, Brody, Long, & Fauber, 1988), decreased academic achievement and concentration problems (Ialongo, Edelsohn, Werthamer-Larsson, Crockett, & Kellam, 1996; Puig-Antich et al., 1993), and increased behavior problems at school, along with poorer relationships with teachers (Puig-Antich et al., 1993).

Although the potential benefit to assessing for psychosocial correlates is clear, how, exactly, they should be assessed is less straightforward. As noted, and as discussed in greater detail below, information gathered from multiple informants is likely to result in discrepant information. The use of a single informant when assessing psychosocial correlates assumes not only that the informant's perspective on family or peer relationships, or the academic environment, is convergent with others' perspectives on these areas, but also that the informant is unbiased in his or her perspective (Cole & McPherson, 1993). These assumptions are of particular relevance when doing clinical work or conducting research with children with depression, as considerable evidence suggests that, like adults, children with depression may demonstrate significant cognitive distortions, particularly regarding conceptualizations of the self and others in social situations, as well as biases in interpersonal information processing (Rudolph, Hammen, & Burge, 1997; Shirk, Van Horn, & Leber, 1997), and decreased perceptions of academic competence (Kendall, Stark, & Adam, 1990).

As with the assessment of depression in children, discussed in greater detail below, the assessment of these common psychosocial and functioning correlates is improved through the use of a multimethod, multi-informant approach. Such an approach should go beyond an overreliance on child self-report by utilizing, for example, observational measures of interpersonal functioning (e.g., Sheeber et al., 1997), as well as including information obtained from multiple informants, such as the child, family members, peers, and/or teachers (e.g., Cole & McPherson, 1993; Rudolph & Clark, 2001).

ISSUES IN THE ASSESSMENT OF DEPRESSION AND RELATED CONSTRUCTS IN CHILDREN AND ADOLESCENTS

Measurement of depression and related constructs in children and adolescents poses some unique challenges that must be taken into account when selecting, implementing, and interpreting the findings of assessment instruments. Aside from methodological considerations, these issues also raise intriguing substantive questions about the nomological network of depression and about assessment of children and adolescents in general. These issues, discussed below in detail, include: (1) cross-informant convergence and specificity, (2) normal developmental change in children's ability to report on their internal states, and (3) understanding depressive phenomena in the context of developmental science on mood, motivation, and cognition in children and adolescents.

Cross-Informant Convergence and Specificity

Depression in children may be assessed by seeking information from a variety of informants, including clinician-administered diagnostic interviews with children and/or parents; rating scales that are completed by clinicians or self-reported through questionnaires with children, parents, teachers, or siblings; peer-nomination inventories; and observational measures. In this section, we provide a brief overview of findings pertaining to different informants, including cross-informant convergence, specificity of informant reports, and predictors of agreement between informants.

Effects of Different Informants

Obtaining information from multiple informants, using multiple assessment methods, is generally considered advantageous for the accurate assessment of psychopathology in children as it results in increased reliability and generalizability of the assessed information. As noted by Cantwell, Lewinsohn, Rohde, and Seeley (1997), obtaining information from multiple informants is particularly important when assessing children, for a number of reasons. Children may not be developmentally capable of accurately and reliably assessing their psychological functioning or may minimize or deny socially undesirable symptoms. Parents may be unaware of internal and nonexpressed symptoms, or of situations in which children may display problematic behavior, such as school. Discrepant reports may be obtained from children, parents, and teachers to the extent that they hold different beliefs regarding what constitutes normative behavior. Finally, children may exhibit different symptoms or behaviors in different settings, producing different behavioral samples for reporters in those distinct contexts.

Low agreement among different informants regarding indices of psychopathology in children is the norm, rather than the exception. In a classic meta-analysis of multi-informant studies of child psychopathology, Achenbach, McConaughy, and Howell (1987) reported a mean cross-reporter correlation of .28 for reports of child behavioral and emotional problems by different informants (e.g., parents and teachers), compared to .22 between self-reports by children and informant report. Recent studies confirm these results (e.g., Crowley, Worchel, & Ash, 1992; Sourander, Helstela, & Helenius, 1999). Furthermore, interrater agreement appears to be particularly poor for internalizing, as opposed to externalizing, problems (Achenbach et al., 1987; Hodges, Gordon, & Lennon, 1990; Kolko & Kazdin, 1993; Sourander et al., 1999; Yeh & Weisz, 2001), perhaps because symptoms of internalizing disorders are more difficult to observe and are generally less disruptive to the family and classroom environment than externalizing disorders, making them less salient to observers.

It is important to note that low interrater agreement may be due to general subjective and situational biases (Berg-Nielsen, Vika, & Dahl, 2003), and, as such, a lack of interrater agreement regarding the child's symptoms does not necessarily reflect inaccuracies on the part of the informants. Rather, it may be due to real differences in child behavior across settings; differences in each informant's perspective on the child, gained through observations of and interactions with the child in different environments and contexts; differences in standards of judgment; and differential effects of each informant on the child's behavior (Schaughency & Rothlind, 1991). Although low interrater agreement is common, evidence suggests that both child- and parent-reports (as well as those from teachers and clinicians) are valid indicators of child psychopathology (Jensen et al., 1999).

In contrast, evidence regarding the relative predictive validity of child, parent, and teacher-reports has been somewhat inconsistent, with some researchers concluding that child- and parent-reports each account for unique variance in predicting relevant outcomes (Ferdinand et al. 2003; Verhulst, Dekker, & van der Ende, 1997) and others suggesting that the use of child- and teacher-reports, as opposed to parent, results in improved prediction of preadolescent depression (Mesman & Koot, 2000). The proper diagnosis of depression or assessment of depressive symptom severity often involves obtaining and integrating information from multiple sources, which may include the child.

Parent-report may also be obtained through diagnostic interviews with parents or parent questionnaires assessing the child's symptoms. Although parents may be less aware of their child's internal states than the child him- or herself, they may nonetheless be able to provide a broader and more stable perspective of the child's depressive symptoms (Cole & Martin, 2005), drawing on observable behavior in the home and family environment, as well as through information gleaned from the child or others, such as teachers or siblings (Tarullo, Richardson, Radke-Yarrow, & Martinez, 1995). When the parent and child complete comparable assessment measures, responses from each may be compared and integrated for a more comprehensive assessment. (Approaches to the combination of information from multiple informants are discussed below.)

Furthermore, and as discussed in greater detail below, information from both mothers and fathers may be useful. Each may provide unique information about the child, depending on his or her perceptions of the child, the amount of time spent with the child, or knowledge of the child's activities both in and outside the home (Verhulst & Van der Ende, 1992). However, the assessing clinician must review discrepant mother, father, and child information carefully. As discussed in detail below, characteristics of the child and his or her parents, as well as the parents' own life circumstances and psychological functioning, may influence parent-report of depressive symptoms in the child.

Teacher-reports allow for yet another perspective on the child's functioning. Along with professional insight into age and developmentally appropriate behaviors, teachers also have the opportunity to observe the child in both structured and unstructured settings, as well as note his or her competence in academic and social realms (Epkins, 1995). Furthermore, as discussed previously, some evidence suggests greater predictive validity of teacher-, as opposed to parent-, report for preadolescent depression (Mesman & Koot, 2000). As might be expected, greater teacher familiarity with the child is associated with greater child–teacher agreement of depressive symptoms (Ines & Sacco, 1992).

Although less frequently utilized, the child's siblings or peers may also provide valuable information. Young children often spend a substantial amount of time with their siblings, and siblings may be particularly useful informants regarding the child's behavior within the family environment. School-age children also spend a majority of each day in the company of their peers, and often participate in a wide range of structured and unstructured activities with them. However, sibling and peer reports may be somewhat unreliable, particularly if the respondents are young ((Epkins & Dedmon, 1999; Younger, 1999); Younger, Schwartzman, & Ledingham, 1985), or, in the case of peers, subject to reputation effects, where the child is rated based on his or her popularity rather than observable behavior (Weiss, Harris, & Catron, 2002).

Several methods may be employed to address discrepancies among informant reports. For example, the "or" approach assumes the presence of a symptom or diagnosis if any informant reports it, whereas the "and" approach requires symptom or diagnosis endorsement by multiple informants. In addition, a number of statistical approaches to aggregating data obtained from different informants have been proposed (e.g., Baillargeon et al., 2001; Kraemer et al., 2003; Rubio-Stipec, Fitzmaurice, Murphy, & Walker, 2003). In general clinical practice, a procedure is usually followed whereby information from multiple informants is integrated by the clinician, using general guidelines for prioritizing discrepant information, such as the preference for self-report regarding internalizing symptoms (Ferdinand, van der Ende, & Verhulst, 2004; Klein, Dougherty, & Olino, 2005). Although such an approach may decrease reliability, as different clinicians may utilize different information, evidence from the adult literature suggests that diagnoses made using such a "best estimate" approach often have high reliability (Klein, Ouimette, Kelly, Ferro, & Riso, 1994).

Given the frequent occurrence of discrepant information, research informing which information to consider and which to disregard is critical. Although low interrater agreement is often the result of situational specificity, wherein the interaction or observation of the child by different informants in different contexts influences their reports (Achenbach et al., 1987), research is beginning to further investigate informant variables that may affect the accurate assessment of depression in children. Variables that have been examined as potentially influencing informant report and interrater agreement include the child's age and sex, the parent's sex, and the psychological functioning of the informant.

In general, research examining parent–child agreement on child depressive symptoms has found that adolescents both report more symptoms than their parents and that parent–child agreement regarding depressive symptoms decreases with age (Achenbach et al., 1987; Handwerk, Larzelere, Soper, & Friman, 1999; Kolko & Kazdin, 1993; Seiffge-Krenke & Kollmar, 1998; Sourander et al., 1999; Tarullo et al., 1995; Verhulst & Van der Ende, 1992; but see also Epkins, 1996; Renouf & Kovacs, 1994). Decreasing child–parent symptom convergence may be the result of reduced parental influence and contact as youths enter into adolescence (Brown, 1990; Sourander et al., 1999). A similar pattern of results is found for adolescent and teacher reports (Stanger & Lewis, 1993; Thomas, Forehand, Armistead,

Wierson, & Fauber, 1990). Decreases in child–teacher convergence may be due to secondary school academic schedules wherein adolescents have classes with multiple teachers for short periods each day (Cantwell et al., 1997), such that each teacher has less experience with the child than would a primary school teacher.

Research examining the effect of the child's sex on interrater agreement has been mixed. Some research finds greater parent agreement with girls' than boys' self-reported depressive symptoms (Epkins & Meyers, 1994; Kazdin, French, & Unis, 1983), perhaps due to an inclination to notice internalizing symptoms more in girls than in boys because of gender stereotyping or because depression is more common in girls than boys. In contrast, some researchers find greater parent–child agreement for internalizing symptoms in boys than in girls (Sourander et al., 1999; Tarullo et al., 1995), which may be the result of a greater focus on sex-atypical disorders. Research examining teacher-report has thus far found no sex differences in teacher–child agreement (Epkins & Meyers, 1994; Ines & Sacco, 1992).

The parent's sex may also influence reports of the child's symptoms, either alone or in interaction with the child's sex. For example, Seiffge-Krenke and Kollmar (1998) found that both parent and child sex significantly influenced parent–child agreement in a sample of adolescents. Specifically, mother– and father–child agreement was higher for daughters than for sons, with father–son agreement particularly low.

This finding may indicate that, although adolescents are increasingly disinclined to confide in their parents, they may nonetheless continue to discuss some personal issues with their mothers, as opposed to their fathers. However, given that research on clinical child and adolescent psychopathology typically involves mothers, to the relative exclusion of fathers (Phares, 1992), very little research has yet been done in this area. The few studies examining interrater agreement in the assessment of depression in children that have included fathers have generally found that mother–father agreement decreases as children age, and that mothers report more symptoms than fathers (Achenbach et al., 1987; Jensen, Traylor, Xenakis, & Davis, 1988; Tarullo et al., 1995, but see also Stanger & Lewis, 1993).

The finding that mothers tend to report more depressive symptoms in their children than do fathers may be a function of maternal adjustment. Research indicates that parental factors, including depression (Briggs-Gowan, Carter, & Schwab-Stone, 1996; Najman et al., 2000; Youngstrom, Loeber, & Stouthamer-Loeber, 2000), as well as family factors, such as high levels of stress or conflict (Kolko & Kazdin, 1993; Seiffge-Krenke & Kollmar, 1998; Youngstrom, Loeber, & Stouthamer-Loeber, 2000), are associated with low agreement on child depressive symptoms between parents and other informants. The underlying mechanisms explaining the effects of parental depression on parents' report of children's symptoms has been controversial, with the main issue being whether parental depression results in greater acknowledgment of depressive symptoms in offspring, or if depression results in cognitive distortions that inflate parental report of child depressive symptoms (Briggs-Gowan et al., 1996; Richters, 1992).

In summary, obtaining multimethod, multi-informant information is optimal for the assessment of depression in children, as such information is more reliable and generalizable than that obtained through single measures. Furthermore, there are potential advantages to obtaining information from multiple informants. Children, parents, teachers, siblings, and peers all may provide unique information regarding the child's internal state or external behavior across different situations. The usefulness of multireporter assessment would be increased by knowledge of how best to integrate information from different reporters. Unfortunately, there is not a body of literature exploring actuarial methods of combining these sources of data for assessing depression in children and adolescents. Absent such empirical guidance, clinicians and researchers alike must be guided by existing knowledge regarding the factors that influence agreement and disagreement across reporters when deciding how to integrate assessment information across informants.

Children's Self-Reports

Given that subjective elements of internalizing disorders may be most validly tapped by obtaining information from youngsters themselves, it is important to consider the skills and limitations children and adolescents possess with regard to reporting on their mood, psychiatric symptoms, and the timing of these experiences. Child-report of depressive phenomena may be obtained through diagnostic interviews or self-report questionnaires. Child-report uniquely accesses aspects of the child's internal, subjective state, which is important for tapping many mood phenomena that are not necessarily evident behaviorally.

As with all self-reported information, child self-report may be subject to respondent or social desirability biases. Child-reports also appear to be somewhat unreliable, particularly for younger children and regarding features of depression such as symptom duration and time of onset (Edelbrock, Costello, Dulcan, Kalas, & Conover, 1985; Schwab-Stone, Fallon, Briggs, & Crowther, 1994). Furthermore, As with adults, child-reports may be influenced by the child's current mood or circumstances (Cole & Martin, 2005) or dependent on the child's level of linguistic ability and cognitive sophistication. Furthermore, given the private nature of internalizing symptoms, the child may have no frame of reference regarding others' mood or depressive experience with which to compare his or her levels of depressive symptoms for normative characteristics (Tarullo et al., 1995).

Very young children's reports of their mood states may be limited by their ability to utilize language relevant to emotion. There are few longitudinal studies of children's use of emotion language in spontaneous speech, but existing data suggest that use of emotion words (but not understanding) is rare prior to the preschool years (Bretherton, Fritz, Zahn-Waxler, & Ridgeway, 1986). Emotion recognition and labeling skills develop considerably across childhood, such that younger children use more global terms to describe their emotions, rather than employing specific terms such as "angry" or "sad" (Widen & Russell, 2003). Therefore, one would expect younger children to be less likely to endorse the specific emotions of depression or irritability than would older children. More basic research on the validity of young children's self-reports of their emotional state would help to guide the development and evaluation of assessment measures for depression in young children.

Developmental Science on Children's Emotions

The assessment of depressive disorders in both children and adolescents, particularly for diagnostic purposes, involves distinguishing normative moods and emotions from pathological emotional experiences. Unfortunately, basic developmental science regarding the developmental trajectory of emotions and moods across childhood and adolescence is very limited, providing little guidance for researchers and clinicians who must make distinctions between normal and abnormal mood experiences. Similarly, the study of depressive disorders in children may also inform our understanding of normal emotional development. Absent such data, clinicians must rely upon a careful assessment of the child's moods and the contexts in which they occur, as well as their understanding of developmental norms.

Assessment Instruments for Measuring Depression in Children and Adolescents

The choice of instrument depends on the purpose of the assessment, the setting in which the assessment occurs, and what aspect of depression is being assessed (e.g., symptoms, diagnosis, risk factors, correlates, impairment). We now review the different types of instruments that may be used in the assessment of depression in children, as well as the appropriateness of each for different assessment purposes or settings, before reviewing some of the more commonly used assessment instruments.

Screening instruments are used to identify individuals at higher likelihood of having a disorder, and may be used in both research and clinical practices. They are particularly useful when a complete assessment is impractical to conduct with a full sample or with each client. Results of screening indicate whether additional assessment is warranted. Many screening instruments assess for multiple types of psychopathology using one instrument. Although a number of the instruments reviewed here could theoretically be used to screen for depression, screening instruments are ideally brief, user-friendly, and easily administered to large numbers of participants or populations by lay interviewers. Given the low base rates of depressive disorders in community samples of children and adolescents (six-month prevalence rates of 1 to 3% in school-aged children, 5 to 6% in adolescents; lifetime prevalence rates of 15 to 20% in adolescents; Garber & Horowitz, 2002; Lewinsohn & Essau, 2002), screening may be particularly important for efficient assessment of the disorder in research on community samples and in large-scale prevention efforts.

Diagnostic interviews are used to determine whether the respondent meets criteria for a particular diagnosis, and may be unstructured, fully structured, or semi-structured. Unstructured interviews, wherein format, duration, focus, and coverage vary by clinician, are subject to missed information, are less comprehensive than structured or semi-structured interviews, and generally result in widely variable information (Klein et al., 2005). Such interviews are, therefore, not typically recommended when assessing for depression in children.

In contrast, fully structured interviews consist of probes/questions that are read exactly as written, with responses recorded without further clarification or interpretation by the interviewer. These interviews are appropriate for administration by lay interviewers, and are useful in epidemiological studies, where the assessment of large numbers of participants may make clinician training prohibitive.

Finally, semi-structured interviews, which utilize clinical knowledge and judgment to evaluate information provided by the respondent, are designed to be administered by appropriately trained and experienced clinicians. Structured and semi-structured interviews may be used to assess mood disorder criteria only, or a broader range of psychopathology. Existing interviews vary in the extent to which they may be used in a modular fashion or the ease with which they may be adapted to assess a narrower range of disorders and related phenomena, such as depressotypic cognitions and schemas. The use of the semi-structured interview format with children as respondents has advantages and disadvantages. This format allows the interviewer to follow up the child's responses in order to ascertain the child's level of understanding of each question or to probe further for clarification (Hodges, 1990). On the other hand, a full diagnostic interview may be long and tiring, particularly for younger children.

Questionnaires are often used to measure depressive symptom severity. Although they are a cost- and time-efficient strategy for obtaining supplemental information from one or more informants, given that questionnaires are less comprehensive than diagnostic interviews, they should not be used as the primary diagnostic instrument. Questionnaires are generally self-administered by the respondent, but they may also be read aloud to younger children. Many questionnaires developed for use with one informant (e.g., the child) are also modified for use with other informants (e.g., parents, teachers, or siblings). Information obtained through comparable questionnaires completed by multiple informants may be easily compared and integrated for a more comprehensive assessment.

Peer-nomination inventories and observational measures may also provide valuable information regarding the child's depressive symptoms and functioning. Peer-nomination inventories typically involve the presentation of a number of behavioral characteristics to each student within a classroom; the student then chooses which of his or her peers best matches each characteristic. The Peer Nomination Inventory of Depression (PNID; Lefkowitz & Tesiny, 1980), for example, is a 19-item sociometric index of depression, happiness, and popularity developed for use with children in grades 3 to 5. Scores reflect peer ratings of the child on each of these three indices.

Observational measures include laboratory or performance-based tasks, which allow for the assessment of depressive symptoms in controlled laboratory settings. These measures are a source of rich observational data, and, depending on what is being assessed by the task (e.g., information-processing, psychological functioning, social interactions with family members or other important social figures), may provide important information regarding the child's functioning in a number of areas. Although observational measures have certain advantages, they are also particularly time consuming, labor intensive, and expensive (Epkins & Dedmon, 1999; Garber & Kaminski, 2000). As such, they are rarely practical for use in clinical settings. For more detailed information regarding specific observational measures, the interested reader is referred to Garber and Kaminski's (2000) review of laboratory and performance-based measures of depression in children.

We now briefly review some of the more commonly used child and adolescent depression assessment instruments (for more comprehensive reviews, see Angold & Fisher, 1999; Brooks & Kutcher, 2001; Myers & Winters, 2002; Silverman & Rabian, 1999). Although there are a number of instruments developed for use with adults that are also widely used with adolescents, the present review is limited to those instruments designed for and used primarily with children and adolescents.

Screening Instruments

Pediatric Symptom Checklist (PSC)

The PSC (Jellinek, Murphy, & Burns, 1986) is a 35-item questionnaire developed for use by pediatric care providers during routine pediatric visits. It assesses internalizing, externalizing, and attention domains, and empirically derived cut-off points assist the pediatric care provider in identifying youths in need of additional psychological evaluation. Originally developed for use with parents regarding their school-age children, the PSC has also been modified for use with youths (Pagano, Cassidy, Little, Murphy, & Jellinek, 2000). In addition, a brief, 17-item version of the PSC, the PSC-17, has been developed for use with parents (Gardner et al., 1999) and youths (Duke, Ireland, & Borowsky, 2005).

The PSC has demonstrated excellent interrater reliability (κ = .82; Murphy, Reede, Jellinek, & Bishop, 1992) and excellent test–retest reliability (r = .80; Navon, Nelson, Pagano, & Murphy, 2001). Research assessing concurrent and criterion validity has demonstrated correlations with clinician diagnosis and other validated measures (Jellinek et al., 1988; Murphy et al., 1992; Navon et al., 2001; Walker, LaGrone, & Atkinson, 1989). Validity for the internalizing subscale of the youth version of the PCS has been demonstrated through moderate correlation with the Child Depression Inventory (CDI; Kovacs, 1992; see below; Pagano et al., 2000). The internalizing subscale of the PSC-17 has also demonstrated validity through correlation with clinician diagnosis and other validated measures of depression (Gardner et al., 1999), as well as evidence of predictive validity (Gardner, Campo, & Lucas, 2004).

Structured and Semi-Structured Diagnostic Interviews

Diagnostic Interview Schedule for Children (DISC)

The DISC (Costello, Edelbrock, Dulcan, Kalas, & Klaric, 1984) is a fully structured interview developed by the National Institute of Mental Health for use with children aged 6 to 17 years. A parent version is also available. The DISC assesses multiple types of psychopathology according to the *Diagnostic and Statistical Manual of Mental Disorders* (the *DSM-IV and International*; American Psychiatric Association [APA], 1994) and International Classification of Diseases (ICD; World Health Organization [WHO], 1993) criteria, including depressive disorders, over the past year. Information regarding the onset and duration of symptoms is also assessed for many items. The DISC has been revised several times, with more recent versions intended to address shortcomings of earlier versions: the DISC-Revised (DISC-R; Shaffer et al., 1993), the DISC-2.1 (Fisher et al., 1993), the DISC-2.3 (Shaffer et al., 1996), and the DISC-IV (Shaffer, Fisher, Lucas, Dulcan, & Schwab-Stone, 2000). Given the highly structured nature of the interview, the DISC may be administered by lay interviewers with only brief training. Administration time of the DISC typically ranges from 1 to 2 hours, depending on the level of psychopathology endorsed by the child.

Although the DISC may be a useful instrument for epidemiological research in that it is easily administered by lay interviewers, it has not demonstrated particularly good reliability and validity. Previous research suggests excellent interrater reliability (*r*s ranging from .94 to 1.00; Costello et al., 1984), poor to good test–retest reliability (κs ranging from .44 to .72; Costello et al., 1984; Edelbrock et al., 1985), poor to excellent internal consistency (αs ranging from .41 to .67; Williams, McGee, Anderson, & Silva, 1989; ICCs ranging from .30 to .81; Edelbrock et al., 1985), and poor to good concordance of MDD diagnoses for child and parent versions (κs ranging from .14 to .50; Costello et al., 1984).

Preliminary results from studies examining the reliability of the most recent version are somewhat more promising (e.g., Shaffer et al., 2000). Research assessing concurrent and criterion validity has likewise been inconsistent. Some research has demonstrated moderate correlation of the depression scale of the DISC with clinician diagnosis and other validated measures of depression (Angold, Costello, Messer, & Pickles, 1995; Costello et al., 1984) and discriminate validity for psychiatric and pediatric referrals (Costello, Edelbrock, & Costello, 1985). In contrast, other studies suggest less than adequate validity when used with clinical samples (Pellegrino, Singh, & Carmanico, 1999; Weinstein, Stone, Noam, Grimes, & Schwab-Stone, 1989).

Diagnostic Interview for Children and Adolescents (DICA)

The DICA (Herjanic & Reich, 1982) was originally developed as a fully structured interview, although the most recent versions, the DICA-R (Reich & Welner, 1988) and the DICA-IV (Reich, 2000), are semi-structured. The DICA-R/IV assesses multiple types of psychopathology according to *DSM–IV* criteria across a lifetime time frame. The DICA-R/IV includes separate interviews for children (aged 6 to 12 years), adolescents (aged 13 to 17 years), and parents. It may be administered by either clinicians or lay interviewers with appropriate training. Administration time of the DICA-R/IV typically ranges from 1 to 2 hours, depending on the level of psychopathology endorsed by the child.

The DICA, particularly the DICA-IV, has demonstrated inconsistent reliability, with evidence of poor to fair interrater reliability (κs ranging from .38 to .47; Granero Perez, Ezpeleta Ascaso, Domenech Massons, & de la Osa Chaparro, 1998), poor to excellent test–retest reliability (κs ranging from .00 to .77; Boyle et al., 1993), and poor to fair concordance of MDD diagnosis for child and parent versions (κs ranging from .21 to .57; Boyle et al., 1993). Preliminary results from studies examining the reliability of the most recent version are somewhat more promising (e.g., Reich, 2000). Research assessing concurrent and criterion validity has demonstrated poor to moderate correlations with clinician diagnosis and other validated measures of depression (Ezpeleta et al., 1997; McClure, Rogeness, & Thompson, 1997).

Child and Adolescent Psychiatric Assessment (CAPA)

The CAPA (Angold, Prendergast et al., 1995) is a semi-structured interview for use with children aged 9 to 17 years. A parent version is also available. The CAPA assesses multiple types of psychopathology according to *DSM–IV* and ICD-10 criteria, including depressive disorders, over the past three months. It also assesses impairment in areas relevant to functioning in family, peer, school, and leisure environments, and has a component allowing for interviewer-based observations of the child's social and affective behavior. The inclusion of an extensive glossary detailing operational definitions of specific symptoms and distress and frequency ratings allows for the administration of the CAPA by either clinicians or lay interviewers with appropriate training. Administration time of the CAPA ranges from 1 to 2 hours, depending on the level of psychopathology endorsed by the child.

Little research evaluating the reliability and validity of the CAPA has yet been conducted, although what does exist is promising. The depression subscale of the CAPA has shown excellent test–retest reliability (κ = .90; ICC = .88; Angold & Costello, 1995). Interrater reliability and internal consistency have not yet been adequately examined. Validity has likewise not yet been adequately assessed, although some research suggests preliminary evidence of validity (Angold & Costello, 2000; Thapar & McGuffin, 1998).

Schedule for Affective Disorders and Schizophrenia for School-age Children (K-SADS)

The K-SADS (Puig-Antich & Chambers, 1978) is a semi-structured interview adapted from the adult Schedule for Affective Disorders and Schizophrenia (SADS; Endicott & Spitzer, 1978). The original K-SADS has been revised several times, resulting in a number of different versions: the K-SADS-Epidemiologic version (K-SADS-E; Orvaschel, Puig-Antich, Chambers, Tabrizi, & Johnson, 1982) assesses both past and current episodes of psychopathology; the K-SADS-Present Episode version (K-SADS-P; Chambers et al., 1985) assesses the child's current state; and the K-SADS-Present and Lifetime version (K-SADS-PL; Kaufman et al., 1997) is an update and combination of the K-SADS-E and the K-SADS-P. The K-SADS is appropriate for use with children aged 6 to 17 or 6 to 18 years, depending on the version used. Each version assesses multiple types of psychopathology according to *DSM–IV* criteria. The administering clinician bases diagnostic decisions on his or her integration of all available sources of information. As such, the K-SADS requires substantial clinical training and experience, and should only be administered by qualified clinicians. Administration time of the K-SADS typically ranges from 30 minutes to 2.5 hours, depending on the level of psychopathology endorsed by the child.

The depression and internalizing components of the K-SADS, particularly the more recent versions, have shown good to excellent interrater reliability (κ = .54; ICCs ranging from .51 to .88; Chambers et al., 1985), excellent test–retest reliability (κs ranging from .90 to 1.00; Kaufman et al., 1997), and good to excellent internal consistency (αs ranging from .68 to .89; Ambrosini, Metz, Prabucki, & Lee, 1989; Chambers et al., 1985). Research assessing concurrent validity has demonstrated moderate correlations with other validated measures of depression (Kaufman et al., 1997; McCauley, Mitchell, Burke, & Moss, 1988). The K-SADS has also demonstrated evidence of predictive validity (McGee & Williams, 1988).

Questionnaires

Children's Depression Rating Scale-Revised (CDRS)

The CDRS (Poznanski & Mokros, 1999) is a clinician-administered observer-rated scale adapted from the adult Hamilton Rating Scale for Depression (Hamilton, 1960). The 17-item CDRS assesses current depressive symptom severity in cognitive, somatic, affective, and psychomotor domains. The CDRS was developed for use with children aged 6 to 12 years (although it is also commonly used with adolescents), and is administered to both the child and a second informant, usually a parent, with the interviewer using clinical judgment to then combine information from each informant. The CDRS may be administered by clinicians or appropriately trained lay interviewers. Administration time of the CDRS typically ranges from 15 to 20 minutes for each informant.

The CDRS has demonstrated inconsistent reliability, with evidence of poor interrater reliability (rs ranging from -.01 to .42; Mokros, Poznanski, Grossman, & Freeman, 1987), excellent test–retest reliability (r = .86; Poznanski et al., 1984), and poor to excellent internal consistency (rs ranging from .38 to .88; Poznanski, Cook, & Carroll, 1979). Research assessing concurrent and criterion validity has demonstrated good to excellent correlations with other validated measures of depression (Shain, Naylor, & Alessi, 1990) and some evidence of discriminate validity (Shain, King, Naylor, & Alessi, 1991), but its sensitivity for assessing change in severity of depression appears less than optimal (Stark, Reynolds, & Kaslow, 1987).

Child Depression Inventory (CDI)

The CDI (Kovacs, 1992) is a self-reported rating scale originally adapted from the adult Beck's Depression Inventory (Beck, Ward, Mendelson, Mock, & Erbaugh, 1961). The 27-item CDI assesses depressive symptom severity over the past two weeks across a broad range of domains, focusing in particular on cognitive symptoms. A 10-item short version of the CDI is also available (Kovacs, 1992). The CDI was developed for use with children aged 7 to 17 years, and it typically takes about 10 to 20 minutes to complete. The CDI has shown poor to excellent test–retest reliability (rs ranging from .38 to .88; Blumberg & Izard, 1986; Kovacs, 1980/1981; Finch, Saylor, Edwards, & McIntosh, 1987; Saylor, Finch, Spirito, & Bennett, 1984; Smucker, Craighead, Craighead, & Green, 1986) and high internal consistency (αs typically over .80; Crowley et al., 1992; Nelson, Politano, Finch, Wendel, & Mayhall, 1987; Smucker et al., 1986). Research assessing concurrent and criterion validity has demonstrated good to excellent correlations with other validated measures of depression (Birleson, 1981; Reynolds, 1987; Shain et al., 1990), although research examining the ability of the CDI to discriminate between depressed and nondepressed youths has been mixed (Costello & Angold, 1988; Lobovits & Handal, 1985; Moretti, Fine, Haley, & Marriage, 1985; Weissman, Orvaschel, & Padian, 1980). The CDI also appears to be a useful instrument for assessing change in severity of depression (Fine, Forth, Gilbert, & Haley, 1991; Garvin, Leber, & Kalter, 1991; Stark et al., 1987).

Mood and Feelings Questionnaire (MFQ)

The MFQ (Angold, Costello et al., 1995) is a 32-item self-reported rating scale developed to assess depressive symptom severity based on *DSM–IV* criteria over the past two weeks. A 13-item short version of the MFQ is also available (Angold, Costello et al., 1995), as well as parent versions of both the full and the short versions. The MFQ was developed for use with children aged 8 to 18 years, and typically takes about 10 minutes to complete.

The MFQ has shown good test–retest reliability (ICCs ranging from .75 to .78; Costello, Benjamin, Angold, & Silver, 1991; Wood, Kroll, Moore, & Harrington, 1995) and excellent internal consistency (αs ranging from .85 to .94; Angold, Costello et al., 1995; Wood et al., 1995), but poor concordance for child and parent versions (rs ranging from .25 to .30; Angold, Costello et al., 1995). Research assessing concurrent and criterion validity has demonstrated poor to moderate correlations with clinician diagnosis and other validated measures of depression (Angold, Costello et al., 1995; Pellegrino et al., 1999; Thapar & McGuffin, 1998; Wood et al., 1995) and evidence of discriminate validity (Kent, Vostanis, & Feehan, 1997; Thapar & McGuffin, 1998). The ability of the MFQ to assess change in depressive symptoms has not yet been adequately investigated, with research conducted thus far mixed (Vostanis, Feehan, Grattan, & Bickerton, 1996; Wood, Harrington, & Moore, 1996).

Reynolds Child Depression Scale (RCDS) and Reynolds Adolescent Depression Scale (RADS)

The RCDS (Reynolds, 1989) and the RADS (Reynolds, 1987) are 30-item self-reported rating scales developed to assess depressive symptoms over the past two weeks based on *DSM–IV* criteria. The RCDS and the RADS were developed for use with children aged 8 to 12 and 13 to 18, respectively, and each typically takes about 10 minutes to complete.

The RCDS and RADS have shown good to excellent test–retest reliability (*r*s ranging from .79 to .86; Baron & DeChamplain, 1990; Reynolds, 1987) and excellent internal consistency (*α*s ranging from .87 to .94; Nieminen & Matson, 1989; Reynolds, 1987; Reynolds & Miller, 1985). Research assessing concurrent and criterion validity has demonstrated good to excellent correlations with clinician diagnosis and other validated measures of depression (Reynolds, 1987; Shain et al., 1990), although the sensitivity of the RCDS and the RADS in detecting depression appears to be somewhat poor (Reynolds, 1987). In addition, although the RCDS and the RADS appear to be somewhat able to assess change in depressive symptoms, other rating scales may be more sensitive in this regard (Reynolds & Coats, 1986; Stark et al., 1987).

FUTURE DIRECTIONS

The assessment of depression in children and adolescents is an area ripe for development. A number of strategies and instruments that have been developed for diagnosis and the measurement of symptom severity demonstrate adequate reliability and validity, and some of the aspects that may influence assessment (i.e., reporter differences) have been identified. However, many instruments in wide use have less than optimal reliability and/or validity, and some depression-related constructs and developmental periods (e.g., preschool years) are not well addressed by existing measures.

Further refinement of existing measures and the construction of new assessment instruments and procedures should be guided by both the needs of the growing research base on depression in children and adolescents, as well as the knowledge generated by the field. First, the existence of cross-reporter differences in information regarding depressive phenomena in children and adolescents calls for a better understanding of how best to integrate information across reporters.

Second, there is a great need for research on predictors of the course of depressive disorders and treatment response in depressed children and adolescents; such information will allow for more refined prediction of outcome and perhaps for advances in treatment matching and planning. This can only occur in the context of refined methods for assessing course and measuring change in depressive symptoms over time.

Third, as research interest in exploring the question of continuity among child, adolescent, and adult depression grows, it will become increasingly important to address issues of how to provide comparable measures of depression across these developmental stages, as well as to test measurement invariance of instruments across developmental periods. Finally, assessment of depressive disorders will primarily benefit from growth in the larger literature on the phenomenology and etiology of depression across the lifespan, as well as that on developmental change in the manifestation of depression at different ages.

REFERENCES

Achenbach, T. M., McConaughy, S. H., & Howell, C. T. (1987). Child/adolescent behavioral and emotional problems: Implications of cross-informant correlations for situational specificity. *Psychological Bulletin, 101*, 213–232.

Ambrosini, P. J., Metz, C., Prabucki, K., & Lee, J. (1989). Videotape reliability of the third revised edition of the K-SADS. *Journal of the American Academy of Child & Adolescent Psychiatry, 28*, 723–728.

American Psychiatric Association. (1994). *Diagnostic and statistical manual of mental disorders* (4th ed.). Washington, DC: American Psychiatric Association.

Angold, A., & Costello, E. J. (1995). A test-retest reliability study of child-reported psychiatric symptoms and diagnoses using the Child and Adolescent Psychiatric Assessment (CAPA-C). *Psychological Medicine, 25*, 755–762.

Angold, A., & Costello, E. J. (2000). The Child and Adolescent Psychiatric Assessment (CAPA). *Journal of the American Academy of Child & Adolescent Psychiatry, 39*, 39–48.

Angold, A., Costello, E. J., & Erkanli, A. (1999). Comorbidity. *Journal of Child Psychology and Psychiatry & Allied Disciplines, 40*, 57–87.

Angold, A., Costello, E. J., Messer, S. C., & Pickles, A. (1995). Development of a short questionnaire for use in epidemiological studies of depression in children and adolescents. *International Journal of Methods in Psychiatric Research, 5*, 237–249.

Angold, A., & Fisher, P. W. (1999). Interviewer-based interviews. In D. Shaffer, C. P. Lucas, & J. E. Richters (Eds.), *Diagnostic assessment in child and adolescent psychopathology* (pp. 34–64). New York: Guilford.

Angold, A., Prendergast, M., Cox, A., Harrington, R., Simonoff, E., & Rutter, M. (1995). The Child and Adolescent Psychiatric Assessment (CAPA). *Psychological Medicine, 25*), 739–753.

Avenevoli, S., Stolar, M., Li, J., Dierker, L., & Merikangas, K.R. (2001). Comorbidity of depression in children and adolescents: Models and evidence from a prospective high-risk family study. *Biological Psychiatry, 49*, 1071–1081.

Baillargeon, R. H., Boulerice, B., Tremblay, R. E., Zoccolillo, M., Vitaro, F. & Kohen, D. E. (2001). Modeling interinformant agreement in the absence of a "gold standard". *Journal of Child Psychology and Psychiatry, 42*, 463–473.

Baron, P., & DeChamplain, A. (1990). Evaluation de la fidelite et de la validite de la version franaise du RADS aupres d'un groupe d'adolescents francophones. [Evaluation of the reliability and validity of the French version of the RADS with francophone adolescents]. Poster presented at the annual convention of the Canadian Psychological Association, Ottawa.

Beck, A. T., Ward, C. H., Mendelson, M., Mock, J., & Erbaugh, J. (1961). An inventory for measuring depression. *Archives of General Psychiatry, 4*, 561–571.

Berg-Nielsen, T. S., Vika, A., & Dahl, A. A. (2003). When adolescents disagree with their mothers: CBCL-YSR discrepancies related to maternal depression and adolescent self-esteem. *Child: Care, Health and Development, 29*, 207–213.

Birleson, P. (1981). The validity of depressive disorder in childhood and the development of a self-rating scale: A research report. *Journal of Child Psychology and Psychiatry, 22*, 73–88.

Birmaher, B., Arbelaez, C, & Brent, D. (2002). Course and outcome of child and adolescent major depressive disorder. *Child and Adolescent Clinics of North America, 11*, 619–638.

Birmaher, B., Ryan, N. D., Williamson, D. E., Brent, D. A., Kaufman, J., Dahl, R. E., et al. (1996). Childhood and adolescent depression: A review of the past 10 years, Part I. *Journal of the American Academy of Child & Adolescent Psychiatry, 35*, 1427–1439.

Blumberg, S. H., & Izard, C. E. (1986). Discriminating patterns of emotions in 10- and 11-year-old children's anxiety and depression. *Journal of Personality and Social Psychology, 51*, 852–857.

Boyle, M. H., Offord, D. R., Racine, Y., Sanford, M., Szatmari, P., Fleming, J. E., et al. (1993). Evaluation of the Diagnostic Interview for Children and Adolescents for use in general population samples. *Journal of Abnormal Child Psychology, 21*, 663–681.

Bretherton, I., Fritz, J., Zahn-Waxler, C., & Ridgeway, D. (1986). Learning to talk about emotions: A functionalist perspective. *Child Development, 57*, 529–548.

Briggs-Gowan, M. J., Carter, A. S., & Schwab-Stone, M. (1996). Discrepancies among mother, child, and teacher reports: Examining the contributions of maternal depression and anxiety. *Journal of Abnormal Child Psychology, 24*, 749–765.

Brooks, S. J., & Kutcher, S. (2001). Diagnosis and measurement of adolescent depression: A review of commonly utilized instruments. *Journal of Child and Adolescent Psychopharmacology, 11*, 341–376.

Brown, B. B. (1990). Peer groups and peer cultures. In S. S. Feldman & G. R. Elliot (Eds.), *At the threshold: The developing adolescent* (pp. 171–196). Cambridge, MA: Harvard University.

Cantwell, D. P., Lewinsohn, P. M., Rohde, P., & Seeley, J. R. (1997). Correspondence between adolescent report and parent report of psychiatric diagnostic data. *Journal of the American Academy of Child & Adolescent Psychiatry, 36*, 610–619.

Carlson, G. A., & Cantwell, D. P (1980). Unmasking masked depression in children and adolescents. *American Journal of Psychiatry, 137*, 445–449.

Carlson, G. A., & Kashani, J. H. (1988). Phenomenology of major depression from childhood through adulthood: Analysis of three studies. *American Journal of Psychiatry, 145*, 1222–1225.

Chambers, W. J., Puig-Antich, J., Hirsch, M., Paez, P., Ambrosini, P. J., Jabrizi, M., et al. (1985). The assessment of affective disorders in children and adolescents by semi-structured interview: Test-retest reliability of the Schedule for Affective Disorders and Schizophrenia for School-Age Children, Present Episode Version. *Archives of General Psychiatry, 42*, 696–702.

Clark, L. A., & Watson, D. (1991). Tripartite model of anxiety and depression: Evidence and taxonomic implications. *Journal of Abnormal Psychology, 100*, 316–336.

Cohen, P., Cohen, J., Kasen, S., Velez, C. N., Hartmark, C., Johnson, J., et al. (1993). An epidemiological study of childhood disorders in late childhood and adolescence: Age and gender-specific prevalence. *Journal of Child Psychology, Psychiatry, and Allied Disciplines, 34*, 851–867.

Cole, D. A., & Martin, N. C. (2005). The longitudinal structure of the Children's Depression Inventory: Testing a latent trait-state model. *Psychological Assessment, 17*, 144–155.

Cole, D. A., & McPherson, A. E. (1993). Relation of family subsystems to adolescent depression: Implementing a new family assessment strategy. *Journal of Family Psychology, 7*, 119–133.

Costello, E. J., & Angold, A. (1988). Scales to assess child and adolescent depression: Checklists, screens, and nets. *Journal of the American Academy of Child & Adolescent Psychiatry, 27*, 726–737.

Costello, E. J., Benjamin, R., Angold, A., & Silver, D. (1991). Mood variability in adolescents: A study of depressed, nondepressed and comorbid patients. *Journal of Affective Disorders, 23*, 199–212.

Costello, E. J., Edelbrock, C. S., & Costello, A. J. (1985). Validity of the NIMH Diagnostic Interview Schedule for Children: A comparison between psychiatric and pediatric referrals. *Journal of Abnormal Child Psychology, 13*, 579–595.

Costello, E. J., Edelbrock, C., Dulcan, M. K., Kalas, R., & Klaric, S. (1984). *Report on the NIMH Diagnostic Interview Schedule for Children (DISC)*. Washington, DC: National Institute of Mental Health.

Crowley, S. L., Worchel, F. F., & Ash, M. J. (1992). Self-report, peer-report, and teacher-report measures of childhood depression: An analysis by item. *Journal of Personality Assessment, 59*, 189–203.

Duke, N., Ireland, M., & Borowsky, I. W. (2005). Identifying psychosocial problems among youth: Factors associated with youth agreement on a positive parent-completed PSC-17. *Child: Care, Health and Development, 31*, 563–573.

Ebata, A. T., & Moos, R. H. (1991). Coping and adjustment in distressed and healthy adolescents. *Journal of Applied Developmental Psychology, 12*, 33–54.

Edelbrock, C., Costello, A. J., Dulcan, M. K., Kalas, R., & Conover, N. C. (1985). Age differences in the reliability of the psychiatric interview of the child. *Child Development, 56*, 265–275.

Egger, H. L., & Angold, A. (2004). The Preschool Age Psychiatric Assessment (PAPA): A structured parent interview for diagnosing psychiatric disorders in preschool children. In R. DelCarmen-Wiggins & A. Carter (Eds.), *Handbook of infant, toddler, and preschool mental health assessment* (pp. 223–243). New York: Oxford University Press.

Endicott, J., & Spitzer, R. L. (1978). A diagnostic interview: The Schedule for Affective Disorders and Schizophrenia. *Archives of General Psychiatry, 35*, 837–844.

Epkins, C. C. (1995). Teachers' ratings of inpatient children's depression, anxiety, and aggression: A preliminary comparison between inpatient-facility and community-based teachers' ratings and their correspondence with children's self-reports. *Journal of Clinical Child Psychology, 24*, 63–70.

Epkins, C. C. (1996). Parent ratings of children's depression, anxiety, and aggression: A cross-sample analysis of agreement and differences with child and teacher ratings. *Journal of Clinical Psychology, 52*, 599–608.

Epkins, C. C., & Dedmon, A. M. M. (1999). An initial look at sibling reports on children's behavior: Comparisons with children's self-reports and relations with siblings' self-reports and sibling relationships. *Journal of Abnormal Child Psychology, 27*, 371–381.

Epkins, C. C., & Meyers, A. W. (1994). Assessment of childhood depression, anxiety, and aggression: Convergent and discriminant validity of self-, parent-, teacher-, and peer-report measures. *Journal of Personality Assessment, 62*, 364–381.

Ezpeleta, L., de la Osa, N., Domenech, J. M., Navarro, J. B., Losilla, J. M., & Judez, J. (1997). Diagnostic agreement between clinicians and the Diagnostic Interview for Children and Adolescents–DICA-R–in an outpatient sample. *Journal of Child Psychology and Psychiatry, 38*, 431–440.

Ferdinand, R. F., Hoogerheide, K. N., van der Ende, J., Heijmens Visser, J., Koot, H. M., Kasius, M. C., et al. (2003). The role of the clinician: Three-year predictive value of parents', teachers', and clinicians' judgment of childhood psychopathology. *Journal of Child Psychology and Psychiatry, 44*, 867–876.

Ferdinand, R. F., van der Ende, J., & Verhulst, F. C. (2004). Parent-adolescent disagreement regarding psychopathology in adolescents from the general population as a risk factor for adverse outcome. *Journal of Abnormal Psychology, 113*, 198–206.

Finch, A. J., Saylor, C. F., Edwards, G. L., & McIntosh, J. A. (1987). Children's Depression Inventory: Reliability over repeated administrations. *Journal of Clinical Child Psychology, 16*, 339–341.

Fine, S., Forth, A., Gilbert, M., & Haley, G. (1991). Group therapy for adolescent depressive disorder: A comparison of social skills and therapeutic support. *Journal of the American Academy of Child & Adolescent Psychiatry, 30*, 79–85.

Fisher, P. W., Shaffer, D., Piacentini, J., Lapkin, J., Kafantaris, L. H., & Herzog, D. B. (1993). Sensitivity of the Diagnostic Interview Schedule for Children, 2nd edition (DISC-2.1) for specific diagnoses of children and adolescents. *Journal of the American Academy of Child & Adolescent Psychiatry, 32*, 666–673.

Fleming, J.E., & Offord, D.R. (1990). Epidemiology of childhood depressive disorders: A critical review. *Journal of the American Academy of Child & Adolescent Psychiatry, 29*, 571–580.

Forehand, R., Brody, G. H., Long, N., & Fauber, R. (1988). The interactive influence of adolescent and maternal depression on adolescent social and cognitive functioning. *Cognitive Therapy and Research, 12*, 341–350.

Garber, J., & Horowitz, J. L. (2002). Depression in children. In I. H. Gotlib & C. L. Hammen (Eds.), *Handbook of depression* (pp. 510–540). New York: Guilford.

Garber, J., & Kaminski, K. M. (2000). Laboratory and performance-based measures of depression in children and adolescents. *Journal of Clinical Child Psychology, 29,* 509–525.

Gardner, W., Campo, J., & Lucas, A. (2004). Validation of the PSC-17 in a primary care sample. *Pediatric Research, 55,* 242A–243A.

Gardner, W., Murphy, M., Childs, G., Kelleher, K., Pagano, M., Jellinek, M., et al. (1999). The PSC-17: A brief pediatric symptom checklist with psychosocial problem sub-scales. A report from PROS and ASPN. *Ambulatory Child Health, 5,* 225–236.

Garvin, V., Leber, D., & Kalter, N. (1991). Children of divorce: Predictors of change following preventive intervention. *American Journal of Orthopsychiatry, 61,* 438–447.

Goodyer, I., Wright, C., & Altham, P. (1990). The friendships and recent life events of anxious and depressed school-age children. *British Journal of Psychiatry, 156,* 689–698.

Goodyer, I., Wright, C., & Altham, P. M. (1988). Maternal adversity and recent stressful life events in anxious and depressed children. *Journal of Child Psychology and Psychiatry, 29,* 651–667.

Gotlib, I. H., & Hammen, C. L. (1992). *Psychological aspects of depression: Toward a cognitive-interpersonal integration.* Chichester, England: Wiley.

Granero Perez, R., Ezpeleta Ascaso, L., Domenech Massons, J. M., & de la Osa Chaparro, N. (1998). Characteristics of the subject and interview influencing the test-retest reliability of the Diagnostic Interview for Children and Adolescents–Revised. *Journal of Child Psychology and Psychiatry, 39,* 963–972.

Hamilton, M. (1960). A rating scale for depression. *Journal of Neurology, Neurosurgery and Psychiatry, 23,* 56–62.

Hammen, C., Adrian, C., Gordon, D., Jaenicke, C., & Hiroto, D. (1987). Children of depressed mothers: Maternal strain and symptom predictors of dysfunction. *Journal of Abnormal Psychology, 96,* 190–198.

Hammen, C., Burge, D., & Stansbury, K. (1990). Relationship of mother and child variables to child outcomes in a high-risk sample: A causal modeling analysis. *Developmental Psychology, 26,* 24–30.

Hammen, C., & Rudolph, K. D. (2003). Childhood mood disorders. In E. J. Mash & R. A. Barkley (Eds.), *Child psychopathology* (2nd ed., pp. 233–278). New York: Guilford.

Handwerk, M. L., Larzelere, R. E., Soper, S. H., & Friman, P. C. (1999). Parent and child discrepancies in reporting severity of problem behaviors in three out-of-home settings. *Psychological Assessment, 11,* 14–23.

Harrington, R., Fudge, H., Rutter, M., Pickles, A., & Hill, J. (1990). Adult outcomes of childhood and adolescent depression—I. Psychiatric status. *Archives of General Psychiatry, 47,* 465 –473.

Herjanic, B., & Reich, W. (1982). Development of a structured psychiatric interview for children: Agreement between child and parent on individual symptoms. *Journal of Abnormal Child Psychology, 10,* 307–324.

Herman-Stahl, M., & Petersen, A. C. (1999). Depressive symptoms during adolescence: Direct and stress-buffering effects of coping, control beliefs, and family relationships. *Journal of Applied Developmental Psychology, 20,* 45–62.

Hodges, K. (1990). Depression and anxiety in children: A comparison of self-report questionnaires to clinical interview. *Psychological Assessment, 2,* 376–381.

Hodges, K., Gordon, Y., & Lennon, M. P. (1990). Parent-child agreement on symptoms assessed via a clinical research interview for children: The Child Assessment Schedule (CAS). *Journal of Child Psychology and Psychiatry, 31,* 427–436.

Ialongo, N., Edelsohn, G., Werthamer-Larsson, L., Crockett, L., & Kellam, S. (1996). Social and cognitive impairment in first-grade children with anxious and depressive symptoms. *Journal of Clinical Child Psychology, 25,* 15–24.

Ines, T. M., & Sacco, W. P. (1992). Factors related to correspondence between teacher ratings of elementary student depression and student self-ratings. *Journal of Consulting and Clinical Psychology, 60,* 140–142.

Jellinek, M. S., Murphy, J. M., & Burns, B. J. (1986). Brief psychosocial screening in outpatient pediatric practice. *Journal of Pediatrics, 109,* 371–378.

Jellinek, M. S., Murphy, J. M., Robinson, J., Feins, A., Lamb, S., & Fenton, T. (1988). Pediatric Symptom Checklist: Screening school-age children for psychosocial dysfunction. *Journal of Pediatrics, 112*, 201–209.

Jensen, P. S., Rubio-Stipec, M., Canino, G., Bird, H. R., Dulcan, M. K., Schwab-Stone, M. E., et al. (1999). Parent and child contributions to diagnosis of mental disorder: Are both informants always necessary? *Journal of the American Academy of Child & Adolescent Psychiatry, 38*, 1569–1579.

Jensen, P. S., Traylor, J., Xenakis, S. N., & Davis, H. (1988). Child psychopathology rating scales and interrater agreement: I. Parents' gender and psychiatric symptoms. *Journal of the American Academy of Child & Adolescent Psychiatry, 27*, 442–450.

Kashani, J. H., & Carlson, G. A. (1987). Seriously depressed preschoolers. *American Journal of Psychiatry, 144*, 348–350.

Kaslow, N. J., Deering, C. G., & Racusin, G. R. (1994). Depressed children and their families. *Clinical Psychology Review, 14*, 39–59.

Kaufman, J., Birmaher, B., Brent, D., Rao, U., Flynn, C., Mordeci, P., et al. (1997). Schedule for Affective Disorders and Schizophrenia for School-Age Children-Present and Lifetime version (K-SADS-PL): Initial reliability and validity data. *Journal of the American Academy of Child & Adolescent Psychiatry, 36*, 980–988.

Kazdin, A. E., French, N. H., & Unis, A. S. (1983). Child, mother, and father evaluations of depression in psychiatric inpatient children. *Journal of Abnormal Child Psychology, 11*, 167–180.

Kendall, P. C., Stark, K. D., & Adam, T. (1990). Cognitive deficit or cognitive distortion of childhood depression. *Journal of Abnormal Child Psychology, 18*, 255–270.

Kent, L., Vostanis, P., & Feehan, C. (1997). Detection of major and minor depression in children and adolescents: Evaluation of the Mood and Feelings Questionnaire. *Journal of Child Psychology and Psychiatry, 38*, 565–573.

Kessler, R.C., Avenevoli, S., & Merikangas, K.R. (2001). Mood disorders in children and adolescents: An epidemiologic perspective. *Biological Psychiatry, 49*, 1002–1014.

Kessler, R.C., McGonagle, K.A., Zhao, S., Nelson, C.V., Hughes, M., Eshleman, S., et al. (1994). Lifetime and 12-month prevalence of *DSM–III–R* psychiatric disorders in the United States: Results from the National Comorbidity Survey. *Archives of General Psychiatry, 51*, 8–19.

Klein, D. N., Dougherty, L. R., & Olino, T. M. (2005). Toward guidelines for evidence-based assessment of depression in children and adolescents. *Journal of Clinical Child and Adolescent Psychology, 34*, 412–432.

Klein, D. N., Ouimette, P. C., Kelly, H. S., Ferro, T., & Riso, L. P. (1994). Test-retest reliability of team consensus best-estimate diagnoses of Axis I and II disorders in a family study. *American Journal of Psychiatry, 151*, 1043–1047.

Kolko, D. J., & Kazdin, A. E. (1993). Emotional/behavioral problems in clinic and non-clinic children: Correspondence among child, parent and teacher reports. *Journal of Child Psychology and Psychiatry, 34*, 991–1006.

Kovacs, M. (1980/1981). Rating scales to assess depression in school-aged children. *Acta Paedopsychiatrica: International Journal of Child and Adolescent Psychiatry, 46*, 305–315.

Kovacs, M. (1992). *The Children's Depression Inventory.* North Tonawanda, NY: Mental Health Systems.

Kovacs, M., & Devlin, B. (1998). Internalizing disorders in childhood. *Journal of Child Psychology and Psychiatry, 39*, 47–63.

Kovacs, M., Gatsonis, C., Paulauskas, S.L., & Richards, C. (1989). Depressive disorders in childhood: IV. A longitudinal study of comorbidity with and risk for anxiety disorders. *Archives of General Psychiatry, 46*, 776–782.

Kraemer, H. C., Measelle, J. R., Ablow, J. C., Essex, M. J., Boyce, W. T., & Kupfer, D. J. (2003). A new approach to integrating data from multiple informants in psychiatric assessment and research: Mixing and matching contexts and perspectives, *American Journal of Psychiatry, 160*, 1566–1577.

Lefkowitz, M. M., & Tesiny, E. P. (1980). Assessment of childhood depression. *Journal of Consulting and Clinical Psychology, 48*, 43–50.

Lewinsohn, P. M., & Essau, C. A. (2002). Depression in adolescents. In I. H. Gotlib & C. L. Hammen (Eds.), *Handbook of depression* (pp. 541–559). New York: Guilford.

Lewinsohn, P. M., Rohde, P., & Seeley, J. R. (1998). Major depressive disorder in older adolescents: Prevalence, risk factors, and clinical implications. *Clinical Psychology Review, 18,* 765–794.

Lobovits, D. A., & Handal, P. J. (1985). Childhood depression: Prevalence using DSM–III criteria and validity of parent and child depression scales. *Journal of Pediatric Psychology, 10,* 45–54.

Lonigan, C. J., Phillips, B. M., & Hooe, E. S. (2003). Relations of positive and negative affectivity to anxiety and depression in children: Evidence from a latent variable longitudinal study. *Journal of Consulting and Clinical Psychology, 71,* 465–481.

Luby, J. L., Heffelmger, A., Mrakotsky, C, Hessler, M. J., Brown, K. M., & Hildebrand, T. (2002). Preschool major depressive disorder: Preliminary validation for developmentally modified *DSM–IV* criteria. *Journal of the American Academy of Child & Adolescent Psychiatry, 41,* 928–937.

Luby, J., Todd, R., & Geller, B. (1996). Outcome of depressive syndromes: Infancy to adulthood. In K. Shulman, M. Tohen, & S. P. Kutcher (Eds.), *Mood disorders across the life span* (pp. 83–100). New York: Wiley.

McCauley, E., Mitchell, J. R., Burke, P. M., & Moss, S. J. (1988). Cognitive attributes of depression in children and adolescents. *Journal of Consulting and Clinical Psychology, 56,* 903–908.

McClure, E., Rogeness, G. A., & Thompson, N. M. (1997). Characteristics of adolescent girls with depressive symptoms in a so-called "normal" sample. *Journal of Affective Disorders, 42,* 187–197.

McGee, R., & Williams, S. (1988). A longitudinal study of depression in nine-year-old children. *Journal of the American Academy of Child & Adolescent Psychiatry, 27,* 342–348.

Mesman, J., & Koot, H. M. (2000). Child-reported depression and anxiety in preadolescence: II. Preschool predictors. *Journal of the American Academy of Child & Adolescent Psychiatry, 39,* 1379–1386.

Messer, S. C., & Gross, A. M. (1995). Childhood depression and family interaction: A naturalistic observation study. *Journal of Clinical Child Psychology, 24,* 77–88.

Mokros, H. B., Poznanski, E., Grossman, J. A., & Freeman, L. N. (1987). A comparison of child and parent ratings of depression for normal and clinically referred children. *Journal of Child Psychology and Psychiatry, 28,* 613–624.

Moretti, M. M., Fine, S., Haley, G., & Marriage, K. (1985). Childhood and adolescent depression: Child-report versus parent-report information. *Journal of the American Academy of Child Psychiatry, 24,* 298–302.

Murphy, J. M., Reede, J., Jellinek, M. S., & Bishop, S. J. (1992). Screening for psychosocial dysfunction in inner-city children: Further validation of the Pediatric Symptom Checklist. *Journal of the American Academy of Child & Adolescent Psychiatry, 31,* 1105–1111.

Myers, K., & Winters, N. C. (2002). Ten-year review of rating scales: II. Scales for internalizing disorders. *Journal of the American Academy of Child & Adolescent Psychiatry, 41,* 634–659.

Najman, J. M., Williams, G. M., Nikles, J., Spence, S., Bor, W., O'Callaghan, M., et al. (2000). Mothers' mental illness and child behavior problems: Cause-effect association or observation bias? *Journal of the American Academy of Child & Adolescent Psychiatry, 39,* 592–602.

Navon, M., Nelson, D., Pagano, M., & Murphy, M. (2001). Use of the Pediatric Symptom Checklist in strategies to improve preventive behavioral health care. *Psychiatric Services, 52,* 800–804.

Nelson, W. M., Politano, P. M., Finch, A. J., Wendel, N., & Mayhall, C. (1987). Children's Depression Inventory: Normative data and utility with emotionally disturbed children. *Journal of the American Academy of Child & Adolescent Psychiatry, 26,* 43–48.

Nieminen, G. S., & Matson, J. L. (1989). Depressive problems in conduct-disordered adolescents. *Journal of School Psychology, 27,* 175–188.

Orvaschel H., Puig-Antich, J., Chambers, W. J., Tabrizi, M. A., & Johnson, R. (1982). Retrospective assessment of prepubertal major depression with the Kiddie-SADS-E. *Journal of the American Academy of Child & Adolescent Psychiatry, 21*, 392–397.

Pagano, M. E., Cassidy, L. J., Little, M., Murphy, J. M., & Jellinek, M. S. (2000). Identifying psychosocial dysfunction in school-age children: The Pediatric Symptom Checklist as a self-report measure. *Psychology in the Schools, 37*, 91–106.

Pellegrino, J. F., Singh, N. N., & Carmanico, S. J. (1999). Concordance among three diagnostic procedures for identifying depression in children and adolescents with EBD. *Journal of Emotional and Behavioral Disorders, 7*, 118–127.

Phares, V. (1992). Where's poppa? The relative lack of attention to the role of fathers in child and adolescent psychopathology. *American Psychologist, 47*, 656–664.

Poznanski, E. O., Cook, S. C., & Carroll, B. J. (1979). A depression rating scale for children. *Pediatrics, 64*, 442–450.

Poznanski, E. O., Grossman, J. A., Buchsbaum, Y., Banegas, M., Freeman, L., & Gibbons, R. (1984). Preliminary studies of the reliability and validity of the Children's Depression Rating Scale. *Journal of the American Academy of Child Psychiatry, 23*, 191–197.

Poznanski, E. O., & Mokros, H. B. (1999). *Children Depression Rating Scale–Revised (CDRS–R)*. Los Angeles: Western Psychological Services.

Puig-Antich J., & Chambers, W. J. (1978). *Schedule for Affective Disorders and Schizophrenia for School-Age Children* (Kiddie-SADS). New York: New York State Psychiatric Institute.

Puig-Antich, J., Kaufman, J., Ryan, N. D., Williamson, D. E., Dahl, R. E., Lukens, E., et al. (1993). The psychosocial functioning and family environment of depressed adolescents. *Journal of the American Academy of Child & Adolescent Psychiatry, 32*, 244–253.

Quiggle, N. L., Garber, J., Panak, W. F., & Dodge, K. A. (1992). Social information processing in aggressive and depressed children. *Child Development, 63*, 1305–1320.

Radke-Yarrow, M. (1998). *Children of depressed mothers: From early childhood to maturity*. Cambridge, UK: Cambridge University Press.

Reich, W. (2000). Diagnostic Interview for Children and Adolescents (DICA). *Journal of the American Academy of Child & Adolescent Psychiatry, 39*, 59–66.

Reich, W., & Welner, Z. (1988). Revised version of the Diagnostic Interview for Children and Adolescents (DICA-R). St. Louis, MO: Department of Psychiatry, Washington University School of Medicine.

Renouf, A. G., & Kovacs, M. (1994). Concordance between mothers' reports and children's self-reports of depressive symptoms: A longitudinal study. *Journal of the American Academy of Child & Adolescent Psychiatry, 33*, 208–216.

Reynolds, W. M. (1987). *Reynolds Adolescent Depression Scale Professional Manual*. Odessa, FL: Psychological Assessment Resources.

Reynolds, W. M. (1989). *Reynolds Child Depression Scale*. Odessa, FL: Psychological Assessment Resources.

Reynolds, W. M., & Coats, K. I. (1986). A comparison of cognitive-behavioral therapy and relaxation training for the treatment of depression in adolescents. *Journal of Consulting and Clinical Psychology, 54*, 653–660.

Reynolds, W. M., & Miller, K. L. (1985). Depression and learned helplessness in mentally retarded and nonmentally retarded adolescents: An initial investigation. *Applied Research in Mental Retardation, 6*, 295–306.

Richters, J. E. (1992). Depressed mothers as informants about their children: A critical review of the evidence for distortion. *Psychological Bulletin, 112*, 485–499.

Rubio-Stipec, M., Fitzmaurice, G. M., Murphy, J., & Walker, A. (2003). The use of multiple informants in identifying the risk factors of depressive and disruptive disorders: Are they interchangeable? *Social Psychiatry and Psychiatric Epidemiology, 38*, 51–58.

Rudolph, K. D., & Clark, A. G. (2001). Conceptions of relationships in children with depressive and aggressive symptoms: Social-cognitive distortion or reality? *Journal of Abnormal Child Psychology, 29*, 41–56.

Rudolph, K. D., Hammen, C., & Burge, D. (1994). Interpersonal functioning and depressive symptoms in childhood: Addressing the issues of specificity and comorbidity. *Journal of Abnormal Child Psychology, 22*, 355–371.

Rudolph, K. D., Hammen, C., & Burge, D. (1997). A cognitive-interpersonal approach to depressive symptoms in preadolescent children. *Journal of Abnormal Child Psychology, 25*, 33–45.

Rudolph, K. D., Kurlakowsky, K. D., & Conley, C. S. (2001). Developmental and social-contextual origins of depressive control-related beliefs and behavior. *Cognitive Therapy and Research, 25*, 447–475.

Ryan, N. D., Puig-Antich, J., Cooper, T., Rabinovitch, H., Ambrosini, P., Davies, M., et al. (1986). Imipramine in adolescent major depression: Plasma level and clinical response. *Acta Psychiatrica Scandinavica, 73*, 275–288.

Saylor, C. F., Finch, A. J., Spirito, A., & Bennett, B. (1984). The Children's Depression Inventory: A systematic evaluation of psychometric properties. *Journal of Consulting and Clinical Psychology, 52*, 955–967.

Schaughency, E. A., & Rothlind, J. (1991). Assessment and classification of Attention Deficit Hyperactive Disorders. *School Psychology Review, 20*, 187–202.

Schwab-Stone, M., Fallon, T., Briggs, M., & Crowther, B. (1994). Reliability of diagnostic reporting for children aged 6–11 years: A test–retest study of the Diagnostic Interview Schedule for Children-Revised. *American Journal of Psychiatry, 151*, 1048–1054.

Seiffge-Krenke, I., & Kollmar, F. (1998). Discrepancies between mothers' and fathers' perceptions of sons' and daughters' problem behaviour: A longitudinal analysis of parent-adolescent agreement on internalising and externalising problem behaviour. *Journal of Child Psychology and Psychiatry, 39*, 687–697.

Shaffer, D., Fisher, P., Dulcan, M. K., Davies, M., Piacentini, J., Schwab-Stone, M. E., et al. (1996). The NIMH Diagnostic Interview Schedule for Children Version 2.3 (DISC-2.3): Description, acceptability, prevalence rates, and performance in the MECA study. *Journal of the American Academy of Child & Adolescent Psychiatry, 35*, 865–877.

Shaffer, D., Fisher, P., Lucas, C. P., Dulcan, M. K., & Schwab-Stone, M. E. (2000). NIMH Diagnostic Interview Schedule for Children Version IV (NIMH DISC-IV): Description, differences from previous versions, and reliability of some common diagnoses. *Journal of the American Academy of Child & Adolescent Psychiatry, 39*, 28–38.

Shaffer, D., Schwab-Stone, M., Fisher, P. W., Cohen, P., Piacentini, J., Davies, M. C., et al. (1993). The Diagnostic Interview Schedule for Children-Revised version (DISC-R): I. Preparation, field testing, interrater reliability, and acceptability. *Journal of the American Academy of Child & Adolescent Psychiatry, 32*, 643–650.

Shain, B. N., King, C. A., Naylor, M., & Alessi, N. (1991). Chronic depression and hospital course in adolescents. *Journal of the American Academy of Child & Adolescent Psychiatry, 30*, 428–433.

Shain, B. N., Naylor, M., & Alessi, N. (1990). Comparison of self-rated and clinician-rated measures of depression in adolescents. *American Journal of Psychiatry, 147*, 793–795.

Sheeber, L., Hops, H., Alpert, A., Davis, B., & Andrews, J. (1997). Family support and conflict: Prospective relations to adolescent depression. *Journal of Abnormal Child Psychology, 25*, 333–344.

Shirk, S. R., Van Horn, M., & Leber, D. (1997). Dysphoria and children's processing of supportive interactions. *Journal of Abnormal Child Psychology, 25*, 239–249.

Silverman, W. K., & Rabian, B. (1999). Rating scales for anxiety and mood disorders. In D. Shaffer, C. P. Lucas, & J. E. Richters (Eds.), *Diagnostic assessment in child and adolescent psychopathology* (pp. 127–166). New York: Guilford.

Smucker, M. R., Craighead, W. E., Craighead, L. W., & Green, B. J. (1986). Normative and reliability data for the Children's Depression Inventory. *Journal of Abnormal Child Psychology, 14*, 25–39.

Sourander, A., Helstela, L., & Helenius, H. (1999). Parent-adolescent agreement on emotional and behavioral problems. *Social Psychiatry and Psychiatric Epidemiology, 34*, 657–663.

Stanger, C., & Lewis, M. (1993). Agreement among parents, teachers, and children on internalizing and externalizing behavior problems. *Journal of Clinical Child Psychology, 22*, 107–115.

Stark, K. D., Reynolds, W. M., & Kaslow, N. J. (1987). A comparison of the relative efficacy of self-control therapy and a behavioral problem-solving therapy for depression in children. *Journal of Abnormal Child Psychology, 15,* 91–113.

Tarullo, L. B., Richardson, D. T., Radke-Yarrow, M., & Martinez, P. E. (1995). Multiple sources in child diagnosis: Parent-child concordance in affectively ill and well families. *Journal of Clinical Child Psychology, 24,* 173–183.

Thapar, A., & McGuffin, P. (1998). Validity of the shortened Mood and Feelings Questionnaire in a community sample of children and adolescents: A preliminary research note. *Psychiatry Research, 81,* 259–268.

Thomas, A. M., Forehand, R., Armistead, L., Wierson, M., & Fauber, R. (1990). Cross-informant consistency in externalizing and internalizing problems in early adolescence. *Journal of Psychopathology and Behavioral Assessment, 12,* 255–262.

Tram, J. M., & Cole, D. A. (2006). A multimethod examination of the stability of depressive symptoms in childhood and adolescence. *Journal of Abnormal Psychology, 115,* 674–686.

Verhulst, F. C., Dekker, M. C., & van der Ende, J. (1997). Parent, teacher and self-reports as predictors of signs of disturbance in adolescents: Whose information carries the most weight? *Acta Psychiatrica Scandinavica, 96,* 75–81.

Verhulst, F. C., & Van der Ende, J. (1992). Agreement between parents' reports and adolescents' self-reports of problem behavior. *Journal of Child Psychology and Psychiatry, 33,* 1011–1023.

Vostanis, P., Feehan, C., Grattan, E., & Bickerton, W.-L. (1996). A randomised controlled out-patient trial of cognitive-behavioural treatment for children and adolescents with depression: 9-month follow-up. *Journal of Affective Disorders, 40,* 105–116.

Walker, W. O., LaGrone, R. G., & Atkinson, A. W. (1989). Psychosocial screening in pediatric practice: Identifying high-risk children. *Journal of Developmental and Behavioral Pediatrics, 10,* 134–138.

Weinstein, S. R., Stone, K., Noam, G. G., Grimes, K., & Schwab-Stone, M. (1989). Comparison of DISC with clinicians' *DSM–III* diagnoses in psychiatric inpatients. *Journal of the American Academy of Child & Adolescent Psychiatry, 28,* 53–60.

Weiss, B., Harris, V., & Catron, T. (2002). Development and initial validation of the Peer-report Measure of Internalizing and Externalizing Behavior. *Journal of Abnormal Child Psychology, 30,* 285–294.

Weissman, M. M., Orvaschel, H., & Padian, N. (1980). Children's symptom and social function self-report scales: Comparisons of mothers' and children's reports. *Journal of Nervous and Mental Disease, 168,* 736–740.

Weisz, J. R., Rudolph, K. D., Granger, D. A., & Sweeney, L. (1992). Cognition, competence, and coping in child and adolescent depression: Research findings, developmental concerns, therapeutic implications. *Development and Psychopathology, 4,* 627–653.

Widen, S. C., & Russell, J. A. (2003). A closer look at preschoolers' freely produced labels for facial expressions. *Developmental Psychology, 39,* 114–128.

Williams, S., McGee, R., Anderson, J., & Silva, P. A. (1989). The structure and correlates of self-reported symptoms in 11-year-old children. *Journal of Abnormal Child Psychology, 17,* 55–71.

Wood, A., Harrington, R., & Moore, A. (1996). Controlled trial of a brief cognitive-behavioural intervention in adolescent patients with depressive disorders. *Journal of Child Psychology and Psychiatry, 37,* 737–746.

Wood, A., Kroll, L., Moore, A., & Harrington, R. (1995). Properties of the Mood and Feelings Questionnaire in adolescent psychiatric outpatients: A research note. *Journal of Child Psychology and Psychiatry, 36,* 327–334.

World Health Organization. (1993). The ICD-10 classification of mental and behavioral disorders: Diagnostic criteria for research. Geneva: World Health Organization.

Yeh, M., & Weisz, J. R. (2001). Why are we here at the clinic? Parent-child (dis)agreement on referral problems at outpatient treatment entry. *Journal of Consulting and Clinical Psychology, 69,* 1018–1025.

Younger, A. J., Schwartzman, A. E., & Ledingham, J. E. (1985). Age-related changes in children's perceptions of aggression and withdrawal in their peers. *Developmental Psychology, 21,* 70–75.

Youngstrom, E., Loeber, R., & Stouthamer-Loeber, M. (2000). Patterns and correlates of agreement between parent, teacher, and male adolescent ratings of externalizing and internalizing problems. *Journal of Consulting and Clinical Psychology, 68,* 1038–1050.

Zahn-Waxler, C., Klimes-Dougan, B., & Slattery, M. J. (2000). Internalizing problems of childhood and adolescence: Prospects, pitfalls, and progress in understanding the development of anxiety and depression. *Development and Psychopathology, 12,* 443–466.

10

Assessment of Bipolar Disorder In Children

STEPHANIE DANNER, MATTHEW E. YOUNG, and MARY A. FRISTAD

Awareness of early-onset bipolar spectrum disorders (BPSD) has grown rapidly in recent years. Parents increasingly approach mental health clinicians questioning whether their children's mood swings constitute BPSD. Childhood-onset BPSD, like other early-onset brain disorders, are associated with worse prognosis and higher levels of interference with functioning than adult-onset BPSD (Kyte, Carlson, & Goodyer, 2006; Perlis et al., 2004). In comparison to those with adult-onset BPSD, children with BPSD experience more difficulties at school, at home, and with peers earlier in their development resulting in less time spent accomplishing developmental goals (Geller, Bolhofner, Craney, Williams, DelBello, & Gunderson, 2000). Some parents describe these children as being difficult from birth and describe significant difficulties with peers in early child care and preschool. Therefore, an accurate timely diagnosis is essential to develop appropriate interventions, the goals of which are to decrease interference and improve functioning across various settings.

In addition to increased awareness of childhood-onset BPSD, controversies about the diagnosis have grown, as well. This chapter presents current trends in the field; recent findings from longitudinal studies concerning the risk, comorbidity, and course of childhood-onset BPSD; a description of bipolar spectrum diagnoses; similarities and differences between child and adult manifestations of BPSD; diagnostic challenges presented by childhood-onset BPSD; and strategies for assessing BPSD. The latter

STEPHANIE DANNER-OGSTON • The Ohio State University
MATTHEW E. YOUNG •
MARY A. FRISTAD •

J.L. Matson et al. (eds.), *Assessing Childhood Psychopathology and Developmental Disabilities*, DOI: 10.1007/978-0-387-09528-8,
© Springer Science+Business Media, LLC 2009

includes a review of multiple informants, screening measures, structured interviews, mood symptom severity scales, a psychosocial history timeline, family history of mental illness, and mood charts. The chapter closes with a vignette illustrating the assessment process and highlighting numerous aspects of the review outlined above.

CONTEMPORARY ISSUES

Trends in the Field

Undoubtedly, the most significant recent trend in the field of childhood-onset BPSD has been increased recognition and diagnosis of this disorder. In the past, manic symptoms were considered extremely rare, if not nonexistent in prepubertal children (Anthony & Scott, 1960). Recently, research on BPSD in children and adolescents has increased dramatically in frequency. For example, a recent search of MEDLINE and PsychInfo databases found 26 journal articles and book chapters on childhood BPSD prior to 1980, 36 in the 1980s, 66 in the 1990s, and 46 in the first two years of this decade (Lofthouse & Fristad, 2004). The diagnosis has received increasing media attention (Lofthouse & Fristad, 2004; Pavuluri, Birmaher, & Naylor, 2005). Public awareness of childhood BPSD has dramatically increased as well. A recent Google Internet search for "childhood bipolar disorder" and "childhood mania" produced 483,000 and 248,000 results, respectively (Leffler & Fristad, 2006). These trends have led some to suggest that BPSD has become a "fad diagnosis," and is being overdiagnosed in children (e.g., Hammen & Rudolph, 2003). This argument may hold some merit, inasmuch as the increase in academic and public interest in BPSD in children and adolescents has advanced faster than clinical training in evidence-based methods of assessment and treatment (Lofthouse & Fristad, 2004). Despite concerns about overdiagnosis, a growing body of evidence suggests that BPSD occurs in children and adolescents more frequently than has been estimated in the past (Youngstrom, Findling, Youngstrom, & Calabrese, 2005).

A community sample of adolescents in Oregon found a lifetime prevalence of 0.12% for Bipolar Disorder-I (BP-I), 1% each for Bipolar Disorder-II (BP-II) and Cyclothymia, and 5.7% with subthreshold symptoms, comorbid conditions, and significant impairment based on self-report of symptoms (Lewinsohn, Klein, & Seely, 1995). This last group, referred to by the authors as "core positive," exhibited levels of impairment similar to the BP-I and BP-II groups (Lewinsohn et al., 1995). The "core positive" group may meet criteria for Bipolar Disorder Not Otherwise Specified (BP-NOS; Lofthouse & Fristad, 2004). The diagnosis of BP-NOS in these "core positive" groups may have increased the incidence of BPSD.

Another trend may also account for some of the increased incidence of childhood BPSD: each generation born after World War II has displayed increased rates and earlier onset of mood disorders (Findling, Kowatch, & Post, 2003). In addition, stimulant and antidepressant medications increasingly have been prescribed to younger children, and can precipitate mood fluctuations in those with a genetic predisposition to mood disorders (Findling et al., 2003). These lines of evidence suggest childhood BPSD may be actually increasing in frequency, rather than the incidence being inflated by overdiagnosis. Diagnostic trends and uncertainty about methods of assessment may lead to overdiagnosis in some settings, whereas lack of recognition of the disorder may simultaneously lead to underdiagnosis in other settings.

Recent Findings

Given the increased interest in childhood BPSD in recent years, questions have been raised about the course of illness. It remains unclear what the long-term outcome is for children. Will their symptom presentation change over time? As they reach adolescence and puberty, will their illness begin to resemble "classic" adolescent- or adult-onset bipolar disorder, or will the atypical symptom presentation characteristic of many children with BPSD (i.e., lack of clearly defined episodes, less likely to meet full diagnostic criteria for Bipolar I Disorder) persist? In an attempt to answer these questions and accurately characterize the phenomenology of BPSD in children and adolescents, researchers have enrolled a large sample (N = 438) of participants in the multisite Course and Outcome of Bipolar Youth (COBY) study (Birmaher et al., 2006; Axelson et al., 2006). Participants in this naturalistic longitudinal study must meet diagnostic criteria for BP-I, BP-II, or an operational definition of BP-NOS (a discussion of the definition is included later in the chapter), and are being followed for a period of up to ten years.

Preliminary findings from the COBY cohort indicate that participants in all diagnostic groups showed high rates of elated mood (i.e., 80% or more). Those diagnosed with BP-NOS most often failed to meet duration criterion for mania, rather than having too few symptoms (Axelson et. al, 2006). Preliminary longitudinal results from a subset of the COBY sample indicate that over a two-year period, participants were symptomatic most of the time. Approximately one-fourth of youth with BP-NOS progressed to a diagnosis of BP-I or BP-II within two years (Birmaher et al., 2006). Comorbid conditions and maternal depression were associated with poorer family functioning among COBY participants (Esposito-Smythers et al., 2006). Participants with childhood-onset, as opposed to adolescent-onset, bipolar disorder were more likely to be male, have lower socioeconomic status, have comorbid Attention-Deficit/Hyperactivity Disorder (ADHD), and were less likely to receive a diagnosis of BP-I or live with both biological parents. Adolescents reporting onset before age 12 also displayed higher rates of anxiety disorders (Rende et al., 2007). Almost one-third of the COBY sample endorsed a lifetime suicide attempt, with older and more severely impaired participants having the highest risk (Goldstein et al., 2005). Family history of mania was not associated with age of onset, but younger onset of illness was associated with significantly higher rates of a number of other mental illnesses in first- and second-degree relatives (Rende et al., 2007).

The COBY study represents an important step in research on child and adolescent BPSD. It provides prospective data on a large cohort of youth, whereas many previous studies have relied on retrospective report of onset (e.g., Geller & Luby, 1997; Perlis et al., 2004). Preliminary results are consistent with studies that have utilized smaller samples (Carlson, Bromet, Driessens, Mojtabai, & Schwartz, 2002; Craney & Geller, 2005; Geller & Tillman, 2005; Geller, Tillman, Craney, & Bolhofner, 2004), suggesting that prepubertal-onset BPSD is associated with high rates of comorbidity, psychosocial impairment, mixed states, and family history of psychopathology.

To extend the knowledge collected by studies such as COBY, researchers at four academic sites (Case Western Reserve University, the Ohio State University, University of Cincinnati, and Western Psychiatric Institute and Clinic) are enrolling participants in the NIMH-funded Longitudinal Assessment of Manic Symptoms (LAMS) study. Children presenting for an evaluation in outpatient clinics are screened with the Parent-General Behavior Inventory-Short Form (Youngstrom, Meyers, et al., 2005; which is discussed later in the screening measures section) for the presence of possible manic symptoms. Children whose parents or guardians rate them above a specified threshold will be followed for a period of up to five years, regardless of their Axis I diagnoses. In fact, because the LAMS study intends to recruit a sample at risk for BPSD, the screening threshold has been set low enough that most children in LAMS do not have any mood disorder diagnoses. Over time, the LAMS study will provide prospective data on the prevalence of manic symptoms in clinical settings and features associated with increased risk of developing BPSD over time. Future data from longitudinal samples such as COBY and LAMS will provide valuable information about the course and outcome of this illness that clinicians can integrate into assessment procedures.

Summary

The field of childhood-onset BPSD has developed at a rapid pace in the past decade. Increased awareness of the disorder has led to more frequent diagnosis. This has led some clinicians and researchers to question whether this trend has gone too far, leading to overdiagnosis of BPSD in children. However, longitudinal studies, such as COBY and LAMS, are underway and will provide critical information needed to clarify the prevalence, clinical characteristics, and long-term outcome of childhood-onset BPSD.

PHENOMENOLOGY OF EARLY-ONSET BPSD

DSM–IV–TR Description of BPSD

The Diagnostic and Statistical Manual–IV–Text Revision (DSM–IV–TR; American Psychiatric Association [APA], 2000) describes two categories of symptoms for the diagnosis of mania/hypomania. There are no distinct criteria for children and adolescents compared to adults. Criterion A is the presence of elevated or irritable mood for a period of at least one week for mania or four days for hypomania. Criterion B describes accompanying symptoms, including: grandiosity; decreased need for sleep; pressured speech; flight of ideas; distractibility; increased goal-directed activity in social, academic, or sexual arenas or psychomotor agitation; and high-risk behaviors.

For a Manic or Hypomanic Episode, the child needs to have either elevated mood and three accompanying symptoms, or irritable mood and four accompanying symptoms. In addition to longer duration, mania causes marked impairment in functioning at home, at school or with peers, may have psychotic features, and/or may require psychiatric hospitalization. Hypomania is associated with a change from baseline functioning, but less severe impairment. A Mixed Episode is diagnosed when criteria for a Major Depressive Episode (except duration) and a Manic Episode are met nearly every day for at least one week and cause marked impairment in functioning (APA, 2000).

The four BPSD can be distinguished by the severity and frequency of depressive and manic symptoms (see Table 10.1). Bipolar Disorder I (BP-I) is the most severe and consists of at least one Manic or Mixed Episode with or without the presence of a Major Depressive Episode or depressive symptoms. Subtypes of BP-I can be distinguished by the type of episode which occurred most recently (Manic, Hypomanic, Mixed, Depressed, or Unspecified). Bipolar Disorder II (BP-II) is the presence of at least one Major Depressive Episode and at least one Hypomanic Episode, without a history of Manic or Mixed episodes. Cyclothymic Disorder is characterized by less intense highs and lows, periods where several hypomanic symptoms are present and periods where several depressive symptoms are present, although not enough to meet a Hypomanic or Major Depressive Episode. Cyclothymic Disorder has a longer duration of at least one year in children and adolescents (two years in adults) with no remittance of symptoms for a period of more than two months. Bipolar Disorder Not Otherwise Specified (BP-NOS) captures the variants of problematic affective highs and lows that do not fit into the other three categories. The longitudinal studies described in the previous section (i.e., COBY and LAMS) have developed an operational definition of BP-NOS. This definition was developed because of equivocal language in the *DSM–IV–TR* definition of BP-NOS, and to document the presence of significant symptom severity, often with short duration, and functional impairment in this diagnostic group (See Table 10.2). This operational definition also aids researchers in monitoring diagnostic "progression" from BP-NOS to Cyclothymia, BP-II, or BP-I.

Table 10.1. Bipolar spectrum disorders

Bipolar I	M (+ D, d, or none)
Bipolar II	hM + D
Cyclothymia	m + d (duration of at least 1 year)

M – Manic Episode, hM – Hypomanic Episode, D – Major Depressive Episode, d – depressive symptoms that do not meet criteria for a Major Depressive Episode , m – manic symptoms that do not meet criteria for a Manic or Hypomanic Episode

Table 10.2. Two Definitions of Bipolar Disorder – Not Otherwise Specified

DSM–IV–TR (APA, 2000)	Operational Definition from Longitudinal Research Studies (COBY[a], LAMS[b])
"The Bipolar Disorder NOS category includes disorders with bipolar features that do not meet criteria for any specific Bipolar Disorder."	A. Intensity: Distinct period of abnormally elevated, expansive, or irritable mood At least 2 additional associated symptoms of mania if elated mood is present *or* at least 3 additional symptoms if irritable Change in functioning (decreased or increased; similar to *DSM–IV* guideline for hypomania) B. Duration of Episode: A total of ≥4 hours within a 24-hour period C. Total Number of Episodes: Lifetime: ≥4 days of above-noted symptom intensity and duration. Days need not be consecutive.

[a]COBY – Course and Outcome of Bipolar Youth
[b]LAMS - Longitudinal Assessment of Manic Symptoms

Childhood- Versus Adult-Onset BPSD

Many children with BPSD do not fit the template for BP-I, BP-II, and Cyclothymic Disorder used for diagnosis in adults and described in DSM–IV–TR. In children, symptom frequency, symptom presentation, typical onset as manic versus depressive, prognosis, and even gender ratios differ from those seen in adults. For adults, decreased need for sleep is almost universal, whereas less than half of children with BPSD experience sleep problems (Biederman et al., 2005; Geller et al., 2004). In contrast to the euphoric, expansive manic episodes frequently seen in adults, children's presenting problems often include outbursts of mood lability, irritability, reckless behavior, and aggression that last hours to days (American Academy of Child Adolescent Psychiatry [AACAP], 2007).

Some children and adolescents experience a waxing and waning of moods that are frequent, intense, and unrelated to environmental events, but lack true "episodes" (Lofthouse & Fristad, 2004). Increased rates of more psychosis, poorer prognosis, slower recovery times, more recurrence of episodes, higher comorbidity, and higher suicide incidence have been reported for youth with BPSD (Findling et al., 2001; Kyte et al., 2006; Lewinsohn et al., 1995). Patel and colleagues (2006) reported more psychomotor retardation, psychotic features, substance use, weight loss, and thought disorder in children compared to adults with BPSD. Also, children with BPSD have more mixed episodes, rapid cycling, and comorbidity with ADHD compared to adults (approximately 75% versus 10–20%; Findling et al., 2001). Childhood-onset BPSD is characterized by having a usual onset of manic or mixed episodes, rather than depression, which is more common in adults with BPSD (Kyte et al., 2006).

Finally, more boys than girls are diagnosed with early-onset BPSD, whereas gender representation is equal in typical-onset BPSD (Biederman et al.). These differences have led some to argue that childhood-onset

BPSD is not the same condition as adult-onset BPSD, but is another disorder altogether. In fact, although several longitudinal studies are in progress, none as of yet has tracked childhood-onset BPSD into adulthood to determine if it progresses into the classic adult disorder (AACAP, 2007), however, many adults with BPSD can identify symptoms they exhibited during their early lives (Lish, Dime-Meenan, Whybrow, Price, & Hirschfeld, 1994; Perlis et al., 2004).

Risk Factors

Risk factors for developing BPSD include having a Major Depressive Disorder, having a family history of affective disorders, or experiencing an antidepressant-induced manic episode. As many as 20 to 48% of youth with childhood-onset major depressive disorder will develop a BPSD (Geller, Fox, & Clark, 1994; Geller, Zimmerman, Williams, Bolhofner, & Craney, 2001). Children whose depressive episodes have rapid onset, psychomotor retardation, and psychotic features are more likely to develop BPSD than those without these characteristics (Kowatch, Youngstrom, et al., 2005; Strober & Carlson, 1982). Also, children with a family history of affective disorders, especially BPSD, have a higher risk of developing BPSD (Geller et al., 1994, 2001; Jones, Tai, Evershed, Knowles, & Bentall, 2006). Children who have experienced an antidepressant-induced manic episode are also more likely to develop BPSD (Baumer, Howe, Gallelli, Simeonova, Hallmayer, & Chang, 2006; Faedda, Baldessarini, Glovinsky, & Austin, 2004; Strober & Carlson, 1982).

Symptom Presentation

As the assessment of depressive disorders is described in a previous chapter, this chapter focuses on assessing manic symptoms and episodes. Diagnosing BPSD in children is difficult. Symptom manifestation is somewhat different for youth compared to adults because of societal and parental limits placed on children's behavior and access to activities (e.g., a credit card for a shopping spree or multiple sexual partners). Many symptoms of mania are developmentally appropriate in specific age groups and/or overlap with other common childhood mental disorders.

Some Criterion B symptoms are present in typically developing children. To determine whether behavior is deviant, one must be familiar with normal social-emotional development. Behavior is pathological when it is not appropriate to the context, represents a change from the child's baseline behavior, and is functionally impairing (Geller, Zimmerman, Williams, DelBello, Frazier, et al., 2002). The FIND criteria, (Kowatch, Fristad et al., 2005, p. 215) Frequency, Intensity, Number, and Duration of symptoms, can assist in determining whether a behavior is abnormal (Table 10.3). Typical and atypical behaviors are described in Table 10.4. Finally, to make a diagnosis of BPSD, manic symptoms have to coalesce over time (Kowatch, Fristad, et al., 2005).

In addition to being familiar with child development themselves, child clinicians need to assess parental knowledge of the same. For example,

Table 10.3. FIND guidelines

Frequency	Symptoms occur most days in a week
Intensity	Symptoms are severe enough to cause extreme disturbance in one domain (home, school, or peers) or moderate disturbance in two or more domains
Number	Symptoms occur three to four times per day
Duration	Symptoms occur 4 or more hours a day, total, not necessarily contiguous

NB: This information is presented in Kowatch, Fristad et al. (2005, p. 215).

a mother who expects her preschooler to practice the piano for an hour without getting up may indeed be frustrated when the child stops every few minutes to pursue other activities. However, the child's behavior is developmentally on target and it is the mother who needs to change her perspective. This mother's report that her child episodically loses attentional capacity should not be taken at face value; rather, behavioral descriptors should be sought so the clinician can apply a developmental filter, as needed. When conducting a comprehensive evaluation (as described below) clinicians need to ask for concrete examples of behavior to place the child's behavior into a developmental context.

Children's manifestation of manic symptoms is modulated not only by their developmental status, but also by their parents' behavior and societal rules. For example, most children possess neither credit cards nor independent means of travel and therefore cannot spontaneously purchase $2,000 worth of tennis outfits. However, they can go to school with prized trading cards and give them all away over recess in an expansively generous manner. A general description and specific examples of each symptom in children and adolescents appear below. Additional examples of children's manic symptoms are provided as "atypical behaviors" in Table 10.4.

Euphoric or Expansive Mood

This symptom is an extreme version of the happy mood a child experiences when looking forward to upcoming events. Nonpathologic euphoric/expansive mood is frequently noted in giddy or silly behavior on Christmas, birthdays, going on vacation, or other special occasions. Pathological euphoria occurs in the absence of one of these triggers or is an intense overreaction to the situation. Euphoric or expansive mood can also result from some medications or illegal drug use. Many children, 87% in one study, experience concurrent elated mood and irritability (Geller, Zimmerman, Williams, DelBello, Bolhofner, et al., 2002).

Irritability

This symptom often manifests as periods of extreme rage or displays of intense aggravation over trivial requests (Kowatch, Fristad, et al., 2005). However, clinicians must be aware that irritability is to children's mental

Table 10.4. Examples of developmentally typical and atypical behaviors

	Typical	Atypical
Elated mood	An 8-year-old who is highly energetic and happy on Thanksgiving Day when he sees his cousins	A 7-year-old who feels he is the luckiest child on earth, that everything is wonderful and happy in his life and acts in an exaggerated manner as a result
Irritability	A 5-year-old who, after a full day of playing, stomps up the stairs when her parents tell her she is being cranky and needs to go to bed	A 10-year-old who runs through the house knocking everything off of tables and throwing toys after his mother tells him to go take a shower
Grandiosity	A 9-year-old child vehemently argues that he is the best runner in his school	An 8-year-old who searches for colleges on the Internet because she plans to start college in the fall rather than 3rd grade
Decreased need for sleep	A 9-year-old cannot sleep the night before his 10th birthday party and is energetic the whole day despite getting 6 hours of sleep, but falls into bed at 7 PM after the party	A 7-year-old who goes to his room for bed at 8 PM, but organizes his toys and draws pictures until 2 AM and wakes up ready for the day at 6 AM
Flight of Ideas	An 8-year-old who jumps from math to gym to art back to math in the description of his school day	A 14-year-old who repeatedly becomes so distracted as he describes events that even friends and family cannot understand him
Distractibility	A 10-year-old who has difficulty focusing on her work and frequently leaves her seat the day before holiday break	A 10-year-old normally calm student cannot remain seated and attentive for 30 minutes and gets up to sharpen her pencil or get a different book every 5 minutes
Increase in goal-directed behavior	A high school student zooms around collecting college information because he is excited about future prospects	A high school student collects college information, starts an art project for professional display, begins repainting his bedroom, and plans a party at his home for the weekend all in a one-hour period
Hypersexuality	A 13-year-old boy who looks at pictures of scantily clad women on the Internet	A 9-year-old boy who touches his teacher's breasts and slaps her bottom A 17-year-old who has four sexual partners in a weekend and wants to have sex several times every day
Involvement in behaviors with a high potential for danger	A 7-year-old, who after seeing BMX bike racing on television, rode his bike at top speed through his quiet neighborhood	An 11-year-old packs and prepares to ride his bike across the United States because he saw a TV story about someone doing this

NB: These behaviors must represent a *change* from baseline functioning, not be caused by drugs or illness, and be associated with functional impairment to count as manic symptoms.

health what fever is to children's physical health. Both indicate the child is not well, but neither is pathognomonic of a particular disorder. Although irritable mood is the most common symptom of mania in children (Geller, Zimmerman, Williams, DelBello, Frazier, et al., 2002), it also can be triggered in healthy children who are hot, hungry, or tired. Additionally, irritability can be part of the symptom constellation of almost every childhood disorder, including Oppositional Defiant Disorder (ODD), ADHD, mood disorders, anxiety disorders, developmental and intellectual delays, and schizophrenia. Qualitative aspects to irritability noted in mania include a vastly disproportionate affective response to a very minute stressor, such as a child smashing all of his mother's ceramic collectibles after she asks him to go get ready for bed.

Grandiosity

This symptom is the belief that one has special talents or abilities ranging from inflated self-confidence to delusions of grandeur. Clinicians need to assess the veracity of the belief, whether the child is engaging in fantasy play, whether he or she can tell the difference between fantasy and reality, and whether the child truly believes the delusion. Asking the child how she knows, for example, that she is a world-renowned ballet dancer can be a way to assess reality testing. Frequently, the answer from an impaired child will be, "Because I just know" (Kowatch, Fristad, et al., 2005).

In addition, the context of the expression of inflated self-esteem should be evaluated. A child who pretends to be a teacher to neighborhood friends after school is significantly different from a child who stands on his desk in class and tells the teacher what the students should be learning and how they should be taught (Kowatch, Fristad, et al., 2005). Likewise, a 5-year-old child who runs through the house with a pillowcase trailing behind him like a cape exclaiming he is Superman is displaying typical behavior whereas a 10-year-old child who claims to be Superman and then attempts to jump out his second story window is atypical.

Decreased Need for Sleep

This symptom is characterized by substantially less sleep (two or more hours) without associated fatigue the following day. Decreased need for sleep should be distinguished from insomnia, commonly found in depressive and anxiety disorders, in which a child has extreme difficulty falling or staying asleep through the night, lays in bed brooding, and wakes up tired the following day (Kowatch, Fristad, et al., 2005). Children with mania are usually out of bed engaged in a variety of activities around the house such as reorganizing the kitchen cupboards, watching inappropriate television shows, or talking on the phone. For example, an 8-year-old girl who, awake and energetic at 3 am, calls everyone in her parents' speed dial several times before being caught and returned to bed only to hop out of bed at 6 am, has a manic decreased need for sleep.

Pressured Speech

This is speech that is often loud, difficult to interrupt, or intrusive and differs from that of an excited, nervous, or angry child who can usually stop the flow of words, especially when the context is not appropriate for the topic (Kowatch, Fristad, et al., 2005). Children who are in a manic state will fail to respect what other people are saying or doing in order to say what is on their mind. For example, a teenager when manic may rush into the room and loudly tell his mother all about the fantastic bike stunt he just did even though she is on the phone having a serious conversation.

Flight of Ideas/Racing Thoughts

These symptoms are the subjective experiences of having too many ideas flowing through one's mind such that they interfere with the child's ability to communicate effectively. Young children, children with lower IQs or expressive language disorders, and children with ADHD may routinely have problems organizing their thoughts into coherent stories or seem like they have too many ideas to express all at once. By way of contrast, children in a manic phase experience a developmentally atypical change from normal functioning. One way to determine this, particularly when an evaluator has just met a child, is to determine if an adult who knows the child well can follow the child's story (Kowatch, Fristad, et al., 2005). Children with racing thoughts can often describe this experience in age-appropriate ways such as, "My thoughts broke the speed limit," or "Too much stuff is flying around up there" (Geller, Zimmerman, Williams, DelBello, Frazier, et al., 2002).

Distractibility

This symptom is a noticeable decrease in the child's ability to tune out events in the environment in order to concentrate on a task. Children with ADHD often have this symptom. To distinguish manic distractibility from that associated with ADHD, the clinician needs to learn what is normal functioning for the child and whether a child's usual ability to focus deteriorates significantly when other manic symptoms are present (Kowatch, Fristad, et al., 2005). Parents and children may need to monitor attentional abilities during a mood episode to be certain about whether there is a change in distractibility associated with mania. As ADHD usually has an earlier age of onset than BPSD, attention levels prior to mood problems often can be assessed. For instance, a child who sits in his seat and fidgets when not experiencing mood problems, but cannot stay seated through classes or even to finish eating dinner during mood disturbances has mood-related distractibility in addition to baseline hyperactivity.

Increased Goal-Directed Activity in Social, Academic or Sexual Arenas/Psychomotor Agitation

These symptoms are changes in the activity level of a child during a manic episode. Increased goal-directed activity is unique to mania and includes starting many different projects (e.g., building a bike ramp, painting a masterpiece, and cleaning his bedroom) or doing a lot of one activity (e.g., a child who is not otherwise very bright and/or self-directed suddenly begins drawing 50 pictures, building extensive block towns, or writing many poems; Kowatch, Fristad, et al., 2005). Highly active or fidgety behavior is common to mania, depression, ADHD, and anxiety disorders. Again, a noticeable increase from baseline accompanied by other manic symptoms helps differentiate the manic symptom from ADHD. Depressed or anxious youth tend to have "nervous habits" such as picking at their clothes or fiddling with objects, whereas manic youth seem driven to engage in the fidgety or active behavior. They may become intensely preoccupied by the desire to do a particular activity or obtain a particular item (e.g., an action figure comparable to ten others on their toy shelf) and almost seem uncomfortable in their own skin unless the craving is satisfied (Kowatch, Fristad, et al., 2005).

Increased Involvement in Pleasurable Activities or Activities with High Potential for Harm

This symptom can be manifested in daredevil activities, uninhibited people-seeking, uncontrolled silliness, and/or hypersexual activity. As a daredevil, a child may try to run across traffic dodging cars or try to drive the family car to a friend's house. Children may talk to anyone they meet or want to go new places to meet people without exercising appropriate caution when they are manic. Exaggerated silliness occurs when the actions are inappropriate to context, such as standing up in the middle of a church service to tell a joke. Again, the silliness has to be extreme for the situation and get the child in trouble at school, at home or with peers. Hypersexuality, as with other symptoms of mania, should reflect a change from the child's typical functioning (e.g., a quiet 10-year-old girl suddenly begins writing sexually provocative notes to multiple boys in her classroom; a 15-year-old boy in a previously monogamous relationship enters into a half-dozen sexual encounters over a weekend). Hypersexual behavior can also be seen in children with a history of sexual abuse, and this should be ruled out before the behavior is attributed to mania. In a study of early-onset BPSD, Geller, Bolhofner, and colleagues (2000) found 43% of their sample presented with hypersexual behavior whereas less than 1% reported sexual abuse. Also, manic hypersexuality has a pleasure-seeking quality to it whereas most abuse-related sexuality has an anxious or compulsive quality that is not associated with enjoyment of sexual urges (Kowatch, Fristad, et al., 2005).

Differential Diagnosis

Medical Causes

Clinicians should also gather information about the physical health, medication history, and drug use of the child/adolescent. Some health problems, such as hyperthyroidism, hypothyroidism, closed or open head injury, multiple sclerosis, systemic lupus erythematosus, temporal lobe epilepsy, and hormonal imbalances can present as major mood disorders (Kowatch, Fristad, et al., 2005). If a child does not have regular medical care or has not had a physical examination for more than a year, the clinician may be wise to recommend a checkup before finalizing a diagnosis.

Furthermore, some medications and illegal drugs can mimic symptoms of mania. Children can have difficulty falling asleep when they begin stimulant medication, which could be mistaken for the early insomnia noted in depressive and anxiety disorders. Some research has linked antidepressants to triggering manic episodes by destabilizing mood (Faedda et al., 2004). Also, parents may describe euthymia in a previously dysthymic youngster as the child being uncharacteristically high in energy, interested in activities, talkative, and requiring less sleep. These symptoms may be merely relief from the symptoms of depression or possibly the start of a manic episode. Coriticosteroid use (e.g., for body building) may lead to increased irritability and even psychosis (Kowatch, Fristad, et al.).

Some illegal drugs cause "highs" (e.g., experiencing elevated energy, talkativeness, grandiosity, flight of ideas, and psychomotor agitation) that could be mistaken for mania or "lows" (e.g., experiencing lack of energy, loss of interest or pleasure in one's usual activities, increased appetite) easily attributed to depression. Even quitting smoking can lead to crankiness and psychomotor agitation that could be mistaken for bipolar symptoms (Kowatch, Fristad et al., 2005).

ADHD

As mentioned earlier, many Criterion B symptoms are present in childhood mental disorders other than BPSD. The essence of ADHD is distractibility, hyperactivity, and impulsive behavior. These could easily be confused with the distractibility, psychomotor agitation, and poor judgment seen in mania. The key difference is the episodic nature of the distractibility and high activity level in mania as opposed to the omnipresence (outside of treatment, both pharmacologic and behavioral) of these characteristics for children with ADHD (Lofthouse & Fristad, 2004).

The child's usual level of activity and attention should be used to determine whether there are periods of distractibility, high energy, and talkativeness above and beyond what is normal for the child. In addition, many children with ADHD are very talkative and have many ideas in their heads at one time, but children with manic behavior have episodes of effusive speech that jumps from one idea to another in a way that can be difficult for others to follow or interrupt (Kowatch, Fristad, et al., 2005). Children with ADHD often get into dangerous situations because they do not think before they act, whereas children experiencing an increase in high-risk behavior are often daredevils who may make extensive plans for their "stunts" without recognizing the inherent danger. The symptoms that seem to best discriminate BPSD from ADHD are euphoric mood, decreased need for sleep, hypersexuality, grandiosity, racing thoughts, and flight of ideas (Geller, Zimmerman, Williams, Bolhofner, et al., 2002).

Disruptive Behavior Disorders

Disruptive behavior disorders also share many characteristics with BPSD. A boy who does not do his chores and instead lays on the couch watching TV all afternoon despite repeated reminders to do his chores, may have symptoms of ODD or fatigue and anhedonia associated with a depressive episode. Again, the episodic nature of the problem can be used as a clue to the associated syndrome. If the child has been cooperative about completing chores until the last few weeks, then this change in behavior may be associated with depression. Conversely, a child who has always resisted doing chores and usually avoids them, while having sufficient energy to engage in social activities, would be better identified as oppositional.

A child who ties balloons to the cat to try to make her "fly" may be showing poor judgment (manic symptom) rather than intentional cruelty to animals (Conduct Disorder [CD] symptom). A high school student who skips a day of school to go audition for the city's orchestra, despite not playing a musical instrument, may be experiencing grandiosity and showing poor judgment (manic symptoms) rather than being truant from school (CD symptom). A teenager who is overzealous in her sexual advances toward a prospective boyfriend may be experiencing a period of hypersexuality (manic symptom) or have the intent to force sexual activity upon another person (CD symptom).

Acute/Posttraumatic Stress Disorder

Some symptoms of Acute or Posttraumatic Stress Disorder (ASD, PTSD) present as BPSD. Sleep problems, irritability, angry outbursts, and difficulty concentrating overlap between the two disorders (APA, 2000). To distinguish ASD and PTSD from BPSD, clinicians need to assess whether there is a history of trauma and if so, collect information about the onset of symptoms relative to the trauma, as well as nonoverlapping symptoms (e.g., reexperiencing, avoidance of stimuli associated with the trauma, and numbing of general responsiveness). When a child's angry outbursts and other problem behaviors started shortly after a traumatic event, and she is having nightmares about the event and avoiding reminders of what happened, she is probably experiencing ASD or PTSD, rather than BPSD. A strategy for careful assessment of the timeline for events and symptoms is discussed below.

Psychosis

Some children and adolescents, 20 to 30% in one sample, with BPSD experience psychotic symptoms during their manic, depressed, or mixed states (Biederman et al., 2005). A rate of psychosis of 60% was noted in a group of bipolar youth age 7 to 16 (Geller, Zimmerman, Williams, DelBello, Bolhofner, et al., 2002). To distinguish whether the child has a separate diagnosis of psychosis, clinicians again should focus on symptom onset and offset using the timeline. If psychotic and affective symptoms always co-occur, the psychotic specifier for BPSD should be used rather than giving a separate diagnosis of psychosis. If the child has heard voices or had delusions outside or before the onset of affective disturbances, a diagnosis of psychosis or schizoaffective disorder should be considered.

Comorbidity

A compounding diagnostic issue is comorbidity. For childhood-onset psychopathology, comorbidity is the rule rather than the exception. That is, when a child has one diagnosis, he or she is at higher risk for having another diagnosis than the general population (Achenbach, 1995; Angold, Costello, & Erkanli, 1999). Comorbidity rates are higher in childhood-onset BPSD than in adult-onset BPSD (AACAP, 2007). In fact, one study found that more than 80% of their early-onset BPSD participants had a comorbid psychiatric condition when their mood was euthymic (Findling, et al., 2001). Comorbidities also help predict functional impairment in children with BPSD (Findling, et al., 2001). Disorders commonly comorbid in children and adolescents with BPSD in order of prevalence include: ADHD, Disruptive Behavior Disorders, Anxiety Disorders, and Substance Abuse.

ADHD

In addition to differential diagnosis, as previously discussed, some children truly have both BPSD and ADHD. The symptom overlap between ADHD and BPSD is discussed above. The rate of comorbid ADHD varies between 11% and 75% in various studies (Pavuluri et al., 2005). Children with BPSD are significantly more likely to have comorbid ADHD (83%) than those with adolescent-onset BPSD (52%, Biederman et al., 2005). Children with both ADHD and BPSD have elevated distractibility and inattention when they are euthymic and these symptoms get significantly worse during a mood episode.

Disruptive Behavior Disorders

Disruptive Behavior Disorders include ODD and CD and are the second most commonly observed comorbid disorders with early-onset BPSD. Rates of ODD fall between 46% and 75% (Kowatch, Youngstrom, et al., 2005). Studies using younger samples reported higher rates of ODD than those using older samples (Kowatch, Youngstrom, et al., 2005). Studies have reported comorbidity rates for CD ranging from 6% to 37% (Pavuluri et al., 2005). Children with BPSD have difficulty regulating their emotions, including their reactions to frustrating situations. When their emotions are out of control during a manic phase, children are more likely to lose their tempers, argue with adults, defy rules, be easily annoyed by others, and feel angry or resentful. These symptoms are sufficient to diagnose a child with ODD if it is not clear that the symptoms are limited to the course of a mood diagnosis (APA, 2000). Some of these symptoms may be present before a full BPSD diagnosis is made or perhaps become a habitual way of reacting and persist beyond mood states. The causal link between childhood BPSD and disruptive behavior disorders warrants further investigation.

Anxiety Disorders

Anxiety Disorders are the third highest comorbid disorders, with rates ranging from 13% to 56% (Pavuluri et al., 2005). Several studies have found no differences in the rates of anxiety disorders between childhood- and adolescent-onset BPSD (Biederman et al, 2005; Findling et al, 2001). Some studies have found links with only specific anxiety disorders (e.g. panic disorder; Birmaher, Kennah, Brent, Ehmann, Bridge, & Axelson, 2002) whereas others have found links with a wide range of anxiety disorders (Harpold et al., 2005). One hypothesis for this overlap, developed from research on adults with BPSD, argues these disorders are linked by the brain structures that cause symptoms of both disorders (Freeman, Freeman, & McElroy, 2002).

Another possible hypothesis regarding increased rates of anxiety disorders in children with BPSD relates to the social problems often experienced as the secondary manifestations of the disorder. For example, if a child, when manic, yells at his teacher in front of the class or punches a classmate with little provocation, he later may be ostracized, rejected, or teased by peers for his out of control behavior. The reputation a child builds can long outlast his manic episode. Children can also appear "moody" to their friends, meaning that an enthusiastic or positive greeting expected from a close friend may not come predictably from a child with BPSD. Likewise, children often tease others who are different from themselves whether in looks, clothing choice, intellectual or physical ability, or physical appearance. Actions and reactions of children with BPSD are likely to be different from their peers in some situations when their mood is dysregulated. The culmination of all of these social forces could lead a child to be more anxious around peers.

Substance Abuse

Finally, the comorbidity of early-onset BPSD with substance use has been reported to range from 0% to 40% (Geller et al., 2001; Pavuluri et al., 2005). In this case, adolescents with BPSD are more likely than children with BPSD to experience comorbid substance use (38% versus 14%, respectively; Biederman et al., 2005). A plausible explanation for the prevalence of substance use among adolescents with BPSD is that substances are being used to self-medicate. This theory has not been investigated in youth, but has been both supported and refuted by research with adults (e.g., Levin & Hennessy, 2004; Grunenbaum et al., 2006). For instance, a child who enjoys the manic highs, but is experiencing a depressive phase may choose to use stimulating drugs like methamphetamine or cocaine to get relief from the depressed mood or experience a "high" similar to their manic phase. In addition, a child who is experiencing a hypomanic phase may take stimulant drugs to elevate his mood further.

Developmental and Intellectual Disabilities

Comorbid BPSD is often missed in children and adolescents with pervasive developmental disorders (PDD) and intellectual disabilities. Research suggests the rate of BPSD may be twice as high in individuals with PDD as in the general population (DeJong & Frazier, 2003). In fact, first-degree relatives of children with autism have an incidence of bipolar disorder of 4.2%, over four times that of the general population (DeJong & Frazier, 2003). The behavioral symptoms of bipolar disorder among children and adolescents with developmental and intellectual disabilities are similar to nondisabled populations (Carlson, 1979). However, some symptoms of bipolar disorder are more difficult to detect in children with developmental and intellectual disabilities, especially if the child has limited expressive language. Caretakers have to look for behavioral indicators of irritable or elated mood, flight of ideas, and grandiosity because these symptoms are usually verbally expressed (Carlson, 1979). When BP and PDD are comorbid, caretakers may notice a higher incidence of self-injurious behavior, apathy, and loss of daily living skills during depressive episodes, and increased verbalizations, overactivity, increased distractibility, and noncompliance during manic episodes (DeJong & Frazier, 2003).

As in other brain disorders, the addition of BPSD to developmental and intellectual disabilities leads to increased problems in functioning. In severely and profoundly mentally retarded adults, those with bipolar disorder exhibited more negative social behavior and verbalizations than those without bipolar disorder (Matson, Terlonge, González, & Rivet, 2006). Kurita and colleagues (2004) found significantly worse nonverbal communication in children with PDD and bipolar disorder compared to children with PDD alone. There were also trends toward higher impairment of relationships with people, poorer auditory responsiveness, and higher Childhood Autism Rating Scale scores, indicating overall higher functional impairment among PDD patients with BPSD (Kurita, Osada, Shimizu, & Tachimori, 2004).

Exacerbation of existing symptoms occurs with the onset of a BPSD, including notable decreases in cognitive functioning, social skills, and communication (DeJong & Frazier, 2003). Recently, Matson and colleagues demonstrated reliability and validity for the manic and depressive scales of the Diagnostic Assessment for the Severely Handicapped-II (DASH-II), used in diagnosing mood disorders in intellectually disabled individuals (Matson, Rush, Hamilton, Anderson, Bamburg, & Baglio, 1999; Matson & Smiroldo, 1997). This measure will help clinicians identify bipolar symptoms in developmentally and intellectually delayed children.

Summary

Diagnosis of early-onset BPSD is complicated by unique symptom presentation due to developmental differences in autonomy and societal limits on behavior. Examples of symptoms noted in children and adolescents with BPSD clarify how the disorder can present. BPSD shares symptoms with several other childhood brain disorders, but it can be differentiated from these disorders by its cyclical pattern of worsening symptoms.

Important disorders to consider when making a differential diagnosis include various medical illnesses, ADHD, disruptive behavior disorders, acute and posttraumatic stress disorder, and psychosis. In addition, many disorders are commonly comorbid with BPSD, including ADHD, disruptive behavior disorders, and anxiety disorders. Substance use and developmental and intellectual disability also co-occur frequently.

Assessment

A relatively recent trend in childhood psychopathology research has been the proliferation of investigations regarding evidence-based assessment and a growing literature that suggests evidence-based diagnoses may be more accurate than diagnoses based on unstructured clinical assessment (Doss, 2005). Making a definitive diagnosis of BPSD in a child is widely regarded as a difficult task given the often atypical presentation of childhood-onset BPSD compared to adult-onset BPSD, the overlap in symptoms of BPSD and other disorders, and the high rates of comorbidity (Bowring & Kovacs, 1992; Geller & Luby, 1997; Pavuluri et al., 2005). Therefore, there is a demand for reliable and valid measures to aid clinicians in the diagnostic process. A screening measure can quickly "rule out" many children who are not experiencing bipolar symptoms and help identify children and adolescents who are in need of a more comprehensive assessment for BPSD.

An evidence-based assessment for BPSD in children should integrate information from multiple informants and utilize multiple methods of data collection, including rating scales, a structured or semi-structured diagnostic interview, a timeline, and an assessment of family history of mood disorders. Measures of current mood symptom severity are also valuable additions, as well as prospective mood monitoring by the parent and/or the child.

Choice of Informants

Although parent-report is often the most valuable data source in assessing BPSD, information from the child and from teachers is often useful (Youngstrom, Findling, et al., 2005). Using multiple informants allows the clinician to learn about the child's functioning in multiple settings. Also, children for whom multiple informants report manic symptoms tend to be more seriously impaired (Carlson & Youngstrom, 2003).

Clinical judgment should be used to determine how much information to collect from the child when completing an assessment. Depending on the child's age, cognitive abilities, insight, and current symptoms, the child may be the primary source of information, or may contribute little (Tillman, Geller, Craney, Bolhofner, Williams, & Zimerman, 2004). Parents or guardians are the best source of information when children are younger, possess less insight, or are more severely impaired. Older children and adolescents can provide valuable information on topics about which parents are less likely to be knowledgeable, such as internalizing symptoms, substance abuse, and sexual activity. However, the child's report of symptoms should not be ignored, even in cases where the child is likely to be a poor reporter. Some children exhibit surprising insight into their mood states, and can provide detailed descriptions of their experiences. For example, a young boy described his manic episode as, "Like I drank 100 cans of Red Bull."

Screening Measures

A large proportion of the research concerning childhood-onset BPSD has been devoted to screening measures. Screening measures provide a convenient first step in identifying cases of childhood BPSD. They are relatively inexpensive to administer and, given the low base rate of childhood BPSD, are useful for identifying cases that warrant more extensive evaluation. Screening measures are not adequate for assigning diagnosis, but are quite effective for "ruling out" a large number of cases.

One potential screening measure for BPSD in children is the Child Behavior Checklist (CBCL; Achenbach & Rescorla, 2001). Results have been mixed, with some research suggesting a CBCL "bipolar profile" consisting of elevations on the Aggression, Attention Problems, and Anxious/Depressed subscales (Mick, Biederman, Pandina, & Faraone, 2003), and other research suggesting that, after controlling for scores on the CBCL Externalizing scale, no other subscales improve identification of BPSD (Youngstrom et al., 2004).

Another screening measure investigated for use with child and adolescent BPSD is the General Behavior Inventory (GBI; Depue, 1987). The GBI contains items related to mania, depression, and mixed states. First developed for use with adults, the GBI has been adapted for parent report (P-GBI), adolescent self-report, (A-GBI; Findling et al., 2002), and teacher-report (T-GBI; Youngstrom, Joseph, & Greene, 2008). A 10-item mania subscale derived from the P-GBI (P-GBI-SF) appears to be quite efficient in identifying children and adolescents with BPSD in research and clinical settings (Youngstrom, Meyers, et al., 2005).

The Mood Disorder Questionnaire (MDQ; Hirschfeld et al., 2000) was developed to screen for bipolar spectrum disorders in adults. It has been adapted for use with adolescents, both as a self-report measure (MDQ-A) and a parent-completed form (P-MDQ). In a clinical sample, the P-MDQ performed better than the MDQ-A at identifying bipolar disorder (Wagner, Hirschfeld, Emslie, Findling, Gracious, & Reed, 2006). The P-GBI-SF appears to outperform both versions of this measure. However, the P-MDQ, used together with the P-GBI-SF, may be most effective in the assessment of younger children (Youngstrom, Meyers, et al., 2005).

As described above, most screening measures used for BPSD in children have been adapted from existing screens used for adult bipolar disorder or general child psychopathology. The Child Bipolar Questionnaire (CBQ) was developed specifically to detect childhood BPSD. Preliminary validation analysis indicates that the CBQ displays high sensitivity and near-perfect specificity (Papolos, Hennen, Cockerham, Thode, & Youngstrom, 2006). However, this study utilized a self-selected Internet sample, which had a high rate of self-identified BPSD. Although a structured interview was used to assign diagnosis in the validity sample, reliability estimates were based on a sample whose diagnosis was not independently verified. Therefore, the CBQ cannot be recommended for clinical use until it is validated in a more representative and independently verified population.

Another measure created specifically to detect childhood BPSD is the Child Mania Rating Scale, parent version (CMRS-P; Pavuluri, Henry, Devineni, Carbray, & Birmaher, 2006). The authors of the CMRS-P intended it to be easy to read and intentionally left out items that poorly discriminated childhood BPSD from other conditions. The CMRS-P demonstrated high internal consistency and test–retest reliability, and factor analysis suggested the scale is unidimensional. Scores on the CMRS-P correlated highly with three measures related to BPSD, and correlated moderately with general scales of psychopathology. With a cut-score of 20, the scale displayed high sensitivity and specificity for BPSD, compared to children with ADHD and healthy control participants (Pavuluri et al., 2006).

The CMRS-P has the potential to be a valuable measure in childhood BPSD assessment, but there are limitations to the findings discussed above. First, interrater reliability estimates were based on a small ($N = 20$) subsample. Also, children whose primary symptom presentation was limited to irritable mood were excluded from the study, and children with BP-NOS were excluded from the evaluation of criterion-related validity. These exclusions make it unclear whether the CMRS-P is effective at identifying children who meet the broad phenotype categories of BPSD. Additional investigation of the CMRS-P in a diagnostically heterogeneous clinical population could allow these limitations to be addressed, and is highly recommended.

The movement to develop more accurate and efficient screening measures represents significant progress in the field of childhood BPSD. Prevalence estimates vary, but generally agree that BPSD occurs less frequently than many other forms of child psychopathology. Screening measures can help detect cases in need of a more lengthy (and expensive) evaluation. Screens also help guard against overdiagnosis by quickly ruling out large numbers of cases. In a clinical setting, a measure with both high sensitivity (to identify cases and assign proper diagnosis) and high specificity (to prevent overdiagnosis and reduce the cost of assessment) is ideal. As a screening questionnaire alone never constitutes an adequate assessment, additional information is needed to corroborate significant scores.

Structured Interviews

Structured assessments are the method used to assign diagnosis in most research studies of childhood BPSD. These instruments ensure standard comprehensive coverage of the symptoms of BPSD and common comorbid conditions. In some cases, especially with more structured assessment measures, they can be administered by nonclinical staff and interpreted by a clinician, which decreases the cost of assessment. In inpatient settings, the use of structured assessments may decrease the frequency of diagnosis of manic episodes. Inpatients diagnosed with manic episodes via a structured interview display higher rates of elated mood and activity, fewer symptoms of depression, and are more likely to meet strictly applied diagnostic criteria for mania (Pogge, Wayland-Smith, Zaccario, Borgaro, Stokes, & Harvey, 2001).

A number of structured and semi-structured assessments are available for use with children. One of the most commonly used, especially in research studies, is the Schedule for Affective Disorders and Schizophrenia for School Aged Children (K-SADS; Kaufman et al., 1997, Puig-Antich & Ryan, 1986). The K-SADS is considered the "gold standard" in empirical studies of child and adolescent BPSD (Nottelmann, et al., 2001). However, the K-SADS requires significant interviewer training and can take several hours to administer to a parent and child (Kaufman et al., 1997), and therefore it is not a practical option in most clinical settings. More structured and concise options include the Diagnostic Interview Schedule for Children (DISC; Shaffer, Fisher, Lucas, Dulcan, & Schwab-Stone, 2000) and the Diagnostic Interview for Children and Adolescents–Revised (DICA-R-C; Reich & Wellner, 1988), however, they are also lengthy and not commonly used in clinical settings.

A promising alternative to these interviews is the Children's Interview for Psychiatric Syndromes, child (ChIPS; Weller, Weller, Rooney, & Fristad, 1999a) and parent (P-ChIPS; Weller, Weller, Rooney, & Fristad, 1999b) editions. The ChIPS and P-ChIPS include *DSM–IV* diagnostic criteria for 20 common Axis I diagnoses, and include ratings of clinical impairment and age of onset for each diagnosis. Administration of the ChIPS or P-ChIPS takes approximately 35 minutes for an outpatient, so the measure is brief enough for general clinical use. Because of its highly structured format, it requires less comprehensive training to administer than many other diagnostic interviews (Rooney, Fristad, Weller, & Weller, 1999). In inpatient children and adolescents, high rates of diagnostic agreement between the ChIPS and the DICA-R-C have been found for major depression, dysthymia, and mania. The ChIPS also significantly agreed with clinician-assigned diagnosis for major depression, dysthymia, and mania (Fristad, Cummins, Verducci, Teare, Weller, & Weller, 1998). Similar rates of agreement were found for mood disorders between the ChIPS and P-ChIPS, and between the P-ChIPS and clinician, in a combined inpatient and outpatient sample (Fristad, Teare, Weller, Weller, & Salmon, 1998).

Mood Symptom Severity Scales

Although structured interviews provide comprehensive coverage of BPSD and comorbid conditions, symptom severity rating scales provide a more focused assessment of BPSD-specific characteristics. The Young Mania Rating Scale (YMRS; Young, Biggs, Ziegler, & Meyer, 1978) was developed as an observational rating measure of manic symptoms for adult inpatients. It has been adapted for use in childhood BPSD as a parent or child interview, a parent questionnaire, and an adolescent self-report questionnaire (Gracious, Youngstrom, Findling, & Calabrese, 2002; Youngstrom, Gracious, Danielson, Findling, & Calabrese, 2003; Youngstrom, et al., 2004; Youngstrom, Meyers, et al., 2005). The YMRS has been criticized for a number of reasons: its initial development as an adult measure;

its inclusion of some symptoms not pertinent to the diagnosis and its exclusion of some basic manic symptoms; and its overweighting the symptom of irritability (Hunt, Dyl, Armstrong, Litvin, Sheeran, & Spirito, 2005).

Another mania-specific rating scale is the K-SADS Mania Rating Scale, (KMRS) which was adapted from the Washington University version of the K-SADS (Geller, Williams, Zimmerman, & Frazier, 1996). Axelson and colleagues (2003) found high interrater reliability and internal consistency for the scale. Hunt and colleagues (2005) found that parent-report on the KMRS discriminated inpatient adolescents with and without a bipolar disorder diagnosis.

In summary, current evidence suggests the KMRS and YMRS are useful as measures of current symptom severity, but their utility as diagnostic tools needs to be evaluated further.

Timeline

Due to the cyclical nature of BPSD, children can present in a number of mood states (i.e., manic, hypomanic, dysphoric, mixed, euthymic). Whether a structured assessment or an unstructured clinical interview is utilized, clinicians must have a working knowledge of mood disorders and diagnostic criteria. If a child presents in a manic or hypomanic episode, diagnosis of BPSD becomes relatively less complicated. However, a careful lifetime history of mood symptoms and episodes is necessary to assign an accurate DSM–IV diagnosis (Youngstrom, Findling, et al., 2005). Comorbid conditions, treatment history and response, psychosocial events, and other information commonly collected in a clinical assessment should also be incorporated.

To aid in collecting this information, our research group has developed guidelines (see Figure 10.1) for information to record and a template for a mood disorder timeline (see Figure 10.2). This timeline has been incorporated into diagnostic assessments in multiple research studies involving children with BPSD and clinical practice with a general clinic-referred sample. Guidelines standardize information collected, and the template's chronological format facilitates the organization of information related to the onset of mood and comorbid symptoms and their course over time. Furthermore, the timeline helps to clarify the number of episodes a child has experienced.

Family History

Collecting a detailed family mental health history is an important part of any assessment of BPSD in a child or adolescent. BPSD is among the most heritable of brain disorders. Genetics accounts for at least 50% of the risk for disorder onset in adults, and likely has an even greater influence in childhood BPSD (Findling et al., 2003). A recent meta-analysis estimated that the presence of bipolar disorder in one parent is associated with a fivefold increase in the risk of bipolar disorder in children (Hodgins, Faucher, Zarac, & Ellenbogen, 2002). This result can be interpreted as a fivefold increase in the odds of a BPSD diagnosis if bipolar

<u>Date of Birth & Current Age</u>
Mark calendar years & ages on timeline to assist
  in determining the relationship in time
  between events

<u>Family Relationships</u>
Mother, father, siblings
Other household members/important adults
  (grandparents, stepparents, aunts/uncles,
  etc.)

<u>Mother's Pregnancy</u>
Medications used during pregnancy
Drug/alcohol/tobacco use
Pregnancy/Labor/delivery complications

<u>Peer Relationships</u>
Number of friends; best/closest friends
Quality & quantity of friendships, activities
  (clubs, sports, etc.)

<u>Major Life Events</u>
Household moves: What age(s)? From where/to
  where? Reason?
Family: Parental divorce or separation, deaths,
  domestic violence, jail, alcohol/drug abuse,
  physical/sexual abuse, accidents
Other

<u>School</u>
What age did child attend preschool?
  Kindergarten?
Grades completed? Any repeated? Why?
School district(s) & school name(s); School
  transitions? Why?
Behavior problems in school/classroom
  functioning
Grades & general functioning in school
Services used (IEP, 504, etc.)

<u>Developmental Milestones</u>
Walking, talking, toilet training (Age reached/On
  time/Delays)
Infant temperament

<u>Child Care</u>
Birth to school age – If parent(s) employed
  who provided child care? After-school
  care?
Who has lived in the household? Any
  changes in caregivers? Why?

<u>Physical Health</u>
Major or chronic illnesses
Medical hospitalizations, surgeries
Serious injuries, etc.
Medication history

<u>Mental Health</u>
When was treatment first sought? Why?
When did various symptoms or behaviors
  begin?
Any other behavioral problems beyond
  presenting problem? (mood, anxiety,
  disruptive behaviors, PDDs, psychosis,
  etc.)
If not spontaneously reported, explain mood
  symptoms & episodes
Dates of mood episode(s) if present
Symptoms present during *each* episode

Figure 10.1. Topics to assess in a mood disorder timeline.

disorder is present in any first-degree relative, an increased risk of half
that magnitude (i.e., 2.5 times) if bipolar disorder is present in a second-
degree relative (Youngstrom, Duax, & Hamilton, 2005). Therefore, a careful assessment of psychopathology in the child's first- and second-degree
biological relatives allows the clinician to estimate the influence of genetic
factors for an individual case. Clearly, clinicians do not possess the time or
resources necessary to contact a child's relatives and assess their mental

Document
- **Above line**: pregnancy, labor and delivery, age in years, calendar years, moves, life stressors, child care arrangements, school placement
- **Below line**: physical health & medical treatment, mental health sx (onset, offset, mood & co-morbid dx) & treatment, functioning (home, school, peers

Pregnancy

Labor & Delivery

Date of Birth

Date of Assessment

Sx Hx

Tx Hx

Current Functioning   Home: School: Peers:

Figure 10.2. Sample blank mood disorder timeline.

health histories directly. Therefore, family history information must be collected from informants such as parents or guardians. There are a number of methods available for collecting family history information, ranging from unstructured clinical interview methods to highly structured interview measures.

One aspect of a family history interview is likely to be familiar to most clinicians: the genogram. Collecting a three-generation genogram should be the first step in collecting family history. Once completed, the clinician can lay it on the desk or table in front of the informant, ensuring they literally "stay on the same page" throughout the collection of the family history. An example of a three-generation genogram for a child with BPSD is provided in Quinn and Fristad (2004).

Many clinicians rely on unstructured interview techniques to gather family history information. Unfortunately, these methods are less accurate than structured interview-based methods. Baker, Berry, and Adler (1987) found that structured interview methods identified over four times as many diagnoses in first-degree and second-degree relatives of inpatient adults, when compared to information collected informally by psychiatric residents. Two structured interview methods that are commonly used in research, the Family History–Research Diagnostic Criteria (FH-RDC; Andreasen, Endicott, Spitzer, & Winokur, 1977) and the Family History Screen (FHS; Weissman, Wickramaratne, Adams, Wolk, Verdeli, & Olfson, 2000), can be adapted easily for clinical use. Both methods probe for the presence of specific symptoms, rather than diagnostic categories. This strategy is advised as informants often are not familiar with or misunderstand diagnostic labels, and may display a tendency to use vague terms such as "nervous breakdown."

The FH-RDC probes for the presence of 14 common diagnoses, can be administered relatively briefly, and has demonstrated adequate reliability and validity (Thompson, Orvaschel, Prusoff, & Kidd, 1982), but it tends to underestimate psychopathology (Andreasen, Rice, Endicott, Reich, & Coryell, 1986) despite performing better than an unstructured interview. The FHS is particularly well suited for clinical use, because it can be administered in approximately 5–20 minutes. It probes for symptoms present in all relatives at once, therefore minimizing administration time (Weissman et al., 2000). However, symptoms endorsed on the FHS may need to be followed up by more specific inquiries if detailed information about relatives' diagnoses is desired. The FH-RDC and FHS are recommended for collecting family history information, because they provide clinicians with reliable and valid data without adding significant time burden to the assessment process.

In spite of the clear evidence that family history is an essential component of any BPSD assessment, clinicians are cautioned not to overestimate the importance of family history. Children with a family history of bipolar disorder are at significantly increased risk for this illness. However, because of the low base rate of BPSD, most of these children will not have BPSD. Thus, clinicians must remember their role is to "diagnose the child, not the family" (Leibenluft, Charney, Towbin, Bhangoo & Pine, 2003). Youngstrom, Duax, and Hamilton (2005) provide clinical strategies for integrating family history information with estimated base rates in a

BPSD assessment. As with screening measures, family history should not be used alone as a diagnostic tool, but as part of a comprehensive assessment. It can aid in calculating a reasonable estimate of the probability of BPSD, but should never be considered a diagnostic criterion.

Mood Charts

Mood charting is a technique frequently used in the assessment and treatment of bipolar disorder. This technique involves the individual, or an informant such as a parent, providing daily ratings of mood states and behaviors such as energy, sleep, and appetite. Mood charting has been successfully implemented with adults (Johnson & Leahy, 2004) and children with bipolar disorder (Fristad & Goldberg-Arnold, 2004). This technique aids assessment of BPSD because it teaches the informant (usually a parent) to more carefully evaluate fluctuations in the child's mood and behavior, and provides the clinician with observations not available in the assessment session. Over the course of treatment, mood charts can be used to evaluate response to pharmacological or psychosocial interventions. The Child and Adolescent Bipolar Foundation (CABF) provides a number of sample mood charts that families of children with BPSD can use (available at http://www.bpkids.org/).

Summary

Evidence-based methods of childhood BPSD assessment include: screening measures, structured and semi-structured interviews, mood symptom severity rating scales, and family history interviews. Other assessment strategies, such as inclusion of multiple informants, a mood disorder timeline, and mood charting, can improve the information obtained by the measures described above. Considered alone, most assessment methods are inadequate for assigning diagnosis. However, a multimethod approach that combines several instruments is an effective assessment strategy. Clinicians currently have a number of effective assessment methods at their disposal, and ongoing research promises to improve the reliability and validity of BPSD diagnosis in children.

CASE VIGNETTE

Austin, a 7-year-old, Caucasian male is a participant in a longitudinal research study examining children with elevated manic symptoms (LAMS). At his baseline assessment, Austin and his mother, Mrs. Reed, were interviewed using screening instruments (P-GBI-SF and P-GBI), a structured interview (K-SADS), mood symptom rating scales (KMRS and Children's Depression Rating Scale-Revised [Poznanski, & Mokros, 1995]; as used in LAMS, ratings on these instruments reflect the severity of various symptom manifestations without regard to the cause of those symptoms, an "unfiltered", or "what you see is what you get" strategy), timeline, and family history (additional information is included in Figure 10.3). After

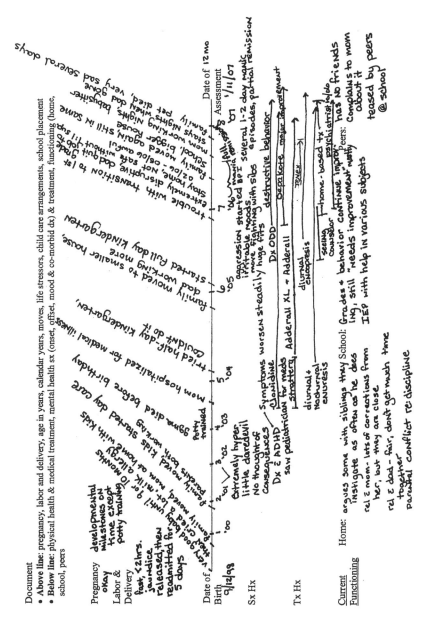

Figure 10.3. Sample completed mood disorder timeline.

reviewing all the evidence collected in an initial comprehensive case review, Austin was diagnosed with:

ADHD Combined type (onset age 3)
ODD (onset age 6, duration 6 months)
Enuresis (both nocturnal and diurnal, onset age 5)
Encopresis (diurnal only, onset age 7)

Baseline Assessment

At the time of the baseline assessment, Austin lived with his biological mother, biological father, three siblings, and one maternal half-sibling. Mrs. Reed was Austin's primary caretaker and a stay-at-home mother. Mrs. Reed described her relationship with Austin as "strained" because she had to punish him often, but stated he felt comfortable talking with her about problems, too. Mr. Reed had a job that required travel and kept him away from home regularly. Austin missed his father and wanted a closer relationship with him. Mrs. Reed reported that she and Mr. Reed disagreed about discipline strategies and whether Austin had a disorder or just needed stricter discipline. Austin physically and verbally fought with his siblings and half-sibling regularly. Austin initiated some of the fights, but his siblings also contributed to their contentious relationships.

According to Mrs. Reed, Austin had been struggling in regular first-grade classes, especially in reading. On his report card, Austin received many grades of "needs improvement" and comments regarding his difficulty staying focused. Austin had a few friends at school, but had some difficulties with peers, including a physical fight about one month after the beginning of school.

Mrs. Reed reported both she and Austin's half-sibling have been diagnosed with Bipolar Disorder. She also noted that three of Austin's maternal second-degree relatives had substance abuse problems and suspected periods of depression.

Austin had been receiving mental health services from a pediatrician, a psychologist, and a psychiatrist. Austin had been seeing his pediatrician for four years about attention problems and difficulty falling asleep for which the pediatrician had prescribed a stimulant and clonidine hydrochloride. Ms. Reed took Austin to therapy due to concerns about Austin's apparent unhappiness and their strained parent–child relationship. At his initial appointment with the psychiatrist, Austin was prescribed guanfacine hydrochloride. At the time of his baseline assessment, Austin had just been assigned a home-based therapist as well.

In addition to symptoms associated with the diagnoses mentioned above, Austin had symptoms of depression and mania (onset age 6, duration 6 months and ongoing). The only threshold depressive symptom was irritability, which affected his functioning at home, but not at school or with peers. Austin had subthreshold (i.e., notable, but nonimpairing) dysphoric mood, insomnia, fatigue, decreased appetite, and feelings of worthlessness. His appetite decrease and insomnia appeared to be associated with an increase in stimulant dosage. During the same 6 months, Mrs. Reed had noted periods of explosive irritability, excessive involvement in risky behaviors, and increased distractibility and subthreshold (i.e., notable, but nonimpairing) pressured speech and flight of ideas. These periods lasted most of the day and occurred several days per month. Mrs. Reed could not describe whether these periods were distinct from periods of depressive symptoms. These symptoms caused problems with peers and family. The mood symptoms described were insufficient in number and duration to warrant a diagnosis of depression or bipolar disorder, but Mrs. Reed was asked to monitor Austin's mood symptoms carefully when the results of the assessment were discussed with her.

Six-Month Follow-Up Interview

Approximately six months later, Mrs. Reed and Austin were seen for a follow-up LAMS assessment. Since the last interview, Austin had experienced his first full manic episode. Mrs. Reed reported that Austin's depressive and manic symptoms reported at their first assessment had continued for two months after the first assessment, then his manic symptoms intensified. Mr. Reed had to quit his job and stay at home to help manage Austin's behavior. Mrs. Reed described Austin's mood as "explosive and labile" during this time, and said he was "out of control." She said that Austin would often calm down for a short period of time, only to "explode again" in an intensely irritable mood and tantrum, with little or no provocation.

Austin's problems with attention and motor hyperactivity intensified during these moods. He talked very quickly, was difficult to interrupt, and his "brain was moving faster than [he] could speak." Mrs. Reed reported Austin needed very little sleep during this time, a few hours per night to feel rested and be highly energetic the next day. She also reported Austin got in more trouble during this time period for doing daredevil tricks on his bike, and once for stealing from a local store. Mrs. Reed reported he needed almost constant one-on-one supervision, and would often try to run out into the street without looking, fight with his siblings, was very difficult to put to bed, and was generally "very disruptive" in the home. After two months of out of control behavior, Austin began taking a mood stabilizer. His mood, behavior, and associated symptoms improved rapidly and markedly. In fact, Mrs. Reed said, Austin went from being the biggest problem in her home to "the least concern" of all her children in less than one month. Austin had enjoyed the last part of the school year and successfully completed first grade. According to both Austin and Mrs. Reed, at the second assessment Austin was not experiencing any depressive or manic symptoms.

Twelve-Month Follow-Up Interview

Approximately six months later, one year after the initial assessment, Mrs. Reed and Austin were interviewed again. Austin continues to take the mood stabilizer and reports minimal depressive symptoms. He is, however, experiencing episodes lasting one to three days in which he meets all criteria for a manic episode except duration. These periods are interfering with

Austin's functioning at home, at school, and with peers. Austin reports he has no friends and is regularly teased at school. Mrs. Reed states Austin frequently complains and feels sad about not having friends, however, Austin reports he does not want friends and he prefers to play by himself. Mrs. Reed attributes Austin's lack of friendships to children recalling his out of control behavior the previous year and disliking his current manic periods and unpredictable mood. Austin's grades are improving, with more "satisfactory" grades than before, but the majority are still "needs improvement." Austin still argues and fights with his siblings and half-sibling on a regular basis, but instigates fewer of the disagreements.

Austin's home-based therapist has terminated services as he was leaving the agency, but Mrs. Reed is hoping to get a new home-based therapist. Austin is seeing a psychiatrist for visits every few months to manage his medications. During the interview, Austin complains he is taking "way too many pills" for problems he does not remember.

Analysis

The careful sequential assessment of Austin's life events and symptoms helped sort out a complicated history and allowed clinicians to be confident that at baseline, Austin did not meet diagnostic criteria for any bipolar spectrum disorder despite symptoms of mood lability and a family history of BPSD (mother and maternal half-sibling), substance abuse, and depression (maternal grandparents and maternal uncle). Longitudinal follow-up revealed the progression from symptoms of depression and mania to a diagnosis of BP-I to full remission to a recurrence of manic symptoms.

Additional aspects of this case study are worth emphasizing. Use of the structured interview in combination with the lifeline helped determine age of onset for various comorbid disorders. For instance, attention problems were noted at age three, whereas oppositional behavior became problematic at age six. Consistent with research concerning childhood BPSD, Austin has several disorders that are commonly comorbid with BPSD—ODD and ADHD—which predated the mood diagnosis. Collection of data from both the parent and the teacher confirmed the presence of depressive symptoms, manic symptoms, attention problems, and oppositional behavior across settings, and documented their interference with Austin's daily functioning.

This case illustrates the importance of obtaining a "streaming video" of the child's lifetime mood history rather than relying on a "snapshot" of the child's current symptom presentation. Had the latter been used, Austin would not have received a BP diagnosis at the 6-month interview and might have been diagnosed with BP-NOS at the 12-month interview. For a therapist working with the family, Mr. and Mrs. Reed's different perspectives on Austin's problems and their impact on the marital relationship would be key considerations. As is common in childhood-onset BPSD, Austin has a genetic loading for mood disorders and a specific loading for bipolar disorder.

As do many children with mood disorders, Austin has multiple treatment providers: pediatrician, psychiatrist, psychologist, and eventually a home-based therapist. Another common pattern is the involvement of the pediatrician or primary care physician when behavior problems first arise. Due to the shortage of child and adolescent psychiatrists, many primary care physicians are managing medications for behavioral and emotional problems. Another common theme for children with BPSD is the difficulty with peers due to unpredictable behavior and inappropriate behaviors around peers at school and in the child's neighborhood. Also, Austin continues to have episodes that meet full manic criteria except for duration after the full manic episode. The rapid cycling and short duration of episodes is characteristic of childhood-onset bipolar disorder.

SUMMARY

Childhood-onset BPSD is a chronic condition associated with significant impairment. Once thought to be exceedingly rare, or even nonexistent, childhood BPSD has recently received increased public, academic, and clinical attention. As a result, BPSD is being identified in settings where it may have been missed years ago. Unfortunately, uncertainty about the clinical presentation of childhood BPSD and limited training in evidence-based childhood BPSD assessment has led to concerns about overdiagnosis. Findings from ongoing longitudinal studies will provide more information about the course and symptom presentation of BPSD in children and adolescents. Research suggests childhood BPSD is more likely to present as a chronic or rapidly changing, rather than episodic, condition. A number of other features, such as high rates of irritability and comorbidity, differentiate childhood BPSD from the "classic" adult presentation of bipolar disorder. Evidence-based assessment practices are essential in assigning a BPSD diagnosis to a child. These include: screening measures, structured interviews, mood symptom rating scales, a psychosocial timeline, and assessment of family history of mood disorders.

REFERENCES

Achenbach, T. M. (1995). Diagnosis, assessment and comorbidity in psychosocial treatment research. *Journal of Abnormal Child Psychology, 23,* 45–65.

Achenbach, T. M., & Rescorla, L.A. (2001). *Manual for the ASEBA school-age forms & profiles.* Burlington, VT: University of Vermont, Department of Psychiatry.

American Academy of Child and Adolescent Psychiatry. (2007). Practice parameter for the assessment and treatment of children and adolescents with bipolar disorder. *Journal of the American Academy of Child and Adolescent Psychiatry, 46,* 107–125.

American Psychiatric Association. (2000). *Diagnostic and statistical manual of mental disorders – IV* (Text revision). Washington, DC: Author.

Andreasen, N. C., Endicott, J., Spitzer, R. L., & Winokur, G. (1977). The family history method using diagnostic criteria: Reliability and validity. *Archives of General Psychiatry, 34,* 1229–1235.

Andreasen, N. C., Rice, J., Endicott, J., Reich, T., & Coryell, W. (1986). The family history approach to diagnosis: How useful is it? *Archives of General Psychiatry, 43,* 421–429.

Angold, A., Costello, E. J., & Erkanli, A. (1999). Comorbidity. *Journal of Child Psychology and Psychiatry, 40,* 57–87.

Anthony, E. J., & Scott, P. (1960). Manic-depressive psychosis in childhood. *Child Psychology and Psychiatry, 1,* 53–72.

Axelson, D., Birmaher, B. J., Brent, D., Wassick, S., Hoover, C., Bridge, J. et al. (2003). A preliminary study of the Kiddie Schedule for Affective Disorders and Schizophrenia for school-age children Mania Rating Scale for children and adolescents. *Journal of Child and Adolescent Psychopharmacology, 13*, 463–470.

Axelson D., Birmaher B., Strober M., Gill, M. K., Valeri, S., Chiapetta, L., et al. (2006). Phenomenology of children and adolescents with bipolar spectrum disorders. *Archives of General Psychiatry, 63*, 1139–1148.

Baker, N. J., Berry, S. L., & Adler, L. E. (1987). Family diagnoses missed on a clinical inpatient service. *American Journal of Psychiatry, 144*, 630–632.

Baumer, F. M., Howe, M., Gallelli, K., Simeonova, D. I., Hallmayer, J., & Chang, K. D. (2006). A pilot study of antidepressant-induced mania in pediatric bipolar disorder: Characteristics, risk factors, and the serotonin transporter gene. *Biological Psychiatry, 60*, 1005–1012.

Biederman, J., Faraone, S. V., Wozniak, J., Mick, E., Kwon, A., Cayton, et al., (2005). Clinical correlates of bipolar disorder in a large, referred sample of children and adolescents. *Journal of Psychiatric Research, 39*, 611–622.

Birmaher, B., Axelson, D., Strober, M., Gill, M. K., Valeri, S., Chiapetta, L., et al. (2006). Clinical course of children and adolescents with bipolar spectrum disorders. *Archives of General Psychiatry, 63*, 175–183.

Birmaher, B., Kennah, A., Brent, D., Ehmann, M., Bridge, J., & Axelson, D. (2002). Is bipolar disorder specifically associated with panic disorder in youths? *Journal of Clinical Psychiatry, 63*, 414–419.

Bowring, M. A., & Kovacs, M. (1992). Difficulties in diagnosing manic disorders among children and adolescents. *Journal of the American Academy of Child & Adolescent Psychiatry, 31*, 611–614.

Carlson, G. A. (1979). Affective psychoses in mental retardates. *Psychiatric Clinics of North America, 2*, 499–510.

Carlson, G. A., Bromet, E. J., Driessens, C., Mojtabai, R., & Schwartz, J. E. (2002). Age at onset, childhood psychopathology, and 2-year outcome in psychotic bipolar disorder. *American Journal of Psychiatry, 159*, 307–309.

Carlson, G. A., & Youngstrom, E. A. (2003). Clinical implications of pervasive manic symptoms in children. *Biological Psychiatry, 53*, 1050–1058.

Craney, J. L., & Geller, B. (2005). A prepubertal and early adolescent bipolar disorder-I phenotype: Review of phenomenology and longitudinal course. *Bipolar Disorders, 5*, 243–256.

DeJong, S., & Frazier, J. A. (2003). Bipolar disorder in children with pervasive developmental disorders. In B. Geller & M. P. DelBello (Eds.), *Bipolar disorder in childhood and early adolescence* (pp. 51–75). New York: Guilford Press.

Depue, R. A. (1987). *General Behavior Inventory (Assessment manual)*. Minneapolis, MN: University of Minnesota.

Doss, A. J. (2005). Evidence-based diagnosis: Incorporating diagnostic instruments into clinical practice. *Journal of the American Academy of Child & Adolescent Psychiatry, 44*, 947–952.

Esposito-Smythers, C., Birmaher, B., Valeri, S., Chiappetta, L., Hunt, J., Ryan, N. et al. (2006). Child comorbidity, maternal mood disorder, and perceptions of family functioning among bipolar youth. *Journal of the American Academy of Child & Adolescent Psychiatry, 45*, 955–964.

Faedda, G. L., Baldessarini, R. J., Glovinky, I. P., & Austin, N. B. (2004). Treatment-emergent mania in pediatric bipolar disorder: A retrospective case review. *Journal of Affective Disorders, 82*, 149–158.

Findling, R. L., Gracious, B. L., McNamara, N. K., Youngstrom, E. A., Demeter, C. A., Branicky, L. A., & Calabrese, J. R. (2001). Rapid, continuous cycling and psychiatric co-morbidity in pediatric bipolar I disorder. *Bipolar Disorders, 3*, 202–210.

Findling, R.L., Kowatch, R.A., & Post, R.M. (2003). *Pediatric bipolar disorder: A handbook for clinicians*. London: Martin Dunitz.

Findling, R. L., Youngstrom, E. A., Danielson, C. K., Delporto-Bedoya, D., Papish-David, R., Townsend, L., et al. (2002). Clinical decision-making using the general behavior inventory in juvenile bipolarity. *Bipolar Disorders, 4*, 34–42.

Freeman, M. P., Freeman, S. A., & McElroy, S. L. (2002). The comorbidity of bipolar and anxiety disorders: Prevalence, psychobiology and treatment issues. *Journal of Affective Disorders, 68*, 1–23.

Fristad, M. A., Cummins, J., Verducci, J. S., Teare, M., Weller, E., & Weller, R. A. (1998). Study IV: Concurrent validity of the DSM–IV revised Children's Interview for Psychiatric Syndromes (ChIPS). *Journal of Child and Adolescent Psychopharmacology, 8*, 227–236.

Fristad, M. A. & Goldberg-Arnold, J. S. (2004). *Raising a moody child: How to cope with depression and bipolar disorder*. New York: Guilford Press.

Fristad, M. A., Teare, M., Weller, E. B., Weller, R. A., & Salmon, P. (1998). Study III: Development and concurrent validity of the Children's Interview for Psychiatric Syndromes-parent version (P-ChIPS). *Journal of Child and Adolescent Psychopharmacology, 8*, 221–226.

Geller, B., Bolhofner, K., Craney, J. L., Williams, M., DelBello, M., & Gunderson, K. (2000). Psychosocial functioning in a prepubertal and early adolescent bipolar disorder phenotype. *Journal of the American Academy of Child and Adolescent Psychiatry, 39*, 1543–1548.

Geller, B., Fox, L. W., & Clark, K. A. (1994). Rate and predictors of prepubertal bipolarity during follow-up of 6- to 12-year-old depressed children. *Journal of the American Academy of Child and Adolescent Psychiatry, 33*, 461–469.

Geller, B., & Luby, J. (1997). Child and adolescent bipolar disorder: A review of the past 10 years. *Journal of the American Academy of Child & Adolescent Psychiatry, 36*, 1168–1176.

Geller B., & Tillman R. (2005). Prepubertal and early adolescent bipolar I disorder: Review of diagnostic validation by Robins and Guze criteria. *Journal of Clinical Psychiatry, 66*, 21–28.

Geller, B., Tillman, R., Craney, J. L., & Bolhofner, K. (2004). Four-year prospective outcome and natural history of mania in children with a prepubertal and early adolescent bipolar disorder phenotype. *Archives of General Psychiatry, 61*, 459–467.

Geller, B., Williams, M., Zimmerman, B., & Frazier, J. (1996). Washington University in St. Louis Kiddie Schedule for Affective Disorders and Schizophrenia (Wash-U-KSADS). St. Louis: Washington University.

Geller, B., Zimmerman, B., Williams, M., Bolhofner, K., & Craney, J. L. (2001). Bipolar disorder at prospective follow-up of adults who had prepubertal major depressive disorder. *American Journal of Psychiatry, 158*, 125–127.

Geller, B., Zimmerman, B., Williams, M., DelBello, M., Bolhofner, K., Craney, J. L., et al. (2002). DSM–IV mania symptoms in a prepubertal and early adolescent bipolar disorder phenotype compared to attention-deficit hyperactive and normal controls. *Journal of Child and Adolescent Psychopharmacology, 12*, 11–25.

Geller, B., Zimmerman, B., Williams, M., DelBello, M., Frazier, J., & Beringer, L. (2002). Phenomenology of prepubertal and early adolescent bipolar disorder: Examples of elated mood, grandiose behaviors, decreased need for sleep, racing thoughts, and hypersexuality. *Journal of Child and Adolescent Psychopharmacology, 12*, 3–9.

Goldstein, T. R., Birmaher, B., Axelson, D., Ryan, N. D., Strober, M. A., Gill, M. K., et al. (2005). History of suicide attempts in pediatric bipolar disorder: Factors associated with increased risk. *Bipolar Disorders, 7*, 525–535.

Gracious, B. L., Youngstrom, E. A., Findling, R. L., & Calabrese, J. R. (2002). Discriminative validity of a parent version of the Young Mania Rating Scale. *Journal of the American Academy of Child & Adolescent Psychiatry, 41*, 1350–1359.

Grunebaum, M. F., Galfalvy, H. C., Nichols, C. M., Caldeira, N. A., Sher, L., Dervic, K., et al. (2006). Aggression and substance abuse in bipolar disorder. *Bipolar Disorders, 8*, 496–502.

Hammen, C., & Rudolph, K. D. (2003). Childhood mood disorders. In E. J. Mash & R. A. Barkley (Eds.), *Child psychopathology* (2nd ed.). New York: Guilford Press.

Harpold, T. L., Wozniak, J., Kwon, A., Gilbert, J., Wood, J., Smith, L., et al. (2005). Examining the association between pediatric bipolar disorder and anxiety disorders in psychiatrically referred children and adolescents. *Journal of Affective Disorders, 88*, 19–26.

Hirschfeld, R. M. A., Williams, J. B. W., Spitzer, R. L., Calabrese, J. R., Flynn, L., Keck, P. E., et al. (2000). Development and validation of a screening instrument for bipolar spectrum disorder: The Mood Disorder Questionnaire. *American Journal of Psychiatry, 157*, 1873–1875.

Hodgins, S., Faucher, B., Zarac, A., & Ellenbogen, M. (2002). Children of parents with bipolar disorder: A population at high risk for major affective disorders. *Child and Adolescent Psychiatric Clinics of North America, 11*, 533–554.

Hunt, J. I., Dyl, J., Armstrong, L., Litvin, E., Sheeran, T., & Spirito, A. (2005). Frequency of manic symptoms and bipolar disorder in psychiatrically hospitalized adolescents using the K-SADS Mania Rating Scale. *Journal of Child and Adolescent Psychopharmacology, 15*, 918–930.

Johnson, S. L., & Leahy, R. L. (Eds.). (2004). *Psychological treatment of bipolar disorder.* New York: Guilford Press.

Jones, S. H., Tai, S., Evershed, K., Knowles, R., & Bentall, R. (2006). Early detection of bipolar disorder: A pilot familial high risk study of parents with bipolar disorder and their adolescent children. *Bipolar Disorders, 8*, 362–372.

Kaufman, J., Birmaher, B., Brent, D., Rao, U., Flynn, C., Moreci, P., et al. (1997). Schedule for Affective Disorders and Schizophrenia for school-age children-present and lifetime version (K-SADS-PL): Initial reliability and validity data. *Journal of the American Academy of Child & Adolescent Psychiatry, 36*, 980–988.

Kowatch, R. A., Fristad, M. A., Birmaher, B., Wagner, K. D., Findling, R. L., Hellander, M., et al. (2005). Treatment guidelines for children and adolescents with bipolar disorder: Child psychiatric workgroup on bipolar disorder. *Journal of the American Academy of Child and Adolescent Psychiatry, 44*, 213–239.

Kowatch, R. A., Youngstrom, E. A., Danielyan, A., & Findling, R. (2005). Review and meta-analysis of the phenomenology and clinical characteristics of mania in children and adolescents. *Bipolar Disorders, 7*, 483–496.

Kurita, H., Osada, H., Shimizu, K., & Tachimori, H. (2004). Bipolar disorders in mentally retarded persons with pervasive developmental disorders. *Journal of Developmental and Physical Disabilities, 16*, 377–389.

Kyte, Z. A., Carlson, G. A., & Goodyer, I. M. (2006). Clinical and neuropsychological characteristics of child and adolescent bipolar disorder. *Psychological Medicine, 3*, 1197–1211.

Leffler, J. M., & Fristad, M. A. (2006) Mood disorders in children and adolescents. In T. G. Plante, (Ed.) *Mental disorders of the new millennium: Behavioral issues (Vol. 1) (pp. 117–137)*. Westport, CT: Praeger /Greenwood.

Leibenluft, E., Charney, D. S., Towbin, K. E., Bhangoo, R. K., & Pine, D. S. (2003). Defining clinical phenotypes of juvenile mania. *American Journal of Psychiatry, 160*, 430–437.

Levin, F. R., & Hennessy, G. (2004). Bipolar disorder and substance abuse. *Biological Psychiatry, 56*, 738–748.

Lewinsohn, P. M., Klein, D. N., & Seely, J. R. (1995). Bipolar disorders in a community sample of older adolescents: Prevalence, phenomenology, comorbidity and course. *Journal of the American Academy of Child and Adolescent Psychiatry, 34*, 454–463.

Lish, J. D., Dime-Meenan, S., Whybrow, P. C., Price, R. A., & Hirschfeld, R. M. (1994). The National Depressive and Manic-Depressive Association (NDMDA) survey of bipolar members. *Journal of Affective Disorders, 31*, 281–294.

Lofthouse, N., & Fristad, M. (2004). Psychosocial interventions for children with early-onset bipolar spectrum disorder. *Clinical Child and Family Psychology Review, 7*, 71–88.

Matson, J. L., Rush, K. S., Hamilton, M., Anderson, S. J., Bamburg, J. W., & Baglio, C. S. (1999). Characteristics of depression as assessed by the Diagnostic Assessment for the Severely Handicapped – II (DASH-II). *Research in Developmental Disabilities, 20*, 305–313.

Matson, J. L., & Smiroldo, B. B. (1997). Validity of the Mania Subscale of the Diagnostic Assessment for the Severely Handicapped – II (DASH-II). *Research in Developmental Disabilities, 18*, 221–225.

Matson, J. L., Terlonge, C., Gonzalez, M. L., & Rivet, T. (2006). An evaluation of social and adaptive skills in adults with bipolar disorder and severe/profound intellectual disability. *Research in Developmental Disabilities, 27*, 681–687.

Mick, E., Biederman, J., Pandina, G., & Faraone, S. V. (2003). A preliminary meta-analysis of the child behavior checklist in pediatric bipolar disorder. *Biological Psychiatry, 53*, 1021–1027.

Nottelmann, E., Biederman, J., Birmaher, B., Carlson, G. A., Chang, K., A., Fenton, W. S., et al. (2001). National Institute of Mental Health research roundtable on prepubertal bipolar disorder. *Journal of the American Academy of Child and Adolescent Psychiatry, 40*, 871–878.

Papolos, D., Hennen, J., Cockerham, M. S., Thode, H. C., & Youngstrom, E. A. (2006). The Child Bipolar Questionnaire: A dimensional approach to screening for pediatric bipolar disorder. *Journal of Affective Disorders, 95*, 149–158.

Patel, N. C., DelBello, M. P., Keck, P. E., Jr., & Strakowski, S. M. (2006). Phenomenology associated with age at onset in patients with bipolar disorder at their first psychiatric hospitalization. *Bipolar Disorders 8*, 91–94.

Pavuluri, M. N., Birmaher, B., & Naylor, M. W. (2005). Pediatric bipolar disorder: A review of the past 10 years. *Journal of the American Academy of Child & Adolescent Psychiatry, 44*, 846–871.

Pavuluri, M. N., Henry, D. B., Devineni, B., Carbray, J. A., & Birmaher, B. (2006). Child mania rating scale: Development, reliability, and validity. *Journal of the American Academy of Child & Adolescent Psychiatry, 45*, 550–560.

Perlis, R. H., Miyahara, S., Marangell, L. B., Wisniewski, S. R., Ostacher, M., DelBello, M. P., et al. (2004). Long-term implications of early onset in bipolar disorder: Data from the first 1000 participants in the systematic treatment enhancement program for bipolar disorder (STEP-BP). *Biological Psychiatry, 55*, 875–881.

Pogge, D. L., Wayland-Smith, D., Zaccario, M., Borgaro, S., Stokes, J., & Harvey, P. D. (2001). Diagnosis of manic episodes in adolescent inpatients: Structured diagnostic procedures compared to clinical chart diagnoses. *Psychiatry Research, 101*(1), 47–54.

Poznanski, E. O., & Mokros, H. B. (1995). *Children's Depression Rating Scale – Revised (CDRS-R) administration booklet*. Pittsburgh, PA: Western Psychological Services.

Puig-Antich, J., & Ryan, N. (1986). The Schedule for Affective Disorders and Schizophrenia for school-age children (Kiddie-SADS)-1986. Pittsburgh: Western Psychiatric Institute and Clinic.

Quinn, C.A., & Fristad, M.A. (2004.) Defining and identifying early onset bipolar spectrum disorder. *Current Psychiatry Reports, 6*, 101–107.

Reich, W., & Wellner, Z. (1988). *Revised version of the Diagnostic Interview for Children and Adolescents*. St. Louis, MO: Washington University School of Medicine, Department of Psychiatry.

Rende, R., Birmaher, B., Axelson, D., Strober, M., Gill, M. K., Valeri, S., et al. (2007). Childhood-onset bipolar disorder: Evidence for increased familial loading of psychiatric illness. *Journal of the American Academy of Child & Adolescent Psychiatry, 46*, 197–204.

Rooney, M. T., Fristad, M. A., Weller, E. B., & Weller, R. A. (1999). *Administration manual for the Children's Interview for Psychiatric Syndromes (ChIPS)*. Washington, D.C.: American Psychiatric Press.

Shaffer, D., Fisher, P., Lucas, C. P., Dulcan, M. K., & Schwab-Stone, M. E. (2000). NIMH Diagnostic Interview Schedule for Children version IV (NIMH DISC-IV): Description, differences from previous versions, and reliability of some common diagnoses. *Journal of the American Academy of Child & Adolescent Psychiatry, 39*, 28–38.

Strober, M., & Carlson, G. (1982). Bipolar illness in adolescents with major depression: Clinical, genetic, and psychopharmalogic predictors in a three- to four-year prospective follow-up investigation. *Archives of General Psychiatry, 39*, 549–555.

Thompson, W. D., Orvaschel, H., Prusoff, B. A., & Kidd, K. K. (1982). An evaluation of the family history method for ascertaining psychiatric disorders. *Archives of General Psychiatry, 39*, 53–58.

Tillman, R., Geller, B., Craney, J. L., Bolhofner, K., Williams, M., & Zimerman, B. (2004). Relationship of parent and child informants to prevalence of mania symptoms in children with a prepubertal and early adolescent bipolar disorder phenotype. *American Journal of Psychiatry, 161*, 1278–1284.

Wagner, K. D., Hirschfeld, R. M. A., Emslie, G. J., Findling, R. L., Gracious, B. L., & Reed, M. L. (2006). Validation of the Mood Disorder Questionnaire for bipolar disorders in adolescents. *Journal of Clinical Psychiatry, 67* (5), 827–830.

Weissman, M. M., Wickramaratne, P., Adams, P., Wolk, S., Verdeli, H., & Olfson, M. (2000). Brief screening for family psychiatric history: The Family History Screen. *Archives of General Psychiatry, 57*, 675–682.

Weller, E. B., Weller, R. A., Rooney, M. T., & Fristad, M. A. (1999a). *Children's Interview for Psychiatric Syndromes (ChIPS)*. Washington, D.C.: American Psychiatric Press.

Weller, E. B., Weller, R. A., Rooney, M. T., & Fristad, M. A. (1999b). *Children's Interview for Psychiatric Syndromes –Parent version (P-ChIPS)*. Washington, D.C.: American Psychiatric Press.

Young, R. C., Biggs, J. T., Ziegler, V. E., & Meyer, D. A. (1978). A rating scale for mania: Reliability, validity and sensitivity. *British Journal of Psychiatry, 133*, 429–435.

Youngstrom, E. A., Duax, J., & Hamilton, J. (2005). Evidence-based assessment of pediatric bipolar disorder, part I: Base rate and family history. *Journal of the American Academy of Child & Adolescent Psychiatry, 44*, 712–717.

Youngstrom, E. A., Findling, R. L., Calabrese, J. R., Gracious, B. L., Demeter, C., Bedoya, D. D., et al. (2004). Comparing the diagnostic accuracy of six potential screening instruments for bipolar disorder in youths aged 5 to 17 years. *Journal of the American Academy of Child & Adolescent Psychiatry, 43*, 847–858.

Youngstrom, E. A., Findling, R. L., Youngstrom, J. K., & Calabrese, J. R. (2005). Toward an evidence-based assessment of pediatric bipolar disorder. *Journal of Clinical Child and Adolescent Psychology, 3*, 433–448.

Youngstrom, E. A., Gracious, B. L., Danielson, C. K., Findling, R. L., & Calabrese, J. (2003). Toward an integration of parent and clinician report on the Young Mania Rating Scale. *Journal of Affective Disorders, 77*, 179–190.

Youngstrom, E. A., Joseph, M. F., & Greene, J. Comparing the psychometric properties of multiple teacher report instruments as predictors of bipolar disorder in children and adolescents. *Journal of Clinical Psychology, 64*, 382–401.

Youngstrom, E. A., Meyers, O., Demeter, C., Youngstrom, J., Morello, L., Piiparinen, R., et al. (2005). Comparing diagnostic checklists for pediatric bipolar disorder in academic and community mental health settings. *Bipolar Disorders, 7*, 507–517.

Part IV

Assessment of Problems
Developmental Disabilities

11

Academic Assessment

GEORGE H. NOELL, SCOTT P. ARDOIN, and KRISTIN A. GANSLE

ACADEMIC ASSESSMENT

Academic demands are central to the lives of children living in the information age and in industrial societies. Schools are the workplaces of children and are the gateways into adult work for most adolescents. Historically, academic concerns are the most common reason that children are referred for special education services within schools and are central to many requests for outpatient services (Lloyd, Kauffman, Landrum, & Roe, 1991). The synergy between children's academic and social/emotional functioning creates a complex interrelationship in which mental health problems can adversely affect children's educational attainment and academic success affects mental health (Johnson, McGue, & Iacono, 2006). Children who suffer from depression, anxiety, or Attention-Deficit/Hyperactivity Disorder (ADHD) are at an apparent disadvantage in attending to, completing, and profiting from instruction. Similarly, children who are at risk for or exhibit conduct problems are at increased risk for poor academic achievement that may result from the interaction of diverse factors (Montague, Enders, & Castro, 2005). The synergy also exists when examined from the opposite perspective. Children who repeatedly fail at school are more likely to exhibit anxiety, depression, negative self-esteem, and conduct problems (Jimerson, Carlson, Rotert, Egeland, & Sroufe, 1997).

When phenomena co-occur, the question of causation naturally arises. Are the client's academic difficulties the result of psychopathology such as a depressive disorder, is the depressive disorder the result of frustration and

GEORGE H. NOELL • Department of Psychology, Louisiana State University, Baton Rouge, LA 70803-5501.
SCOTT P. ARDOIN • Louisiana State University
KRISTIN A. GANSLE • University of South Carolina

J.L. Matson et al. (eds.), *Assessing Childhood Psychopathology and Developmental Disabilities*, DOI: 10.1007/978-0-387-09528-8,
© Springer Science+Business Media, LLC 2009

chronic failure at school, or are both concerns the result of a third factor? The limitations of correlational and epidemiological research likely preclude a strong determination of a causal connection between psychopathology and academic performance. Additionally, the ways psychopathology and academic attainment interact may be substantively idiographic. For some children, psychopathology may create substantive barriers to academic achievement; for others, psychopathological symptoms may be largely the result of chronic negative environmental events resulting from academic failure that are nearly inescapable due to mandatory school attendance. Although parents and teachers may view psychopathology as causing academic concerns, for some children academic concerns may be an important stressor contributing to psychopathology (Jimerson et al., 1997; Kelley, Reitman, & Noell, 2002).

Given the central nature of education in the lives of children, comprehensive psychological assessment for children typically will include assessment of the client's educational context and attainment, thus, the inclusion of this chapter in a volume devoted to the assessment of psychopathology. This chapter is organized around the assumption that clinicians will seek answers to the same questions relevant to diagnosis and treatment selection that have been discussed extensively elsewhere as an organizing heuristic for behavioral and psychological assessment (e.g., Haynes & O'Brien, 2000).

First, is there a problem, and if so, what is the nature of that problem (diagnosis)? Second, if there is an academic problem, what should be done to ameliorate that problem (treatment specification)? Although these two questions provide a simple powerful heuristic for organizing the psychological assessment of academic performance, the real challenge arises in the details. The selection of specific measurement tools, observation occasions, and integration of data that vary in their technical quality inevitably will create substantial challenges for the design, execution, and interpretation of the assessment (Messick, 1995).

The following sections of this chapter describe three fundamental issues relevant to the assessment of academic functioning. The first section describes selected diagnostic considerations relevant to academic concerns. Primary consideration is devoted to diagnosis under the Individuals with Disabilities Education Improvement Act of 2004 (IDEA) due to the central importance of schools to the treatment of academic concerns and based on the assumption that users of this volume are more conversant with the *Diagnostic and Statistical Manual of Mental Disorders* (*DSM–IV–TR*, American Psychiatric Association, 2000).

The second section of the chapter describes a number of assessment methodologies developed to move beyond traditional norm-referenced tests to direct, low-inference quantification of academic behavior. Broadly these assessments can be described as direct observational procedures and curriculum based assessments. They are utilized for diagnosis, treatment selection, and progress monitoring.

The final section describes a general case problem-solving approach for addressing academic concerns. The authors wish to acknowledge at the outset that space limitations preclude a comprehensive treatment of the issues surrounding academic assessment relevant to psychopathology and developmental disabilities. Indeed, many journals and complete volumes are devoted to academic diagnosis, assessment, and treatment each year. This chapter provides an overview of selected issues in these domains as they relate to the assessment of childhood psychopathology and developmental disabilities.

DIAGNOSTIC CONSIDERATIONS

The two primary authoritative sources for diagnosis of academic concerns used in the United States are the Diagnostic and Statistical Manual of Mental Disorders (DSM–IV–TR, American Psychiatric Association [APA], 2000), now in its fourth edition, and Public Law 108–446, commonly known as the Individuals with Disabilities Education Improvement Act of 2004 (IDEA). These diagnostic systems emphasize an intraindividual approach, suggesting that the disorder resides within the child rather than the environment or a person environment interaction. Despite the intuitive appeal of this approach for many, diagnostic work based on these approaches typically gives minimal consideration to the possibility that inadequate instruction and/or environmental disadvantage are substantially the cause of a child's academic underachievement (Gresham & Gansle, 1992).

It is important to acknowledge that IDEA does explicitly acknowledge environmental disadvantage as a condition that precludes diagnosis of a learning disability; however, the extent to which this is commonly assessed or integrated into assessment in practice is unclear. It is also important to recognize that diagnosis from either *DSM–IV–TR* and IDEA have little if any treatment utility for academic concerns. They are nosological rather than functional. However, diagnosis is frequently necessary to allow children access to treatment in schools and community settings.

Academic problems are a common feature of many of the diagnoses first identified in infancy, childhood, adolescence, or in school settings. For example, children diagnosed with any of the Pervasive Developmental Disorders (e.g., Autistic Disorder, Childhood Disintegrative Disorder, Asperger's Disorder), Posttraumatic Stress Disorder, Schizophrenia, Conduct Disorder, or Serious Emotional Disturbance are likely to demonstrate problems with academic achievement. However, academic concerns will likely be secondary to these concerns and treatment is more likely to be focused on social emotional functioning than academic attainment. This chapter focuses primarily on concerns for which academic performance and attainment are the central issues.

Although used for different purposes and in different settings, *DSM-IV-TR* and educational diagnoses that stem from IDEA share some features that may allow practitioners across schools and community clinics to communicate efficiently and effectively. They each seek to address ability and its relationship to achievement in reading, mathematics, and written expression. *DSM–IV–TR* and educational diagnoses differ with respect to the diagnoses that may be made as well as specificity of their features. Children who struggle with academics in the general curriculum traditionally have been assessed using standardized, norm-referenced tests in clinical or school settings. These instruments generally have technical properties appropriate to and adequate for diagnostic use.

Diagnostic and Statistical Manual of Mental Disorders, 4th Edition, Text Revision (DSM–IV–TR)

Mental Retardation

Due to the pervasive nature of the impairments resulting from mental retardation, academic concerns can take on a more central or secondary focus. For many individuals functioning in the mild range of mental retardation, academic concerns may be of central importance. Common diagnostic requirements for MR include intellectual functioning that is approximately two standard deviations (or more) below the mean (IDEA, DSM–IV–TR; APA, 2000). Given the measurement error inherent in all assessment, DSM–IV–TR cautions that individuals with scores some-what above the diagnostic boundary may still qualify for the diagnosis if additional indicators are significantly impaired. Similarly, individuals with scores more than two standard deviations below the mean may not qualify if additional diagnostic indicators are not significantly impaired (APA).

Second, the individual must have concurrent deficits in adaptive functioning in at least two skill areas. *DSM–IV–TR* defines adaptive functioning as "how effectively individuals cope with common life demands and how well they meet the standards of personal independence expected of someone in their particular age group, sociocultural background, and community setting" (p. 42). Adaptive functioning skills include all areas relevant to social independence, such as communication and social skills, work and community involvement, academic skills, and health and safety (APA, 2000).

Third, the onset of the disorder must be before the age of 18 years. It is possible for the initial MR diagnosis to be made after the age of 18, but there must be evidence of onset prior to that age.

Learning Disorders

In DSM–IV–TR, when an individual's achievement in reading, mathematics, or written expression on individually administered standardized tests is substantially below what is expected given the individual's age, education, or intelligence, a Learning Disorder may be diagnosed. Substantially below is defined as a discrepancy between achievement and Intellectual Quotient (IQ) that must be more than two standard deviations. However, DSM-IV-TR does allow for smaller discrepancies under certain conditions, such as questionable IQ scores due to difficulties in testing, other mental disorders or medical conditions that may compromise testing, and ethnic or cultural background factors.

Reading Disorder, Mathematics Disorder, and Disorder of Written Expression may be diagnosed when a discrepancy is found between IQ and achievement in one or more of those academic areas. For a diagnosis to be made, the disorder must have an important negative impact on academic achievement or daily living skills. Specific learning disorders may be based on a breakdown in a basic skill within the domain such as reading fluency, calculation, or composition.

Attention-Deficit/Hyperactivity Disorder

Attention-Deficit/Hyperactivity Disorder (ADHD) may be diagnosed within DSM–IV–TR when a child displays a pattern of inattention and/or impulsivity/hyperactivity to a degree that appreciably exceeds that of their same-aged peers, with symptoms present before the age of seven years, in at least two settings (APA, 2000). It must affect the individual's functioning in social, academic, or occupational contexts. Unlike the Specific Learning Disorders, there is no specific qualification criterion for the diagnosis. The word "often" is common to all specific behavioral diagnostic criteria (e.g., "Is often forgetful in daily activities," APA, p. 92). Clinicians are not instructed to determine a specific difference between the child's scores on an instrument compared to typically developing children. Individuals with ADHD may be diagnosed as predominantly hyperactive/impulsive, predominantly inattentive, or combined. When the individual has major symptoms of ADHD but specific criteria for ADHD subtypes are not met, ADHD Not Otherwise Specified may be diagnosed.

INDIVIDUALS WITH DISABILITIES EDUCATION IMPROVEMENT ACT OF 2004 (IDEA)

Children in the United States are entitled to a free and appropriate public education in the least restrictive environment that is appropriate to their individual needs (IDEA, 2004). Children with disabilities must receive a diagnosis of those disabilities within the due process provisions of IDEA and applicable case law, using nondiscriminatory multifactored evaluation (IDEA) in order to receive special services under IDEA. Diagnostic evaluations are completed with the expressed purpose of ascertaining eligibility for and providing services to children with disabilities. Eligibility must be determined based on the presence of a disability defined in IDEA and by state law, and the documentation of need for special services to remediate the educational deficits caused by the disability. Once eligibility has been established and a service plan designed and implemented, schools receive federal funding based on the level of service provided to students with disabilities.

Under IDEA, disabilities for which special education services may be provided are identified in one or more of 13 categories. As with *DSM–IV–TR*, the diagnoses available for use by multidisciplinary teams (MDTs) in schools address concerns about children that have an impact on their educational achievement; however, many of them require planning for issues in addition to academic achievement (e.g., Deaf-blindness, Other Health Impairment, or Emotional Disturbance). For this chapter, assessment for diagnoses whose primary focus is academic is addressed. Although the educational diagnostic categories are broadly delineated in federal legislation

(IDEA, 2004), each state determines the specific operational diagnostic criteria for use in its jurisdiction. It is also worth noting that states vary widely in terms of the qualifications of the examiners that are required in order for data to contribute to a MDT determination. Typically, assessor qualifications focus on educational licenses or certifications.

Mental Retardation

IDEA defines Mental Retardation (a.k.a., Mental Disability) as "significantly subaverage general intellectual functioning, existing concurrently with deficits in adaptive behavior and manifested during the developmental period, that adversely affects a child's educational performance" (IDEA, 2004). Although IDEA does not define "significantly subaverage intellectual functioning," leaving that determination to the states, an IQ score approximately two standard deviations below the mean is considered such by the American Association on Mental Retardation (AAMR, 2002), a leader in advocacy, policy, and research for individuals with MR. Not all education agencies, however, choose to use two standard deviations as the IQ criterion for the diagnosis, and the degree to which a child's intellectual functioning must deviate from the mean differs according to the agency setting the policy.

Adaptive behavior is "the collection of conceptual, social, and practical skills that people have learned so they can function in their everyday lives" (AAMR, 2002). Adequate adaptive behavior may be inferred from the degree to which individuals function independently, taking expectations of age and culture into account. Although *DSM-IV-TR* further classifies MR by severity, IDEA does not provide similar categories. Services are made available to students according to need, and those needs are established using descriptions of current levels of educational performance and goals and objectives for future performance (IDEA, 2004).

Specific Learning Disabilities

IDEA (2004) describes Specific Learning Disability (SLD) as "a disorder in one or more of the basic psychological processes involved in understanding or in using language, spoken or written, that may manifest itself in the imperfect ability to listen, think, speak, read, write, spell, or to do mathematical calculations." It may include disorders such as dyslexia, brain injury, and developmental aphasia. The seven areas that may be affected by the disability are a much broader application of SLD than the three areas (Reading Disorders, Mathematics Disorders, Disorders of Written Expression) used by DSM–IV–TR, despite the lack of clear empirical support for all seven areas as distinct SLDs (Fletcher et al., 2002). Exclusionary criteria for the diagnosis indicate that other factors such as visual, hearing, motor problems, MR, emotional disturbance, and environmental, cultural, or economic disadvantage may not be responsible for the learning problem (IDEA, 2004). Although this is spelled out in the federal definition, research on identification practices has demonstrated that in the face of criteria that exclude students from receiving special services for some of the very reasons they need assistance in the first place, MDTs identify large numbers of students who fail to meet eligibility criteria as SLD (Lyon, 1996; MacMillan, Gresham, & Bocian, 1998; Shaywitz, Shaywitz, Fletcher, & Escobar, 1990).

Whereas *DSM–IV–TR* defines the disorder concretely as the discrepancy between ability and achievement, IDEA describes SLD as a disorder in psychological processes. The resulting diagnostic process for SLD focuses on processes that cannot be observed directly and may be logically inconsistent (Gresham, 2002). The original IDEA indicated that children labeled as SLD must have a "severe discrepancy" between ability and achievement (U. S. Office of Education, 1977, p. 65083). Over the years, the federal government has proposed a variety of formulas for determining discrepancy and all have been challenged (Heward, 2006). This is likely due to a number of documented problems with these formulas (Fletcher, Francis, Morris, & Lyon, 2005; Fletcher et al., 2002; Fletcher et al., 1998, 1989, 2005; Kavale, 2002).

Given the problems associated with discrepancy formulas, a burgeoning literature describes a range of alternatives including different discrepancy formulas and response to intervention models (see Gresham, 2002; Kavale, 2002); however, none has gained widespread acceptance in the policy, research, and practice communities. The current IDEA mentions neither discrepancy nor specific criteria for determining the diagnosis. The states, then, are left to operationalize the definition. This, in turn, has led to substantial heterogeneity between states and LEAs in the criteria and procedures for classifying children with learning disabilities (Kavale, 2002; MacMillan & Siperstein, 2002; Ysseldyke, 2001).

Despite these differences, however, the most common practice for identifying SLD is to determine whether a severe discrepancy exists between achievement predicted by individually administered measures of intellectual ability and actual achievement (Heward, 2006; Mercer, Jordan, Allsopp, & Mercer, 1996), that severe discrepancy, of course, being defined at the state or local level.

Attention-Deficit/Hyperactivity Disorder

Despite the relationship between ADHD and achievement problems (Biederman et al., 1999), IDEA does not include ADHD as one of its diagnoses. Modifications and accommodations for ADHD may be made on the child's Individual Education Program (IEP) if the child has been determined eligible and receives special services for another disability. Some students have received a diagnosis of Other Health Impaired (OHI) under IDEA as a result of ADHD symptoms; however, the applicability of OHI to ADHD varies based on the operational definition employed in each state. The key issue from the federal definition of OHI in IDEA is the possibility that a chronic medical condition can cause problems with alertness which has been interpreted by some to include the attention problems that are part of the core of ADHD. Accommodations and modifications for students with ADHD may also be provided through Section 504 of the Rehabilitation Act of 1973, provided the disability is not sufficiently severe to warrant the provision of special education services.

TRADITIONAL DIAGNOSTIC ASSESSMENT TOOLS

The poor treatment utility of the instruments and procedures traditionally used to make diagnostic determinations for academic concerns have been previously discussed at length (Gresham & Witt, 1997; Shinn, 1989). Academic assessment that leads to diagnosis frequently lacks an empirical basis for guiding treatment recommendations. Assessment practices that were developed primarily for treatment selection and progress monitoring are discussed later in the chapter. Diagnostic assessments under both DSM–IV–TR and IDEA have emphasized the use of individually administered standardized tests of intelligence and achievement. Although group tests of intelligence and achievement are less expensive, the magnitude of the implications of assessment outcomes has argued for using instruments that generally are regarded as producing the most accurate assessment results.

Tests of Intelligence

Standardized tests of intelligence commonly are used for diagnoses of MR and for SLD, as, in most cases, the child's level of intellectual functioning must be established before a diagnosis may be assigned and/or educational services provided. Tests of intelligence are norm-referenced; they are designed to convey information about the individual's performance as compared to a large representative sample of other children (with and without disabilities) of the same age. They are given in the same way to every person to whom the test is administered as an effort to control for variations in test scores due to testers. Although there are other quality tests available, the Wechsler Intelligence Scale for Children (3rd ed., Wechsler, 1991) and the Stanford–Binet (4th ed., Thorndike, Hagen, & Sattler, 1986) are the two intelligence tests in widest use (Heward, 2006).

Measures of Adaptive Behavior

Systematic assessment of adaptive behavior is important for determining supports needed for success in the person's environment (Rush & Francis, 2000; Schalock, 1999), as well as establishing deficits concomitant with those in intellectual functioning for diagnosing MR (AAMR, 2002; DSM–IV–TR, American Psychiatric Association, 2000; IDEA, 2004). In most cases, an informant who is familiar with the client answers questions in the form of an interview or a questionnaire. The AAMR Adaptive Behavior Scale has different forms that describe behavior either in school (ABS-S, Lambert, Nihira, & Leland, 1993) or in residential and community settings (ABS-RC, Nihira, Leland, & Lambert, 1993). The Vineland Adaptive Behavior Scales (Sparrow, Balla, & Cicchetti, 1984) measure a wide range of adaptive behaviors in the communication, daily living skills, socialization, and motor skills domains, using either interviews or a questionnaire for classroom teachers. The Scales of Independent Behavior-Revised(SIB-R, Bruininks, Woodcock, Weatherman, & Hill,

1996) is a norm-referenced assessment of 14 areas of adaptive behavior and 8 areas of problem behavior, and is designed to be used with individuals of all ages.

Measures of Achievement

Standardized tests of achievement are routinely given to children to determine SLD; and in educational contexts, may be given to children with MR to determine their present levels of functioning in specific academic areas. Traditionally, for diagnostic purposes, achievement is measured using standardized tests of achievement in order to establish a discrepancy between IQ and achievement. Standardized tests of achievement routinely are used within educational contexts to document educational impairment for other disorders such as OHI or Severe Emotional Disturbance.

Standardized individually administered tests of educational achievement appear to be the most ubiquitous element of diagnostic assessment under IDEA. Some achievement tests are designed to measure achievement in one area of academic functioning, such as the KeyMath-Revised/ Normative Update (Connolly, 1997, norms; 1988, content), which provides scores for Basic Concepts, Operations, and Applications; the Test of Written Language, 3rd edition (TOWL-III, Hammill & Larsen, 1996), which has eight subtest scores in a variety of areas from Spelling to Style to Conventions; and the Gates-MacGinitie Reading Tests (4th ed., MacGinitie, MacGinitie, Maria, & Dreyer, 2000), which measures a variety of skills from letter-sound correspondence to vocabulary to comprehension.

Others measure overall achievement, and may take the form of group achievement tests administered to a group of students in a classroom, such as the Iowa Tests of Basic Skills (ITBS, Hoover, Hieronymus, Frisbie, & Dunbar, 1996) or individual achievement tests that are administered to one student at a time, such as the Woodcock–Johnson III Tests of Achievement (Woodcock, McGrew, & Mather, 2001).

Rating Scales

Additional measures commonly are used to gather information from individuals familiar with children's behavior in home and school settings. Rating scales provide norm-referenced comparisons of a child's behavior to that of same-aged peers. These instruments generally ask teachers, parents, the child, or other individuals who spend time with the child to rate the frequency with which he or she engages in specific behaviors. Some rating scales are directed at specific diagnoses, such as the Conners' Rating Scales-Revised (Conners, 1997), which focuses on behaviors relevant to ADHD diagnosis. Rating scales that most commonly are used in schools, however, sample a wide range of behaviors, such as the Child Behavior Checklist (Achenbach & Edelbrock, 1991), and the Behavior Assessment System for Children-Revised (Reynolds & Kamphaus, 1998).

Summary Diagnostic Assessment

Standardized norm-referenced tests provide clinicians with an estimate of a student's skills relative to a national normative sample. Although these tests have established utility for making diagnostic determinations, generally they are inadequate for academic intervention planning or monitoring. Tests typically contain very few items specific to any skill due to the broad surveys they provide and the assessment of academic attainment as a psychological construct. Thus, norm-referenced tests generally fail to provide information regarding clients' proficiency in particular skills and as a result are substantially deficient for treatment planning (Deno, 1985). In addition, norm-referenced assessments do not consider variables that are well established as critical to educational attainment such as the quality of instruction. They appear to assume a normative or generic school experience that may be irrelevant to the education of the client.

Comparing an individual's skills to others who have received the same instruction provides a better indication of whether the student may be having difficulty with learning. Furthermore, norm-referenced tests are poor choices for monitoring intervention effects because of the cost of administration, practice effects, and insensitivity to small changes in student performance (D. Marston, Fuchs, & Deno, 1986). Given these three limitations of norm-referenced tests, it is important that alternative measures are used when evaluating student skills, developing intervention plans, and monitoring the effects of intervention.

DIRECT ACADEMIC ASSESSMENT: CURRICULUM-BASED ASSESSMENT

Curriculum-based assessments (CBA) can provide clinicians with data to evaluate a client's skills, identify instructional needs, monitor the client's response to changes in instruction, and test potential interventions. It is increasingly important that clinicians are familiar with these measures as the amendments to IDEA of 2004 dramatically increase the likelihood that schools will use CBA to identify clients in need of intervention, to monitor their response to intervention, and to diagnose disability under a response to intervention (RTI) model. Several approaches have been described for the direct behavioral assessment of academic skills including multiple models of CBA (Shapiro, 1996), curriculum-based measurement (CBM; Shinn, 1989), and curriculum-based evaluation (CBE; Howell & Nolet, 2000). These approaches vary in terms of the comprehensiveness of the assessment model (e.g., including or failing to examine instruction), the comparative points used for decision making (norm- or criterion-referenced), and the extent to which the approach provides a global outcome measure model versus a model for the breakdown and analysis of specific skills.

Although entire books have been devoted to CBA, CBE, and CBM (see the sources above), the approaches commonly share the fluency-based measures originally developed within CBM. The consideration of direct behavioral assessment measures herein focuses on the measures developed within CBM due to their wide adoption beyond CBM, utility in making a range of decisions, and well-established psychometric properties. CBM was initially developed in the early 1970s in response to the need for identification and intervention materials that were simple, efficient, and cost-effective (Deno, 1985). Common characteristics of CBM and CBA include: (1) measurement that is direct, (2) brief administration procedures, (3) procedures that allow for frequent and repeated use, and (4) procedures that enable progress to be monitored systematically using graphs and charts (Frisby, 1987). The following sections describe selected measures used within CBM.

Curriculum-Based Measurement (CBM)

CBM is described in the literature as a method for measuring student proficiency in the curriculum (Deno, 1985; Shinn, 1989). CBM typically focuses on long-term instructional goals and is often referred to as a global outcome measure. It combines components of traditional and alternative assessment models, and it relies on standardized measurement methods (Fuchs & Deno, 1992). Extensive evidence exists demonstrating the reliability, validity, and sensitivity of CBM procedures in the areas of reading, writing, mathematics, and spelling (Ardoin et al., 2004; Fuchs, Fuchs, Hamlett, & Allinder, 1989; Fuchs et al., 1994; Gansle et al., 2004).

CBM in Reading

The curriculum-based measure most familiar to educators is probably oral reading fluency (CBM-ORF). The Reading First Assessment Panel designated CBM-ORF procedures as having sufficient evidence for identifying students in need of intervention and for monitoring their progress (Francis et al., 2002). Extensive evidence exists demonstrating its reliability and validity in predicting overall reading achievement as well as comprehension skills. CBM-ORF procedures are administered individually. Students are given one minute to read a narrative text, while the examiner records errors made by the student. If students hesitate on a word for three seconds, the word is provided and recorded as an error by the examiner. Other words scored as errors include words mispronounced given the context of the story and not self-corrected and skipped words. The primary dependent measure is the number of words read correctly within one minute. When universal screening procedures are conducted (see below) it is advised that three probes are administered to students and their median performance is used. When conducting frequent progress monitoring, typically only one probe is administered during each session (Hosp, Hosp, & Howell, 2007).

CBM Maze

The maze is another global measure of reading fluency that has undergone extensive scrutiny. Although shown to be a reliable and valid predictor of reading achievement, evidence indicates that CBM-ORF is a better measure of reading achievement than is the maze (Ardoin et al., 2004).

However, the maze can be administered to groups or computer technology can be used. Administering a maze involves providing a narrative text to clients; however, every seventh word following the first sentence is deleted and replaced with three options, only one of which is a correct word. Examinees are allowed three minutes to read the text silently and circle the correct words within each set. The dependent measure is the number of correct words circled (Hosp et al., 2007).

CBM Prereading Measures

Several prereading measures exist that have been shown to have adequate reliability and validity including letter identification, letter sound identification, and nonsense word fluency (Kaminski & Good III, 1996). Other relatively new measures, often referred to as DIBELS (Dynamic Indicators of Early Literacy Skills), are used by many schools but have not undergone the same level of scrutiny yet as existing CBM (Good & Kaminski, 2002). Readers can access detailed information regarding DIBELS prereading measures as well as the probes at http://dibels.uoregon.edu/.

CBM in Mathematics

The majority of research in CBM mathematics has focused on evaluating and monitoring basic math calculation skills. These probes can be developed either to assess one skill or to assess multiple skills. Generally, when monitoring performance across an extended period of time, multiple skill probes are used. Probes can be administered either individually or in groups. Examinees are provided two minutes to complete as many problems as they can and are encouraged to put an "X" through any problem that they do not know how to complete. Rather than scoring responses to a problem as simply correct or incorrect, each digit written is counted as either correct or incorrect. Thus, if an answer to 5 + 5 is 12, one digit correct is scored for the 1 in the tens column (Thurber, Shinn, & Smolkowski, 2002).

CBM Mathematics Concepts and Applications

Minimal research exists evaluating the reliability and validity of CBM mathematics concepts and application probes; however, this body of literature is growing and seems promising. These probes include multiple skills sampled from across the curriculum. The limit for these probes varies from two to five minutes. Similar to CBM basic calculation procedures, the probes can be administered to groups or individually and students may earn partial credit (i.e., digits correct) rather than simply scoring each answer as correct or incorrect (Connell, 2006; Fuchs et al., 1994).

CBM in Written Expression

Compared to reading or mathematics, the assessment of written expression is more challenging (Gansle, VanDerHeyden, Noell, Resetar, & Williams, 2006). Standardized CBM procedures involve providing a story starter (e.g., My best memory is when ...), allowing the student one minute to think about what to write, and three minutes to write. Among the most common measures that are technically adequate are total words written, correct word sequences, and words spelled correctly. Total words written counts the number of words written by the student; correct spelling and the relationship of the words to each other or to standard English is not assessed (Shinn, 1989). Correct word sequences involve counting pairs of words that are spelled correctly and grammatically correct within the context of the sentence (Shinn, 1989). Words spelled correctly counts the total number of correctly spelled words considered in isolation (Shinn, 1989). Although these fluency or production-dependent measures (Jewell & Malecki, 2005) have been determined technically adequate (Deno, Marston, & Mirkin, 1982; Deno, Mirkin, & Marston, 1980; Gansle, Noell, VanDerHeyden, Naquin, & Slider, 2002, Marston & Deno, 1981; Videen, Deno, & Marston, 1982), there has been research to support the validity of production-independent measures such as percentage of words spelled correctly (Tindal & Parker, 1989), as well as accurate production indices like correct minus incorrect word sequences (Espin, Shin, Deno, Skare, Robinson, & Benner, 2000).

Difficulties with CBM writing include the fact that an infinite number of correct responses is possible for every prompt, the extent to which validated measures reflect what is considered "good writing" varies (Gansle, Gilbertson, & VanDerHeyden, 2006), and the time necessary to score CBM written expression probes varies according to the measures chosen (Gansle et al., 2002).

Advantages of CBM

CBM offers several advantages over traditional norm-referenced test-based assessment. First, CBM materials are inexpensive. Although Deno and other pioneers in the area originally suggested that measures should be derived from the curriculum in which a student is being taught, subsequent research has suggested that it was not necessary that materials be sampled from the curriculum (Fuchs & Deno, 1992, 1994). Since that time various companies have made available CBM materials that are available at modest or no cost (e.g., Dynamic Indicators of Early Literacy Skills, AimsWeb, www.interventioncentral.com). Second, CBM procedures require minimal time to administer and score and have demonstrated technical adequacy. Third, the emphasis on fluency, along with accuracy information, permits differentiation between students who are at an acquisition, fluency building, and mastery stage of learning (Binder, 1996). Measuring fluency also facilitates the graphing of student data across time and avoids common ceiling effects.

A fourth advantage of CBM is the relative ease with which multiple equivalent level forms can be developed. Having multiple equivalent forms, that can be administered and scored quickly, permits frequent progress monitoring in the school and/or clinic. These procedures allow for continual evaluation of the effectiveness of instruction and intervention. Studies have found that students make greater academic gains when their teachers use CBM progress monitoring data to guide their instruction decisions

(National Center on Student Progress Monitoring, 2006; Stecker & Fuchs, 2000). Fifth, CBM can serve multiple purposes including: (a) universal screenings, (b) intervention plan design, (c) progress monitoring, and (d) contributing to special education entitlement determination within a problem -solving/RTI model. The fact that CBM can provide reliable and valid information at multiple levels for multiple purposes should result in more resources being available for intervention/treatment with relatively less time needed for collecting assessment data.

CBM for Universal Screening

Universal screening involves the administration of quick, reliable, and valid assessments to all students in a class/grade/school. Using CBM procedures, a class can be screened in the areas of reading, mathematics, and writing. Students' performance can be quickly scored, entered into a spreadsheet, and provided to teachers on the day of administration. Given the cost and time efficiency of CBM, CBM universal screenings can be conducted multiple times across the academic year using probes that are of equivalent difficulty.

Assessing students multiple times with equivalent probes provides data regarding growth as well as current level of performance. Repeated universal screening data permit examination of schools, classrooms, and individuals relative to normative and criterion-based benchmarks for performance and learning (Noell, Gilbertson, VanDerHeyden, & Witt, 2005). This approach permits isolation of the appropriate target for intervention at the school, classroom, or individual level. If the concerns evident for the referred child are also evident for most peers it appears that intervention would most profitably be targeted at the school or classroom level rather than the individual level.

Universal screening data also can be evaluated at the individual level by comparing an individual's current performance and rate of growth to his or her peers who have received similar instruction. Examining how a student compares to his/her peers, allows one to examine the possibility that poor achievement is systemic rather than an individual student problem (Ardoin, Witt, Connel, & Koenig, 2005). Researchers have demonstrated that CBM measures can reliably predict which first-grade students are likely to fail state mandated tests administered in third grade (Good, Simmons, & Kame'enui, 2001; Silberglitt & Hintze, 2005).

Fortunately, the evidence suggests that if provided with intense instruction, using empirically supported procedures, many students at risk for failing state mandated tests and developing later academic problems can catch up to their peers (Coyne, Kame'enui, Simmons, & Harn, 2004; Vellutino, Scanlon, Small, & Fanuele, 2006). Recognizing that those students whose level of achievement is discrepant from their peers commonly continue to fall further behind their peers if not provided with intervention services further emphasizes the need for assessment that can detect trend as well as level (Stanovich, 1986; Torgesen, 2002).

Although typically it is impossible for professionals outside the school to collect universal screening data, a growing number of schools are collecting CBM universal screening data on a triannual basis that can be of great utility to clinicians outside the school. Objective data from standardized assessment such as CBM allow for comparison of a client's performance to peers as well as contributing to evaluation of variables external to the client. Comparing a client's performance to an expected level of performance that is based upon his or her peers provides an indication of whether low levels of performance are specific to the client or are shared by many peers and thus may result from environmental factors.

Providers of CBM materials such as DIBELS (Good, 2004) generally provide criterion scores for student performance across grades and at multiple times across the academic year for predicting which students are at risk for failing state mandated tests. If clinicians do not have access to school-wide data, recommended levels of performance provided by companies that provide CBM materials can be beneficial for predicting a client's success as well as for establishing goals for progress monitoring purposes.

Entitlement and Diagnostic Determination using CBM

With the passage of IDEA 2004, schools may use a response to intervention model in determining students' special education eligibility for Learning Disabilities. Ideally, implementation of RTI models will increase the early identification of students at risk of developing academic problems, reduce the number of students referred for and who are in need of special education services, and reduce the overrepresentation of minorities in special education.

Although several models of RTI exist, the general premise of RTI is that a student's eligibility for special education is based upon the student's response to interventions whose efficacy has been supported by prior research. Students' response to general education is measured, followed by assessment of their response to interventions of increasing intensity.

Students who fail to respond adequately to the regular education curriculum, often referred to as tier 1, are provided with supplemental intervention, which is generally referred to as tier 2. Their response to tier 2 instruction is monitored and if data suggest that a student is not responding adequately to tier 2 instruction, more intense intervention is provided. Should a student not make adequate gains with intense intervention special education eligibility is considered.

A primary source of the data used when making the diagnostic decision is the data collected reflecting the student's progress while being provided with varying levels of intervention (Fuchs & Fuchs, 1998; Vaughn & Fuchs, 2003). Fuchs and Fuchs recommend that a dual discrepancy model be used for making special education entitlement decisions. This approach compares student performance to the level of peers based on CBM universal screening data as well as examining the rate of growth from progress monitoring data.

INTERVENTION: MOVING FROM IDENTIFYING PROBLEMS TO ACTING ON THEM

Assessments that end with the identification of educational concerns have extremely limited utility. Although it may give some a sense of understanding or control to have a name for the problem, a rich literature suggests that identifying academic problems and expecting existing environmental resources such as special education to successfully ameliorate them is unrealistic (Kavale & Forness, 1999). If assessment is going to lead to an improvement in the clients' functioning it will need to lead to an effective treatment plan that is implemented. In simple terms, we need to move from naming the problem to doing something about it.

Academic concerns are similar to other areas of developmental psychopathology in that behavior is determined by a complex interaction of biological and environmental factors. Although this initially can seem an overwhelmingly complex web of causal and mediating factors to assess, it is important to recognize a practical reality. Although behavior may be the result of a complex interaction of many variables, it is frequently quite sensitive to current environmental conditions (e.g., Iwata, Vollmer, & Zarcone, 1990). Stated differently, although a client's poor writing skills may be the result of a complex interplay of schooling, family, and constitutional factors, it may be quite feasible to teach the client how to write competently by directly instructing him or her (e.g., Walker, Shippen, Alberto, Houchins, & Cihak, 2005).

This final section of the chapter describes a general case heuristic for devising academic interventions. The heuristic is organized around six critical questions to be answered in a case conceptualization model for academic concerns. The six questions discussed are:

1. What is the mismatch between the client's academic performance and current expectations?
2. Does the student have the skills necessary to meet academic expectations?
3. Are there environmental conditions that reduce the client's success in meeting academic expectations?
4. How can an effective treatment plan be devised based on individual and environmental assessment data?
5. How can the therapist cause the treatment to be implemented?
6. How should the treatment effects best be monitored?

1. What is the mismatch between the client's academic performance and current expectations?

Referrals regarding academic performance do not arise in a vacuum and may be usefully conceptualized as a mismatch between environmental expectations and behavior. The problem is not necessarily that the client reads 46 words correct per minute (WCPM) in grade-level texts per se, but that students at his school commonly are expected to read 70–100 WCPM by the middle of fifth grade. Additionally, the client's low reading rate can be expected to interfere with reading comprehension and task completion.

The critical challenge at this stage of the assessment process is moving from global concerns to specific target behaviors that can be acted on. Common initial concerns such as failing mathematics or poor reading skills may capture the heart of the referral source's concern without being sufficiently specific to develop a treatment plan. Obviously, defining the difference between expected and actual performance requires asking two preliminary questions. What is it that the client does and what is it he or she is expected to do? If a prior diagnostic assessment was completed, data gathered as part of that assessment may or may not contribute to answering these questions.

Although defining behavior and expectations is conceptually simple, it is practically complex for at least two reasons. First, for most clinicians the point of contact is with the parents; however, they are virtually never the origin of the mismatch between academic performance and expectations. The mismatch almost always will occur between the client and her or his teacher(s). The authors would argue that any psychological assessment of an academic concern that does not include interviews of the client's teachers and observations in school is incomplete.

Second, in many cases, teachers will express their concerns in the global terms that are part of common discourse, "He is not working up to his potential," or "She is failing math." The critical need at this stage of the assessment for treatment process is to move beyond broad generalizations to specifics. What, specifically, must the student need do to work up to his potential or pass her math class? This specification of expectations ideally should be stated in objective measurable terms such as completing weekly quizzes with at least 70% accuracy or completing multiplication and division facts with 100% accuracy at a rate of 30 facts per minute.

The final stage of clarifying the mismatch between actual and expected performance is typically easier than clarifying the expectations, that is, specifying the current performance. The critical thing to bear in mind in this regard is that the problem is not performance on a standardized test of achievement, but performance in the school. What is the client doing and how that is discrepant from expectations? Arriving at specific statements regarding how the client's actual performance differs from the expected performance will set the occasion for additional detailed assessment of the referral concern.

2. Does the student have the skills necessary to meet academic expectations?

Examination of the second and third questions is designed to provide clinicians with a useful hypothesis as to why the client is not meeting instructional expectations. In this context "useful" is used to connote a focus on variables that can be modified to improve the client's functioning. Although it may be the case that intellectual disability is contributing to mathematics failure, that is not something that psychologists have technology to change. On the other hand, we can help arrange environments that increase motivation, teach needed skills, and limit competing stimulation.

Once assessment has identified how the client's behavior is discrepant from expectations, the next stage of the assessment should focus on what the client knows how to do. The fact that a client does not produce acceptable academic products does not mean that the client does not know how to do so (e.g., Duhon et al., 2004). It may well be the case that the client has the requisite skills, but that there is an absence of reinforcement for completing academic tasks or that reinforcement for other behaviors is more potent (e.g., Martens & Houk, 1989).

Prior research has demonstrated relatively simple procedures for differentiating between students who lack sufficient motivation and those who lack basic skills (Noell, Freeland, Witt, & Gansle, 2001). A sample of academic performance is obtained under typical or standardized conditions, which is followed by a repeat assessment with equivalent materials but providing a salient reward contingency for improved performance. Researchers have found that some clients' performances will improve substantially under reward conditions, suggesting primarily a motivational issue rather than a skill deficit (Noell et al.). Additionally, the data demonstrated that relatively brief assessments of motivational issues were predictive of participants' response to intervention. It is important to acknowledge that in the range of presentations that clinicians are confronted with for some clients, a timed test with a reward contingency may not be optimal (e.g., highly anxious clients). However, the conceptual model of reassessing performance under conditions that are optimized for that client to obtain an estimate of skills should be broadly applicable.

If the client does not perform well enough to be judged competent in contexts that have been optimized to obtain a maximal rather than a typical performance, a more detailed assessment of his or her skills is needed. The detailed assessment will focus on the collection of skills that make up the terminal behavior that is the focus of the assessment. The individual steps that are needed to complete the target behavior as well as the prerequisite skills that are needed are collectively described as the subordinate skills. A description of subordinate skills is commonly available in curriculum guides used in schools.

Additionally, clinicians also may choose to complete their own task analyses of the target skill or consult published sources. For example, a writing assignment might be broken down into brainstorming a topic, outlining, drafting, reviewing for clarity of thought, revision for clarity/organization, reviewing for mechanics, and final revision. Detailed information regarding conducting task analyses and developing functionally relevant interventions is beyond the scope of the chapter; however, several resources are available (e.g., Hosp & Ardoin, in press; Hosp, Hosp, & Kurns, in press; Witt, Daly, & Noell, 2000).

Once the relevant academic skills have been identified, assessment should focus on describing the client's accuracy and fluency for each subordinate skill. For example, a student whose target behaviors included addition facts might be asked to read numbers, write numbers, and respond orally to fact operations to isolate key component skills. In this context it typically is most efficient to assess the subordinate skills in a context optimized for performance (e.g., no distractions, contingencies for performance) so that the current maximal performance can be immediately identified. The assessment should yield both accuracy and fluency data that will be critical in the development of intervention planning.

Once accuracy and fluency data for each subordinate skill have been obtained, the next stage of the assessment process should compare those data to standards for competent performance. Unfortunately, clinicians frequently do not have access to accuracy and fluency standards for each relevant subordinate skill. For example, a ready guide is not available for the fluency with which seventh-grade students should solve systems of two three-term equations for two unknowns or how quickly they should provide the functions for all parts of the cell. In this context there is a natural draw toward focusing on accuracy alone. However, fluency is a critical part of many academic skills and often is absolutely necessary for competent performance in many areas.

For example, students who read slowly are more likely to exhibit poor comprehension and difficulty with task completion (Francis et al., 2002). Similarly, fluency with basic operations and writing skills has been linked to success with more advanced academic skills in those domains. The continuum from slow accurate responding to fluent responding also forms the basis for the Instructional Hierarchy (IH) which provides a very useful general case organizational heuristic for developing academic interventions (Haring & Eaton, 1978). The link between accuracy, fluency, and subordinate skills is discussed below in more detail in the section dealing with intervention design.

3. Are there environmental conditions that reduce the client's success in meeting academic expectations?

Any academic assessment that does not examine the current schooling context is incomplete. The context for the client's behavior, the demands, and the expectations are all provided by the school. Numerous environmental conditions that can influence academic performance are observable by visiting classrooms. For example, proximity to the teacher has been found to be beneficial for children with ADHD under some conditions (Granger, Whalen, Henker, & Cantwell, 1996). This might cause one to question why a referred client with ADHD was sitting at the back of the classroom. Similarly, conditions such as crowding, distracting noises, and disruptive behavior by other students can all contribute to poor performance and have been found to differentially affect disabled students (Dockrell & Shield, 2006). Simply visiting and observing the classes the client attends can provide invaluable information about instructional routines, demands, and the classroom context.

Ideally, classroom observations should collect information regarding the antecedents and consequences to the student's appropriate and inappropriate behavior. Such data provide information not only regarding the target student's behavior, but also the behavior of teachers and peers, who may have a substantial influence on the client's behavior. A variety of studies has demonstrated the utility of understanding the pattern of classroom interactions in devising effective interventions for students with or without significant psychopathology (e.g., Martens, 1992; Martens & Houk, 1989; Umbreit, 1995). The data also can be examined to determine the extent to which the client is provided with modeling, opportunities to practice, and corrective feedback for academic performance. It can be quite useful to collect a sample of representative peer data to determine the degree to which the client is an outlier or is typical of the behavior in the classroom (see Witt et al., 2000).

4. How can an effective treatment plan be devised based on the assessment data?

Typically, initial intervention design will consider salient environmental factors whose modification may help the client meet expectations. For example, observing that a distractible client is sitting at the back of the classroom would suggest moving the client to the front of the classroom. Similarly, if observation revealed that the client receives consistent adult and peer attention for off-task and disruptive behavior, initial intervention might focus on shifting the availability of attention from off-task behaviors to work completion (e.g., Northup et al., 1995; Umbreit, 1995). If observation revealed that common classroom routines do not make clear what the expectations and timelines are for assigned work, it may be possible to work with teachers to assure that the client or all students receive this information in a consistent clear format. Classroom-based intervention is a particularly critical element of intervention design when conditions in the classroom substantially limit the client's ability to benefit from instruction, irrespective of individualized intervention outside the classroom. It is also important to acknowledge, that in some cases, no obvious barriers to the client's success will be identified in the classroom.

In most instances, idiographic assessment identifies targets for individualized academic intervention for children and youth referred for academic concerns. Academic assessment results will be described as generally suggesting one of four hypotheses, each of which suggests a particular approach to intervention. First, and perhaps most encouragingly, assessment data may indicate that the student completes academic tasks exceeding criterion levels of accuracy and fluency under optimized conditions such as a reward contingency. This assessment-derived demonstration of previously unobserved skills has been described as a performance deficit, as contrasted with a skill deficit (Noell et al., 2001). The critical elements for the successful treatment of performance deficits include the reduction of reinforcement for alternative behaviors and the increase of reinforcement for the target behavior (Duhon et al., 2004; Martens & Houk, 1989; Noell et al.).

Shifting contingencies to support adaptive behavior can be achieved through many procedures including goal setting with contingencies, school-home notes, and/or self-monitoring systems. Additionally, taking reasonable actions to reduce the clients' access to reinforcers associated with off-task behavior is desirable. The key to intervention for performance deficits is the shifting of environmental contingencies to support use of skills the client possesses.

In other instances, the assessment of the target concerns will reveal deficient skills in either the target skill or subordinate skills, for which the obvious course of action is to program supplemental instruction that will strengthen these skills so that the client can meet educational expectations.

The conceptual heuristic provided by the Instructional Hierarchy (IH, Haring & Eaton, 1978) provides an organizational framework for intervening on academic skill problems that has proven successful. The IH describes the initial stages of skill acquisition as progressing from establishing accuracy to developing fluency. Although establishing accuracy has intuitive appeal and as a result is commonly attended to, the development of fluency frequently receives inadequate attention. Fluency with skills has been demonstrated to contribute to diverse positive outcomes including the skill application and task persistence (Binder, 1996).

Accuracy

Accurate responding is established by programming a sufficient number of complete learning trials (CLT). A complete learning trial minimally consists of programming a discriminative stimulus for the target responses (e.g., an addition problem), an opportunity for response, and feedback on the accuracy of the response. It is critical that the lag between a response and instructor feedback be short enough that clients can learn from the feedback. Generally, younger clients and those who are in the initial stages of learning a skill need more immediate feedback.

Additionally, for early acquisition, extra environmental support for initial correct responding commonly is required. This can take diverse forms, but typically includes a prompt such as a model or physical guidance (Demchak, 1990). A number of prompting procedures have been demonstrated to be successful such as cover-copy-compare, constant time delay, and least-to-most prompting (Skinner, Bamberg, Smith, & Powell, 1993; Wolery et al., 1992). In contexts in which consultation leads to a desire to increase access to CLTs for many students, procedures such as choral responding (Heward, Courson, & Narayan, 1989) and reciprocal peer tutoring (Fantuzzo, King, & Heller, 1992) have been employed extensively and successfully at a classroom level to increase CLTs for all students.

Constant time-delayed prompting (Wolery et al., 1992) is an instructional approach that facilitates correct responding while minimizing student errors. Constant time-delayed prompting begins by presenting students with an instruction demand such as a spelling word, a mathematics operation, or sight word. Following a predefined delay period (e.g., four seconds; Cybriwsky & Schuster, 1990) a model of the correct response is presented if the student has not responded. Procedures for responding to incorrect responses have varied across studies including ignoring incorrect responding and corrective feedback with modeling. Constant time delay is an efficient procedure for establishing accurate responding that is easily taught and relatively easily implemented. Detailed procedural descriptions of constant time-delayed prompting are available in a number of sources (see Wolery et al., 1992 or Handen & Zane, 1987).

Fluency

Once students can respond accurately they will commonly need systematic instruction to develop fluency. The core element of developing fluency is sufficient practice that emphasizes quick responding. The immediacy of feedback for each response is less important at this stage of learning because the student should be responding at or near 100% correct before moving on to fluency building. Instructional feedback should shift to a rate-based assessment of performance and provide informative markers regarding the client's progress toward fluency goals. It is important to consider building motivational elements into fluency-building exercises as they are hard work and can be perceived by some clients as tedious (Noell et al., 1998).

Integration and Generalization

For many clients, intervention should move beyond discrete skills to more elaborate behaviors. Frequently, clients need direct instruction regarding how to integrate component skills to complete more complex tasks. Integrating subordinate skills can be particularly challenging for complex tasks such as essay writing or completing mathematics application problems. Intervention providing modeling of skill integration, strategy instruction, and self-monitoring skills have been used successfully to aid skill integration (Davis & Hajicek, 1985; Dunlap & Dunlap, 1989; Howell & Nolet, 2000). A model can help clients generalize and integrate skills by making it clear to them how they can combine their skills and abilities to solve new challenges.

Strategy instruction teaches the client how to combine previously mastered skills to create a problem-solving process and frequently includes "verbal mediation" in which the students talk themselves through the process of solving the problem (Davis & Hajicek). Self-monitoring is similar to strategy instruction in that the emphasis is on providing students with new organizational skills to help them mediate the use of their subordinate skills. Self-monitoring as an instructional strategy commonly includes providing clients a written guide that cues them how to complete the task and training on how to self-monitor.

5. How can the therapist cause the treatment to be implemented?

The reality that a consulting psychologist or other mental health care provider is virtually never the person providing academic intervention greatly increases the risk that intervention plans will not be implemented. Researchers examining intervention in schools as well as research with parents suggests that treatment implementation and/or utilization are far from assured and can be extremely problematic (Noell, Witt, et al., 2005). The school-based literature examining treatment plan implementation has repeatedly demonstrated poor and deteriorating implementation in the absence of systematic follow-up (Noell, Witt, et al., 2005). The critical elements that have been demonstrated effective in sustaining implementation have been objective assessment of implementation with the intervention's permanent products, graphing implementation and student outcome, and feedback to the treatment agent on implementation (see Noell, 2008, for a review). This model appears to be practical in many contexts treating psychopathology. The intervention agent can be asked to bring the work products in for a weekly review and consultation regarding the academic intervention as well as other pertinent issues can be provided.

6. How should the treatment effects best be monitored?

Multiple studies have demonstrated that monitoring a student's performance across time and making instructional decisions based upon those data result in greater academic gains for students than when teachers do not have access to CBM progress monitoring data (National Center on Student Progress Monitoring, 2006; Stecker & Fuchs, 2000). CBM progress monitoring procedures generally entail administering a CBM probe twice weekly and plotting the data in time series fashion.

One of two procedures typically is used for evaluating the data and determining whether intervention modifications are needed. The most common approach uses a goal line plotted on the graph. This goal line is established with its origin at the median point of the first three data points collected and the endpoint located at the desired level of fluency at projected end of intervention for that skill. The desired terminal rate can be determined based on a published criterion, local norm, or research-based norms (see Hosp et al., 2007 for researched based norms). Typically, if four consecutive data points fall below the goal line, intervention modification is suggested (Marston & Tindal, 1996).

A procedure used less frequently is to calculate a slope based upon sufficient data and make modifications if the growth rate is less than desired. Although ten data points are considered sufficient by many for evaluating intervention effectiveness (Good & Shinn, 1990), recent research suggests that substantially more data are needed in order to accurately predict a client's growth rate (Christ, 2006; Christ & Silberglitt, in press). Regardless of the procedure used for evaluating intervention effectiveness, caution should be taken when evaluating data based upon less than 15 data points across seven weeks, and confidence intervals should be placed around slope estimates (Christ, 2006).

SUMMARY AND CONCLUSION

Assessment of academic concerns is driven by the same assessment questions as the assessment of childhood psychopathology more broadly: what is the problem and what can be done about it? At a practical level, the question of problem specification frequently will include both diagnostic considerations and more molecular examination of academic skills. Diagnosis may be the referral sources' initial concern and also may be necessary to obtain services for the client. However, current diagnostic systems for academic concerns (IDEA and DSM–TV–TR) lack treatment utility (Gresham & Gansle, 1992). Current diagnoses are not sufficiently detailed to guide treatment selection.

In addition, the types of instruments that commonly are used to make diagnostic determinations have very limited treatment utility due to the limited coverage of specific skills at any given level (Marston et al., 1986). Also, many achievement instruments assess academic skill at the level of broad constructs (e.g., broad reading or mathematics) rather than specific skills (e.g., completes addition facts at 95% accuracy and 25 digits correct per minute). Under IDEA, newer approaches to diagnosis in schools using CBM within RTI models potentially can use data that have both treatment utility and diagnostic utility.

Moving to the second question, treatment specification, typically occasions a shift in assessment methods to specific behaviors and expectations within the school context. CBM and similar direct, low inference, and rate-based measures of academic behavior have demonstrated both treatment utility and adequate reliability and validity (Ardoin et al., 2004; Fuchs, Fuchs, Hamlett, & Allinder, 1989; Fuchs et al., 1994; Gansle et al., 2004). Additionally, consideration of classroom expectations and environmental factors that may be influencing achievement can provide a contextualized assessment picture that can lead to a useful case formulation and treatment plan.

Intervention planning for academic concerns typically begins by operationally defining the ways in which the client's performance fails to meet expectations. This, in turn, should lead to assessment of the specific skills the client possesses in some detail. Assessment typically should also examine the possibility that motivation plays a pivotal role in poor current functioning and that environmental factors adversely affect academic performance. This should lead to an intervention plan based on the specific needs of the client at his or her current stage of skill acquisition. The final and potentially most critical element for assuring effective services for children exhibiting academic concerns and psychopathology is assuring that services are delivered as designed and that meaningful progress monitoring data are collected to guide ongoing program modification.

REFERENCES

Achenbach, T. M., & Edelbrock, C. S. (1991). *Manual for the Child Behavior Checklist.* Burlington, VT: University of Vermont, Department of Psychiatry.

American Association on Mental Retardation (2002). *Definition of mental retardation.* Retrieved February 20, 2007, from the AAMR website: http://www.aamr.org/Policies/faq_mental_retardation.shtml.

American Psychiatric Association. (2000). *Diagnostic and statistical manual of mental disorders* (4th ed., text revision). Washington, DC: Author.

Ardoin, S. P., Witt, J. C., Connell, J. E., & Koenig, J. (2005). Application of a three-tiered response to intervention model for instructional planning, decision making, and the identification of children in need of services. *Journal of Psychoeducational Assessment, 23,* 362–380.

Ardoin, S. P., Witt, J. C., Suldo, S. M., Connell, J. E., Koenig, J. L., Resetar, J. L., & Slider, N. J. (2004). Examining the incremental benefits of administering a maze and three versus one curriculum-based measurement reading probe when conducting universal screening. *School Psychology Review, 33,* 218–233.

Biederman, J., Faraone, S. V., Mick, E., Williamson, S., Wilens, T. E., Spencer, T. J., Weber, W., Jetton, J., Kraus, I., Pert, J., & Zallen, B. (1999). Clinical correlates of ADHD in females: Findings from a large group of girls ascertained from pediatric and psychiatric referral sources. *Journal of the American Academy of Child & Adolescent Psychiatry. 38,* 966–975.

Binder, C. (1996). Behavioral fluency: Evolution of a new paradigm. *The Behavior Analyst, 19*, 163–197.

Bruininks, R. H., Woodcock, R. W., Weatherman, R. F., & Hill, B. K. (1996). *Scales of Independent Behavior—Revised*. Itasca, IL: Riverside.

Christ, T. J. (2006). Short term estimates of growth using curriculum-based measurement of oral reading fluency: Estimates of standard error of the slope to construct confidence intervals. *School Psychology Review, 35*, 128–133.

Christ, T. J., & Silberglitt, B. (in press). Curriculum-based measurement of oral reading fluency: The standard error of measurement. *School Psychology Review*.

Connell, J. E., Jr. (2006). Constructing a math applications, curriculum-based assessment: An analysis of the relationship between applications problems, computation problems and criterion-referenced assessments. Ann Arbor, MI: ProQuest Information & Learning.

Conners, C. K. (1997). *Conners' Rating Scales-Revised*. North Tonawanda, NY: Multi-Health Systems.

Connolly, A. J. (1997, norms; 1988, content). *KeyMath-revised/Normative update*. Bloomington, MN: Pearson Assessments.

Coyne, M. D., Kame'enui, E. J., Simmons, D. C., & Harn, B. A. (2004). Beginning reading intervention as inoculation or insulin: First-grade reading performance of strong responders to kindergarten intervention. *Journal of Learning Disabilities, 37*, 90–104.

Cybriwsky, C. A., & Schuster, J. W. (1990). Using constant time delay procedures to teach multiplication facts. *RASE: Remedial and Special Education, 11*, 54–59.

Davis, R. W., & Hajicek, J. O. (1985). Effects of self-instructional training and strategy training on a mathematics task with severely behaviorally disordered students. *Behavioral Disorders, 10*, 275–282.

Demchak, M. (1990). Response prompting and fading methods: A review. *American Journal on Mental Retardation, 94*, 603–615.

Deno, S. L. (1985). Curriculum-based measurement: The emerging alternative. *Exceptional Children, 52*, 219–232.

Deno, S. L., Marston, D., & Mirkin, P. K. (1982). Valid measurement procedures for continuous evaluation of written expression. *Exceptional Children, 48*, 368–371.

Deno, S. L., Mirkin, P. K., & Marston, D. (1980). *Relationships among simple measures of written expression and performance on standardized achievement tests* (Research Report No. 22). Minneapolis, MN: University of Minnesota, Institute for Research on Learning Disabilities.

Dockrell, J. E., & Shield, B. M. (2006). Acoustical barriers in classrooms: The impact of noise on performance in the classroom. *British Educational Research Journal, 32*, 509–525.

Duhon, G. J., Noell, G. H., Witt, J. C., Freeland, J. T., Dufrene, B. A., & Gilbertson, D. N. (2004). Identifying academic skill and performance deficits: The experimental analysis of brief assessments of academic skills. *School Psychology Review, 33*, 429–443.

Dunlap, L. K., & Dunlap, G. (1989). A self-monitoring package for teaching subtraction with regrouping to students with learning disabilities. *Journal of Applied Behavior Analysis, 22*, 309–314.

Espin, C., Shin, J., Deno, S. L., Skare, S., Robinson, S., & Benner, B. (2000). Identifying indicators of written expression proficiency for middle school students. *Journal of Special Education, 34*, 140–153.

Fantuzzo, J. F., King, J. A., & Heller, L. R. (1992). Effects of reciprocal peer tutoring on mathematics and school adjustment: A component analysis. *Journal of Educational Psychology, 84*, 331–339.

Fletcher, J. M., Espy, K. A., Francis, D. J., Davidson, K. C., Rourke, B. P., & Shaywitz, S. E. (1989). Comparison of cutoff and regression-based definitions of reading disabilities. *Journal of Learning Disabilities, 22*, 334–338.

Fletcher, J. M., Francis, D. J., Morris, R. D., Lyon, G. R. (2005). Evidence-based assessment of learning disabilities in children and adolescents. *Journal of Clinical Child and Adolescent Psychology, 34*, 506–522.

Fletcher, J. M., Francis, D. J., Shaywitz, S. E., Lyon, G. R., Foorman, B. R., Stuebing, K. K, & Shaywitz, B. A. (1998). Intelligent testing and the discrepancy model for children with learning disabilities. *Learning Disabilities Research and Practice, 13,* 186–203.

Fletcher, J. M., Lyon, G. R., Barnes, M., Stuebing, K. K., Francis, D. J., Olson, R. K., & Shaywitz, S. E., & Shaywitz, B. A. (2002). Classification of learning disabilities: An evidence-based evaluation. In R. Bradley, L. Danielson, & D. P. Hallahan (Eds.) *Identification of learning disabilities: Research to practice* (pp. 185–250). Mahwah, NJ: Lawrence Erlbaum.

Francis, D. J., Fuchs, L. S., Good, R. H., III, O'Connor, R. E., Simmons, D. C., Tindal, G., & Torgesen, J. K. (2002). Analysis of reading assessments instruments for K-3: Results by grade. Retrieved August 24, 2003, from http://idea.uoregon.edu/assessment/analysis_results/se_lists/assess_grade.pdf.

Frisby, C. (1987). Alternative assessment committee report: Curriculum-based assessment. *CASP Today, 36,* 15–26.

Fuchs, L. S., & Deno, S. L. (1992). Effects of curriculum within curriculum-based measurement. *Exceptional Children, 58,* 232–242.

Fuchs, L. S., & Deno, S. L. (1994). Must instructional useful performance assessment be based in the curriculum? *Exceptional Children, 61,* 15–24.

Fuchs, L. S., & Fuchs, D. (1998). Treatment validity: A unifying concept for reconceptualizing the identification of learning disabilities. *Learning Disabilities Research and Practice, 13,* 204–219.

Fuchs, L. S., Fuchs, D., Hamlett, C. L., & Allinder, R. M. (1989). The reliability and validity of skills analysis within curriculum-based measurement. *Diagnostique, 14,* 203–221.

Fuchs, L. S., Fuchs, D., Hamlett, C. L., Thompson, A., Roberts, P. H., Kubek, P., & Stecker, P. M. (1994). Technical features of a mathematics concepts and applications curriculum-based measurement system. *Diagnostique, 19,* 23–49.

Gansle, K. A., Gilbertson, D. N. & VanDerHeyden, A. M. (2006). Elementary school teachers' perceptions of curriculum-based measures of written expression. *Practical Assessment Research & Evaluation, 11(5),* 1–17. Available online: http://pareonline.net/getvn.asp?v=11&n=5.

Gansle, K. A., Noell, G. H., VanDerHeyden, A. M., Naquin, G. M., & Slider, N. J. (2002). Moving beyond total words written: The reliability, criterion validity, and time cost of alternate measures for curriculum-based measurement in writing. *School Psychology Review, 31,* 477–497.

Gansle, K. A., Noell, G. H., Vanderheyden, A. M., Slider, N. J., Hoffpauir, L. D., Whitmarsh, E. L., & Naquin, G. M. (2004). An examination of the criterion validity and sensitivity to brief intervention of alternate curriculum-based measures of writing skill. *Psychology in the Schools, 41,* 291–300.

Gansle, K. A., VanDerHeyden, A. M., Noell, G. H., Resetar, J. L., & Williams, K. L. (2006). The technical adequacy of curriculum-based and rating-based measures of written expression for elementary school students. *School Psychology Review, 35,* 435–450.

Good, R. H., III, & Kaminski, R. A. (2002). *Dynamic Indicators of Basic Early Literacy Skills* (6th ed.). Eugene, OR: Institute for the Development of Educational Achievement. Available: http://dibels.uoregon.edu.

Good, R. H., III, & Shinn, M. R. (1990). Forecasting accuracy of slope estimates for reading curriculum-based measurement: Empirical evidence. *Behavioral Assessment, 12,* 179–193.

Good, R. H., III, Simmons, D. C., & Kame'enui, E. J. (2001). The importance and decision making utility of continuum of fluency-based indicators of foundational reading skills for third grade high-stakes outcomes. *Scientific Studies of Reading, 5,* 257–288.

Good, R. H., III. (2004). Using the Dynamic Indicators of Basic Early Literacy (DIBELS). Retrieved May 10th, 2004, from http://dibels.uoregon.edu/index.php.

Granger, D. A., Whalen, C. K., Henker, B., & Cantwell, C. (1996). ADHD boys' behavior during structured classroom social activities: Effects of social demands, teacher proximity, and methylphenidate. *Journal of Attention Disorders, 1,* 16–30.

Gresham, F. M. (2002). Responsiveness to intervention: An alternative approach to the identification of learning disabilities. In R. Bradley, L. Danielson, & D. P. Hallahan (Eds.) *Identification of learning disabilities: Research to practice* (pp. 467–519). Mahwah, NJ: Lawrence Erlbaum.

Gresham, F. M., & Gansle, K. A. (1992). Misguided assumptions of DSM–III–R: Implications for school psychological practice. *School Psychology Quarterly, 7,* 79–95.

Gresham. F. M., & Witt, J. C. (1997). Utility of intelligence tests for treatment planning, classification, and placement decisions: Recent empirical findings and future directions. *School Psychology Quarterly, 12,* 249–267.

Hammill, D. D., & Larsen, S. C. (1996). *Test of written language* (3rd ed.). Austin, TX: Pro-Ed.

Handen, B. L., & Zane, T. (1987). Delayed prompting: A review of procedural variations and results. *Research in Developmental Disabilities, 8,* 307–330.

Haring, N. G., & Eaton, M. D. (1978). Systematic procedures: An instructional hierarchy. In N. G. Haring, T. C. Lovitt, M. D. Eaton & C. L. Hansen (Eds.), *The fourth R: Research in the classroom.* Columbus, Ohio: Charles E. Merrill.

Haynes, S. N., & O'Brien, W. H. (2000). *Principles and practices of behavioral assessment.* New York: Kluwer Academic/Plenum.

Heward, W. L. (2006). *Exceptional children: An introduction to special education* (8th ed.). Upper Saddle River, NJ: Pearson Education.

Heward, W. L., Courson, F. H., & Narayan, J. S. (1989). Using choral responding to increase active student response during group instruction. *Teaching Exceptional Children, 21,* 72–75.

Hoover, H. D., Hieronymus, A. N., Frisbie, D. A., & Dunbar, S. B. (1996). *Iowa tests of basic skills.* Itasca, IL: Riverside.

Hosp, J. L., & Ardoin, S. P. (in press). Assessment for instructional planning. *Assessment for Effective Intervention.*

Hosp, M. K., Hosp, J. L., & Howell, K. W. (2007). *The ABCs of CBM: A practical guide to curriculum-based measurement.* New York: Guilford Press.

Howell, K. W., & Nolet, V. (2000). *Curriculum-based evaluation: Teaching and decision making* (3rd ed.). Belmont, CA: Wadsworth.

Individuals with Disabilities Education Improvement Act of 2004, 20 U.S.C. § 1400 *et seq.*

Iwata, B. A., Vollmer, T. R., & Zarcone, J. R. (1990). The experimental (functional) analysis of behavior disorders: Methodology, applications, and limitations. In A. C. Repp & N. N. Singh (Eds.), *Perspectives on the use of nonaversive and aversive interventions for persons with developmental disabilities* (pp. 301–330). Sycamore, IL: Sycamore.

Jewell, J., & Malecki, C. K. (2005). The utility of CBM written language indices: An investigation of production-dependent, production-independent, and accurate-production scores. *School Psychology Review, 34,* 27–44.

Jimerson, S., Carlson, E., Rotert, M., Egeland, B., & Sroufe, L. A. (1997). A prospective, longitudinal study of the correlates and consequences of early grade retention. *Journal of School Psychology, 35,* 3–25.

Johnson, W., McGue, M., Iacono, W. G. (2006). Genetic and environmental influences on academic achievement trajectories during adolescence. *Developmental Psychology, 42,* 514–532.

Kaminski, R. A., & Good III, R. H. (1996). Toward a technology for assessing basic early literacy skills. *School Psychology Review, 25,* 215–227.

Kavale, K. A. (2002). Discrepancy models in the identification of learning disability. In R. Bradley, L. Danielson, & D. P. Hallahan (Eds.), *Identification of learning disabilities: Research to practice* (pp. 369–426). Mahwah, NJ: Lawrence Erlbaum.

Kavale, K. A., & Forness, S. R. (1999). Effectiveness of special education. In C. R. Reynolds & T. B. Gutkin (Eds.), *The handbook of school psychology* (3rd ed., pp. 984–1024). New York: Wiley.

Kelley, M. L., Reitman, D., & Noell, G. H. (2002). *Practitioner's guide to empirically based measures of school behavior.* New York: Kluwer Academic/Plenum.

Lambert, N., Nihira, K., & Leland, H. (1993). *AAMR adaptive behavior scales—School: 2nd ed.* Austin, TX: Pro-Ed.

Lloyd, J. W., Kauffman, J. M., Landrum, T. J., & Roe, D. L. (1991). Why do teachers refer pupils for special education? An analysis of referral records. *Exceptionality, 2,* 115–126.

Lyon, G. R. (1996). Learning disabilities. *The Future of Children: Special Education for Students with Disabilities, 6,* 56–76.

MacGinitie, W., MacGinitie, R., Maria, R. K., & Dreyer, L. G. (2000). *Gates–MacGinitie reading tests* (4th ed.). Itasca, IL: Riverside.

MacMillan, D. L., Gresham, F. M., & Bocian, K. M. (1998). Discrepancy between definitions of learning disabilities and school practices: An empirical investigation. *Journal of Learning Disabilities, 31,* 314–326.

MacMillan, D. L., & Siperstein, G. N. (2002). Learning disabilities as operationally defined by schools. In R. Bradley, L. Danielson, & D. P. Hallahan (Eds.), *Identification of learning disabilities: Research to practice* (pp. 287–333). Mahwah, NJ: Lawrence Erlbaum.

Marston, D., & Deno, S. L. (1981). *The reliability of simple, direct measures of written expression* (Research Report No. 50). Minneapolis, MN: University of Minnesota, Institute for Research on Learning Disabilities.

Marston, D., & Tindal, G. (1996). Best practices in performance monitoring. In A. Thomas & J. Grimes (Eds.), *Best Practices in School Psychology III.* Bethesda, MD: NASP Publications.

Marston, D., Fuchs, L. S., & Deno, S. I. (1986). Measuring pupil progress: A comparison of standardized achievement tests and curriculum-related measures. *Diagnostique, 11,* 71–90.

Martens, B. K. (1992). Contingency and choice: The implications of matching theory for classroom instruction. *Journal of Behavioral Education, 2,* 121–137.

Martens, B. K., & Houk, J. L. (1989). The application of Hernstein's law of effect to disruptive and on-task behavior of a retarded adolescent girl. *Journal of the Experimental Analysis of Behavior, 51,* 17–27.

Mercer, C. D., Jordan, L., Allsopp, D. H., & Mercer, A. R. (1996). Learning disabilities definitions and criteria used by state education departments. *Learning Disability Quarterly, 19,* 217–232.

Messick, S. (1995). Validity of psychological assessment. *American Psychologist, 50,* 741–749.

Montague, M., Enders, C., & Castro, M. (2005). Academic and behavioral outcomes for students at risk for emotional and behavioral disorders. *Behavioral Disorders, 31,* 84–94.

National Center on Student Progress Monitoring. (2006). What are the benefits of progress monitoring? Retrieved October 02, 2006, from www.studentprogress.org.

Nihira, K., Leland, H., & Lambert, N. (1993). *AAMR adaptive behavior scales—Residential and community: 2nd ed.* Austin, TX: Pro-Ed.

Noell, G. H. (2008). Research examining the relationships among consultation process, treatment integrity, and outcomes. In W. P. Erchul & S. M. Sheridan (Eds.) *Handbook of research in school consultation: Empirical foundations for the field.* Mahwah, NJ: Lawrence Erlbaum. pp. 323–342.

Noell, G. H., Freeland, J. T., Witt, J. C., & Gansle, K. A. (2001). Using brief assessments to identify effective interventions for individual students. *Journal of School Psychology, 39,* 335–355.

Noell, G. H., Gansle, K. A., Witt, J. C., Whitmarsh, E. L., Freeland, J. T., LaFleur, L. H., Gilbertson, D. A. & Northup, J. (1998). Effects of contingent reward and instruction on oral reading performance at differing levels of passage difficulty. *Journal of Applied Behavior Analysis, 31,* 659–664.

Noell, G. H., Gilbertson, D. N., VanDerHeyden, A. M., & Witt, J. C. (2005). Eco-Behavioral Assessment and Intervention for Culturally Diverse At-Risk Students. In C. L. Frisby & C. R. Reynolds (Eds.) *Comprehensive handbook of multicultural school psychology* (pp. 904–927). Hoboken, NJ: John Wiley & Sons.

Noell, G. H., Witt, J. C., Slider, N. J., Connell, J. E., Gatti, S. L., Williams, K. L., Koenig, J. L., Resetar, J. L., & Duhon, G. J. (2005). Treatment implementation following behavioral consultation in schools: A comparison of three follow-up strategies. *School Psychology Review, 34,* 87–106.

Northup, J., Broussard, C., Jones, K., George, T., Vollmer, T. R., & Herring, M. (1995). The differential effects of teacher and peer attention on the disruptive classroom behavior of three children with a diagnosis of attention deficit hyperactivity disorder. *Journal of Applied Behavior Analysis, 28*, 227–228.

Rehabilitation Act of 1973, as amended, 29 U.S.C. § 794 (Section 504).

Reynolds, C. R., & Kamphaus, R. W. (1998). *Behavior assessment system for children-Revised.* Circle Pines, MN: American Guidance Service.

Rush, A. J., & Francis, A. (Eds.). (2000). Expert consensus guideline series: Treatment of psychiatric and behavioral problems in mental retardation. *American Journal of Mental Retardation, 105*, 159–228.

Schalock, R. L. (Ed.). (1999). *Adaptive behavior and its measurement: Implications for the field of mental retardation.* Washington, DC: American Association on Mental Retardation.

Shapiro, E. S. (1996). *Academic skills problems: Direct assessment and intervention (2nd ed.).* New York: Guilford.

Shaywitz, S. E., Shaywitz, B. A., Fletcher, J. M., & Escobar M. D. (1990). Prevalence of reading disability in boys and girls: Results of the Connecticut Longitudinal Study. *Journal of the American Medical Association, 264*, 998–1002.

Shinn, M. R. (1989). *Curriculum-based measurement: Assessing special children.* New York: Guilford Press.

Silberglitt, B., & Hintze, J. M. (2005). Formative assessment using CBM-R cut scores to track progress toward success on state-mandated achievement test: A comparison of methods. *Journal of Psychoeducational Assessment, 23*, 304–325.

Skinner, C. H., Bamberg, J. W., Smith, E. S., & Powell, S. S. (1993). Cognitive cover, copy, and compare: Subvocal responding to increase rates of accurate division responding. *RASE: Remedial and Special Education, 14*, 49–56.

Sparrow, S. S., Balla, D. A., & Cicchetti, D. (1984). *Vineland adaptive behavior scales.* Circle Pines, MN: American Guidance Service.

Stanovich, K. E. (1986). Matthew effects in reading: Some consequences of individual differences in the acquisition of literacy. *Reading Research Quarterly, 21*, 360–407.

Stecker, P. M., & Fuchs, L. S. (2000). Effecting superior achievement using curriculum-based measurement: The importance of progress monitoring. *Learning Disabilities Research & Practice, 15*, 128–134.

Thorndike, R. L., Hagen, E. P., & Sattler, J. M. (1986). *Technical manual, the Stanford-Binet intelligence scale: 4th ed.* Chicago, IL: Riverside.

Thurber, R. S., Shinn, M. R., & Smolkowski, K. (2002). What is measured in mathematics tests? Construct validity of curriculum-based mathematics measures. *School Psychology Review, 31*, 498–513.

Tindal, G., & Parker, R. (1989). Assessment of written expression for students in compensatory and special education programs. *Journal of Special Education, 23*, 169–183.

Torgesen, J. K. (2002). The prevention of reading difficulties. *Journal of School Psychology, 40*, 7–26.

U. S. Office of Education. (1977). Procedures for evaluating specific learning disabilities. *Federal Register, 42*, 65082–65085.

Umbreit, J. (1995). Functional assessment and intervention in a regular classroom setting for the disruptive behavior of a student with attention deficit hyperactivity disorder. *Behavioral Disorders, 20*, 267–278.

Vaughn, S., & Fuchs, L. S. (2003). Redefining learning disabilities as inadequate response to instruction: The promise and potential problems. *Learning Disabilities Research & Practice, 18*, 137–146.

Vellutino, F. R., Scanlon, D. M., Small, S., & Fanuele, D. P. (2006). Response to intervention as a vehicle for distinguishing between children with and without reading disabilities: Evidence for the role of kindergarten and first-grade interventions. *Journal of Learning Disabilities, 39*, 157–169.

Videen, J., Deno, S., & Marston, D. (1982). *Correct word sequences: A valid indicator of proficiency in written expression* (Research Report No. 84). Minneapolis, MN: University of Minnesota, Institute for Research in Learning Disabilities.

Walker, B., Shippen, M. E., Alberto, P., Houchins, D. E., & Cihak, D. F. (2005). Using the expressive writing program to improve the writing skills of high school students with learning disabilities. *Learning Disabilities Research & Practice, 20*, 175–183.

Wechsler, D. (1991). *Wechsler intelligence scale for children, 3rd ed.*, San Antonio, TX: Psychological Corporation.

Witt, J. C., Daly, E. J., III, & Noell, G. H. (2000). *Functional assessments: A step-by-step guide to solving academic and behavior problems.* Longmont, CO: Sopris West.

Wolery, M., Holcombe, A., Cybriwsky, C., Doyle, P. M., Schuster, J. W., Ault, M. J., & Gast, D. L. (1992). Constant time delay with discrete responses: A review of effectiveness and demographic, procedural, and methodological parameters. *Research in Developmental Disabilities, 13,* 239–266.

Woodcock, R. W., McGrew, K. S., & Mather, N. (2001). *Woodcock–Johnson tests of achievement* (3rd ed.). Itasca, IL: Riverside.

Ysseldyke, J. (2001). Reflections on a research career: Generalizations from 25 years of research on assessment and instructional decision making. *Exceptional Children, 67,* 295–309.

12

Behavioral Assessment of Self-Injury

TIMOTHY R. VOLLMER,
KIMBERLY N. SLOMAN,
and CARRIE S.W. BORRERO

INTRODUCTION

Self-injurious behavior (SIB) is a behavior disorder that can range in severity from self-inflicted mild bruising and abrasions, to life-threatening tissue damage (Carr, 1977). The focus of this chapter is on SIB displayed by individuals with developmental disabilities (DD), including autism. Although SIB occurs in psychiatric patients (e.g., self-mutilation) and in some otherwise typically developing adolescents and adults (e.g., self-cutting), these variations of SIB are not the focus here. In addition, this chapter focuses on assessment rather than treatment. Finally, the specific focus is behavioral assessment rather than medical, biological, or psychiatric (diagnostic) assessment.

The numerous forms (topographies) of SIB described in clinical reports and scientific publications include self-hitting, head banging, self-biting, self-scratching, self-pinching, self-choking, eye gouging, hair pulling, and many others (Iwata et al., 1994b). Although there are clear genetic and biological correlates with the disorder (e.g., Lesch & Nyhan, 1964), the majority of SIB appears to be learned behavior. Not including tics and related behavior, most of human behavior can be compartmentalized as either operant or reflexive (and respondent) behavior. There is no empirical evidence that SIB occurs in a fashion similar to a tic or nervous twitch.

TIMOTHY R. VOLLMER • Psychology Department, University of Florida, Gainesville, Florida 32611, 352-392-0601 ext. 280, vollmera@ufl.edu
KIMBERLY N. SLOMAN • Department of Psychology, University of Florida, Gainesville, FL 32611
CARRIE S.W. BORRERO • Kennedy Krieger Institute, Johns Hopkins university Meidcal School, Baltimore, MD 21205

J.L. Matson et al. (eds.), *Assessing Childhood Psychopathology and Developmental Disabilities*, DOI: 10.1007/978-0-387-09528-8,
© Springer Science+Business Media, LLC 2009

The vast majority of evidence suggests that SIB is operant behavior controlled by either automatic (nonsocially mediated) or socially mediated consequences. There is some evidence that a minority of SIB could be reflexive, but that evidence is indirect and not the focus of this chapter. The only evidence to date supporting SIB as reflexive behavior is found in the research on biting by various species that occurs in response to severe aversive stimulation (e.g., Hutchinson, 1977). Specifically, laboratory research has shown that many species of animals, including humans, will bite down on virtually whatever is available when certain kinds of aversive stimulation such as shock or loud noise are presented. Conceivably then, some self-biting might occur in response to either unconditioned or conditioned aversive stimuli.

The clearest evidence supports the notion that SIB is operant behavior strengthened (reinforced) by consequences to the behavior. The behavior is often so severe and so disturbing that care providers tend to act immediately and decisively to end an episode or bout of self-injury. Although well meaning, actions to end an episode of SIB might inadvertently reinforce the behavior. For example, one common care provider response is to give attention in the form of reprimands or comfort statements when severe behavior occurs (e.g., Sloman et al., 2005; Thompson & Iwata, 2001).

Social attention might serve as a source of socially mediated positive reinforcement for the SIB. Research has shown that even reprimands can serve as positive reinforcement, despite a clear intent of the care provider to scold or punish the behavior (e.g. Fisher, Ninness, Piazza, & Owen-DeSchryver, 1996). Other care providers may be inclined to comfort or nurse the individual following episodes of SIB (e.g., Fischer, Iwata, & Worsdell, 1997). Similarly, care providers may attempt to figure out what the individual "is upset about" and begin handing over tangible items including food, drinks, favorite toys or activities (e.g., Marcus & Vollmer, 1996).

Conversely, escape from or avoidance of social interaction might serve as a source of socially mediated negative reinforcement for SIB. A common response of care providers is to move away from and terminate ongoing activity when SIB occurs, thus allowing escape or avoidance of an interaction that normally would have ensued. For example, dozens of behavioral assessment studies have shown that escape and avoidance of instructional activities, self-care activity, and daily living activity can reinforce SIB (e.g., Iwata, Pace, Kalsher, Cowdery, & Cataldo, 1990; Steege et al., 1990; Vollmer, Marcus, & Ringdahl, 1995). Similarly, some studies have shown that escape from close proximity during medical examinations (Iwata et al., 1990) or even during regular social interaction can reinforce SIB.

Not all SIB is reinforced by the actions of other people. In some cases, SIB produces its own source of reinforcement, independent of the social environment. In fact, some individuals with SIB will sit in a room alone for extended time periods engaging in repetitive SIB, even though the behavior produces no social reaction. In these cases, SIB is maintained by automatic reinforcement, meaning that no social mediation is required for the reinforcement. The specific sources of automatic reinforcement are not as well understood as the specific sources of socially mediated reinforcement, but there is some evidence that SIB can be automatically reinforced by pain attenuation (e.g., Fisher et al., 1998), attenuation of itching skin (e.g., Cowdery, Iwata, & Pace, 1990), pleasing self-stimulation (e.g., Lovaas, Newsom, & Hickman, 1987), and production of endogenous opiates (e.g., Sandman et al., 1983), among other possible sources.

One general purpose of a behavioral assessment of SIB is to identify which types of reinforcement are maintaining SIB in a given case. It cannot be assumed that SIB that looks similar in two different individuals serves the same function for both individuals. Conversely, similar forms of reinforcement can maintain SIB that looks very different in topography (e.g., head hitting by one individual and self-biting by another individual). Even one form of SIB displayed by a single person can serve multiple functions (Smith, Iwata, Vollmer, & Zarcone, 1993). Complications such as these underscore the need for individualized behavioral assessments. Typically, assessment components aimed at identifying the operant function of SIB involve some combination of interviews and checklists given to care providers, direct observation by a trained observer, or a functional analysis in which hypothesized reinforcers are tested. Identifying the specific source of reinforcement has powerful implications for treatment. For example, if SIB is reinforced by social attention, care providers can be taught to minimize attention following SIB and to reinforce some alternative attention-getting behavior.

A second general (but related) purpose of a behavioral assessment of SIB is to identify situations correlated with the occurrence of SIB. If SIB is most likely to occur during particular activities or kinds of activities, an intervention or further assessment may be focused on that particular activity or set of activities. Interviews and checklists, direct observation, and functional analyses are also used for this purpose.

A third general purpose of a behavioral assessment of SIB is to provide a baseline of the severity of the behavior in terms of response rate or tissue damage incurred. In so doing, the effects of behavioral or medical treatments can be compared to the period prior to intervention. Again, interviews and checklists, direct observation, and functional analyses are used for this purpose. In addition, severity charts and scales can be used to document changes in wound appearance (self-injury trauma (SIT) scale; Iwata, Pace, Kissel, Nau, & Farber, 1990) and wound size (Wilson, Iwata, & Bloom, in press).

This chapter is divided into sections describing behavioral assessment formats for SIB. The first section describes variations of interview and checklist approaches to assessment. The second section describes variations of descriptive analysis methods conducted via direct observation of SIB. The third section describes variations of functional analysis methods. The fourth section describes variations of severity scales and charts. All sections include a discussion of advantages and disadvantages of assessment formats.

INDIRECT ASSESSMENTS

Indirect assessments are used to identify relevant characteristics of SIB, without directly observing the behavior. The assessment typically occurs at a different time and place from the actual occurrence of the self-injury.

Indirect assessments rely on reports in the form of records (e.g., school discipline referrals, medical records), interviews (e.g., O'Neil, Horner, Albin, Sprague, Storey, & Newton, 1997), questionnaires (e.g., Lewis, Scott, & Sugai, 1994), checklists (e.g., Van Houten & Rolider, 1991), or rating scales (e.g., Durand & Crimmins, 1988). Table 12.1 lists several commonly used forms of indirect assessment questionnaires, checklists, and rating scales. The information gathered from indirect assessments may be used to develop treatments for self-injury or to provide a foundation for a more direct assessment. In weighing benefits and limitations of indirect assessments, most practitioners recommend that they should not be used as a sole source of information, but rather in conjunction with direct assessment methods (e.g., Zarcone, Rodgers, Iwata, Rourke, & Dorsey, 1991).

The primary advantage of indirect assessments is that they offer a time-efficient alternative to direct assessment methods (e.g., descriptive and experimental analyses). In most cases, the assessment can be administered within 15 minutes. This is in contrast to most direct assessment methods, which may take several days or even weeks to complete. Second, the assessments may be administered by individuals who require relatively little training on the methods. This is in contrast to direct assessment procedures that may require sophisticated professionals to implement. Third, indirect assessments may be useful when SIB is too dangerous to allow in a direct assessment (e.g., severe forms of pica, forceful head banging). This is in contrast to procedures that require direct observation or possibly even temporary exacerbation of the SIB. Fourth, the behavior could occur too infrequently to reliably observe. Thus, direct assessment via behavioral observation is not an option for some cases of SIB. Fifth, indirect assessments may provide some preliminary information, such as operational definitions or correlated environmental events, that will be needed to conduct subsequent direct assessments. Collectively, these advantages of indirect assessments suggest there is some utility to the general method. Nonetheless some limitations of the approach should also be considered.

The primary limitation of indirect assessments is that all information is correlational, even if accurately reported by the respondent. For example, a respondent might report that SIB frequently produces attention. However, recent research has shown the dangerous behavior commonly produces

Table 12.1. Commonly used Indirect assessment methods

Child Behavior Checklist (CBCL)	Achenbach (1991)
Aberrant Behavior Checklist (ABC)	Aman et al. (1985)
Motivational Assessment Scale (MAS)	Durand & Crimmins (1988)
Functional Analysis Screening Tool (FAST)	Iwata & DeLeon (1996)
Problem Behavior Questionaire (PBQ)	Lewis, Scott, & Sugai (1994)
Functional Assessment for Multiple Causality	Matson et al. (2003)
Questions About Behavioral Function (QABF)	Matson & Vollmer (1995)
Functional Assessment Interview (FAI)	O'Neill, et al. (1997)
Behavior Problems Inventory (BPI)	Rojahn et al. (2001)

attention from careproviders (Thompson & Iwata, 2001) even if the attention is not serving as reinforcement for the behavior (St. Peter et al., 2005). In short, dangerous behavior such as SIB is likely to induce various social reactions by care providers. By merely identifying those common consequences to behavior, a behavioral assessment falls short of necessarily identifying cause and effect variables.

A secondary limitation of indirect assessments involves the reliance on human report, especially when the human report is given long after the SIB event or events have occurred. In short, the information obtained may not be accurate. There are several factors that may contribute to the inaccuracy of indirect assessments. First, the individual providing the information (respondent) may not be able to recall all of the relevant information about the behavioral episode or episodes. Second, the respondent may not have enough experience with the behavior. For example, a staff member may only work with a client for a limited time and therefore has only observed a few instances of the behavior. Third, the respondent may provide biased responses. For example, a teacher may report that a student is consistently reprimanded following SIB (with the teacher believing that is the correct response), but fails to report that the student also consistently receives a break from academic tasks (believing that to be an incorrect response). Such erroneous information might lead to a false hypothesis regarding attention as reinforcement while ignoring the possible hypothesis of escape from academic tasks as reinforcement.

Indirect assessments should be conducted with informants who are commonly present when the behavior occurs and who are familiar with the person who engages in the SIB. In most cases, the indirect assessments are conducted with the individual's parents, teachers, or other caregivers. During indirect assessments, informants are generally asked questions related to the form and patterns of the SIB, possible antecedent (events that tend to occur prior to SIB) and consequent events (events that tend to occur as a result of SIB). Numerous indirect assessment methods exist and range from unstructured interviews to standardized psychometric instruments. A majority of these indirect assessments attempt to identify possible sources of reinforcement for problem behavior including social positive reinforcement (e.g., access to attention, access to preferred items or activities), social negative reinforcement (e.g., avoidance of academic tasks, escape from other people), and automatic/sensory reinforcement or reinforcement that is not socially mediated (e.g., sensory stimulation, attenuation of painful stimuli).

For example, in the Motivation Analysis Rating Scale (MARS) designed by Weiseler, Hanson, Chamberlain, and Thompson (1985) informants are asked to rate statements such as "When the self-injurious behavior occurs, the resident is trying to get something he wants." The Motivational Assessment Scale (MAS) developed by Durand and Crimmins (1988) includes several questions aimed at identifying relevant events that precede the problem behavior. For example, the informant is asked to rate questions such as "Does the behavior occur when any request is made of this person?" or "Does the behavior occur when you take away a favorite toy, food, or activity?" Affirmative answers to these questions may indicate that the behavior is influenced by escape from tasks and access to tangible reinforcers, respectively. Other indirect assessments, such as the Questions About Behavioral Function (QABF) include components to identify both antecedent and consequent events (e.g., Matson & Vollmer, 1995).

By comparing assessment results from two independent informants (interrater reliability), or with the same informant over time (test–retest reliability), the reliability of indirect measures may be assessed. For instance, the assessment could be administered to both a parent and a teacher and then the outcomes would be compared. Or, for example, the assessment could be administered to the teacher at one point in time and then again at another point in time. The reliability studies on indirect assessments have yielded mixed results (e.g., Durand & Crimmins, 1988; Andorfer, Miltenberger, Woster, Rotvedt, & Gaffaney, 1994; Zarcone, et al. 1991).

Durand and Crimmins (1988) administered the MAS to classroom teachers of students who engaged in severe problem behavior including self-injury. The authors compared the outcomes from two teachers and then calculated correlation coefficients based on the results. These coefficients were calculated using the overall responses to the questions rather than on a question-by-question basis. The authors reported a high level of interrater reliability (e.g., correlation coefficients ranging from .62 to .90). Zarcone et al. (1991) conducted a replication of the study with both teachers and direct care staff of 55 individuals who engaged in self-injury. In addition to the overall correlation coefficient calculation, Zarcone et al. evaluated point-to-point correspondence between responses to specific questions. The authors reported low correlation coefficients for both reliability measures. In fact, only 15% of the sample had correlation coefficients above .80.

It is important to consider that low reliability scores do not necessarily reflect a failure of the assessment method. It is possible that the self-injury occurs under different circumstances for different people. Therefore, it is possible that two informants respond differently, but both are accurate. This might especially be the case when the assessment is administered in two different environments (e.g., school and home). It is equally possible that test–retest reliability is confounded by changes in behavioral function over time (Lerman, Iwata, Smith, Zarcone, & Vollmer, 1994). For example, it is possible that behavior that was once reinforced by access to attention is now reinforced by escape from instructional activity. Collectively, these considerations suggest that the reliability of indirect assessments may be improved by administering the assessment within a small time window, to individuals in the same environment who both have a lot of experience with the behavior.

Other studies have evaluated the validity of indirect assessments by comparing outcomes to the results from direct assessments (e.g., functional analyses) or treatment analyses (e.g., Matson, Bamburg, Cherry, & Paclawskyj, 1999). For example, a study by Andorfer, Miltenberger, Woster, Rortvedt, and Gaffaney (1994) compared the results from structured interviews to analogue functional assessments and found correspondence between the two assessment methods. Validity analyses of the MAS have produced mixed results. Durand and Crimmins (1988) compared the results from the MAS to analog functional assessments, using direct assessment procedures described by Carr and Durand (1985) as the point of comparison. The authors reported that the MAS accurately predicted the results from the functional analyses for eight out of eight participants. In contrast, a study by Crawford, Brockel, Schauss, and Miltenberger (1992) found poor validity between the MAS and both functional analyses and direct observations.

The level of validity of indirect assessments may be related to the characteristics of the problem behavior. For example, Paclawskyj, Matson, Rush, Smalls, and Vollmer (2001) reported low validity scores between the QABF and analogue functional analyses. However, the authors attributed the results in part to difficulties with the functional analysis methodology. That is, the problem behavior was low-frequency/high-intensity in nature and was not observed in the function analysis conditions. Although functional analysis is widely viewed as the "acid test" for behavioral function, it is not clear it is best suited as a point of comparison for low rate behavior because the nonoccurrence of behavior during the functional analysis necessarily leads to a "no match" between the indirect and direct assessment.

To summarize, indirect assessments can provide useful information for subsequent direct assessments and for subsequent treatment recommendations. In addition, indirect assessments may be a useful option when the problem behavior is not conducive to direct assessment techniques, such as with extremely low rate SIB or extremely dangerous forms of SIB. Numerous studies have examined the reliability and validity of indirect assessments but further research is warranted to improve the utility of these assessments. More specifically, additional research may help to determine the conditions under which these assessments yield clear and accurate results. Finally, outcomes of indirect assessments should be viewed with caution due to the idiosyncrasies of subjective human report.

DESCRIPTIVE ANALYSIS

Descriptive analysis refers to the observation of behavior, usually during naturally occurring interactions (Bijou, Peterson, & Ault, 1968; Iwata, Kahng, Wallace, & Lindberg, 2000). Descriptive analyses are frequently used as one component of a comprehensive assessment of SIB and, in turn, as a basis for developing interventions to decrease SIB and to increase replacement behavior. This approach has been applied in a variety of settings including classrooms (e.g., Doggett et al., 2001; Ndoro, Hanley, Toger & Heal, 2006; Sasso et al., 1992; VanDerHeyden, Witt, & Gatti, 2001), residential settings (e.g., Lerman & Iwata, 1993; Mace & Lalli, 1991), and inpatient settings (e.g., Borrero, Vollmer, Borrero, & Bourret, 2005; Vollmer, Borrero, Wright, Van Camp, & Lalli, 2001). The descriptive analysis approach is used for a variety of response forms such as bizarre speech (Mace & Lalli, 1991), disruption, and aggression (e.g., Vollmer et al., 2001), but the approach is applicable in the assessment of SIB. In this section we describe three commonly used approaches to descriptive analysis: direct observation, scatterplots, and antecedent-behavior-consequence (A-B-C) recording.

Direct Observation

One approach to descriptive analysis is to have the professional assessor directly observe behavior in the natural setting. One formal assessment tool that has been frequently used for this purpose is the Functional Assessment Observation (FAO) designed by O'Neill, Horner, Albin, Sprague, Storey, and Newton (1997). When using the FAO, an observer collects data (using a "paper and pencil method") on various topographies of behavior, predictors of behavior (e.g., demands, difficult task, transitions, etc.), perceived functions of behavior (e.g., "get/obtain" and "escape/avoid" items or activities), and actual consequences for behavior. Subsequent analyses of data collected may provide information regarding the potential function of SIB, and to assist with treatment recommendations. Of course, when collecting data based on naturalistic observations, a number of events typically occur at the same time, and it may be difficult to capture all of the events using a paper and pencil data collection method.

In recent years, much of the research on direct observation methods has involved continuous recording using computerized data collection programs, which allows a large number of events and behavior to be scored during the observation. The results of a direct observation with computerized data are often analyzed by calculating the number of events that occur antecedent and subsequent to the behavior assessed (e.g., Forman, Hall & Oliver, 2002; Mace & Lalli, 1991; Oliver, Hall, & Nixon, 1999; & Ndoro et al., 2006), with the most frequent antecedents and consequences considered as potential establishing operations and reinforcers. The general approach of using computerized assessment methodology is limited insofar as many practitioners do not have resources available for this purpose.

There are several potential advantages to using direct observation as an SIB assessment component. First, direct observation provides a means of obtaining a true baseline of SIB levels occurring in the natural environment. Having a true baseline should aid in subsequent decision making about the efficacy or lack thereof of behavioral treatment or other forms of treatment (such as medical treatment). Second, direct observation may aid in developing operational definitions of the SIB. Third, idiosyncratic antecedent events or behavioral consequences might be identified. Fourth, direct observation may be practical in some settings where experimental manipulation of variables is not possible. For example, in some schools it is considered undesirable for a child to be pulled out of class for a lengthy assessment; yet, a descriptive analysis can occur in the classroom itself. A fifth potential advantage is that some severe forms of SIB cannot be allowed to occur in a functional analysis, especially if the functional analysis has a chance of temporarily increasing SIB rates. Although it might be argued that the same severe SIB should not be allowed to occur during direct observation either, an ethical argument can be made that the behavior does in fact occur already in the natural setting and a descriptive analysis can be kept very short if it is used mainly to capture baselines or to develop operational definitions.

If an eventual goal is to conduct a functional analysis of SIB, but SIB is extremely severe, a practitioner may wish to identify precursor behavior that is highly correlated with the occurrence of SIB. Descriptive analyses may be useful in identifying such precursors (Smith & Churchill, 2002). Recently Borrero and Borrero (2008) conducted descriptive analyses to identify precursors to more severe problem behavior, and subsequently assessed both via functional analyses (Iwata et al. 1982/1994). Results reported by Borrero and Borrero and Smith and Churchill showed that precursors to more severe problem behavior (e.g., vocalizations that reliably preceded SIB) were members of the same operant class as SIB (i.e., served the same operant function).

The principle limitation of a descriptive analysis in the form of direct observation (or any type of descriptive analysis for that matter) is that in the absence of experimental manipulation, functional relations between SIB and hypothesized variables cannot be confirmed. In fact, at times high correlations identified in a descriptive analysis are misleading. For example, St. Peter, Vollmer, Bourret, Borrero, Sloman, and Rapp (2005) showed via descriptive analysis that various forms of problem behavior were highly correlated with adult attention, but when a functional analysis was conducted it was shown that adult attention did not reinforce the SIB. Thus, high positive correlations between SIB and consequent events does not equate to identification of a reinforcer.

The severity of SIB makes it highly likely that care providers will in some way attend to the behavior (although the attention may be functionally irrelevant to the behavior). On the other hand, some SIB may only intermittently produce attention or other reinforcers (yielding a low correlation between SIB and the reinforcer), but such relations could represent lean variable ratio (VR) or variable interval (VI) schedules of reinforcement. For example, if a parent attends to SIB one out of every ten times it occurs on average, the behavior could be reinforced on a VR 10 schedule. Thus, as with indirect assessments, descriptive analyses should be conducted in conjunction with functional analyses when possible to tease out correlation/causation distinctions (e.g., Arndorfer et al., 1994; Desrochers et al., 1997; Ellingson et al., 1999).

It could be argued that, given the correlation/causation problem, why conduct a direct observation as a form of descriptive analysis at all? Why not skip directly to a functional analysis (described later in this chapter)? The answer is that the purpose of the direct observation would be to identify common situations in which the behavior occurs, to develop operational definitions, to gather baseline data, and so on (see advantages of direct observation). In addition, further utility of direct observation as a form of descriptive analysis is discussed below. The purpose of the functional analysis would be to identify reinforcers maintaining behavior. It is important to note that direct observation may provide some hints about reinforcers maintaining behavior, but the true purpose of such an approach should be to gather the kinds of miscellaneous information about the environmental context that would not ordinarily emerge in a functional analysis. Thus, in our view, the purposes of a descriptive analysis and of a functional analysis are different.

If both a direct observation (as descriptive analysis) and a functional analysis are used to identify the operant function of behavior, the results of these methods too often do not match. Thus, reinforcer identification via descriptive analysis is considered (at least by us) to be an inappropriate usage of the method. Whereas previously common usage of the descriptive analysis was as a prelude to a functional analysis (e.g., Mace & Lalli, 1991; Lerman & Iwata, 1993), a more recent usage of the direct observation during a descriptive analysis is just the opposite: to evaluate what reinforcement contingencies might look like in the natural environment once reinforcers have already been identified via functional analysis.

In short, data obtained via direct observation can provide a means to quantify details of naturally occurring social interactions that might strengthen SIB. For example, descriptive data may be evaluated to compare probabilities during naturally occurring interactions (e.g., the probability of attention given SIB vs. the overall probability of attention; Vollmer et al., 2001) or to evaluate dynamic moment-to-moment changes in the probability of various environment–behavior relations via lag sequential analysis (e.g., Emerson et al., 1995; Samaha et al., in press).

Descriptive data may also be used to identify parameters of reinforcement for both SIB and replacement behavior, including the rate, duration, probability, quality, and delay to reinforcement (e.g., Borrero et al., 2005). Conceivably such information could be critical to obtain as a baseline from which to compare the effects of care provider training. For example, in some cases SIB must be reinforced (such as when a care provider must block attention-maintained SIB). As a result, the probability of attention following SIB may be very close to 1.0, but the care provider could improve the relative parameters of reinforcement for replacement behavior. Table 12.2 shows hypothetical data on reinforcement parameters for SIB reinforced by attention. The left two columns show the reinforcement parameters for SIB and replacement behavior prior to training and the right two columns show the reinforcement parameters after training.

Table 12.2.

Replacement Parameter	SIB	Replacement Behavior	SIB	Replacement Behavior
Rate	.95 per min	.12 per min	.3 per min	.95 per min
Duration	30 s	3 s	5 s	40 s
Probability	1.0	.1	.2	.99
Delay	0 s	20 s	45 s	0 s

Hypothetical data on reinforcement parameters for SIB reinforced by attention. The left two columns show the reinforcement parameters for SIB and replacement behavior prior to training and the right two columns show the reinforcement parameters after training.

Scatterplot

At times it is either inconvenient or not possible for a professional psychologist or behavior analyst to directly observe SIB. In such cases, care providers such as staff, parents, and teachers are asked to collect data, usually in some simplified and manageable format that would not require extensive training or time consumption. One example is the scatterplot technique. Touchette, MacDonald, and Langer (1985) used a scatterplot to estimate the frequency of problem behavior across days and weeks to identify patterns in responding. The scatterplot method usually involves a grid data sheet that allows for the recording of data in specified time intervals (e.g., 30-min intervals through school hours) that correspond to the individual's daily schedule. Typically, the frequency of behavior is scored as either "no occurrence" (or leaving the box blank), "low-rate responding" (e.g., drawing stripes in the box), and "high-rate responding" (e.g., filling in the box). Prior to completing the scatterplot, low- and high-rate responding must be defined on an individual basis. Figure 12.1 shows an example of a scatterplot data sheet.

After the scatterplot is completed, it may be possible to see patterns in responding, such as behavior occurring at a certain time of day or during a specific activity. In fact, Touchette et al. (1985) used the scatterplot to identify times of day associated with SIB and aggression and then made changes in the programmed schedule for participants, resulting in a decrease in problem behavior. Although it was not highlighted by Touchette et al, another potential advantage of a scatterplot is that it yields a visual display to estimate the occurrence of behavior both before and after the initiation of SIB treatment. Thus, advantages of the scatterplot method include ease of implementation, possible identification of SIB allocation by time of day or activity, and possible use as an estimate of baseline SIB occurrences.

Despite the possible advantages, there are some limitations to the scatterplot to consider. First, just as with any descriptive analysis method, only behavior–environment correlations can be obtained (rather than cause–effect relations). Second, although it may be fairly simple to complete the grid, the method may not be sensitive to changes in high-rate SIB. For example, if during baseline high-rate SIB occurs 20 or more times during a 30-min interval, the scatterplot might look the same following treatment even when a 50% reduction in behavior is obtained. Third, although identification of temporal patterns is a common usage of scatterplots, clear outcomes may be relatively rare. Kahng et al. (1998) evaluated completed scatterplots for 15 individuals (those individuals for whom acceptable reliability data were obtained) and found that out of the 15 scatterplots no reliable temporal patterns of responding were identified via visual analysis.

A-B-C Recording

The A-B-C method is another relatively simple approach that is most often conducted by care providers, after a modicum of training, in the natural environment. The A-B-C method involves recording potential antecedents to and consequences of behavior, as suggested by Skinner's

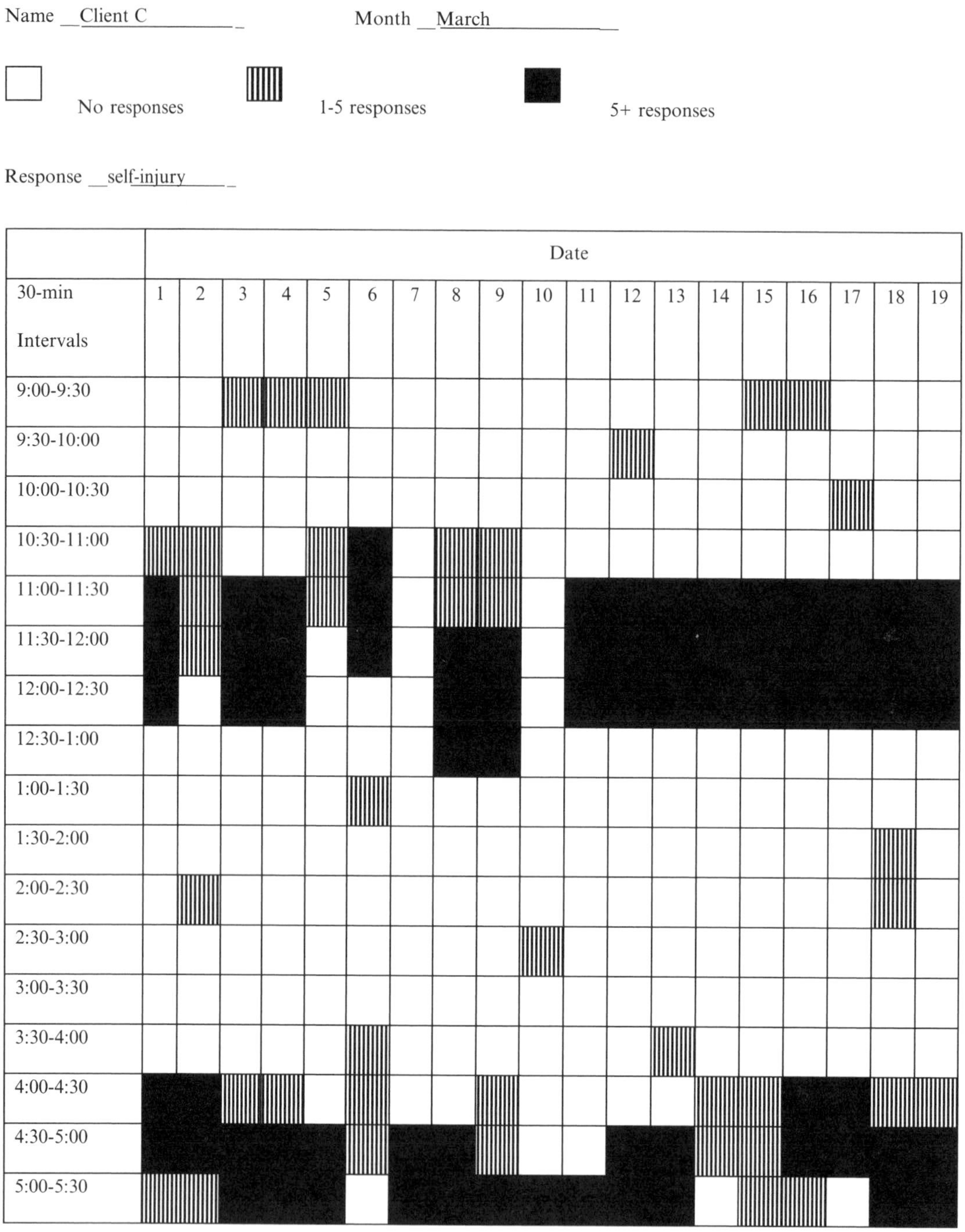

Name __Client C_____ _   Month __March_____

Name __Client C__ Month __March__
□ No responses   ▥ 1-5 responses   ■ 5+ responses

Response __self-injury____ _

Figure 12.1. Completed scatterplot sheet. Dates are listed horizontally and 30-minute intervals are listed vertically. The different patterns denote different frequencies of self-injury for the particular interval.

three-term contingency (Skinner, 1953). Simple A-B-C data sheets typically use narrative recording, and include a definition of the behavior, and columns where the observer should record what happened before and after the behavior. The space for recording antecedents and consequences can be left open ended (see Figure 12.2), or might contain multiple options in order to focus the responses of the observer (see Figure 12.3).

The primary advantage of the A-B-C method is the ease of implementation. A second advantage is that if behavior is low-rate, a professional observer is not likely to see the behavior. Thus, having a care provider record instances of behavior allows the professional to obtain some level of information in the absence of direct observation. The potential disadvantages include possible problems with data reliability (given that observers are not professionally trained observers) and possible problems with the type of information reported. Although very little research has been conducted using parents and staff as observers, our experience has been that a wide range of descriptions are recorded on A-B-C sheets, and those descriptions are not always technically sound and do not always represent observable environmental events.

Instructions: When an instance of SIB occurs, record the activity/event that occurred prior to the behavior, and the activity/event that occurred following the behavior.				
Date and Time SIB occurred	Description of SIB	What occurred before SIB?	What occurred after SIB?	Additional Comments

Figure 12.2.   An example of a simple A-B-C recording sheet.

Date and Time	Description of SIB	What occurred before SIB? (Please check)	What occurred after SIB? (Please check)	Additional Comments
		____ Instructions	____ Instructions ended	
		____ Item Removed	____ Instructions cont.	
		____ No Attention	____ Reprimand	
		____ Close Proximity	____ Medical Attention	
		____ Diverted Attention	____ No Attention	
		____ No Specific Event	____ Item Presented	
		____ Other	____ No Specific Event	
			____ Other	
		____ Instructions	____ Instructions ended	
		____ Item Removed	____ Instructions cont.	
		____ No Attention	____ Reprimand	
		____ Close Proximity	____ Medical Attention	
		____ Diverted Attention	____ No Attention	
		____ No Specific Event	____ Item Presented	
		____ Other	____ No Specific Event	
			____ Other	
		____ Instructions	____ Instructions ended	
		____ Item Removed	____ Instructions cont.	
		____ No Attention	____ Reprimand	
		____ Close Proximity	____ Medical Attention	
		____ Diverted Attention	____ No Attention	
		____ No Specific Event	____ Item Presented	
		____ Other	____ No Specific Event	
			____ Other	
		____ Instructions	____ Instructions ended	
		____ Item Removed	____ Instructions cont.	
		____ No Attention	____ Reprimand	
		____ Close Proximity	____ Medical Attention	
		____ Diverted Attention	____ No Attention	
		____ No Specific Event	____ Item Presented	
		____ Other	____ No Specific Event	
			____ Other	

Figure 12.3.   An example of an A-B-C recording sheet with multiple options for antecedent and consequent events.

Functional Analysis

The term functional analysis as it relates to SIB assessment refers to specific procedures to identify relationships between antecedent and consequent events and behavior. Functional analysis differs from other forms of behavioral assessment in that it not only involves direct observation and repeated measurement of behavior, but also involves an experimental manipulation of environmental variables. That is, antecedent events (e.g., restriction of preferred items, presentation of demands) are controlled, and consequent events (e.g., delivery of preferred items, termination of demands) are provided contingent upon problem behavior in order to test hypotheses about the operant function of behavior. Functional analyses have been conducted for almost every type of SIB that has been reported in the literature, including head banging (Iwata, Pace, Cowdery, & Miltenberger, 1994), hand mouthing or biting (Goh et al., 1994), scratching (Cowdery, Iwata, & Pace, 1990), pica (Piazza, Hanley, & Fisher, 1996), and eye poking (Lalli, Livezey, & Kates, 1996), among many others.

The presentation of potential reinforcing events for SIB may seem counterintuitive upon initial consideration for assessment and treatment purposes. Why would the professional want to make the behavior worse? A medical analogy that helps make sense of the assessment logic is to consider the purpose of an allergy test: the allergist intentionally exposes the patient to hypothesized allergens and then evaluates the response to those hypothesized allergens. Analogously, in the assessment of SIB, a functional analysis is conducted as a means of exposing an individual, albeit temporarily, to possible environmental factors causing SIB. The functional analysis approach is considered the best practice for identifying environmental variables affecting problem behavior, at least when behavior occurs at a high enough rate to be observed during relatively short duration sessions and when an individual is not placed in immediate and severe danger (Hanley, Iwata, & McCord, 2003).

Typically, a functional analysis includes conditions to serve as analogues for typical situations in the individual's natural environment. Thus, the individual is not being exposed to situations he or she does not already experience on a day-to-day basis. Functional analyses may lead to effective interventions because the treatment can be based on known functional properties of the SIB rather than being based on a priori assumptions, potentially spurious correlations (St. Peter et al., 2005), or verbal report. A complete functional analysis of behavior may also prevent the implementation of treatments that are contraindicated to the function of problem behavior (e.g., Iwata et al., 1994). For example, timeout might actually reinforce escape maintained SIB.

Because SIB is such a dangerous behavior disorder, several considerations must be addressed before conducting functional analyses. For example, if there is risk of immediate tissue damage or trauma, medical personnel should be consulted. Medical personnel can help evaluate whether the SIB is amenable to a functional analysis, and also help to determine appropriate session termination criteria if the SIB becomes too severe (Iwata et al., 1982/1994). There may be cases when the characteristics of the behavior (e.g., frequency or topography) are determined to be inappropriate for a functional analysis. For example, the behavior may occur at low rates (e.g., once per day) or the behavior may be too dangerous (e.g., pica with sharp metallic objects) to expose to a functional analysis. For these cases, other assessment methods (e.g., indirect assessments) or variations of traditional functional analyses may be more appropriate.

Although the functional analysis of SIB has been a hallmark of behavior analysis for many years (e.g., Lovaas and Simmons, 1969), Iwata et al. (1982/1994) presented the first empirical demonstration of functional analysis methodology designed specifically as an assessment method. Iwata et al. conducted functional analyses for nine children who engaged in SIB. The assessment results pointed to clear variables maintaining SIB for six of the nine participants. The methodology described by Iwata et al. has served as the standard model for a majority of subsequent functional analysis studies and clinical applications. Functional analyses are commonly conducted in highly controlled settings, such as inpatient hospital settings, so that all relevant environmental variables (e.g., delivery of attention) can be regulated. However, functional analyses have also been conducted in other environments such as the client's home or school (e.g., Northup et al., 1994).

Most functional analyses include three test conditions and one control condition. The purpose of the control condition is to evaluate the effects of an environment in which little SIB is expected to occur (Iwata et al., 1982/94). In the control condition, the client is typically given free access to preferred items and the therapist delivers attention on a time-based schedule. Additionally, no demands are placed on the client. The purpose of two of the test conditions is to evaluate the sensitivity of SIB to common socially mediated consequences such as positive reinforcement (such as adult attention or contingent access to preferred tangible items) and negative reinforcement (such as escape from instructional activity or self care routines).

There is also usually a test condition for automatically reinforced behavior, or behavior that occurs in the absence of socially medicated consequences (e.g., the client is left alone in a room in order to evaluate whether the behavior persists in the absence of socially mediated consequences.) Each session (whether test or control) typically lasts 5 to 15 minutes. The presentation of conditions is usually alternated randomly in a multielement experimental design (Sidman, 1960). However, other design variations have been used including the repeated measurement of SIB in reversal designs (e.g., Vollmer, Iwata, Duncan, & Lerman, 1993b) and alternation of one test and control condition at a time (pairwise design; Iwata, Duncan, Zarcone, Lerman, & Shore, 1994).

In most functional analysis conditions, the consequence is provided for each occurrence of problem behavior (a continuous reinforcement schedule, or CRF). For example, in the "attention" condition (described below) the adult therapist provides a reprimand, comfort statement, or some other form of attention every time SIB occurs. Some researchers have argued that CRF leads to better discrimination of test conditions and therefore yields clear assessment results (Iwata, Vollmer, & Zarcone, 1990). However, some researchers have used intermittent reinforcement schedules in order to more closely mimic consequences as they are delivered in the natural environment (e.g., Lalli & Casey, 1996). Whatever the reinforcement schedule, a common feature of functional analyses is that data are collected on the rates of SIB for the purposes of comparison in each of the conditions. The response patterns in each of the test conditions are then compared to the control condition. A higher rate of responding in a particular test condition indicates a possible source of reinforcement. Some of the most frequently used functional analysis conditions are described below.

Care provider attention has been shown to be one of the most common consequences for problematic behavior, including SIB, displayed by individuals with developmental disabilities (e.g., Thompson & Iwata, 2001).

In the attention condition, the client has access to preferred items or activities and the therapist engages in work or other activities away from the client. Some variations of this condition involve a "diverted" attention component in which the therapist attends to other individuals in the environment, and not the client. When an instance of SIB occurs, the therapist turns toward the client and provides brief attention. Higher rates of self-injury in the attention condition relative to the control condition would suggest that SIB is reinforced by attention. The upper panel of Figure 12.4 shows hypothetical results of a functional analysis showing reinforcement via attention.

An attempt should be made to match the type of attention delivered in the functional analysis to the type of attention commonly provided in the client's natural environment. For example, some care providers are more likely to reprimand SIB whereas other care providers are more likely to provide comfort or soothing conversation after SIB. Some studies have shown that the form of attention may influence the reinforcing value of attention as reinforcement for problem behavior (e.g., Fisher, Ninness, Piazza, & Owen-DeSchryver, 1996; Piazza, et al., 1999). For example, Piazza et al. found that for some participants verbal reprimands were actually more potent reinforcers than praise statements. Thus, consideration of the form of attention should be addressed prior to implementing a social positive reinforcement test condition.

Another form of social positive reinforcement is the delivery of preferred toys, food, or activities. In natural interactions, these items are sometimes given to clients after SIB as a means to distract or appease the client, but the result is an inadvertent reinforcement effect. The test condition for this type of reinforcement is sometimes called the "tangible" condition. In the tangible condition, the therapist provides attention to the client but access to highly preferred items or activities is restricted. When SIB occurs, the therapist allows access to the items for a short period of time. Higher rates of SIB in the tangible condition, relative to the control condition would suggest that SIB is reinforced by access to tangible items. The second panel of Figure 12.4 shows hypothetical results for behavior reinforced by tangibles.

The tangible condition is typically included in the functional analysis if other assessments (e.g., caregiver interviews, direct observations) have determined that access to tangibles is a common consequence for the problem behavior. Otherwise, one concern is the inclusion of tangible condition may lead to a false positive functional analysis outcome (e.g., Shirley, Iwata, & Kahng, 1999). For example, Shirley et al. conducted functional analyses of hand mouthing for one participant and found that elevated rates of hand mouthing occurred across two test conditions, including the tangible condition. However, direct observations in the participant's natural environment showed that presentation of preferred items never followed hand mouthing. However, it is important to note that there may be some utility to including a tangible condition even if that is not how SIB is currently maintained for a given individual: that is, it could be argued that SIB is at least sensitive to tangible reinforcement and, therefore, clear recommendations could be made to avoid contingent delivery of tangibles as a consequence to SIB.

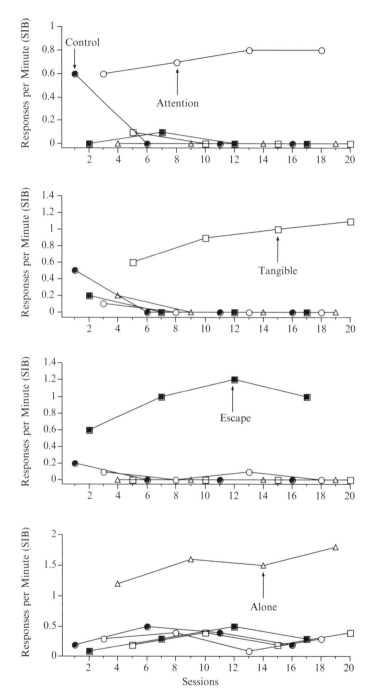

Figure 12.4. Hypothetical functional analysis outcomes. For all of the panels, the attention condition is represented by the open circles, the tangible condition is represented by the open squares, the escape condition is represented by the closed squares, the alone condition is represented by the open triangles, and the play condition is represented by the closed circles. (Upper Panel) Functional analysis outcome for self-injury maintained by access to attention. (Upper Middle Panel) Functional analysis outcomes for self-injury maintained by access to tangibles. (Lower Middle Panel) Functional analysis outcome for self-injury maintained by escape from demands. (Lower Panel) Functional analysis outcome for self-injury maintained by automatic reinforcement.

Escape from demands (e.g., academic tasks, self-care routines, chores) is another common consequence for SIB. In fact, Thompson and Iwata (2001) evaluated common consequences for various topographies of problem behavior and found that escape from demands was the most common consequence for SIB among adults with developmental disabilities living in a residential facility. To improve the validity of the functional analysis outcomes, the demand context should be similar to demands that the individual experiences in the natural environment. The type of demand presented may affect the functional analysis outcomes. For example, a client may readily comply with academic tasks but may engage in SIB during self-care tasks. Using only academic tasks in the escape condition of the functional analysis would yield inaccurate results (i.e., a false negative).

In the escape condition (also called the "demand" condition), the therapist presents demands to the client using a three-step prompting sequence. The prompting sequence first begins with a verbal instruction. If the client does not comply within a specified time period (usually five or ten seconds), the therapist performs a model or demonstration of the correct response. If the client again does not comply within a specified time period, the therapist physically guides him or her to comply. If compliance occurs at any point in the sequence, the therapist provides brief praise and then restarts the prompting sequence. This sequence continues unless the client engages in SIB. If SIB occurs, the therapist turns away from the client and provides a brief break from the instructional activities. Higher rates of responding in the escape condition relative to the control condition would suggest that SIB is reinforced by escape from demands. The third panel of Figure 12.4 shows hypothetical results for SIB reinforced by escape.

The most common type of social negative reinforcement is escape from demands or instructional activities. However, in some cases, the mere proximity of another person may evoke self-injury. A variation of the escape condition, known as "social escape", has also been conducted in functional analyses (e.g., Iwata, Pace et al. 1994). In this condition, the therapist is in close proximity to the client and may provide attention. If SIB occurs, the therapist moves away from the client for a brief period of time. Higher rates in the social escape condition relative to the control condition indicate that behavior is reinforced by escape or avoidance of close social or physical proximity.

In some cases SIB may persist in the absence or independent of social consequences. This type of reinforcement has been referred to as automatic reinforcement because the behavior produces its own reinforcement in the form of sensory stimulation or pain attenuation. The meaning of "automatic" is simply to imply that no social mediation is responsible for reinforcement of the behavior; it is not an explanation of the actual source of reinforcement. An epidemiological study by Iwata and colleagues (1994) showed that over 25% of 152 participants' SIB were maintained by automatic reinforcement.

An alone or no consequence condition is typically used to test if behavior is automatically reinforced. In these conditions, the client is either left alone in a room and observed through a one-way mirror, or remains in the room with a therapist who provides no programmed consequences for SIB. Higher rates in the alone or no consequence condition relative to the control condition suggests that behavior is maintained by automatic reinforcement. Undifferentiated responding, or responding that is high in all conditions including the control condition, may also suggest that behavior is maintained by automatic reinforcement, especially if the SIB does not extinguish following repeated alone or no consequence sessions (e.g., Vollmer, Marcus, Ringdahl, & Roane, 1995). The lower panel of Figure 12.4 shows hypothetical results for SIB maintained by automatic reinforcement.

Carr and Durand (1985) presented another variation of functional analysis methodology with four children who engaged in problem behavior, including SIB, in a school setting. Only antecedent events (i.e., presentation of attention and demands) were manipulated and no consequent events were programmed. Two experimental conditions and one control condition were included. One experimental condition evaluated the effects of low rates of antecedent teacher attention on problem behavior. Higher rates in this condition relative to the control condition suggested that behavior was sensitive to access to attention (i.e., the participants were motivated to increase attention levels under conditions of low attention). The other test condition evaluated the effects of presenting difficult demands on problem behavior. Higher rates in this condition relative to the control condition suggested behavior was sensitive to escape from demands (i.e., the participants were motivated to decrease demand difficulty under conditions of high demand). Results from Carr and Durand showed this method produced clear results for all four participants. In addition, treatments based on the results of the functional analysis were presented and showed decreases in disruptive behavior for all participants.

Carr and Durand's variation of functional analysis may have advantages over traditional functional analyses because no programmed consequences are delivered, so problem behavior is not intentionally reinforced. However, there may be some limitations to this methodology. First, because consequent events are not manipulated, there is no empirical demonstration of cause-and-effect relationships between reinforcement and behavior. Second, it is possible that behavior would extinguish, or stop occurring during the sessions without the presentation of maintaining consequent events (i.e., reinforcers). Third, the antecedent manipulations may not be noticeable enough to produce differences across conditions. That is, this method requires the participant to be sensitive to slight changes such as delivery of attention once every 10s in the control condition compared to delivery of attention once every 30s in the attention condition (Fischer, Iwata, & Worsdell, 1997). Finally, this antecedent type of functional analysis fails to test for other possible sources of reinforcement such as access to preferred items or activities and automatic reinforcement.

Overall, a clear advantage of functional analysis as an SIB assessment is that functional relations between the behavior and environment are demonstrated. This is an advantage over descriptive analyses, where only correlations can be identified and it is an advantage over verbal reports and checklists because it is based on experimental logic and direct behavioral observation.

Despite the utility of functional analyses, several potential limitations have been reported. One putative limitation of functional analysis methodology is the time required to complete the assessment. In some settings, time constraints may preclude a thorough functional analysis. However, some studies have evaluated the efficacy of brief functional analyses (e.g., Cooper, Wacker, Sasso, Reimers, & Donn, 1990; Cooper et al., 1992; Derby, et al., 1992; Harding, Wacker, Cooper, Millard, & Jensen-Kovalan, 1994; Northup et al., 1991). For example, Northup et al. (1991) conducted brief functional analyses in an outpatient clinic setting with three individuals who engaged in aggressive behavior. In some cases, the time to conduct the assessment was limited to 90 minutes. The assessments involved one to two brief 10-minute exposures to functional analysis conditions similar to Iwata et al. (1994). For some participants, responding was differentially higher in the test conditions than the control condition. In addition, implementation of a treatment resulted in high rates of appropriate behavior and low rates of problem behavior.

Derby et al. (1992) conducted a large-scale study to evaluate the efficacy of brief functional analyses. Results from 79 brief functional analyses were summarized and showed that only 63% of the participants engaged in the problem behavior during the functional analysis. Maintaining variables were identified for 74% of the participants who did exhibit problem behavior during the brief assessment. Thus, brief functional analyses may only be effective for a limited number of individuals. In addition, data analysis techniques such as minute-by-minute evaluations can reduce the assessment duration in some cases (e.g., Vollmer, Marcus, Ringdahl, & Roane, 1995).

A second potential limitation of functional analysis is that it may be inappropriate for some types of behavior. For instance, the topography of SIB may be too severe to expose to functional analysis conditions. However, in these cases, it may be possible to identify precursor behavior (i.e., behavior that reliably precedes the self-injury) and conduct functional analyses of these responses. For example, Smith and Churchill (2002) conducted functional analyses of both SIB and precursor behavior for four participants and showed that the function of SIB could be inferred by conducting functional analyses of precursor behavior.

Functional analyses may also be inappropriate for behavior that occurs infrequently (e.g., once per day). However, varying the duration or structure of conditions of the functional analysis may better accommodate low-rate behavior. For example, it may be possible to identify specific times of the day that the behavior occurs and then conduct the functional analysis during these times. Furthermore, the time allotment for each condition can be increased from the typical 10 to 15 minutes to longer time periods (e.g., one to two hours) to adequately assess the behavior. Kahng, Abt, and Schoenbacher (2001) reported the successful assessment and treatment of low rate behavior using extended-time functional analysis methods for one participant in a hospital inpatient setting.

Another potential limitation is when functional analyses result in undifferentiated response patterns. This may occur for several reasons: the SIB may be automatically reinforced, the SIB may be multiply controlled (i.e., reinforced by more than one general type of consequence), the individual may not be discriminating the test conditions, or there may be carryover effects from one test condition to another. Although problematic, the issue of undifferentiated outcomes can be resolved in some cases, depending on the reason for the undifferentiated outcome. For example, undifferentiated results produced by automatic reinforcement can be identified by running numerous consecutive alone sessions to see if SIB extinguishes (e.g., Ellingson et al., 2000).

Undifferentiated results produced by multiple controls can be identified by sequentially implementing treatments to address one hypothesized operant function and then another (Smith, Iwata, Vollmer, & Zarcone, 1993). Undifferentiated outcomes produced by discrimination failures can be overcome by enhancing (distinguishing) stimulus features of the test conditions, such as therapist, therapist clothing color, and so on (Conners et al., 2000). Undifferentiated results produced by carryover effects from one condition to another can be identified by carefully evaluating within-session response patterns (Vollmer, Iwata, Duncan, & Lerman, 1993a). For example, Vollmer et al. found that sessions following attention sessions produced an apparent extinction burst of SIB that yielded similar overall session means but distinct response patterns that pointed to attention as a source of reinforcement.

Thus, functional analysis is a robust method for assessing SIB. In addition, the use of functional analysis techniques has resulted in the development of effective, function- based treatments. The results from several studies show that functional analysis methodology can be adapted for special situations in which traditional functional analysis methods either cannot be conducted or somehow produce unclear results. Nonetheless, more research on functional analysis is needed. Some of the most obvious assessment-related research questions remain unanswered as of this writing; for example, does a functional analysis lead to overall better treatment effects than would have occurred if a reasonably educated professional implemented intervention after a modicum of direct observation?

RESPONSE PRODUCTS

When assessing SIB through direct observation and functional analysis methods, results are presented using rate or interval recording methods. It is also sometimes useful to assess response severity or intensity and its corresponding response products (Marholin & Steinman, 1977). Response products involve measuring the outcome of a response rather than the rate of the response itself (Miltenberger, 2001). By definition, SIB suggests that physical damage has been caused by the response (Iwata et al., 1990). The type of injury caused by the response may differ depending on the topography of the response (e.g., self-biting, hitting head on a hard surface, skin-picking).

The principal advantage of an evaluation of SIB response products comes when assessing a response for which rate of responding does not indicate the level of damage caused by SIB. For example, if an individual hits his or her head on a hard surface, low-rate responding may still be problematic if such SIB causes substantial physical harm. A second advantage is that a baseline response product (injury) measurement provides a point of comparison when a goal of a SIB intervention is not merely to reduce SIB, but to reduce its associated sequelae (i.e., injury itself).

A third potential advantage of SIB response product measurement is that, in some cases, responses may only occur covertly (e.g., Grace, Thompson, & Fisher, 1996; Rapp et al., 1999); that is, responses occur either when the individual is alone or when the individual cannot be observed. Thus, response products of SIB may be the only evidence that the response has occurred and assessments of physical damage may be the only source of information regarding the severity and occurrence of a response. Although self-cutting displayed by otherwise typically developing adolescents is not a focus of this chapter, such SIB typically occurs covertly and might only be assessed via response products. Assessing response products for self-cutting therefore represents a promising future application.

Research on SIB response products has provided useful tools for the assessment of SIB severity (e.g., Iwata, Pace, Kissel, Nau, & Farber, 1990; Wilson, Iwata & Bloom, in press), including during SIB treatment (e.g., Carr & McDowell, 1980; Grace, Thompson, & Fisher, 1996). Iwata et al. (1990b) developed the Self-Injury Trauma (SIT) scale to classify and quantify damage resulting from various topographies of SIB, including the location, number, severity, and type of injury. The researchers developed the scale to provide objective measurements of these variables, and experimentally validated the reliability of 50 completed scales by assessing interobserver agreement (IOA) for all variables. Results showed that IOA calculated for the SIT scale was always above 89%, and, for some variables, including location of injuries, type of injuries, severity of injuries, the overall agreement was at least 94%.

Advantages of this instrument include the objective nature of the scale, and its applicability to assess various aspects of injury. Disadvantages of the instrument include the lack of rate measures and difficulty in assessing internal injuries. Thus, as recommended by Iwata et al. (1990b), the instrument should be used in conjunction with direct observations of the behavior and other medical evaluation.

Grace et al. (1996) conducted an assessment and treatment of severe SIB exhibited by an adult diagnosed with developmental disabilities with SIB response products serving as a dependent variable. The participant often engaged in SIB (i.e., skin picking, head banging, and inserting objects in his nose and ears), that was rarely observed. However, the SIB response products were observed (i.e., bleeding, objects observed in his nose and ears). In the study, nurses completed physical exams and documented existing physical injuries, as well as new ones. One specific dependent measure was the percentage of exams with new injuries. A subsequent treatment analysis was conducted and resulted in a decrease in the occurrence of new injuries.

Chapman, Fisher, Piazza, and Kurtz (1993) have applied a relatively novel approach to the use of response products, as applied to a particularly challenging form of self-injury. As a component of this study, Chapman et al. applied blue residue to pill bottles (containing colored placebos). In conjunction with direct observation, the researchers assessed pill bottle manipulation (correlated with pill ingestion) based on blue residue that appeared on the participant's hands and clothing. A treatment that involved differential reinforcement and ultimate elimination of the blue residue successfully reduced self-injury.

More recently, Wilson et al. (in press) used a computerized measurement of wound surface areas (WSA) to assess SIB. They compared the computerized method of measurement of WSA, using digital photographs, to the transparency method of measurement and found that the results were similar for both methods. Then the researchers compared the computerized measurement method to direct observation to determine if both methods were successful in identifying changes in the levels of SIB during assessment and treatment conditions. Results showed that both methods indicated changes in the levels of SIB, and suggested that the computerized method for measuring response products may not only enhance the results of direct observation, but may be used as a primary dependent variable for SIB.

As mentioned previously, there are some limitations to using response products as the dependent variable when assessing SIB. Perhaps the most apparent limitation associated with using permanent products (alone), is the extent to which the "cause" of the injury can be adequately inferred. For example, an individual with an extensive history of self-injury may present with bruising as result of a fall, or as a result of self-injury. Thus, interpretations based on response products should be interpreted cautiously, and preferably should be used in conjunction with direct observation when possible. Although it is important and often necessary to determine the extent of the physical damage caused by SIB, response products do not provide any information regarding the rate of self-injury, and may not identify particular situations or conditions under which self-injury occurs. An additional limitation pointed out by Iwata et al. (1990) suggests that the SIT and similar methods merely provide a physical description of the injury on the surface of the skin, and do not measure internal injuries. Additional medical assessments may be indicated to provide such information, such as x-rays, CT scans, ultrasounds, and so on.

CONCLUSIONS

Self-injury is a complex and severe behavior disorder displayed by individuals with developmental disabilities. A large body of research suggests that SIB is learned (operant) behavior sometimes reinforced by other people and sometimes reinforced automatically. The purpose of a behavioral assessment is to identify where and when the SIB is most likely and least likely to occur and to identify possible sources of reinforcement for the behavior. Assessment methods include indirect techniques such as checklists and questionnaires, descriptive analysis, functional analysis, and response product measurement. Although each assessment type has its own set of strengths and limitations, some combination of assessment components is usually recommended and rarely should any single assessment type by used in isolation.

An idealized behavioral assessment of SIB would include first a set of interviews with relevant care providers; second, direct observation by a professional coupled with simple data collection by care providers; third, a functional analysis of hypothesized sources of reinforcement; and fourth, an evaluation of response products (injury) caused by the behavior. Collectively, the information obtained would serve as an empirical basis to address perceptions of relevant care providers, idiosyncracies of the SIB in the natural environment, cause and effect relations, and the extent of tissue damage caused by the behavior.

REFERENCES

Achenbach, T. M. (1991). *Manual for the Child Behavior Checklist/4-18 and 1991 Profile.* Burlington, VT: University of Vermont, Department of Psychiatry.

Aman, M. G., Singh, N. N., Stewart, A. W., & Field, C. J. (1985). The aberrant behavior checklist: A behavior rating scale for the assessment of treatment effects. *American Journal of Mental Deficiency, 89,* 485–491.

Arndorfer, R. E., Miltenberger, R. G., Woster, S. H., Rortvedt, A. K., & Gaffaney, T. (1994). Home-based descriptive and experimental analysis of problem behaviors in children. *Topics in Early Childhood Special Education, 14,* 64–87.

Bijou, S. W., Peterson, R. F., & Ault, M. H. (1968). A method to integrate descriptive and experimental field studies at the levels of data and empirical concepts. *Journal of Applied Behavior Analysis, 1,* 175–191.

Borrero, C. S. W., & Borrero, J. C. (2008). Descriptive and experimental analyses of potential precursors to problem behavior. *Journal of Applied Behavior Analysis, 41,* 83–96.

Borrero, C. S. W., Vollmer, T. R., Borrero, J. C., & Bourret, J. (2005). A method of evaluating parameters of reinforcement during parent–child interactions. *Research in Developmental Disabilities, 26,* 577–592.

Carr, E. G. (1977). The motivation of self-injurious behavior: A review of some hypotheses. *Psychological Bulletin, 84,* 800–816.

Carr, E. G., & Durand, V. M. (1985). Reducing problem behavior through functional communication training. *Journal of Applied Behavior Analysis, 18,* 111–126.

Carr, E. G., & McDowell, J. J. (1980). Social control of self-injurious behavior of organic etiology. *Behavior Therapy, 11,* 402–409.

Chapman, S., Fisher, W., Piazza, C. C., & Kurtz, P. F. (1993). Functional assessment and treatment of life-threatening drug ingestion in a dually diagnosed youth. *Journal of Applied Behavior Analysis, 26,* 255–256.

Conners, J., Iwata, B. A., Kahng, S., Hanley, G. P., Worsdell, A. S., & Thompson, R. H. (2000). Differential responding in the presence and absence of discriminative stimuli during multielement functional analyses. *Journal of Applied Behavior Analysis, 33,* 299–308.

Cooper, L., Wacker, D., Sasso, G., Reimers, T., & Donn, L. (1990). Using parents as therapists to assess the appropriate behavior of their children: Application to a tertiary diagnostic clinic. *Journal of Applied Behavior Analysis, 23,* 285–296.

Cooper, L. J., Wacker, D. P., Thursby, D., Plagmann, L. A., Harding, J., Millard, T., & Derby, M. (1992). Analysis of the effects of task preferences, task demands, and adult attention on child behavior in outpatient and classroom settings. *Journal of Applied Behavior Analysis, 25,* 823–840.

Cowdery, G. E., Iwata, B. A., & Pace, G. M. (1990). Effects and side effects of DRO as treatment for self-injurious behavior. *Journal of Applied Behavior Analysis, 23,* 497–506.

Crawford, J., Brockel, B., Schauss, S., & Miltenberger, R. G. (1992). A comparison of methods for the functional assessment of stereotypic behavior. *Journal of the Association for Persons with Severe Handicaps, 17,* 77–86.

Derby, K. M., Wacker, D. P., Sasso, G., Steege, M., Northup, J., Cigrand, K., & Asmus, J. (1992). Brief functional assessments techniques to evaluate aberrant behavior in an outpatient setting: A summary of 79 cases. *Journal of Applied Behavior Analysis, 25,* 713–721.

Desrochers, M. N., Hile, M. G., & Williams-Mosely, T. L. (1997). Survey of functional assessment procedures used with individuals who display mental retardation and severe problem behaviors. *American Journal on Mental Retardation, 101,* 535–546.

Doggett, A. R., Edwards, R. P., Moore, J. W., Tingstrom, D. H., Wilczynski, S. M. (2001). An approach to functional assessment in general education classroom settings. *School Psychology Review, 30,* 313–328.

Durand, V. M. & Crimmins, D. B. (1988). Identifying the variables maintaining self-injurious behavior. *Journal of Autism and Developmental Disorders, 18.* 99–117.

Ellingson, S. A., Miltenberger, R. G., & Long, E. S. (1999). A survey of the use of functional assessment procedures in agencies serving individuals with developmental disabilities. *Behavioral Interventions, 14,* 187–198.

Ellingson, S. A., Miltenberger, R. G., Stricker, J. M., Garlinghouse, M. A., Roberts, J., Galensky, T. L., & Rapp, J. T. (2000). Analysis and treatment of finger sucking. *Journal of Applied Behavior Analysis, 33,* 41–52.

Emerson, E., Thompson, S., Reeves, D., & Henderson, D. (1995). Descriptive analysis of multiple response topographies of challenging behavior across two settings. *Research in Developmental Disabilities, 16,* 301–329.

Fischer, S. M., Iwata, B. A., & Worsdell, A. S. (1997). Attention as an establishing operation and as reinforcement during functional analyses. *Journal of Applied Behavior Analysis, 30,* 335–338.

Fisher, W. W., Bowman, L. G., Thompson, R. H., Contrucci, S. A., Burd, L., & Alon, G. (1998). Reductions in self-injury produced by transcutaneous electrical nerve stimulation. *Journal of Applied Behavior Analysis, 31,* 493–496.

Fisher, W. W., Ninness, H. A. C., Piazza, C. C., & Owen-DeSchryver, J. S. (1996). On the reinforcing effects of the content of verbal attention. *Journal of Applied Behavior Analysis, 29,* 235–238.

Forman, D., Hall, S., & Oliver, C. (2002). Descriptive analysis of self-injurious behavior and self-restraint. *Journal of Applied Research in Intellectual Disabilities, 15,* 1–7.

Goh, H., Iwata, B. A., Shore, B. A., DeLeon, I. G., Lerman, D. C., Ulrich, S. M., & Smith, R. G. (1995). An analysis of the reinforcing properties of hand mouthing. *Journal of Applied Behavior Analysis, 28,* 269–283.

Grace, N. C., Thompson, R., & Fisher, W. W. (1996). The treatment of covert self-injury through contingencies on response products. *Journal of Applied Behavior Analysis, 29,* 239–242.

Hanley, G. P., Iwata, B. A., & McCord, B. E. (2003). Functional analysis of problem behavior: A review. *Journal of Applied Behavior Analysis, 36,* 147–185.

Harding, J., Wacker, D. P., Cooper, L. J., Millard, T., & Jensen-Kovalan, P. (1994). Brief hierarchical assessment of potential treatment components with children in an outpatient clinic. *Journal of Applied Behavior Analysis, 27,* 291–300.

Hutchinson, R.R. (1977). By-products of aversive control. In W.K. Honig & Staddon (Eds.), *Handbook of operant behavior* (pp. 415–431). Englewood Cliffs, NJ: Prentice-Hall.

Iwata, B., & DeLeon, I. (1996). *The functional analysis screening tool.* Gainesville, FL: The Florida Center on Self-Injury, University of Florida.

Iwata, B. A., Dorsey, M. F., Slifer, K. J., Bauman, K. E., & Richman, G. S. (1994a). Toward a functional analysis of self-injury. *Journal of Applied Behavior Analysis, 27,* 197–209. (Reprinted from *Analysis and Intervention in Developmental Disabilities, 2,* 3–20, 1982.)

Iwata, B. A., Duncan, B. A., Zarcone, J. R., Lerman, D. C., & Shore, B. A. (1994b). A sequential, test-control methodology for conducting functional analyses of self-injurious behavior. *Behavior Modification, 18,* 289–306.

Iwata, B. A., Kahng, S., Wallace, M. D., & Lindberg, J. S. (2000). The functional analysis model of behavioral assessment. In J. Austin & J. E. Carr (Eds.), *Handbook of applied behavior analysis* (pp. 61–89). Reno, NV: Context Press.

Iwata, B. A., Pace, G. M., Cowdery, G. E., & Miltenberger, R. G. (1994). What makes extinction work: An analysis of procedural form and function. *Journal of Applied Behavior Analysis, 27,* 131–144.

Iwata, B. A., Pace, G. M., Dorsey, M. F., Zarcone, J. R., Vollmer, T. R., Smith, R. G., et al. (1994). The functions of self-injurious behavior: An experimental-epidemiological analysis. *Journal of Applied Behavior Analysis, 27,* 215–240.

Iwata, B. A., Pace, G. M., Kalsher, M. J., Cowdery, G. E., & Cataldo, M. F. (1990). Experimental analysis and extinction of self-injurious escape behavior. *Journal of Applied Behavior Analysis, 23,* 11–27.

Iwata, B. A., Pace, G. M., Kissel, R. C., Nau, P. A., & Farber, J. M. (1990). The self-injury trauma (SIT) scale: A method for quantifying surface tissue damage caused by self-injurious behavior. *Journal of Applied Behavior Analysis, 23,* 99–110.

Iwata, B. A., Vollmer, T. R., & Zarcone, J. R. (1990). The experimental (functional) analysis of behavior disorders: Methodology, applications, and limitations. In A. C. Repp & N. N. Singh (Eds.), *Perspectives on the use of non-aversive and aversive interventions for persons with developmental disabilities* (pp. 301–330). Sycamore, IL: Sycamore.

Kahng, S., Abt, K. A., & Schonbachler, H. E. (2001). Assessment and treatment of low-rate high-intensity problem behavior. *Journal of Applied Behavior Analysis, 34,* 225–228.

Kahng, S. W., Iwata, B. A., Fischer, S. M., Page, T. J., Treadwell, K. R. H., Williams, D. E., et al. (1998). Temporal distributions of problem behavior based on scatter plot analysis. *Journal of Applied Behavior Analysis, 31,* 593–604.

Lalli, J. S., & Casey, S. D. (1996). Treatment of multiply controlled problem behavior. *Journal of Applied Behavior Analysis, 29,* 391–396.

Lalli, J. S., Livezey, K., & Kates, K. (1996). Functional analysis and treatment of eye poking with response blocking. *Journal of Applied Behavior Analysis, 29,* 129–132.

Lerman, D. C., & Iwata, B. A. (1993). Descriptive and experimental analysis of variables maintaining self-injurious behavior. *Journal of Applied Behavior Analysis, 26,* 293–319.

Lerman, D. C., Iwata, B. A., Smith, R. G., Zarcone, J. R., & Vollmer, T. R. (1994). Transfer of behavioral function as a contributing factor in treatment relapse. *Journal of Applied Behavior Analysis, 27,* 357–370.

Lesch, M., and Nyhan, W. L. (1964). A familial disorder of uric acid metabolism and central nervous system function. *American Journal of Medicine 36,* 561–570.

Lewis, T. J., Scott, T. M., & Sugai, G. (1994). The problem behavior questionnaire: A teacher-based instrument to develop functional hypotheses of problem behavior in general education classrooms. *Diagnostique, 19,* 103–115.

Lovaas, I., Newsom, C., & Hickman, C. (1987). Self-stimulatory behavior and perceptual reinforcement. *Journal of Applied Behavior Analysis, 20,* 45–68.

Lovaas, O. I., & Simmons, J. Q. (1969). Manipulation of self-destruction in three retarded children. *Journal of Applied Behavior Analysis, 2,* 143–157.

Mace, F. C., & Lalli, J. S. (1991) Linking descriptive and experimental analyses in the treatment of bizarre speech. *Journal of Applied Behavior Analysis, 24,* 553–562.

Marcus, B. A., & Vollmer, T. R. (1996). Combining noncontingent reinforcement and differential reinforcement schedules as treatment for aberrant behavior. *Journal of Applied Behavior Analysis, 29,* 43–51.

Marholin, D., & Steinman, W. M. (1977). Stimulus control in the classroom as a function of the behavior reinforced. *Journal of Applied Behavior Analysis, 10,* 465–478.

Matson, J. L., Bamburg, J. W., Cheery, K. E., & Paclawskyj, T. R. (1999). A validity study on the questions about behavioral function (QABF) scale: Predicting treatment success for self-injury, aggression, and stereotypies. *Research in Developmental Disabilities, 20,* 163–175.

Matson, J. L., Kuhn, D. E., Dixon, D. R., Mayville, S. B., Laud, R. B., Cooper, C. L., et al. (2003) The development and factor structure of the Functional Assessment for Multiple Causality (FACT). *Research in Developmental Disabilities, 24,* 485–495.

Matson, J. L., & Vollmer, T. R. (1995). *User's guide: Questions About Behavioral Function (QABF).* Baton Rouge, LA.: Scientific.

Miltenberger, R. G. (2001). *Behavior modification: Principles and procedures.* Belmont, CA: Wadsworth.

Ndoro, V. W., Hanley, G. P., Tiger, J. H., & Heal, N. A. (2006). A descriptive assessment of instruction-based interactions in the preschool classroom. *Journal of Applied Behavior Analysis 39,* 79–90.

Northup, J., Wacker, D. P., Berg, W. K., Kelly, L., Sasso, G., & DeRaad, A. (1994). The treatment of severe behavior problems in school settings using a technical assistance model. *Journal of Applied Behavior Analysis, 27*, 33–48.

Northup, J., Wacker, D., Sasso, G., Steege, M., Cigrand, K., Cook, J., & DeRaad, A. (1991). A brief functional analysis of aggressive and alternative behavior in an out-clinic setting. *Journal of Applied Behavior Analysis, 24*, 509–522.

O'Neill, R. E., Horner, R. H., Albin, R. W., Sprague, J. R., Storey, K., & Newton, J. S. (1997). *Functional assessment and program development for problem behavior: A practical handbook* (2nd ed.). Pacific Grove, CA: Brooks.

Oliver, C., Hall, S., & Nixon, J. (1999). A molecular to molar analysis of communicative and problem behavior. *Research in Developmental Disabilities, 20*, 197–213.

Paclawskyj, T. R., Matson, J. L., Rush, K. S., & Smalls, Y. (2001). The validity of the questions about behavioral function (QABF). *Journal of Intellectual Disabilities, 45*, 484–494.

Piazza, C. C., Bowman, L. G., Contrucci, S. A., Delia, M. D., Adelinis, J. D., & Goh, H. (1999). An evaluation of the properties of attention as reinforcement for destructive and appropriate behavior. *Journal of Applied Behavior Analysis, 32*, 437–449.

Piazza, C. C., Hanley, G. P., & Fisher, W. W. (1996). Functional analysis and treatment of cigarette pica. *Journal of Applied Behavior Analysis, 29*, 437–449.

Rapp, J. T., Miltenberger, R. G., Galensky, T. L., Ellingson, S. A., & Long, E. S. (1999). A functional analysis of hair pulling. *Journal of Applied Behavior Analysis, 32*, 329–337.

Rojahn, J., Matson, J. L., Lott, D., Esbensen, A. J., & Smalls, Y. (2001). The Behavior Problems Inventory: An instrument for the assessment of self-injury, stereotyped behavior, and aggression/destruction in individuals with developmental disabilities. *Journal of Autism and Developmental Disorders, 6*, 577–588.

St. Peter, C. C., Vollmer, T. R., Bourret, J. C., Borrero, C. S. W., Sloman, K. N., & Rapp, J. T. (2005). On the role of attention in naturally occurring matching relations. *Journal of Applied Behavior Analysis, 38*, 429–443.

Samaha, A. L., Vollmer, T. R., Borrero, C., Sloman, K., & St. Peter, C. (in press). Analyses of response-stimulus sequences in descriptive observations. *Journal of Applied Behavior Analysis.*

Sandman, C. A., Datta, P. C., Barron, J., Hoehler, F. K., Williams, C., & Swanson, J. M. (1983). Naloxone attenuates self-abusive behavior in developmentally disabled clients. *Applied Research in Mental Retardation, 4*, 5–11.

Sasso, G. M., Reimers, T. M., Cooper, L. J., Wacker, D., Berg, W., Steege, M. et al. (1992). Use of descriptive and experimental analyses to identify the functional properties of aberrant behavior in school settings. *Journal of Applied Behavior Analysis, 25*, 809–821.

Shirley, M. J., Iwata, B. A., & Kahng, S. (1999). False–positive maintenance of self-injurious behavior by access to tangible reinforcers. *Journal of Applied Behavior Analysis, 32*, 201–204.

Sidman, M. (1960). *Tactics of scientific research.* New York: Basic Books.

Skinner, B. F. (1953). *Science and human behavior.* New York: Macmillan.

Sloman, K. N., Vollmer, T. R., Cotnoir, N. M., Borrero, C. S. W., Borrero, J. C., Samaha, A. L., et al. (2005). Descriptive analysis of caregiver reprimands. *Journal of Applied Behavior Analysis, 38*, 373–383.

Smith, R. G., & Churchill, R. M. (2002). Identification of environmental determinants of behavior disorders through functional analysis of precursor behaviors. *Journal of Applied Behavior Analysis, 35*, 125–136.

Smith, R. G., Iwata, B. A., Vollmer, T. R., & Zarcone, J. R. (1993). Experimental analysis and treatment of multiply controlled self-injury. *Journal of Applied Behavior Analysis, 26*, 183–196.

Steege, M. W., Wacker, D. P., Cigrand, K. C., Berg, W. K., Novak, C. G., Reimers, T. M., Sasso, G. M., & DeRaad, A. (1990). Use of negative reinforcement in the treatment of self-injurious behavior. *Journal of Applied Behavior Analysis, 23*, 459–467.

Thompson, R. H., & Iwata, B. A. (2001). A descriptive analysis of social consequences following problem behavior. *Journal of Applied Behavior Analysis, 34*, 169–178.

Touchette, P. E., MacDonald, R. F., & Langer, S. N. (1985). A scatter plot for identifying stimulus control of problem behavior. *Journal of Applied Behavior Analysis, 18*, 343–351.

VanDerHeyden, A. M., Witt, J. C., & Gatti, S. (2001). Descriptive assessment method to reduce overall disruptive behavior in a preschool classroom. *School Psychology Review, 30,* 548–567.

Van Houten, R. and Rolider, A. (1991). Research in Applied Behavior Analysis. In J. L. Matson & J. A. Mulick (Eds). *Handbook of mental retardation* (2nd ed.). New York: Pergamon Press.

Vollmer, T. R., Borrero, J. C., Wright, C. S., Van Camp, C., & Lalli, J. S. (2001). Identifying possible contingencies during descriptive analyses of severe behavior disorders. *Journal of Applied Behavior Analysis, 34,* 269–287.

Vollmer, T. R., Iwata, B. A., Duncan, B. A., & Lerman, D. C. (1993a). Within-session patterns of self-injury as indicators of behavioral function. *Research in Developmental Disabilities, 14,* 479–492.

Vollmer, T. R., Iwata, B. A., Duncan, B. A., & Lerman, D. C. (1993b). Extensions of multielement functional analyses using reversal-type designs. *Journal of Developmental and Physical Disabilities, 5,* 311–325.

Vollmer, T. R., Marcus, B. A., & Ringdahl, J. E. (1995). Noncontingent escape as treatment for self-injurious behavior maintained by negative reinforcement. *Journal of Applied Behavior Analysis, 28,* 15–26.

Vollmer, T. R., Marcus, B. A., Ringdahl, J. E., & Roane, H. S. (1995). Progressing from brief to extended experimental analyses in the evaluation of aberrant behavior. *Journal of Applied Behavior Analysis, 28,* 561–576.

Weiseler, N. A., Hanson, R. H., Chamberlain, T. R., & Thompson, T. (1985). Functional taxonomy of stereotypic and self-injurious behavior. *Mental Retardation, 23,* 230–234.

Wilson, D. M., Iwata, B. A., and Bloom, S. E. (in press). Evaluation of a computer-assisted technique for measuring wound severity. *Journal of Applied Behavior Analysis.*

Zarcone, J. R., Rodgers, T. A., Iwata, B. A., Rourke, D. A., & Dorsey, M. F. (1991). Reliability analysis of the motivation assessment scale: A failure to replicate. *Research in Developmental Disabilities, 12,* 349–360.

13

Autism Spectrum Disorders and Comorbid Psychopathology

JESSICA A. BOISJOLI and JOHNNY L. MATSON

Autism spectrum disorders (ASD) are a group of disorders that are typically first diagnosed in childhood. These disorders are characterized by a triad of impairments that often require specialized intervention and treatment throughout childhood and oftentimes into adulthood. In addition to the three major impairments of ASD (i.e., socialization, communication, and restricted interests and repetitive behaviors), co-occurring behavioral challenges and psychopathology are also evident and even occur at higher rates than in the general population (Gillberg & Billstedt, 2000). The aim of this chapter is to review the assessment of ASD and comorbid psychopathology.

AUTISM SPECTRUM DISORDERS

Over the past 60 years since Leo Kanner (1943) first wrote of 11 children he termed as having "autistic disturbance of affective contact" there has been and continues to be an impressive amount of research and interest on the topic. The deficit reported by Kanner to be present in all of the 11 children was "a disability in relating themselves in the ordinary way to people and situations from the beginning of life" (p. 242). At the same time as Kanner's initial research on children with autism, Hans Asperger (1991), an Austrian physician, also wrote of 4 children that he reported as having an "autistic psychopathy". All of the observed children had impairments in the areas of nonverbal communication, social adaptation, and special

JESSICA A. BOISJOLI and JOHNNY L. MATSON • Department of Psychology, Louisiana State University, Baton Rouge, LA 70803.

J.L. Matson et al. (eds.), *Assessing Childhood Psychopathology and Developmental Disabilities*, DOI: 10.1007/978-0-387-09528-8,
© Springer Science+Business Media, LLC 2009

interests, and evinced idiosyncrasies in verbal communication, intellectualization of affect, clumsiness and poor body awareness, and conduct problems. What both Kanner and Asperger were studying were children with ASD.

Core Features of ASD

Since the earliest research in the field of ASD, a common theme has been the triad of impairments. These impairments encompass the following domains: socialization, communication, and behavior (i.e., resistance to change, repetitive movements). An overview of these core features of ASD follows.

Socialization

A key feature in people with ASD is their inability to relate to other people. Typically developing babies learn throughout the first months of life to socialize with those in their environment. Infants look at the face of a caregiver, make eye contact, and vocalize. Historical accounts from parents have indicated that infants with ASD fail to socially smile, engage in eye contact, and other social behaviors appropriate for their developmental level (Volkmar, 1987). By about six to nine months, typically developing children begin to share attention with other people. This phenomenon is referred to as "joint attention" and entails looking at a person and then either looking at or pointing to an object of interest in order to coordinate attention. Many children with ASD fail to master the use of eye gaze and gestures to share attention with another person. Because joint attention is a social skill that is typically acquired at such a young age, impairment in joint attention is one of the first symptoms noticed in infants with ASD (Osterling & Dawson, 1994).

Although some social functioning may improve as children develop (Rutter & Garmezy, 1983), deficits in social skills are lifelong and continue into adulthood (Matson, Baglio, Smirolodo, Hamilton, & Packlowskyj, 1996). Intellectual disability (ID) co-occurs in a large number of individuals with ASD, and individuals with the more severe forms of ID typically have greater deficits in social skills. ID coupled with symptomotology of ASD then results in much greater deficits in this domain (Njardvic, Matson, & Cherry, 1999). Njardvik and colleagues (1999) studied the differences in social skills between participants with Autistic Disorder (AD), Pervasive Developmental Disorder Not Otherwise Specified (PDD-NOS; a less severe variant of ASD), and ID only.

Social skills deficits were most severe in people with AD, followed by those with PDD-NOS, and then ID. Additionally, significant differences were found between the skills of people with AD and those with just ID. Fewer differences were found between participants with PDD-NOS and those with AD and those with ID only. These results are consistent with current literature, characterizing ASD as a disorder of social skills with more severe deficits in social skills in people with AD and less severe deficits in individuals with PDD-NOS.

Language and Communication

Early research on ASD suggested that about half of the individuals with a diagnosis would never acquire speech (Rutter, 1978). However, this estimate may be decreasing due to more accurate methods of diagnosis, earlier diagnosis, and early intervention (Klinger, Dawson, & Renner, 2003). Some people with autism never develop speech and for those who do, many never acquire functional speech. For many individuals with ASD who do have language, their speech may be abnormal, involving echolalia and pronoun reversal (Rutter & Bartak, 1971). Furthermore, for the children who develop language, their speech may be of unusual rhythm, stress, intonation, or volume when compared to other children with ID (Lord et al., 2000).

In addition to the deficits in verbal communication, people with ASD also have marked difficulties with nonverbal communication. Eye contact/ gaze and nodding in response to a request or to gain attention from a person are often impaired. Deficits in nonverbal communication also encompass their awareness of other people's nonverbal communication, such as facial expression and body language. For example, a person with ASD may engage in monologues about a particular area of interest without noticing the listener's obvious lack of interest displayed through body language, such as yawning or looking away.

For people with ASD, deficits in communication overlap with the deficits in socialization. The social context of language is referred to as pragmatics. Although some people with ASD develop language, their use of language in conversations and in a social context is lacking. Deficiencies in social interactions such as maintaining, joining, and ending conversations, are often noted.

Behavior

The third hallmark characteristic of individuals with ASD encompasses behavioral excesses. Restricted areas of interest, repetitive behaviors, and insistence on sameness are observed in people with ASD. Many children with ASD have circumscribed interests that are more intense than normal. These interests may consume the child, not allowing time for much else. Also characteristic of people with ASD are repetitive behaviors called stereotypies. These behaviors are motor movements such as whole body rocking, hand flapping, or other unusual, repetitive hand movements. These behaviors are rhythmic in nature and appear purposive. Lastly, an insistence on sameness is often observed in this population. People with ASD may demand that the arrangement of furniture in a room remain unchanged, insist on the same route always being taken to the store, or engaging in rituals. Insistence on these factors is characteristic of people with ASD and can be a source of distress (Kanner, 1951).

Differential Diagnosis

Symptoms of ASD vary from person to person along a continuum of severity. The most severe form is what many people refer to as "classic autism" or AD according to the *Diagnostic and Statistical Manual Fourth Edition: Text Revision* (*DSM–IV–TR*; American Psychiatric Association [APA], 2000) and the least severe being PDD-NOS. In order to differentiate between the disorders of the spectrum, severity and the age of onset of symptoms are considered as well as the individual's cognitive functioning, particularly in the diagnosis of Asperger's syndrome (AS). However, there is much debate regarding the use of these criteria to differentiate between diagnoses on the autism continuum (Matson & Minshawi, 2006).

Not until the introduction of the *DSM–III* (APA, 1986) was autism officially recognized as a disorder distinct from childhood schizophrenia (Cohen, Paul, & Volkmar, 1987). Autism now fell under a broader category of Pervasive Developmental Disorders (PDD), often referred to as ASD in the literature (APA, 1986). A problem arose in the autism subdomain where it was termed Early Infantile Autism because deficits persist into adulthood. The *DSM–IV* (APA, 1994) renamed the diagnosis AD, which still fell under the umbrella of PDD. The PDD are comprised of five disorders that are all characterized by impairments beginning in childhood, involving deficits with socialization, communication, and restricted behaviors. The five PDD are AD, Childhood Disintegrative Disorder, Rett's Disorder, PDD-NOS, and AS.

Children diagnosed with AD show symptoms prior to the age of three years and have more severe deficits in the triad of impairments. Socially, these children are often described as aloof and may only approach others to satisfy needs (Wing & Attwood, 1987). These children are also likely to have more severe deficits in communication and more repetitive behaviors. In addition, there is a higher prevalence of ID in people with AD as well as a poorer outcome when compared to children with higher cognitive ability and less severe symptoms, such as those with AS (Klin & Volkmar, 1995). Fombonne (2003) reviewed prevalence studies of AD since 1987 and estimated the prevalence to be approximately 10/10,000 people.

The first reference to a disorder characterized by regression after seemingly normal development was by Theodore Heller in 1908. The disorder referred to as Heller's syndrome or "dementia infantalis" is now termed Childhood Disintegrative Disorder (CDD). Children with CDD regress around the age of three to four years, losing previously gained skills and behaviors. The regression begins with mood problems, speech loss, incontinence, and regression of other skills (Volkmar, 1992). One study conducted in India reported a prevalence rate of CDD at .45% in a clinic population, a mean age of onset of 3.76 years for a sample that was 83% male (Malhorta & Gupta, 2002). However, the sample size of participants presenting with CDD was low ($n = 12$), therefore limiting the generalizability of results. When compared to the amount of research on AD, research involving CDD is quite scarce.

Similar to the defining feature of CDD (i.e., age of onset after apparently normal development), Rett's Disorder is another PDD that is characterized by regression in development. The difference, however, is that this disorder is primarily observed in females, and the time of normal development is shorter than found with CDD: months as opposed to years. Additionally, Rett's Disorder has traceable genetic causes on an X-linked gene.

The infants have typical development until the 6th to 18th month of life when there is a slowing down or regression in social skills, head growth deceleration, and loss of functional use of the hands along with an emergence of stereotypic "hand wringing," with the regression continuing until about the third year of life (Van Acker, 1991).

More recently, researchers have suggested that the early development of infants affected with Rett's Disorder may actually be deviant in terms of posture and body movement (Burford, Kerr, & Macleod, 2003), contradicting the implication that these children had normal development prior to the regression. Additionally, Rett's Disorder once believed to only affect females, has been reported in males, although infrequently (Budden, Dorsey, & Steiner, 2005).

Rett's Disorder is believed to be quite rare with few studies published on its prevalence. One study conducted in Sweden placed the prevalence of this disorder at .65/10,000 girls (Hagberg, 1985) and another study in Australia placed the prevalence at .72/10,000 females (Leonard, Bower, & English, 1997). Failure to recognize the symptoms of Rett's Disorder may contribute to an underestimation of its prevalence with one researcher suggesting that this disorder may account for up to one-third of the cases of females with progressive developmental disabilities (Hagberg, 1985).

For people who do not meet the full criteria for a diagnosis of AD, although still evincing qualitative impairments in the core features of ASD, a diagnosis of PDD-NOS is applied. However, reliable criteria for diagnosing PDD-NOS is still elusive (Towbin, 1997). Instead, the diagnosis of PDD-NOS is made when criteria for other categories of ASD are not met (Tidmarsh & Volkmar, 2003). A study by Chakrabarti and Fombonne (2005), using a birth cohort from the years 1991 to 1998, found a prevalence rate of 31.4 per 10,000 diagnosed with PDD-NOS. Furthermore, PDD-NOS is the most commonly diagnosed disorder along the autism spectrum, yet it remains one of the least studied (Matson & Boisjoli, 2007).

Although many people with ASD also have ID, some have average or above average intellectual functioning. One diagnosis on the autism spectrum not commonly associated with ID is AS. However, some researchers have suggested that AS may also occur in people with mild ID to Borderline Intellectual Functioning (Strum, Fernell, & Gillberg, 2004). AS is characterized by most researchers as average or above average intelligence, impairments in socialization and communication, and restricted interests and repetitive behaviors. The prevalence of AS was estimated by Fombonne (2003) to be 2.5/10,000 people; one quarter the prevalence of AD.

One criterion differentiating AS from a "high functioning" autism (i.e. AD with cognitive functioning in the average range) according to the *DSM–IV–TR* is language development. In the more classic autism, a marked delay in language acquisition is observed in both those with low and high intellectual functioning. In people with AS this delay is not evident. Language is acquired at a developmentally normal rate or possibly even earlier, with some children evincing hyperlexia (Nation, Clarke, Wright, Williams, & Patterns, 2006). Although there have been some studies on differentiating between the disorders along the ASD continuum, considerable research is still needed.

Assessment/Diagnosis

The *DSM–IV–TR* (APA, 2000) is a diagnostic schedule used to classify psychological disorders. The *DSM–IV–TR* requires the presentation of qualitative impairments in social interaction, communication, and/or restricted patterns of interest for a diagnosis of a PDD. As stated earlier, the five PDD classified in the *DSM–IV–TR* are AD, AS, PDD-NOS, and the two less common disorders, Rett's Disorder and Childhood Disintegrative Disorder.

AD is characterized by deficits in the areas of socialization, communication, and repetitive behaviors/restricted interests. For a diagnosis of AD, the person must possess at least two impairments in social interaction, at least one impairment in communication, and exhibit at least one behavioral excess, with a total of six criteria exhibited. Additionally, deficits in social interaction, language, or symbolic/imaginative play need to be evident prior to the age of 36 months. See Table 13.1 for a complete list of *DSM–IV–TR* criteria for AD (APA, 2000).

No specific criteria for the diagnosis of PDD-NOS are provided in the *DSM–IV–TR*. The manual states that for a diagnosis of PDD-NOS, severe impairments in social interaction and either deficits in communication or occurrence of stereotyped behaviors/restricted pattern of interests need to be present. That is, the individual did not meet sufficient criteria for a diagnosis of AD or AS although still exhibiting deficits in socialization and communication or behavior. This diagnosis is used as a residual category for disorders that do not fit in any of the other categories. Nonetheless, the person should still exhibit symptoms consistent with the description of a PDD.

To make a diagnosis of AS using the *DSM–IV–TR*, criteria are similar to that of AD with one important distinction: impairment in the communication

---

Table 13.1. *DSM–IV–TR* (APA, 2000) criteria for a diagnosis of Autistic Disorder

A total of at least 6 of the following deficits/impairments needs to be displayed for a diagnosis of Autistic Disorder and the person must possess at least two impairments
- In social interaction including impairment
- In multiple nonverbal behaviors
- Failure to develop peer relationships (appropriate to developmental level)
- Lack of spontaneous seeking to share enjoyment
- Lack of social and emotional reciprocity

At least one of the following impairments in communication
- Delay in, or total lack of, the development of spoken language
- In individuals with adequate speech, marked impairment in the ability to initiate or sustain a conversation with others
- Stereotyped and repetitive or idiosyncratic language
- Lack of varied, spontaneous make-believe play or social imitative play appropriate to the developmental level

At least one of the following behavioral excesses
- Preoccupation with one or more stereotyped and restricted patterns of interest that is abnormal in either intensity or focus
- Apparent inflexible adherence to specific, nonfunctional routines or rituals
- Stereotyped and repetitive motor mannerisms
- Persistent preoccupation with parts of objects

Additionally, deficits in social interaction, language, or symbolic/imaginative play need to be evident prior to the age of 36 months.

domain is not present. The individual needs to meet at least two of the criteria in the socialization domain and at least one criterion in the behavior domain. Additionally, the deficits must cause a clinically significant impairment in important areas of functioning (e.g., social, occupational), and there must be no clinically significant delay in language, cognitive development, self-help skills, adaptive behavior, and curiosity with his or her environment. It is important to note that the person cannot meet criteria for another PDD in order to be diagnosed with AS.

According to the *DSM–IV–TR*, there are separate criteria for a diagnosis of Rett's Disorder. Rett's Disorder is diagnosed if the person meets each of the following criteria: (1) apparently normal prenatal and perinatal development; (2) apparently normal psychomotor development through the first 5 months after birth; and (3) normal head circumference at birth. After the period of normal development, each of the following also must be met: (1) deceleration of head growth between the ages of 5 and 48 months; (2) loss of previously acquired purposeful hand skills between the ages of 5 and 30 months with the subsequent development of stereotyped hand movements (e.g., hand-wringing or hand washing); (3) loss of social engagement early in the course (although social interaction often develops later); (4) appearance of poorly coordinated gait or trunk movements; and (5) severely impaired expressive and receptive language development with severe psychomotor retardation.

Childhood Disintegrative Disorder, like Rett's Disorder, has a distinct set of criteria under the PDD category. Criteria from the *DSM–IV–TR* include: (1) apparently normal development for at least the first 2 years after birth as manifested by the presence of age-appropriate verbal and nonverbal communication, social relationships, play, and adaptive behavior; (2) clinically significant loss of previously acquired skills (before age 10 years) in at least two of the following areas: (a) expressive or receptive language, (b) social skills or adaptive behavior, (c) bowel or bladder control, (d) play, or (e) motor skills; and (3) abnormalities of functioning in at least two of the following areas: (a) qualitative impairment in social interaction (e.g., impairment in nonverbal behaviors, failure to develop peer relationships, lack of social or emotional reciprocity), (b) qualitative impairments in communication (e.g., delay or lack of spoken language, inability to initiate or sustain a conversation, stereotyped and repetitive use of language, lack of varied make-believe play), or (c) restricted, repetitive, and stereotyped patterns of behavior, interests, and activities, including motor stereotypes and mannerisms.

Rating Scales

Childhood Autism Rating Scale (CARS)

One of the most commonly used scales to detect ASD in children is the CARS (Schopler, Reichler, & Renner, 1988). This test was initially developed to differentiate between children having an ASD or ID diagnosis that were referred to the Treatment and Education of Autistic and related Communication handicapped CHildren (TEACCH; Schlopler et al., 1988) in North Carolina. The scale is intended for people over the age of 2 years. Fifteen independent subscales comprise the CARS. The subscales include: relating to people; imitation; emotional response; body use; object use; adaptation to change; visual response; listening response; taste, smell, and touch response and use; fear or nervousness; verbal communication; nonverbal communication; activity level; level and consistency of intellectual response; and general impressions.

The rater scores the individual on a scale from 1 to 4, with "1" indicating normal for the child's age and "4" indicating severely abnormal. Psychometrics of the CARS are good, with rater agreement of .71, and test–retest at 12 months having yielded nonsignificant changes in means from the first assessment. Validity studies indicate good criterion-related validity with $r = .80$ correlation with clinical judgments. Additionally, the scale was able to correctly predict 100% group membership for children with ASD and those with ID. Potential limitations of the CARS are that some expertise with ASDs is required for accurate administration. Furthermore, symptoms represented in the CARS do not directly match *DSM–IV–TR* criteria. This discrepancy may in part be due to the fact that the CARS was developed prior to the *DSM–IV–TR*. Using the CARS, one is able to differentiate between severities of ASD. However, the scale does not provide diagnoses along the spectrum of autistic disorders.

Autism Behavior Checklist (ABC)

The ABC (Krug, Arick, & Almond, 1980) is a rating scale designed for use by teachers and others without extensive experience with ASD. The scale was developed as a screen and consists of 57 items. The informant rates the child along five subscales: sensory, relating, language, socialization and self-help, and body and object use, using dichotomous scoring (i.e., yes or no). Each item is weighted on a four-point continuum. Reliability studies have shown adequate results for interrater reliability and good internal consistency (Krug et al., 1980). Additionally, the scale appears to be effective in discriminating children diagnosed with an ASD and those with developmental or learning disabilities that do not fall along the ASD spectrum (Wadden, Bryson, & Rodger, 1991). Weaknesses of the measure are that it does not make diagnoses along the autism spectrum nor according to criteria of the *DSM–IV–TR*.

Checklist for Autism in Toddlers (CHAT)

Different from the previously discussed assessments of ASD, the CHAT (Baron-Cohen, Cox, Baird, Swettenham, & Nighingale 1996) was designed to be used by pediatricians as a screener at toddlers' 18-month checkups. The screener assesses three areas: pretend play, joint attention by pointing, and monitoring of gaze. The parent answers yes/no to nine questions and the pediatrician answers five questions based on observation. For use as a population screen, the scale has been shown to have low sensitivity when only including the high-risk group, but improves when including children with medium risk (Baron-Cohen et al., 1996). Sensitivity improved and specificity was excellent when both groups were considered (Baron-Cohen et al., 1996). Other studies using the CHAT with children who were older showed good levels of sensitivity and specificity (Scambler, Rogers, & Wehner, 2001). One weakness of the CHAT is that data are not available on the effectiveness of the CHAT in differentiating children with ASD and those with other forms of psychopathology (Matson & Minshawi, 2006).

Interviews/Observations

Autism Diagnostic Interview-Revised (ADI-R)

Another popular tool used to assess ASD is the ADI-R (Lord, Rutter, & Le Couteur, 1994). The ADI-R was a revision of the original Autism Diagnostic Interview (ADI). The revision overcame some of the shortcomings of the ADI, such as only diagnosing children under the age of five years and decreasing administration time (Lord et al., 1994). The ADI-R is in an interview format with parents/caretakers serving as informants. This measure is intended for use with children with a mental age of at least 18 months and extends into adulthood. The ADI-R has proved to have good psychometrics with interrater reliability ranging from .62 to .89 (Lord et al., 1994). The ADI-R diagnoses along *DSM–IV* criteria. However, some drawbacks are that the ADI-R relies solely on parent-report, is lengthy and time consuming to administer, and it requires a clinician that is experienced with ASD.

Autism Diagnostic Observation Schedule (ADOS)

In 1989, Lord and colleagues developed a scale to focus on discriminating among groups of children with ASD, ID, and typically developing children based on social and communicative behaviors. The ADOS is designed for toddlers through adults. However, the authors caution that for children below the nonverbal developmental age of 12–18 months, concern should be taken when interpreting the results, particularly when scores near the cut-off point. Four modules comprise the ADOS with each used for people with differing levels of verbal fluency. The ADOS is observation-based rather than informant-based. The child is placed in situations requiring her to request help, engage in symbolic play, take turns, perform simple tasks, tell a story, discuss tasks that occurred earlier in the assessment, and discuss social and emotional situations. The child is rated on each task by the examiner as within normal limits, infrequent or possible abnormality, or definite abnormality.

The criteria for an ASD using the ADOS are based on the World Health Organization, *International Classification of Diseases*, 10th edition (ICD-10; WHO, 1992) criteria. Reliability of the scale is reported to be good, with individual items between .61 and .92 (Lord et al., 1989). Validity was also reportedly good as the tool is successful in differentiating between children with and without ASD. Weaknesses of the scale are that separately, the communication and social subscales were not able to classify groups, and the scale does not measure behavioral deficits and excesses.

Screening Tool for Autism in Two-Year-Olds (STAT)

The STAT was developed in 1997 by Stone and Ousley as a screening measure to identify the symptoms of ASD in two-year-olds. Health care/service providers administer an interactive assessment to determine if the child is in need of further evaluation (Stone, Coorod, & Ousley, 2000). This brief assessment consists of 12 items assessing play, attention, imitation, and requesting items with binary scoring: pass or fail. Sensitivity and specificity estimates were acceptable at .83 and .86 respectively (Stone et al., 2000). Stone and associates (2004) conducted further psychometric analyses on the measure showing excellent test–retest and interobserver agreement. Additionally, the STAT was validated using the ADOS. High agreement was observed when classifying children as "high risk" (Stone et al., 2004). One weakness of this measure is that it is not as effective in identifying children diagnosed with PDD-NOS, only classifying 35% of these children as "high risk."

Measures for Differential Diagnosis

Diagnoses of ASD are increasing and research on the topic is flourishing. However, experts in the field of ASD cannot agree on the criteria that constitute each of the three more commonly diagnosed ASD: AD, AS, and PDD-NOS. Although the *DSM–IV–TR* delineates criteria for each of these disorders (or the absence of enough criteria for a diagnosis of AD or AS in the case of PDD-NOS), the research community disputes the validity of using the criteria and suggest clinical judgment as the "gold standard" in diagnosing these disorders (Volkmar et al., 1994). Rett's Disorder has a clear symptom pattern and genetic link, making diagnosis straightforward, and the rarity of Childhood Disintegrative Disorder and the suggestion that the disorder may not be distinct from AD (Rapin, 1997) has resulted in little attention to these two disorders in the literature. However, attempts have been made to design measures to differentially diagnose along the autism continuum. These efforts are reviewed next.

Autism Spectrum Disorder-Diagnostic for Children (ASD-DC)

The ASD-DC (Matson & Gonzalez, 2007c) is a new, informant-based measure used to assess symptoms of ASD as well as differentiate between three of the five ASDs: AD, AS, and PDD-NOS. The ASD-DC is used along with two other measures (i.e., ASD-CC and ASD-BPC) which assess comorbid psychopathology and behavior problems and are discussed in more detail in this chapter. The informants are parents/caretakers who are instructed to compare the child to a typically developing child, the same age, and rate each item on a Likert-type scale: 0, "not different; no impairment"; 1, "somewhat different; mild impairment"; or 2, "very different; severe impairment." The items of the ASD-DC were generated through a review of the current literature and diagnostic guidelines for ASD, critical incidents reported by experienced clinicians, and expert review (Matson & Gonzalez, 2007c).

Initial studies of the ASD-DC have shown promising results, with good to excellent interrater and test–retest reliability correlations and excellent internal consistency at .99 (Matson, Gonzalez, Wilkins, & Rivet, in press). Additionally, the measure is successful in differentiating between children with ASD and controls (Matson, Gonzalez, Wilkins, & Rivet, 2007). Validity studies are currently under way.

Diagnostic Interview for Social and Communication Disorders (DISCO)

The DISCO (Wing, Leekam, Libby, Gould, & Larcombe, 2002) is a semi-structured interview used to assist in the diagnosis of ASD as well as other disorders of socialization and communication. Items on the DISCO request information regarding developmental history and current behavior. The format of the interview is semi-structured in that the interviewer does not have a set sample of questions. The interviewer continues to ask questions in order to gain ample information to make a rating for the item. This measure also allows for the collection of other information provided during the evaluation to be used towards the scoring of DISCO items. The interview covers the following areas: development, motor skills, self-care, communication, social interaction, imitation, imagination, skills, stereotypies, sensory response, routines and resistance to change, emotions, activity patterns, maladaptive behaviors, sleep, catatonic, and quality of socialization.

Interrater reliability is reportedly high (Leekam, Libby, Wing, Gould, & Taylor, 2002). This measure has proved to be valid in the diagnosis of ASD (Leekam et al., 2002), however, the authors caution the use of the measure in this manner. They note that the scale was not designed to provide categorical diagnoses as diagnoses are based on the collective information provided in the evaluation, not just the information provided from the DISCO. Consequently, a clinician experienced with ASD may be needed to administer this measure.

In addition to measures designed to differentially diagnose along the autism spectrum, there are also measures that attempt to diagnose a specific ASD, not including AD. Such measures assess for Rett's Disorder and AS. A brief review of these measures follows.

Rett's Disorder Assessment

Rett Syndrome Behavior Questionnaire (RSBQ)

One measure specific to differentiating individuals with the more severe forms of ID, AD, and those with Rett's Disorder is the RSBQ (Mount, Charman, Hastings, Reilly, & Cass, 2002). This scale was designed to identify behavioral phenotypes that are more specific to people with Rett's Disorder (Mount et al., 2002). The RSBQ is a 45-item informant-based measure with a total of eight empirically derived subscales. The subscales measure general mood, breathing problems, hand behaviors, repetitive face movements, body rocking and expressionless face, night-time behaviors, fear/anxiety,

and walking/standing. The scale has good reliability with intraclass correlations for the total score and all subscales >.70 and good internal consistency (Mount et al, 2002). In addition, sensitivity and specificity were 86.3%
and 86.8%, respectively, for differentiating between people with Rett's Disorder and others with severe/profound ID. However, additional studies are
warranted to further assess the validity of the RSBQ.

Asperger's Syndrome Assessments

Matson and Boisjoli (2008) conducted a review of existing measures
and their psychometric properties for AS. Although there are a sizable
number of scales designed to assess this disorder, very little research has
been conducted on many of the scales, only about one to three published
studies per scale (Matson & Boisjoli, 2008). Such a low number of soundly
studied scales may be due in part to problems in defining what AS is and
how it differs from AD (Matson, 2007a).

As already mentioned, a number of measures of AS exist, however, with
little empirical support. Some of the more studied measures are the Gilliam
Asperger's Disorder Scale (GADS; Gilliam, 2001), the Childhood Asperger's
Syndrome Test (CAST; Scott, Baron-Cohen, Bolton, & Brayne, 2002), and
the Krug Asperger's Disorder Index (KADI; Krug & Arick, 2003). One major
weakness of each of these measures is that they may actually only differentiate people on the autism spectrum according to cognitive abilities rather
than provide categorical diagnoses along the spectrum (i.e., the ability to
differentiate between people who have below-average cognitive abilities and
those with average or above). Additional research on the measurement of AS
and distinguishing it from other disorders, including AD, is greatly needed.

Dual Diagnosis/Comorbidity

Comorbidity is the co-occurrence of more than one form of psychopathology occurring in the same person (Matson & Nebel-Schwalm, 2007).
Although research in the area of comorbid conditions in typically developing children is beginning to flourish, research investigating other psychological disorders occurring along with ASD is generally lacking. Numerous
reasons exist as to why this clinical population has received very little
attention. The current literature points to the high co-occurrence of ID
and ASD, the heterogeneity in symptoms in people with ASD, psychopathology symptoms manifesting differently in this population (Matson
& Nebel-Scwalm, 2007), and the possible overlap of ASD symptoms with
other forms of psychopathology all contributing to the sparse amount of
research on the topic. These issues, particularly in conjunction, make
diagnosis of comorbid psychopathology problematic.

The most common dual diagnosis for people with ASD is ID. A study
done by Chakrabarti and Fombonne (2001) reported on a sample of 97
children, all diagnosed with an ASD. Twenty-five point eight percent
(25.8%) of their sample was diagnosed with some form of ID. A more recent
review of epidemiological data by Fombonne (2003) looked at 20 studies
conducted between 1966 and 2001 and found the median proportion of

participants with an ID was 70%. When ID was broken down by severity, 30% of the participants had mild to moderate ID and 40% had severe to profound levels of ID (Fombonne, 2003). Due to changing criteria for diagnosis of a PDD (i.e., AS included as a PDD since the *DSM–IV* [APA, 1994]), more sophisticated tools to identify the disorders and at an earlier age, and more children receiving early intervention services, all may have an impact on the often debated prevalence of co-occurring ASD and ID.

The focus of this chapter is the assessment of comorbid psychopathology and ASD, however, comorbidity of ID and ASD is an important consideration due to the difficulty in diagnosing psychopathology in people with ID. With such a large incidence of people with ASD having comorbid ID, whether it is 25% or 75%, imposes complications with the identification of other co-occurring conditions. Children with ID typically have limited verbal abilities, and therefore, diagnosing other forms of psychopathology using more traditional, self-report/parent-report methods, has obvious limitations. Together with a diagnosis of ASD, the task of identification becomes even more daunting. Thus, there is a lack of research on comorbid disorders of children with ASD with and without ID as well as specific assessment measures for identifying co-occurring psychopathology.

Research, albeit limited, has focused on the more common disorders, such as anxiety and depression, finding a higher incidence in people with ASD (Attwood, 1998; Howlin, 1997; Ghaziuddin, Ghaziuddin, & Greden, 2002; Tantum, 2000). With the inadequate evidence, there is need for better measures and comprehensive research on comorbid disorders that appear to occur with ASD. Such disorders as Attention-Deficit/Hyperactivity Disorder, Conduct Disorder, Obsessive Compulsive Disorder, Phobia, Tic Disorder, Affective Disorders, and feeding difficulties have all been reported to either share symptoms or possibly co-occur with this population (Attwood, 1998; Gadow & DeVincent, 2005; Gilmour, Hill, Place, & Skuse, 2004; Goldstein & Schwebach, 2004; Kinnell, 1985; Loveland & Tunlai-Kotoski, 1997; Matson & Love, 1990; Volkmar, Klin, & Cohen, 1997); however, the research is scarce. Psychopathology that appears to more commonly occur in children with ASD is briefly reviewed.

Attention-Deficit/Hyperactivity Disorder

Attention-Deficit/Hyperactivity Disorder (ADHD) is characterized, according to the *DSM–IV–TR*, as a pattern of inattention and hyperactivity-impulsivity that is more severe and occurs more frequently than in a typically developing individual of the same developmental level (APA, 2000). The presentation of the impairing symptoms needs to be present prior to seven years of age. However, the diagnosis of an ASD is exclusionary for a diagnosis of ADHD according to the *DSM–IV–TR*. Little research has been published regarding the relationship between ADHD and ASD (Loveland & Tunali-Kotoski, 1997). This lack of attention may be due in part to the exclusion criteria for an ADHD diagnosis as well as that symptoms of ADHD may be characteristic of ASD (Volkmar, Klin, & Cohen, 1997). People with ASD often exhibit either hyper- or hypoactive behavior (i.e., behavior rarely within normal limits; Gillberg & Billstedt, 2000).

A study by Goldstein and Schwebach (2004), using a retrospective chart review, compared children with ASD meeting diagnostic criteria for ADHD, to children with a diagnosis of just ADHD with no ASD diagnosis, and to a third group of children diagnosed with ASD alone. The authors found a clinically distinct group of children diagnosed with ASD who met criteria for ADHD compared to children with just a diagnosis of ASD. The children with ASD displayed symptoms of ADHD similar to those diagnosed with ADHD only (Goldstein & Schwebach, 2004). This research lends itself to the suggestion that ADHD may co-occur with ASD.

Conduct Disorder

Just as with people with ASD, individuals with Conduct Disorder also display social impairments. Conduct Disorder is identified by the *DSM–IV–TR* as behavior that violates the basic rights of others or some societal norms (APA, 2000). These behaviors include aggression toward others, destruction of property, deceitfulness or theft, and serious violations of rules. Researchers have found evidence that there are children identified as having Conduct Disorder, who also meet criteria for an ASD (Gilmour, Hill, Place, Skuse, & 2004). Although these two groups share some features, Gilchrist and colleagues (2001) successfully differentiated between adolescents with AS and high-functioning AD and those with Conduct Disorder based on measures of ASD (i.e., ADOS and ADIR) and IQ. The participants with Conduct Disorder had a different IQ profile compared to both of the ASD groups and displayed reciprocal communication and less social impairment (Gilchrist et al., 2001).

In addition to research investigating differences between individuals with Conduct Disorder and ASD, research on comorbidity in children has not been conducted with this population to date. This scarcity in the literature of Conduct Disorder in this population may also be due in part to the difficulty in determining if the individual engaged in the behaviors with the intent to do harm to another person. With many children with ASD also having ID and/or limited verbal abilities, it may be a challenge to differentiate between this form of psychopathology and a learned maladaptive behavior. Considerably more research on the topic is warranted.

Anxiety

Anxiety is characterized by worry and is reportedly common to people with ASD (Attwood, 1998). According to the *DSM–IV–TR*, Anxiety Disorders are broken down into numerous other disorders, such as Panic Disorder, Agoraphobia, Specific Phobia, Social Phobia, Obsessive-Compulsive Disorder, Posttraumatic Stress Disorder, and Generalized Anxiety Disorder, among others (APA, 2000). Tantum (2000) reported that panic, social anxiety, and obsessive-compulsive characteristics appear to be the most commonly evinced symptoms of anxiety in people with ASD. Additionally, Muris and colleagues (1998) reported on a sample of children with ASD with 84.1% of the children meeting criteria for an anxiety disorder. Obsessive Compulsive Disorder and Phobia in relation to ASD are reviewed below.

Obsessive Compulsive Disorder

Characteristics of Obsessive Compulsive Disorder (OCD), such as repetitive actions or words, may present as or resemble the behavioral excesses of people with ASD. Defined by the *DSM–IV–TR*, obsessions or compulsions recur and are time consuming and distressing to the individual affected (APA, 2000). People with ASD may discuss a particular topic exhaustively, require the physical environment remain exact, or insist on a particular ritual or dialogue be carried out. The preoccupations or rituals characteristic of people with ASD can be confused with the obsessions or compulsions evinced by people with OCD. However, the difference is that people with OCD are typically distressed by the behavior, whereas the person with ASD is not (Wing & Attwood, 1987). Although this distinction, the behavior causing distress or enjoyment, is made in the "typical" adult population, with children it is more complicated. The *DSM–IV–TR* states that with children, distress does not need to be evident for a diagnosis of OCD, due to a lack of cognitive awareness, therefore making diagnosis of symptoms more complicated and often difficult to tease apart. This complication may be even more so for the child with ASD. Better scales to measure the traits of OCD are needed along with more research on the prevalence of OCD co-occurring with ASD, as knowledge in this area is lacking.

Phobia

The *DSM–IV–TR* categorizes Specific Phobias as those that are a persistent fear and avoidance that is excessive or unreasonable, cued by the presence or anticipation of a specific object or situation (APA, 2000). Exposure to the phobic stimulus will provoke an immediate anxiety response, such as an anxiety attack. However, in the case of children with a Specific Phobia, the anxiety response may be in the form of crying, tantrums, "freezing," or clinging. For adults, there needs to be awareness that the fear is excessive or unreasonable; however, just as with criteria for OCD, this awareness does not need to be evident in children.

Characteristic of many children with ASD is the presence of phobias. Matson and Love (1990) conducted a study that found children with ASD to have a higher incidence of phobias compared to typically developing, age-matched peers. Children with ASD had more phobias related to animals, as well as medical and particular situations.

Additionally, Evans, Canavera, Kleinpeter, Maccubbin, and Taga (2005) were able to replicate these findings while including a group of children with Down syndrome along with control children matched on both mental and chronological age. These researchers investigated whether fears that are common to children with ASD are just characteristic of the disorder, a separate comorbid condition, or a natural progression of fears developmentally. The authors found that the children with ASD had a different pattern of fears and anxiety compared to mental and chronologically age matched peers.

Tic Disorder

Tic disorders, like OCD, share some commonalities with symptoms of ASD. As defined by the *DSM–IV–TR*, a tic is a sudden vocalization or motor movement that is recurrent and stereotyped (APA, 2000). Repetitive and stereotyped behaviors, diagnostic criteria for ASD, can vary in topography and may be difficult to differentiate from a tic. In some cases the distinction can be made, as tics tend to be involuntary where stereotypies appear to be more intentional. Tics are sudden and disrupt the flow of speech and are not as rhythmic in nature as stereotypies (Baron-Cohen, Mortimore, Moriarty, Izaguirre, & Robertson, 1999). Additionally, people who display tics may appear distressed whereas a person exhibiting a stereotypy may appear amused (Lainhart, 1999).

Tics also appear to occur on a continuum of severity and topography, making differentiation in this population more difficult (Golden, 1978). However, researchers have reported that tic disorders can be diagnosed and are common to children with ASD (Gadow & DeVincent, 2005; Gadow, DeVincent, Pomeroy, & Azizian, 2004). Furthermore, Gadow and DeVincent (2005) reported that children with ASD, who also exhibited signs of tics and ADHD, were also more likely to have other psychiatric symptoms and more severe expressions of ASD. In addition, these researchers found no differences in the co-occurring tic symptoms in the children with or without ASD. These results suggest that a tic disorder is distinguishable from the stereotypic characteristics of ASD presenting similarly to typically developing children who evince tics.

Affective Disorders

Depression is a common comorbid disorder in people with ASD (Loveland & Tunlai-Kotoski, 1997). Researchers have also reported that people with ID have a higher incidence and prevalence of depression (Kazdin, Matson, & Senatore, 1983). However, depression is difficult to diagnose in people with ID as the topography of the symptoms may change with the severity of ID, a complicating factor when the child also has ASD.

A review was conducted by Smiley and Cooper (2003) investigating possible behavioral equivalents of depression in people with severe and profound ID. The authors found that in individuals with depression, there were increases in agitation, self-injury, skill loss, increased social withdrawal, or isolation, and an increase in somatic complaints (Smiley & Cooper, 2003). In addition, due to the limitation in expressive language, these symptoms are generally reported by a caretaker or other third party as changes in behavior (Ghaziuddin & Greden, 1998).

With ASD being comprised of deficits in communication, diagnosing depression in children with ASD and ID often poses a challenge. As of late, researchers have attempted to investigate the co-occurrence of the two forms of psychopathology, ASD and depression. Ghaziuddin, Tsai, and Ghaziuddin (1992), for example, reported an occurrence rate of comorbid depression in children with AD at 2%, and in those with AS as high as 30%. Additionally, a number of studies found much higher rates of depression when considering AS alone (Ghaziuddin, Ghaziuddin, & Greden, 2002; Lainhart, 1999). Due to the limited measures of depression for this population, Ghaziuddin and Greden (1998) looked at the family history of people with ASD and prevalence of depression. The authors used *DSM–III-R* criteria and found that 77% of the children who had a diagnosis of depression also had a family member with the disorder.

Eating/Feeding Disorders

Even in Leo Kanner's (1943) first account of children with "autistic disturbance of affective contact," eating problems were noted. Three feeding disorders are noted in the *DSM–IV–TR*: Pica, Rumination, and Feeding Disorder of infancy or early childhood (APA, 2000). Pica is the ingestion of nonfood items such as string, paint chips, cigarette butts, leaves, and feces. The prevalence of Pica in people with ASD has been suggested by researchers to be higher than in people with Down syndrome, 60% compared to 4%, respectively (Kinnell, 1985). Rumination is another feeding disorder recognized by the *DSM–IV–TR* and is characterized by the repeated regurgitation and chewing of food, without evidence of gastrointestinal illness or medical condition. Additionally, for people with ID and/or ASD the rumination needs to be severe enough to warrant attention. The last eating disorder defined by the *DSM–IV–TR* is Feeding Disorder of Infancy or Childhood. Individuals with this disorder have gone for one month or more without eating adequately, resulting in no weight gain or weight loss. Again, this behavior cannot be the result of a gastrointestinal illness or medical condition.

In addition to the feeding disorders classified in the *DSM–IV–TR*, children with ASD often exhibit other difficulties that interfere with mealtime. Such behaviors are food selectivity (for food type and/or texture) and food refusal (Ahearn, Castine, Nault, & Green, 2001). Ahearn and colleagues (2001) conducted a study investigating the feeding difficulties of children with ASD. The authors found that more than half of the participants displayed low levels of food acceptance including selectivity and refusal.

ASSESSMENT OF COMORBID PSYCHOPATHOLOGY

Researchers have shown evidence of comorbid psychopathology in individuals with ASD (Evans, Canavera, Kleinpeter, Maccubbin, & Taga, 2005; Ghaziuddin et al., 1992; Kinnell, 1985; Matson & Love, 1990; Morgan, Roy, & Chance, 2003). As mentioned previously, identifying symptoms and characteristics of psychopathology in people with limited verbal abilities poses an obvious difficulty with regard to diagnosis. Additionally, in people with multiple disabilities, symptoms of comorbid disorders may be displayed topographically different from the typical population. Due to the complexity of the target population, few measures are available to screen and/or assess additional Axis I disorders in children with ASD.

Currently there are numerous measures used to assess typically developing children for symptoms of psychopathology. However, these

measures have not been validated for the use with children diagnosed with
ASD (Leyfer et al., 2006) and may not be appropriate due to variations in
symptom profiles of ASD children relative to the general population. Measures used with typically developing children are generally based on *DSM*
criteria, thus posing obvious problems when used with children who may
have deficits in verbal abilities and limited cognitive functioning (Einfield
& Aman, 1995).

Einfield and Aman (1995) proposed some recommendations for empirically developing a taxonomy of psychological symptoms for people with ID.
Such recommendations include modification to the current diagnostic
system, the *DSM–IV–TR*, to account for the specific characteristics of people
with developmental disabilities (i.e., Should it be considered stealing
when the person does not understand the concept of ownership?); using
multivariate statistics; examining biomedical markers in individuals and
comparing them to people without ID (for our purposes, individuals without ASD) with the particular disorder; investigating family history; probing
with the use of pharmacology; and neuroimaging and comparing to individuals with known disorders in the general population.

These recommendations could prove fruitful in the diagnosis of comorbid disorders in the ASD population as well; however, many of the strategies can be time consuming, expensive, and potentially dangerous (i.e.,
prescribing psychotropic medications unnecessarily). High rates of ASD
and the very serious, debilitating nature of the condition, particularly
when comorbid psychopathology is present, make scale development for
differential diagnosis essential. A compelling argument for such an assessment method exists although few measures of comorbid psychopathology
for children with ASD have been developed to date. Due to the difficulties
with assessing and diagnosing this population, clinicians are often left to
rely on informant-based measures, particularly rating scales. The best
available instruments are reviewed below.

Screening Measures

Broadband or disorder-specific measures can be used to assess comorbidity in this population. Specific measures assess a particular disorder.
Broadband measures are used to screen across numerous disorders, where
elevations would indicate further examination is warranted, possibly with
a disorder-specific measure. Broadband measures are discussed.

Autism Spectrum Disorders-Comorbidity for Children (ASD-CC)

The ASD-CC (Matson & Gonzalez, 2007b) is a new, informant-based
measure that assesses children with a current diagnosis of ASD for psy-
chopathologies that are more commonly found to occur with ASD based
on available literature (Ghaziuddin et al., 1992; Kinnell, 1985; Matson &
Love, 1990; Morgan et al., 2003). The ASD-CC is used in conjunction with
two other measures, the ASD-DC and the Autism Spectrum Disorders-
Behavior Problems in Children (ASD-BPC; Matson & Gonzalez, 2007a),
as a comprehensive assessment battery. Each of the 84 items loads onto

one of seven subscales of psychopathology. The subscales are depression, conduct, attention-deficit/ hyperactivity, tics, obsessions/compulsions, phobia, and eating. Sample items include: appearance of physical stress, easily becomes angry, is always on the go, and engages in repetitive behaviors to reduce stress. Informants are parents or caretakers who know the child well and are instructed to rate each item to the extent that it has been recent problem: "0 = not a problem or impairment; not at all"; "1 = mild problem or impairment"; "2 = severe problem or impairment"; or "X = does not apply or don't know". The psychometrics properties of the measure are currently under investigation.

Early Childhood Inventory-4 (ECI-4) and Child Symptom Inventory-4 (CSI-4)

These scales are parent- and teacher-report measures that assess psychopathology in children. The ECI-4 (Sprafkin & Gadow, 1996) is used with children ages 3 through 5 years and the CSI-4 (Gadow & Sprafkin, 1998) is used for children ages 5 through 12. The following disorders are assessed by the ECI-4: ADHD, Oppositional Defiant Disorder, Conduct Disorder, Generalized Anxiety Disorder, Social Phobia, Separation Anxiety Disorder, OCD, Specific Phobia, Selective Mutism, Major Depressive Disorder, Dysthymia, Reactive Attachment Disorder, Pervasive Developmental Disorder, Asperger's Disorder, Motor Tics, Vocal Tics, and Posttraumatic Stress Disorder. Problems in eating, sleeping, and elimination are also assessed.

The ECI-4 has shown adequate criterion validity for ADHD, Oppositional Defiance Disorder, and PDD, adequate test–retest reliability, and predictive validity (Sprafkin, Volpe, Gadow, Nolan, & Kelley, 2002).

The CSI-4 assess the following disorders, ADHD, Oppositional Defiant Disorder, Conduct Disorder, Separation Anxiety, Generalized Anxiety, Social Phobia, Specific Phobia, Depression, Dysthymia, Asperger's Disorder, Pervasive Developmental Disorder, Schizophrenia, OCD, Posttraumatic Stress Disorder, Motor Tics, and Vocal Tics. The parent version contains 97 items and the teacher version contains 77 items. Items are scored on a 4-point Likert-type scale. Both measures, the ECI-4 and the CSI-4, are based on *DSM–IV* criteria.

These measures have been used to assess psychopathology in children with ASD. Gadow and DeVincent (2005) used the ECI-4 and the CSI-4 to assess ADHD and tics in children. Weisbrot and colleagues (2005) assessed anxiety in children with ASD and compared them to children with anxiety and without an ASD diagnosis. The researchers found that children with ASD and anxiety presented symptoms similar to the children with anxiety and no ASD diagnosis. This measure may be useful in diagnosing comorbid disorders in children with ASD; however, the measure has yet to be validated with this population.

Nisonger Child Behavior Rating Forms (NCBRF)

The NCBRF (Aman, Tasse, Rojahn, & Hammer, 1996) is a modification of an earlier scale, the Child Behavior Rating Form (Edlebrock, 1985) which was designed for typically developing children. The targeted population for the NCBRF is children with ID. The modifications included changes in scoring, rewording of items to make them more easily understood, and the addition of 16 items to the measure. There are separate, but similar, parent and teacher forms. Validity studies using the Aberrant Behavior Checklist (ABC) showed large positive correlations for subscales of the measures, and interrater agreement for parents and teachers was high with alpha levels of .87 and .85 respectively (Aman et al., 1996). Although not as high, agreement between parents and teachers was still adequate at .51.

Lecavalier and colleagues (2004) conducted a study on the factor structure of the NCBRF with a population of children with ASD. Through exploratory factor analysis, a five-factor solution was obtained. The factors included conduct problem, insecure/anxious, hyperactive, self-injury/stereotypic, and self-isolated-ritualistic (Lecavalier et al., 2004). This factor structure was somewhat different from the original study in that the Aman and associates (1996) study found a six-factor solution to be optimal with participants with ID, where Lecavalier and associates chose five factors as optimal as the sixth factor "fell out" (Lecavalier et al., 2004).

Diagnostic Interview Schedule for Children (DISC)

The DISC (Schwab-Stone, et al., 1993) is an interview that has two versions that can be completed by the parent/caretaker or the child. The parent version is for children ages 6 years through 17 years, and the child-report is used with children ages 9 years through 17 years. The DISC assesses disorders in the broad areas of mood, anxiety, substance abuse, behavior, and other (e.g., eating and elimination disorders, tics, and schizophrenia). Using the DISC with non-ASD populations, the measure has shown to have adequate interrater and test–retest reliability (Schwab-Stone et al., 1993; Schaffer et al., 1993). Validity of the DISC has also been established (Piacentini et al., 1993). The DISC was used in a study by Muris and colleagues (1998) to assess anxiety in a sample of children with ASD. The anxiety section of the DISC assesses the following disorders: Simple Phobia, Social Phobia, Agoraphobia, Panic Disorder, Separation Anxiety Disorder, Avoidant Disorder, Overanxious Disorder, and OCD. However, the psychometric properties of the measure have not been established with the ASD population.

Autism Comorbidity Interview-Present and Lifetime Version (ACI-PL)

More recently, Leyfer and colleagues (2006) adapted the Kiddie Schedule for Affective Disorders and Schizophrenia, which is designed for typically developing children, for children with ASD. For the new scale, the ACI-PL added sections to establish the child's baseline by asking the informants to provide information on the child "at his/her best." Also, for each section that assesses psychopathology, additional items were added to address symptoms that may manifest differently by people with ASD according to caregivers. The Major Depressive Disorder, OCD, and ADHD subscales had kappa values above .70 for interrater agreement (Leyfer et al., 2006). Validity studies also proved adequate for ADHD and depression diagnoses with sensitivity at 100% and specificity ranging from 83% to 93.7%.

Developmental Behavior Checklist (DBC)

The DBC (Einfeld & Tonge, 1995) is another measure used with children with ID to assess psychopathology along 96 items. Ninety-five of the 96 items are rated on a three-point scale and summed to give a Total Behavior Problem Score. This score is used to provide a general score of psychopathology for the individual. The initial analyses on this measure resulted in good reliability as well as validity (Einfeld & Tonge, 1995). Through principle components analysis, a five-factor solution resulted with the following subscales, disruptive, self-absorbed, communication disturbance, anxiety, autistic relating, and antisocial. However, the DBC has been studied with children with ID, not specifically ASD.

Additional Modes of Assessment

Using more than one mode of measurement when assessing children with ASD is desirable in most contexts. In addition to the rating scales, clinicians should do a thorough review of the child's records as well as behavioral observations (Rush, Bowman, Eidman, Toole, & Mortenson, 2004). A review of records may reveal patterns of symptoms that may be useful in the determination of psychopathology and treatment course. Behavioral observation by an experienced clinician is also beneficial. The clinician can assist in distinguishing between symptoms of a comorbid disorder, a common characteristic of ASD, or a learned maladaptive behavior. For example, in the case of tics and symptoms of OCD, these topographically similar symptoms need a trained eye to discern them. Also of great importance are assessments of maladaptive behaviors. Severity, duration, and intensity should be considered when assessing treatment efficacy.

A new measure, the ASD-BCA is a scale designed to assess maladaptive behaviors that more commonly occur in children with ASD, such as self-injury, aggression, and other disruptive behavior. This measure is used in conjunction with the ASD-DC and the ASD-CC. Furthermore, a functional assessment should be conducted so as to determine the variables that may be maintaining the behaviors, in addition to the co-occurring psychopathology. One popular measure used to assess behavioral function, is the Questions About Behavior Function (QABF; Matson & Vollmer, 1995).

Another important consideration when assessing people with limited verbal skills is the person's family history. Oftentimes certain forms of psychopathology are highly heritable and research on the families of people with ASD and comorbid psychopathology also shows higher levels of psychopathology, such as with depressive symptoms and obsessive compulsive behaviors (Ghaziuddin & Greden, 1998; Hollander, King, Delaney, Smith, & Silverman, 2003).

In addition to the ratings of psychopathology, record review, family history, behavioral observations, and maladaptive behavior, ratings of adaptive behavior and social skills are also important to assess (Reiss, 1993). Ratings of adaptive behavior can be obtained by using measures such as the Vineland Adaptive Behavior Scales (Sparrow, Balla, & Cicchetti, 1984) or the AAMR Adaptive Behavior Scales: Second Edition (ABS-2; Lambert, Nihira, & Leland, 1993). Additionally, social skills should be assessed. The Matson Evaluation of Social Skills in Youngsters (MESSY; Matson, 2007b) is a measure of appropriate and inappropriate social skills in children, normed according to age. A thorough investigation of many facets of an individual's life should provide clinicians with information to assist in the diagnosis of comorbid psychopathology. Discussed throughout this chapter, people with ASD and/or ID, having limited verbal abilities, may express symptoms of psychopathology differently than the general population making assessing a wide area of skills and behaviors essential.

CONCLUSION

This chapter covers the assessment of ASD and the more commonly occurring comorbid conditions. Furthermore, we have discussed the limited number of measures used to assess psychopathology in this population. Experts in the field are still debating the characteristics of and differential diagnosis within ASD. Without clear delineation of the core symptoms of the disorder, diagnosing comorbid disorders is troublesome.

ASD are a group of disorders that alone have a substantial impact on the development of the child with regards to learning, personal relations, and family functioning. ASD coupled with an additional Axis I diagnosis can have debilitating effects on the individual. It is important for clinicians, community professionals, and parents to be aware of the possibility of additional diagnoses. Appropriate referrals to specialized clinicians are necessary for accurate diagnosis and to distinguish these disorders from the more common characteristics of ASD. With these children at a higher risk for comorbidity, broadband screening may be the most efficient method for assessing symptoms for such a wide range of disorders.

Through accurate identification of the core symptoms of ASD and of comorbid psychopathology, these children can receive individualized treatment appropriate for their diagnosis, whether it be therapy or pharmacological or both. Although awareness, funding, and research are increasing with regard to the identification and intervention for ASD, wholesale application in clinical practice lags far behind recommended service provision based on empirical literature.

REFERENCES

Ahearn, W. H., Castine, T., Nault, K., & Green, G. (2001). An assessment of food acceptance in children with autism or Pervasive Developmental Disorder - Not Otherwise Specified. *Journal of Autism and Developmental Disorders, 31*, 505–512.

Aman, M. G., Tassé, M. J., Rojahn, J., & Hammer, D. (1996). The Nisonger CBRF: A Child Behavior Rating Form for children with developmental disabilities. *Research in Developmental Disabilities, 17,* 41–57.

American Psychiatric Association. (1986). *Diagnostic and statistical manual of mental disorders* (3rd ed.). Washington, DC: Author.

American Psychiatric Association. (1994). *Diagnostic and statistical manual of mental disorders* (4th ed.). Washington, DC: Author.

American Psychiatric Association. (2000). *Diagnostic and statistical manual of mental disorders* (4th ed., Text Revision). Washington, DC: Author.

Asperger, H. (1991). "Autistic Psychopathy" in childhood. In Frith, U. (Ed.). *Autism and Asperger syndrome* (pp. 37–92). Cambridge, U.K.: Cambridge University Press.

Attwood, T. (1998). Asperger's syndrome: A guide for parents and professionals. Philadelphia: Kingsley.

Baron-Cohen, S., Cox, A., Baird, G., Swettenham, J., & Nighingale, N. (1996). Psychological markers in the detection of autism in infancy in a large population. *British Journal of Psychiatry, 168,* 158–163.

Baron-Cohen, S, Mortimore, C., Moriarty, J., Izaguirre, J., & Robertson, M. (1999). The prevalence of Gilles de la Tourette syndrome in children and adolescents with autism. *Journal of Child Psychology and Psychiatry, 40,* 213–218.

Budden, S. S., Dorsey, H. C., & Steiner, R. D. (2005). Clinical profile of a male with Rett Syndrome. *Brain and Development, 27,* S69–S71.

Burford, B., Kerr, A. M., & Macleod, H. A. (2003). Nurse recognition of early deviation in development in home videos of infants with Rett disorder. *Journal of Intellectual Disability Research, 47,* 588–596.

Chakrabarti, S. & Fombonne, E. (2001). Pervasive developmental disorders in preschool children. *Journal of the American Medical Association, 285,* 3093–3099.

Chakrabarti, S. & Fombonne, E. (2005). Pervasive developmental disorders in preschool children: Confirmation of high prevalence. *American Journal of Psychiatry, 162,* 1133–1141.

Cohen, D. J., Paul, R., & Volkmar, F. R. (1987). Issues in classification of pervasive developmental disorders and associated conditions. In D.J. Cohen & Donnellan, A. M. (Eds.), *Handbook of autism and pervasive developmental disorders.* New York: John Wiley & Sons.

Evans, D. W., Canavera, K., Kleinpeter, F. L., Maccubin, E. & Taga, K. (2005). The fears, phobias, and anxieties of children with autism spectrum disorders and Down Syndrome: Comparisons with developmentally and chronologically age-matched children. *Child Psychiatry and Human Development, 36,* 3–26.

Edelbrock, C. S. (1985). Child Behavior Rating Form. *Psychopharmalogical Bulletin, 21,* 835–837.

Einfeld, S. L. & Aman, M. G. (1995). Issues in the taxonomy of psychopathology in mental retardation. *Journal of Autism and Developmental Disorders, 25,* 143–167.

Einfeld, S. L. & Tonge, B. J. (1995). The Developmental Behavior Checklist: The development and validation of an instrument to assess behavioral and emotional disturbance in children and adolescents with mental retardation. *Journal of Autism and Developmental Disorders, 25,* 81–104.

Fombonne, E. (2003). Epidemiological surveys of autism and other pervasive developmental disorders: An update. *Journal of Autism and Developmental Disorders, 33,* 365–382.

Gadow, K. D. & DeVincent, C. J. (2005). Clinical significance of tics and attention-deficit hyperactivity disorder (ADHD) in children with pervasive developmental disorder. *Journal of Child Neurology, 20,* 481–488.

Gadow, K. D., DeVincent, C. J., Pomeroy, J., & Azizian, A. (2004). Psychiatric symptoms in preschool children with PDD and clinic comparison samples. *Journal of Autism and Developmental Disorders, 34,* 379–393.

Gadow, K.D. & Sprafkin, J. (1998). Child Symptom Inventory-4 screening manual. Stony Brook, NY: Checkmate Plus.

Ghaziuddin, M., Ghaziuddin, N., & Greden, J. (2002). Depression in persons with autism: Implications for research and clinical care. *Journal of Autism and Developmental Disorders, 32,* 299–306.

Ghaziuddin, M. & Greden, J. (1998) Depression in children with autism/pervasive developmental disorders: A case-control family history study. *Journal of Autism and Developmental Disorders, 28,* 111–115.

Ghaziuddin, M., Tsai, L., Ghaziuddin, N. (1992). Comorbidity of autistic disorder in children and adolescents. *European Child and Adolescent Psychiatry, 1,* 643–649.

Gillberg, C. & Billstedt, E. (2000). Autism and Asperger syndrome: Coexistence with other clinical disorders. *Acta Psychiatr Scand, 102,* 321–330.

Gilliam, J. E. (2001). *Gilliam Asperger's Disorder Scale.* Austin, Texas: Pro-Ed.

Gilchrist, A., Cox, A., Rutter, M., Green, J., Burton, D., & Le Couteur, A. (2001). Development and current functioning in adolescents with Asperger Syndrome: A comparative study. *Journal of Psychology and Psychiatry, 42,* 227–240.

Gilmour, J., Hill, B., Place, M., & Skuse, D.H. (2004). Social communication deficits in conduct disorder: A clinical and community survey. *Journal of Child Psychology and Psychiatry,45,* 967–978.

Golden, G.S. (1978). Tics and Tourette's: A continuum of symptoms? *Annals of Neurology, 4,* 145–148.

Goldstein, S., & Schwebach, A.J. (2004). The comorbidity of Pervasive Developmental Disorder and Attention Deficit Hyperactivity Disorder: results of a retrospective chart review. *Journal of Autism and Developmental Disorders, 34,* 329–339.

Hagberg, B. (1985). Rett's syndrome: Prevalence and impact on progressive severe mental retardation in girls. *Acta Paediatr Scand, 74,* 405–408.

Hollander, E., King, A., Delaney, K., Smith, C.J., & Silverman, J.M. (2003). Obsessive-compulsive behaviors in parents of multiplex autism families. *Psychiatry Research, 117,* 11–16.

Howlin, P. (1997). Psychiatric disturbances in adulthood. In P. Howlin (Ed.), *Autism: Preparing for adulthood,* pp.216–35. London: Routledge.

Kanner, L. (1943). Autistic disturbances of affective contact. *The Nervous Child, 2,* 217–250.

Kanner, L. (1951). The conception of wholes and parts in early infantile autism. *American Journal of Psychiatry, 108,* 23–26.

Kazdin, A. E., Matson, J. L., & Senatore, V. (1983). Assessment of depression in mentally retarded adults. *American Journal of Psychiatry, 140,* 1040–1043.

Kinnell, H. G. (1985). Pica as a feature of autism. *British Journal of Psychiatry, 147,* 80–82.

Klin, A. & Volkmar, F. R., (1995). Asperger's Syndrome Guidelines for assessment and *diagnosis.* Learning Disabilities Association of America.

Klinger, L.G., Dawson, G., & Renner, P. (2003). Autistic disorder. In E. Marsh & R. Barkley (Eds.), *Child psychopathology* (2nd ed.). New York: Guilford Press.

Krug, D. A., & Arick, J. R. (2003). *Krug Asperger's Disorder Index.* Autsin, Texas: Pro-Ed.

Krug, D. A., Arick, J. R. & Almond, P., (1980). Behavior checklist for identifying severely handicapped individuals with high levels of autistic behavior. *Journal of Child Psychology and Psychiatry, 21,* 221–229.

Lainhart, J.E. (1999). Psychiatric problems in individuals with autism, their parents and siblings. *International Review of Psychiatry, 11,* 278–298.

Lambert, N., Nihira, K., & Leland, H. (1993). *AAMR Adaptive Behavior Scales: Second Edition (ABS-2).* Austin, TX: Pro-Ed.

Leonard, H., Bower, C., & English, D. (1997). The prevalence and incidence of Rett syndrome in Australia. *European Child and Adolescent Psychiatry, 6*(1), 8–10.

Lecavalier, L., Aman, M. G., Hammer, D., Stoica, W., & Mathews, G. L. (2004). Factor analysis of the Nisonger Child Behavior Rating Form in children with autism S spectrum disorders. *Journal of Autism and Developmental Disorders, 34,* 709–721.

Leekam, S. R., Libby, S. J., Wing, L., Gould, J., & Taylor, C. (2002). The Diagnostic Interview for Social and Communication Disorders: Algorithms for ICD-10 childhood autism and Wing and Gould autistic spectrum disorder. *Journal of Child Psychology and Psychiatry, 43,* 337–342.

Leyfer, O. T., Folstein, S. E., Bacalman, S., Davis, N. O., Dinh, E., Morgan, J., et al. (2006). Comorbid psychiatric disorders in children with autism: Interview development and rates of disorders. *Journal of Autism and Developmental Disorders, 36,* 849–861.

Lord, C., Risi, S., Lambrecht, L. Cook, E. H., Lenthal, B. C, DiLavore, P. C., et al. (2000). The Autism Diagnostic Observation-Generic: A standard measure of social and communication deficits associated with the spectrum of autism. *Journal of Autism and Developmental Disorders, 30,* 205–223.

Lord, C., Rutter, M., Goode, S., Heemsbergen, J., Jordan, H., Mawhood, L., et al. (1989). Autism Diagnostic Observation Schedule: A standardized observation of communicative and social behavior. *Journal of Autism and Developmental Disorders, 19,* 185–212.

Lord, C., Rutter, M., Le Couteur, A. (1994). Autism Diagnostic Interview-Revised: A revised version of a diagnostic interview for caregivers of individuals with possible pervasive developmental disorders. *Journal of Autism and Developmental Disorders, 24,* 659–685.

Loveland, K. A. & Tunali-Kotoski, B. (1997). The school-age child with autism. In D. J. Cohen, & F. R. Volkmar, (Eds.), *Handbook of autism and pervasive developmental disorders.* New York: John Wiley & Sons.

Malhorta, S. & Gupta, N. (2002). Childhood disintegrative disorder re-examination of the current concept. *European Child & Adolescent Psychiatry, 11,* 108–114.

Matson, J. L. (2007a). Current status of differential diagnosis for children with autism spectrum disorders. *Research in Developmental Disabilities, 28,* 109–118.

Matson, J. L. (2007b). The Matson Evaluation of Social Skills with Youngsters – Revised (MESSY-R). Worthington, OH: International Diagnostic Systems.

Matson, J. L., Baglio, C. S., Smirolodo, B. B., Hamilton, M., & Packlowskyj, T. (1996). Characteristics of autism as assessed by the Diagnostic Assessment for the Severely Handicapped-II (DASH-II). *Research in Developmental Disabilities, 17,* 135–143.

Matson J. L. & Boisjoli, J. A. (2008). Strategies for assessing Asperger's Syndrome: A critical review of data based methods. *Research in Autism Spectrum Disorders, 2*(2), 237–248.

Matson, J. L. & Boisjoli, J. A. (2007). Differential diagnosis of PDDNOS in children. *Research in Autism Spectrum Disorders, 1,* 75–84.

Matson, J. L., & González, M. L. (2007a). *Autism spectrum disorders – Behavior problems – Child version.* Baton Rouge, LA: Disability Consultants.

Matson, J. L., & González, M. L. (2007b). *Autism spectrum disorders – Comorbidity – Child version.* Baton Rouge, LA: Disability Consultants.

Matson, J. L., & González, M. L. (2007c). *Autism spectrum disorders – Diagnosis – Child version.* Baton Rouge, LA: Disability Consultants.

Matson, J. L., Gonzalez, M. L., Wilkins, J., & Rivet, T. T. (2007). Reliability of the Autism Spectrum Disorder-Diagnosis for Children (ASD-DC). *Journal of Developmental and Physical Disabilities, 19,* 565–577.

Matson, J. L. & Love, S. R. (1990). A comparison of parent-reported fear for autistic and non-handicapped age-matched children and youth. *Australian and New Zealand Journal of Developmental Disabilities, 16,* 349–357.

Matson, J. L., & Minshawi, N. F. (2006). Early intervention for autism spectrum *disorders: A critical analysis.* Oxford, UK: Elsevier Science.

Matson, J. L. & Nebel-Schwalm, M. (2007). Comorbid psychopathology with autism spectrum disorder in children: An overview. *Research in Developmental Disabilities, 28,* 341–352.

Matson, J. L. & Vollmer, T. (1995). Questions *About Behavioral Function (QABF).* Baton Rouge, LA: Disability Consultants. Translated into Italian.

Morgan, C. N., Roy, M., & Chance, P. (2003). Psychiatric comorbidity and medication use in autism: A community survey. *Psychiatric Bulletin, 27,* 378–381.

Mount, R. H., Charman, T., Hastings, R. P., Reilly, S., & Cass, H. (2002). The Rett Syndrome Behavior Questionaire (RSBQ): Refining the behavioral phenotype of Rett syndrome. *Journal of Child Psychology and Psychiatry, 43,* 1099–1110.

Muris, P., Steerneman, P., Merckelbach, H., Holdrinet, I.,& Meesters, C. (1998). Comorbid anxiety symptoms in children with pervasive developmental disorders. *Journal of Anxiety Disorders, 12,* 387–393.

Nation, K., Clarke, P., Wright, B., Williams, C. & Patterns (2006). Patterns of reading ability in children with autism spectrum disorder. *Journal of Autism and Developmental Disorders, 36,* 911–919.

Njardvik, U., Matson, J. L., Cherry, K. E. (1999). A comparison of social skills in adults with autistic disorder, pervasive developmental disorder not otherwise specified, and mental retardation. *Journal of Autism and Developmental Disorders, 29,* 1999.

Osterling, J. & Dawson, G. (1994). Early recognition of children with autism: A study of first home video tapes. *Journal of Autism and Developmental Disorders, 24,* 247–257.

Piacentini, J., Shaffer, D., Fisher, P., Schwab-Stone, M., Davies, M., Gioia, P. (1993). The Diagnostic Interview Schedule for Children-revised version (DISC-R): III. Concurrent criterion validity. . *Journal of the American Academy of Child and Adolescent Psychiatry, 32,* 658–665.

Rapin, I. (1997). Classification and causal issues in autism. In D. J. Cohen & F. R. Volkmar (Eds.), *Handbook of autism and pervasive developmental disorders* (2nd ed., pp.847–867). New York: John Wiley & Sons.

Reiss, S. (1993). Assessment of psychopathology in persons with mental retardation. In J. L. Matson & R. P. Barrett (Eds.), *Psychopathology in the mentally retarded* (2nd ed., pp. 17–39). Needham Heights, MA: Allyn & Bacon.

Rush, K. S., Bowman, L. G., Eidman, S. L., Toole, L. M., & Mortenson, B. P. (2004). Assessing psychopathology in individuals with developmental disabilities. *Behavior Modification, 28,* 621–637.

Rutter, M. (1978).Diagnosis and definition. In M. Rutter & E. Schopler (Eds.), *Autism: A reappraisal of concepts and treatment.* New York: Plenum Press.

Rutter, M. & Bartak, L. (1971). Causes of infantile autism. *Journal of Autism and Childhood Schizophrenia, 1,* 1, 20–32.

Rutter, M. & Garmezy, N. (1983). Developmental psychopathology. In E. M. Hetherington (Ed.), *Handbook of child psychology, Vol. 4.* New York: Wiley.

Scambler, D., Rogers, S. J., & Wehner, E. A. (2001). Can the checklist for autism in toddlers differentiate young children with autism from those with developmental delays? *Journal of the American Academy of Child & Adolescent Psychiatry, 40,* 1457–1463.

Schopler, E., Reichler, R. J., & Renner, B. R. (1988). *The Childhood Autism Rating Scale (CARS).* Los Angeles: Western Psychological Services.

Schwab-Stone, M., Fisher, P., Piacentini, J., Schaffer, D., Davoes, M., & Briggs, M. (1993). The Diagnostic Interview Schedule for Children-revised version (DISC-R): II. Test-retest reliability. *Journal of the American Academy of Child and Adolescent Psychiatry, 32,* 651–657.

Shaffer, D., Schwab-Stone, M., Fisher, P., Cohen, P., Piacentini, J., Davies, M., Connors, K., & Rgier, D. (1993). The Diagnostic Interview Schedule for Children-revised version (DISC-R):I. Preparation, field testing, interrater reliability, and acceptability. *Journal of the American Academy of Child and Adolescent Psychiatry, 32,* 643–650.

Scott, F. J., Baron-Cohen, S., Bolton, P., & Brayne, C. (2002). The CAST (Chldhood Asperger Syndrome Test): Preliminary development of a UK screen for mainstream primary-school age children. *Autism, 6,* 9–31.

Smiley, E. & Cooper, S. A. (2003). Intellectual disabilities, depressive episode, diagnostic criteria and Diagnostic Criteria for Psychiatric Disorders for Use with Adults with Learning Disabilities/Mental Retardation (DC-LD). *Journal of Intellectual Disabilities, 47,* Supplement 1, 62–71.

Sparrow, S., Balla, D., & Cicchetti, D. V. (1984). *The Vineland Adaptive Behavior Scales (Survey Form).* Circle Pines, MN: American Guidance Service.

Sprafkin, J. & Gadow, K.D. (1996). Early Childhood Symptom Inventories manual. Stony Brook, NY: Checkmate Plus.

Sprafkin, J, Volpe, R. J., Gadow, K. D. Nolan, E. E., Kelly, K. (2002). A *DSM–IV*–referenced screening instrument for preschool children: The Early Childhood Inventory-4. *Journal of the American Academy of Child & Adolescent Psychiatry, 41,* 604–612.

Stone, W. L., Coonrod, E. E., & Ousley, O. Y. (2000). Screening Tool for Autism Two-Year-Olds (STAT): Development and preliminary data. *Journal of Autism and Developmental Disorders, 30,* 607–612.

Stone, W. L., Coonrod, E. E., Turner, L. M., & Pozdol, S. L. (2004). Psychometric properties of the STAT for early autism screening. *Journal of Autism and Developmental Disorders, 34,* 691–701.

Stone, W. L., & Ousley, O. Y. (1997). *STAT Manual: Screening tool for autism in two-year-olds.* Unpublished manuscript, Vanderbilt University.

Strum, H., Fernell, E., & Gillberg, C. (2004). Autism spectrum disorders in children with normal intellectual levels: Associated impairments and subgroups. *Developmental Medicine and Child Neurology, 46*, 444–447.

Tantum, D. (2000). Psychological disorder in adolescents and adults with Asperger syndrome. *Autism, 4*, 47–62.

Tidmarsh, L. & Volkmar, F. (2003). Diagnosis and epidemiology of autism spectrum disorders. *The Canadian Journal of Psychiatry, 48*, 517–525.

Towbin, K. (1997). Pervasive developmental disorders not otherwise specified. In D. J. Cohen and F. R. Volkmar (Eds.), *Handbook of autism and pervasive developmental disorders* (2nd ed.). New York: Wiley.

Van Acker, R. (1991). Rett Syndrome: A review of current knowledge. *Journal of Autism and Developmental Disabilities, 21*, 381–406.

Volkmar, F. R. (1987). Social Development. In Cohen, D.J. & Donnellan (Eds.) *Handbook of Autism and Pervasive Developmental Disorders*. New York: John Wiley & Sons.

Volkmar, F. R. (1992). Childhood disintegrative disorder: Issues for *DSM–IV. Journal of Autism and Developmental Disorders, 22*, 4, 625–642.

Volkmar, F. R., Klin, A., & Cohen, D. J. (1997). Diagnosis and classification of autism and related conditions: Consensus and issues. In D. Cohen and F. Volkmar (Eds.), *Handbook of autism and pervasive developmental disorders* (2nd ed.). New York: John Wiley and Sons, Inc.

Volkmar, F. R., Klin, A., Siegel, B., Szatmari, P., Lord, C., et al., (1994). Field trial for autistic disorder in *DSM–IV. American Journal of Psychiatry, 151*, 1361–1367.

Wadden, N.P.K., Bryson, S.E., & Rodger, R.S. (1991). A closer look at the Autism Behavior Checklist: Discriminant validity and factor structure. *Journal of Autism Developmental Disorders, 21*, 529–542.

Weisbrot, D. M., Gadow, K. D., & DeVincent, C. J. (2005). The presentation of anxiety in children with pervasive developmental disorders, *Journal of Child and Adolescent Psychopharmacology, 15*, 477–496.

Wing, L. & Attwood, A. (1987). Syndromes of autism and atypical development. In D. J. Cohen, & Donnellan (Eds.) *Handbook of autism and pervasive developmental disorders*. New York: John Wiley & Sons.

Wing, L. R., Libby, S. J., Gould, J., & Larcomb, M. (2002). The Diagnostic Interview for Social and Communication Disorders: Background, inter-rater reliability and clinical use. *Journal of Child Psychology and Psychiatry, 43*, 307–325.

Wing, L., Leekam, S. R., Libby, S. J., Gould, J., & Larcombe, M. (2002). The Diagnostic Interview for Social and Communication Disorders: Background, inter-rater reliability and clinical use. *Journal of Child Psychology and Psychiatry, 43*(3), 307–325.

World Health Organization (1992). *International classification of diseases* (10th ed.). Geneva, Switzerland: Author.

Part V

Behavioral Medicine

14

Assessment of Eating Disorder Symptoms In Children and Adolescents

NANCY ZUCKER, RHONDA MERWIN, CAMDEN ELLIOTT, JENNIFER LACY, and DAWN EICHEN

The most recent diagnostic classification system delineated by the American Psychiatric Association (*DSM–IV*; American Psychiatric Association, 2000) is not sensitive to the expression of disordered eating in children and adolescents (Cooper, Watkins, Bryant-Waugh, & Lask, 2002). The issues are complex. First, symptom expression in children and adolescents may manifest differently than in adults due to developmental influences on cognition, affect, and physical maturation. Second, children and adolescents may require different symptom thresholds for diagnosis given the sensitivity and importance of nutritional health for these age groups. Indeed, malnourishment may have permanent negative effects on cognitive and emotional functioning, sexual maturation, and physical growth, damage that may be particularly pronounced during this sensitive developmental period (Oninla, Owa, Onayade, & Taiwo, 2007). The end result of these challenges is that clinicians may fail to detect children and adolescents in need of intervention, the failure to detect lower symptom thresholds may have permanent negative health consequences, diminished sensitivity to the age-related expression of symptoms may interfere with appropriate treatment formulation, and the failure to consider developmental nuances may prevent the advance of a meaningful research agenda. This chapter is intended to address

NANCY ZUCKER, RHONDA MERWIN, CAMDEN ELLIOTT, JENNIFER LACY, and DAWN EICHEN • Department of Psychiatry and Behavioral Sciences, Duke University Medical Center, Duke University.

J.L. Matson et al. (eds.), *Assessing Childhood Psychopathology and Developmental Disabilities*, DOI: 10.1007/978-0-387-09528-8,
© Springer Science+Business Media, LLC 2009

these important issues by proposing strategies for assessment that consider developmentally sensitive manifestations of eating disturbance in children and adolescents for the purposes of diagnosis and case formulation.

ORGANIZATION OF THIS CHAPTER

There is considerable debate about the most effective manner to delineate patterns of eating disturbance (ED). At one extreme exist proponents of a transdiagnostic approach to eating disorder classification (Fairburn, Cooper, & Shafran, 2003). Advocates of this approach challenge the validity of syndromes for eating disorder diagnosis and emphasize the clinical reality of significant diagnostic crossover, that is, individuals who initially meet criteria for one eating disorder diagnosis, such as anorexia nervosa (AN), and subsequently meet criteria for an alternative disorder, such as bulimia nervosa (BN).

Of additional challenge to strict categorical diagnosticians is the high rates of individuals (estimates range from 30–50% of individuals who present for treatment) who fall into the diagnostic category eating disorder not otherwise specified (ED-NOS). For children and adolescents, this percentage is even more daunting: 40–60% of children and adolescents fall into this nebulous classification abyss (Peebles, Wilson, & Lock, 2006; Turner & Bryant-Waugh, 2004).

This category, which includes the provisional diagnosis of binge eating disorder, was intended to capture individuals with eating disturbance that resulted in clinical impairment, although the frequency (e.g. engaging in purgative behavior at a rate lower than required for a diagnosis of bulimia nervosa) or diagnostic threshold (e.g. although losing a significant amount of weight, the amount of weight lost overall did not meet the diagnostic threshold for anorexia nervosa) was not sufficient to meet criteria for a full syndrome disorder. Rather, a dimensional approach could, perhaps, have individuals all receive a diagnosis of "eating disorder" and then characterize the expression of various symptoms (e.g. dietary intake; extreme weight loss behaviors) to result in a symptom profile for each patient (Beaumont, Garner, & Touyz, 1994). Advocates of a transdiagnostic or more dimensional approach suggest this strategy could accommodate developmental challenges such as lower symptom thresholds and unique clinical presentations in younger ages.

At the other extreme are researchers and clinicians who recognize both the pragmatic reality of stringent diagnostic classification to facilitate healthcare insurance reimbursement and from the research perspective, to facilitate precise phenotypic descriptions to propagate genetic research. Although there have been impressive epidemiological (Wade, Crosby, & Martin, 2006) and sophisticated statistical attempts to address this complicated issue (Wonderlich, Joiner, Keel, Williamson, & Crosby, 2007), no satisfactory answers have been achieved. In this chapter, we take a dimensional approach given the limited knowledge base of symptom expression in young children and adolescents. As the appropriate delineation of syndromes specific to young children and adolescents remains to be firmly adjudicated, we err on the conservative side and approach diagnosis by examining eating disorder symptoms in isolation and comment on developmental and motivational challenges to assessment.

CONSIDERATION OF MEDICAL SEVERITY

Prior to the assessment of psychological status, a medical exam is essential to determine the appropriate intensity of care (Rome et al., 2003). This chapter assumes that prior to a mental health assessment, a thorough medical exam has been undertaken. The purpose of this exam is to determine whether, based on medical compromise, a child or adolescent needs immediate medical intervention or whether treatment can proceed on an outpatient basis. Indeed, starvation has pervasive effects on all bodily systems, and extreme weight loss behaviors such as self-induced vomiting may result in abrupt alterations in body homeostasis (e.g. dehydration, electrolyte imbalance) that may demand immediate medical attention (Walsh, Wheat, & Freund, 2000). Furthermore, some symptoms of disordered eating, such as extreme weight loss, are also seen as a side effect of undiagnosed medical conditions (e.g., Type I diabetes mellitus). A medical exam is needed to rule out any medical sequelae contributing to current symptomatology. Also, a mental health clinician should educate himself about these medical sequelae not only so he can be alerted to behavioral warning signs, but also so the family and patient can be educated about the severe nature of the problem being assessed.

As entire chapters have been devoted to the impact of eating disturbance on physical health and typical growth patterns, we restrict our chapter to recommendations (Mitchell, Pomeroy, & Adson, 1997). Thus, it is highly recommended that a thorough medical evaluation precede any psychological assessment, that contact with the evaluating physician and review of medical records precede the psychological evaluation, and finally, that this physician remain an active and informed part of the treatment process.

GENERAL CONSIDERATIONS

Although in general the assessment of children and adolescents poses unique challenges due to limitations in cognitive and emotional development, the assessment of eating disturbance in younger ages may be particularly difficult. Complex cognitive processes such as abstract reasoning and risk perception continue to evolve throughout adolescence (Boyer, 2006). Unfortunately, complexities of many eating disorder diagnostic symptoms require such advanced capacities. For example, children and adolescents with eating disturbance may lack appreciation of the impact of their behaviors on health (Couturier & Lock, 2006). Rather than being construed as active denial (one of the symptoms of the disorder of anorexia nervosa), this limited perception may reflect developmental limitations on higher-order cognitive processes such as the ability to integrate emotional consequences into complex decisions (Boyer, 2006). Thus, young patients may not appreciate the dangerous consequences of extreme weight loss behaviors.

Children and adolescents may have difficulty describing and understanding emotional experience. Alexithymia (Zonnevylle-Bender et al., 2004) and poor interoceptive awareness (Fassino, Piero, Gramaglia, & Abbate-Daga, 2004) have been documented in adults with eating disorders, deficits that may be compounded by neurocognitive development. By definition, alexithymia connotes limited ability to decipher or distinguish bodily signals of emotion from other somatic signals (Lane et al., 1996). In children, this deficit may potentially be exacerbated by normative developmental limitations on emotion regulation and abstract reasoning. Thus, rather than appreciating the emotional significance of bodily signals, eating disorder symptoms in children may be verbalized as somatic complaints (e.g., rather than anxiety, children may identify stomach discomfort or sensitivity).

Unfortunately, an additional challenge may be parents' understanding or acceptance of mental health symptoms. A stomachache may be far easier for parents to understand and endorse relative to an eating disorder. Thus, assessment of parental attitudes towards mental illness will need to be integrated into the clinician's clinical formulation, including the manner in which the illness is presented to the family. Findings from the medical evaluation are essential to differentiate the role of psychological processes on physical symptom exacerbation.

Children and adolescents with eating disorders may not wish to be in treatment. Unlike many individuals who experience distress from their psychiatric symptoms, individuals with eating disturbance often do not wish to be relieved of their disorder (Vitousek, Watson, & Wilson, 1998). In fact, eating disorder symptoms are often referred to as *ego syntonic* (Vitousek et al., 1998). A particular perplexity in the assessment of children with AN, for example, is that they often feel quite energetic despite their severe state of malnutrition. Furthermore, self-imposed rules regarding food restriction may reduce guilt and therefore be experienced as comforting (Rieger & Touyz, 2006). Thus, a clinician may need to assess other areas of functioning such as friendships and related social isolation, patterns that often increase with eating disorder symptoms, to highlight the impact of the disorder on quality of life (Rieger & Touyz, 2006). Both expected developmental limitations on cognitive functions combined with the challenging presentation of eating disturbance increase the complexity of assessment and highlight the imperative inclusion of family members in this process.

FAMILY INVOLVEMENT IN EATING DISORDER ASSESSMENT

Mimicking the legacy of the "schizophrenogenic mother" in schizophrenia (Hartwell, 1996) and the "refrigerator mother" in autism (Bettelheim, 1967), parents of children with an eating disorder have received undue blame in the etiology of their child's illness (Whitney & Eisler, 2005). Certain family patterns or dynamics such as the psychosomatic family delineated by

Minuchin and colleagues were viewed as contributory to disorder expression and maintenance (Minuchin, Rosman, & Baker, 1978). An unfortunate result of this history is that families with a child with an eating disorder were often excluded from both assessment and treatment. In contrast, the most empirically validated treatment for adolescent AN to date views parents as a necessary and crucial part of the intervention process (Steiner & Lock, 1998). Thus, in seemingly a complete reversal, the active involvement of parent perspectives regarding changing family dynamics since disorder onset provides a pivotal foundation to frame a clinical intervention.

Parents provide crucial information for the evaluation of eating disturbance in children or adolescents. Individuals with eating disorders often lack insight into the severity of their illness, a factor that may inhibit accurate assessment of eating disorder symptomatology and serve as a barrier to subsequent treatment (Couturier & Lock, 2006). Discrepancies between parent- and child-report may accentuate areas in which the child or adolescent lacks understanding of the nature of her symptoms. Furthermore, parents may be more reliable historians of stressors that may have increased the likelihood of subsequent eating disturbance.

For example, although the specificity of trauma for subsequent eating disturbance continues to be debated, converging evidence highlights the onset of eating disturbance following a significant life event (Schmidt, Tiller, Blanchard, Andrews, & Treasure, 1997), including during a key developmental transition such as adolescence. More specifically, the role of sexual and emotional trauma in increasing the risk of later eating disturbance has received particular attention (Steiger & Bruce, 2007). Although not specific to the development of eating disturbance, a review by Steiger and Bruce (2007) highlights the importance of considering multiple levels of analysis (e.g., genetic, trait, developmental, and environmental) to understand the impact of life events.

They cite that a specific functional polymorphism of the serotonergic system is associated with particular behavioral patterns and characterological traits (i.e., affective instability and impulsivity). Individuals with bulimic symptoms who are both carriers of this genetic variant and have experienced childhood sexual abuse endorsed more pronounced sensation-seeking and attachment disturbance. Such findings highlight that although not increasing the specific risk for eating disorder symptoms, the presence of these characterological profiles may serve as setting events that synergistically interact with traumatic life experiences to promote the development of psychopathology (as cited in Steiger & Bruce, 2007). Understanding changes in the child's eating patterns relative to a significant life event may help in the formulation of hypotheses on the adaptive functions of eating disorder symptoms.

SUGGESTIONS FOR CLINICAL INTERVIEW

The following questions may help elicit relevant information. "Many children experience life events or changes as stressful. We have also learned that in many children who develop eating disturbance, there may have been particularly upsetting circumstances in their past. Learning more about these events can greatly improve our treatment planning. Can you describe important events your child experienced during the year preceding any signs of disturbance? For example, is there a person or animal that died, other deaths, losses, or a family move? To your knowledge is there any history of emotional, physical, or sexual abuse? By emotional abuse, this can be someone at school who bullied or teased your child or it can be more personal such as a family member or someone well known to your child. Physical abuse and sexual abuse are both sometimes described when a child is displaying symptoms of psychopathology. Do you have any concerns that any significant or unsettling events may have occurred?"

Family Characteristics and Environment

As the family is increasingly responsible for the management of their child's illness, assessment should focus on factors that would complicate the execution of this task. For example, specific patterns of family communication, such as expressed emotion, have been reported to affect treatment progress (Eisler et al., 1997). Expressed emotion (EE) connotes a pattern of critical communication whereby family members blame the ill child for his illness (Vaughn & Leff, 1976). Notably, adolescents with disordered eating from critical families are more likely to drop out of family therapy (Szmukler, Eisler, Russell, & Dare, 1985), and high levels of maternal criticism are predictive of poor treatment outcome (van Furth et al., 1996).

Furthermore, ED families that present with high levels of criticism show less progress in treatment than families with more positive EE scores. In fact, EE measures of criticism, hostility, and warmth for individuals with ED who did not improve with treatment actually worsened over the course of a six-month treatment period, and differed significantly from families with a child with an ED who made progress during treatment (Le Grange, Eisler, Dare, & Hodes, 1992). In sum, these findings indicate that levels of EE in eating-disordered families may be predictive of treatment outcome and may change as treatment progresses (Le Grange et al., 1992). Accordingly, assessing the nature of family EE (Table 14.1) and aiming to reduce parental hostility and criticism at the beginning of treatment may prove efficacious in contributing to a positive treatment outcome.

In addition to understanding the way the family interacts as a unit, assessment should also examine the dyads within the family. Gathering knowledge about the strength of the parents' marriage and the characteristics of sibling interactions may inform treatment options, as difficulties within these relationships may create additional barriers to successful recovery or prevent the child with an eating disturbance from getting adequate support at home. This information may also identify ways to use family members most efficiently during the process of recovery. Examples of assessment tools include the Stress Index for Parents of Adolescents (SIPA; Abidin, 2004) and the Family Adaptability and Cohesion Evaluation Scales (FACES; Olson, 2000) and are effective self-assessment tools to characterize the nature of interaction patterns (see Table 14.1).

Table 14.1. *Selected Eating Disorder Assessment Tools*

Name of Measure	Type	Construct Assessed	Strengths & Weaknesses
Eating Disorder Examination (EDE, Fairburn & Cooper, 1993; Peterson et al., 2007)	Interview and self-report versions available	Dietary restraint, concerns regarding eating, shape, and body weight	Interview format is one of most frequently used measures; Extensive reliability and validity data; Quantifies symptoms, provides useful subscale scores; Child (EDE-C) and adolescent (EDE-A) versions available. The adolescent version is validated. Less data on the psychometric properties of EDE-C and questionnaire format (EDE-Q).
Eating Disorder Inventory (EDI, Garner, Olmstead, & Polivy, 1983)	Self-report	ED symptoms, including body dissatisfaction. Also assesses related features, such as interoceptive deficits, inter- and intrapersonal dysfunction, perfectionism	Comprehensive measure; Currently in its third edition; The second iteration of the EDI has been specifically adapted for use with children (EDI-C, Eklund, Paavonen, & Almqvist, 2005). Adolescent norms for the EDI-2 are available.
Body image measures			
Body Image Assessment-Children (BIA-C, Veron-Guidry & Williamson, 1996)	Schematic Figure Drawings	Satisfaction with current body size and shape, accuracy of body size estimation	1-week reliability, Pearson $r = .67–.79$; Evidence of concurrent validity: Discrepancy between current and ideal body size, as measured by the BIA correlated significantly with severity of ED symptoms; Norms for male and female children ages 8–13 available.
Body Rating Scale (BRS, Sherman et al., 1995)	Schematic Figure Drawings	Satisfaction with current body size and shape, accuracy of body size estimation	Psychometrically similar to the Figure Rating Scale, however has advantage of increased face validity for young people with the use of adolescent female figures; Pearson Product Moment Correlation Coefficient between BSR and other body scales, $r = .81–.95$; females only.
Children's Body Image Scale (CBIS, Truby & Paxton, 2002)	Schematic Figure Drawings	Body satisfaction and perceptual accuracy in pre-pubescent children	Easily administered and visual image requires less abstract reasoning and verbal fluency; Uses real life images of male and female children between ages 7–12 with known BMI; Evidence measure is not appropriate for use with younger boys (7–8 y/o).
Somatomorphic Matrix (Cafri & Thompson, 2004)	Contour Drawn Silhouettes	Body satisfaction and perceptual accuracy	Includes both adiposity and muscularity dimensions; Easily administered via computer; Evidence of construct validity; however, Current versions have poor reliability.

(continued)

Table 14.1. (continued)

Name of Measure	Type	Construct Assessed	Strengths & Weaknesses
Body Shape Questionnaire (BSQ, Cooper, Taylor, Cooper, & Fairburn, 1987; Rosen et al., 1996)	Self-report	Preoccupation and distress related to body size and shape, experience of "feeling fat"	Original version is 34 items, a validated 14-item brief version is also available (Dowson, 2001). Reliability and validity studies with adult samples only; however, BSQ has been used with school-aged children.
Body Esteem Scale (BES, Mendelson & White, 1982)	Self-report	Body satisfaction, weight and size concerns	Child, adolescent and adult versions available; Spilt-half reliability for a sample of males and females age 8.5–17.4, .85; Equally appropriate for boys and girls.
Drive for Muscularity Scale (McCreary & Sasse, 2000)	Self-report	Attitudes and behaviors related to satisfaction with muscular appearance	Measure created with sample of 16–24 year-olds. Assesses components of male body image (BI) not assessed by traditional measures; Internal consistency .78–.84. Evidence of discriminant validity: uncorrelated with measures that assess drive for thinness.
Body Checking Questionnaire (BCQ, Reas & Grilo, 2004)	Self-report	Body checking behaviors (e.g., pinching fat). Includes 3 subfactors: body checking related to overall appearance, specific body parts, and idiosyncratic checking rituals.	Test–retest reliability = .94. Subfactors have good internal consistency (.83–.92). Evidence of construct validity: correlated with measures of body satisfaction and eating disorder symptoms. Found to differentiate ED patients and normal controls
Situational Inventory of Body Image Dysphoria (SIBID, Cash 2002b)	Self-report	Degree to which particular situations or activities evoke negative feelings about one's body	Good psychometric properties for both the long and short form. Short form: 1-month reliability, $r = .80–.86$; Correlated with other measures of BI disturbance and psychological maladjustment .5–.6)
Body Image States Scale (BISS, Cash et al., 2002)	Self-report	Dissatisfaction with body and appearance at a particular moment in time	Approaches BI as a state rather than a trait, capturing fluctuations in body experience and satisfaction; Brevity of the measure makes it easy to administer. Acceptable psychometric properties.
Digital photograph of image in mirror; Projected to be life size (Shafran & Fairburn, 2002)	Dynamic Assessment Technique	Body satisfaction and size estimation	Decreases reliance on memory and other executive functions; Provides experience that most closely approximates real life encounters with one's physical image. No information available regarding reliability or use with children.
Family functioning SIPA/PSI (Abidin, 2004)	Self-report	Levels of total parenting stress; Adolescent, parenting, and life factors contributing to total stress; The nature of the parent–child and marital relationships	The SIPA is used for adolescents (11–19 years) and the PSI is used for children (1 month–12 years); normative comparisons available

Table 14.1. (continued)

Name of Measure	Type	Construct Assessed	Strengths & Weaknesses
FACES IV (Olson, 2000)	Self-report	General family functioning, with an emphasis on family cohesion, flexibility, and communication skills	Specifically designed to identify dysfunctional areas of family functioning and help with treatment planning for families
Family Assessment Measure-III (FAM III, Skinner, Steinhauer, & Santa-Barbara, 2003)	Self-report	Family strengths and weaknesses in the family unit as a whole, dyads within the family, and the individual's perception of their role and functioning within the family	Normative data available for families of AN and BN patients
Family History Research Diagnostic Criteria (FH-RDC, Andreasen et al., 1977)	Self-report	Measure of family psychiatric history	Most reliable standardized method for assessing family history of psychiatric disturbance; results must be interpreted with caution, as underreporting commonly occurs
Family History Assessment (Andreasen et al., 1977)	Self-report	Brief screening for family psychiatric history; measures informant and their first-degree relatives	Less valid than the FH-RDC, but more time efficient; most valid for assessing major depression, anxiety disorders, substance dependence, and suicide attempts; effectiveness increases when more than one family member is assessed

The family environment can serve as both an asset and liability for the promotion of messages and values regarding health, eating, and body image. Current research indicates that parents can have both a positive and negative influence on children's eating behaviors (Ackard & Neumark-Sztainer, 2001). Haworth-Hoeppner (2000) suggests that consistent conversation in the home regarding weight reinforces cultural messages that value the importance of thinness, and parental encouragement to diet is predictive of unhealthy dieting behaviors in eighth- and ninth-grade girls (Dixon, Adair, & O'Connor, 1996; Haworth-Hoeppner, 2000). In contrast, Ackard and Neumark-Sztainer (2001) found eating disorder behaviors in individuals with bulimia to be inversely proportional to the frequency of family meals. One hypothesis is that family meals can increase healthy family interaction and provide an opportunity for parents to model healthy eating behaviors. Accordingly, gathering information about the structure of mealtimes and the importance of health may reveal familial influences to draw upon during treatment, as well as potential negative aspects that should be targeted for change.

Suggestions for Assessment

What magazines would I find around your living room if I were to look in your home right now? What TV shows are watched and who monitors this decision? Are there rules about clothing, how people have to look when they leave the house? How important are family meals/family dinners in your home? Does your family ever take bike rides or walks together? Who decides what food is in the refrigerator/cupboards? Are certain types of foods not allowed or seen as "bad foods"? Who does the grocery shopping? Who orders at restaurants and how do you decide where to go?

Family Psychiatric History

Another issue to address in the initial assessment is the psychiatric history of the parents and their extended family. The presence of mental illness in parents and family members both greatly informs potential treatment options while complicating illness management. Given the burgeoning responsibilities imparted to parents for the management of their child, the presence of mental illness in either or both parents may greatly compromise their ability to manage their child's severe state and may necessitate additional strategies. Unfortunately, the presence of an individual with an eating disorder increases the risk that a family member will be diagnosed with an eating disorder (Strober, Freeman, Lampert, Diamond, & Kaye, 2000), anxiety disorder (Bulik, 1995), affective disorder (Lilenfeld et al., 1998), and/or substance abuse (Lilenfeld et al., 1998). In particular, parents should be questioned about their own eating habits, as research demonstrates that eating disorders are often seen in first-degree relatives of patients (Lilenfeld et al., 1998). Assessment of family psychiatric history can be bolstered via self-report measures, such as the Family History Assessment (Andreasen Endicott, Spitzer, & Winokur, 1977) (See Table 14.1). Understanding family history of psychiatric illness can help inform potential barriers to the parents' ability to manage their child's illness.

Assessment of Eating Disorder Symptoms

Body Weight: Definition and Significance of Construct

Extreme weight loss is arguably the defining feature of individuals with anorexia nervosa. Unlike the considerable overlap in symptoms of disordered eating across syndromes (e.g., purgative behavior is seen both in individuals diagnosed with bulimia nervosa and anorexia nervosa), extreme weight loss is unique to the disorder of AN. As defined in the current diagnostic system authored by the American Psychiatric Association (2000), this criterion is defined as determined weight loss leading to body weight at or above a minimally normal weight for age and height. Examples include a level 85% or less than expected or, in children, a failure to gain weight during a period of growth leading to a body weight less than 85% of expected.

Although the assessment of this feature would seem straightforward, there is considerable dissention regarding the sensitivity of current guidelines to define clinical severity (Hebebrand, Casper, Treasure, & Schweiger, 2004). A further issue complicating diagnosis is the debate and clinical relevance of focusing on an individual's specific weight value relative to an individual's history of weight change. In response to these challenges, there have been several proposed alternatives to distinguishing severe weight loss in children and adolescents.

The clinical validity of current weight criteria in defining symptom severity has been challenged by studies with adult research samples. Although research conducted in adult samples is of only marginal utility in guiding clinical decision-making in AN, this work is notable in demonstrating the poor validity of current cut-offs. For example, McIntosh et al. (2004) examined the clinical validity of strict body mass index (BMI; < 17.5) relative to lenient criteria (BMI 17.5–19) for AN (McIntosh et al., 2004). Of importance, no group differences were reported on physical measures (other than BMI) including blood pressure, history of amenorrhea, weight loss history, body temperature, or heart rate. Similar findings were reported on self-report measures of eating disorder psychopathology with the exception of body image discrepancy (McIntosh et al., 2004).

Individuals in the lenient group described a larger discrepancy between their current weight and their ideal weight. This evidence has been further bolstered by multisite studies comparing the clinical severity of AN to subthreshold AN (all symptoms of AN but weight along with either menstrual dysfunction or cognitive criteria of AN) indicating no reliable differences in clinical features or degree of impairment (Crow, Agras, Halmi, Mitchell, & Kraemer, 2002). As weight loss in children and adolescents may have more severe impact due to the potentially negative effects on growth and development (Peebles et al., 2006), these results question both the sensitivity and interpretative power of current weight cut-offs in the determination of clinical severity.

Developmental Considerations

Several authors have recommended the use of body mass index centiles as a more developmentally sensitive alternative to percentage ideal body weight. As highlighted by Hebebrand et al. (2004), a criterion of 85% ideal body weight corresponds to a body mass index (BMI) roughly between the fifth and tenth BMI centile in the United States, with the BMI index of ≤ 17.5 (kg/m^2) providing a more conservative provision for defining weight. BMI is a widely adapted indicator of nutritional status as it provides an index of weight per height (Bray, 1998). Of importance, consideration of both the 85 percentile as well as the BMI criterion of 17.5 kg/m^2 corresponds to different levels of severity across the growth trajectory ironically being more stringent at sensitive developmental ages for diagnoses (Hebebrand et al., 2004). For example, although the tenth centile for adult females is a BMI value of 18.9 (kg/m^2), a weight that crosses the threshold of healthy leanness, a sixteen-year-old of this weight classification would have a BMI value of 17.5 (kg/m^2), in accordance with a more strict diagnostic criterion.

To highlight the potential severity of this issue, Peebles, Wilson, and Lock (2006) compared the clinical presentation of 109 children under the age of 13 years to 850 patients from ages 13–18 years old. Despite exhibiting a shorter duration of illness, children exhibited a more rapid rate of weight loss resulting in a lower ideal body mass index at clinical presentation relative to their older peers. These results highlight the insufficiency of current weight loss criteria for children. One solution proposed by Hebebrand et al. (2004) is the use of the tenth BMI centile as a conservative, but sensitive indicator of diagnostic severity.

An alternative diagnostic strategy is the consideration of weight and height trends such as deviation from previous growth and sexual maturity trajectories and/or percentage of weight loss (Workgroup for the Classification of Eating Disorders in Children and Adolescents, 2007). Such a strategy not only has the advantage of considering each individual within the context of his own developmental history, but by considering both growth and maturational indices, can provide several mechanisms to evaluate potentially serious changes. Thus, rather then define severity based on a clinical cut-point, consideration of change from previous growth velocity may provide a more clinically meaningful index of severity.

Assessment Methods

The growth charts established by the Center for Disease Control (CDC) (2002) not only provide a sensitive indicator of clinical reality, they can be implemented as a powerful visual tool to communicate the severity of weight loss to a reluctant clinical audience. It is important to note that these charts were not established as standards of health (Center for Disease Control, 2002). Rather, these charts reflect the current state of body weight regulation at the population level. Thus, if the health of the population is changing, than values considered relative to the population have different meanings at different times. However, at the level of the individual, CDC growth charts provide a sensitive visual clinical tool intended to facilitate more rapid detection of changes in previous growth velocity. Thus, a clinician should consider plotting an individual's weight and height history so trends can be readily perceived.

For both parents and their children with disordered eating, the clinical severity of recent weight loss is often not readily discerned. Subtle changes in weight are not easily detectable when a family member is seen on a daily basis. Compounding this problem, unlike a serious medical illness, children and adolescents with disordered eating often feel "fine." Thus, the dramatic graphic illustration of a changing growth pattern may be one of the most effective manners to demonstrate to both the child and the child's parent the severity of current nutritional habits.

There is little guiding evidence about the frequency and strategy of regular body mass assessments. For children and adolescents with disordered eating, the numbers on the scale function as exposures to noxious stimuli (Vitousek, 2002). The anxiety-provoking nature of weighing is potentially exacerbated by the concrete thinking style often described in individuals with AN, in which randomly designated weight values are deemed fat or slender. Combined, the child or adolescent has difficulty appreciating the value of weight trends, that is, the need to interpret a series of weight values over time to make meaningful conclusions about the trajectory of change. Rather, children may become exceedingly agitated about a natural body weight fluctuation and may exacerbate food restriction in response to an invalid interpretation of their body weight value.

In support of these considerations, empirically validated strategies for body mass assessment come from treatment studies. For example, in the Maudsley Model of family therapy, the most empirically valid treatment strategy for the treatment of adolescent AN (Lock, Le Grange, Agras, & Dare, 2001), weekly weighing occurs only in the therapist's office with only the adolescent and therapist. The weight is then communicated to the family by the therapist so that the previous strategies undertaken by the family towards weight gain can be evaluated. Given the importance of the family for their child's weight management, and their need for data to guide their behavior, this strategy is clinically useful. Furthermore, it provides an opportunity for the therapist to address misinterpretations regarding the meaning of subtle weight fluctuations. Thus, weekly weighing in the presence of the therapist rather than at home reflects the most empirically valid standard of practice.

Differential Diagnosis

Unexpected or severe weight loss is often encountered in relation to physical illness thus further substantiating the importance of the initial medical exam to rule out medical causes for body mass change (Mitchell & Crow, 2006). There would seem to be a difference between the intentional weight loss associated with an eating disorder and the potentially accidental weight loss that may accompany a physical illness, however, in practice the issue is not straightforward. Sometimes both factors are at play in that the initial cause of weight loss may be the result of accidental physical factors, but the maintenance, exacerbation, or persistence of severe weight loss is a result of behavioral factors.

For example, weight loss is a frequent harbinger of Type I diabetes, an autoimmune disorder of the endocrine system with a frequent age of onset in childhood reflecting the body's failure to produce and utilize the insulin necessary to metabolize glucose (Eisenbarth, Polonsky, & Buse, 2003). Although the weight loss that predates diabetes diagnosis and treatment reflects this endocrine abnormality, in fact, adolescents with diabetes may exhibit an increased likelihood of a diagnosis of an eating disorder (Colton, Olmsted, Daneman, Rydall, & Rodin, 2004). Of importance, the presence of eating disorder symptomatology may manifest as a failure to adhere to proscribed medical recommendations resulting in poor glycemic control. Thus, a careful medical diagnosis must distinguish comorbid medical conditions that may instigate or contribute to nutritional deprivation from behavioral factors that may maintain unhealthy weight regulation.

Sensitivity to somatic experience is a further issue that complicates the differentiation of physical from psychological disorder. The issue of sensory sensitivity is relatively unexplored in children and adolescents with eating disturbance relative to other childhood diagnoses such as pervasive developmental disorders. An exception is a classification system specifically designed to address the unique diagnostic needs of children and adolescents referred to as the *Great Ormand Street Criteria* (Nicholls, Chater, & Lask, 2000). Within this diagnostic system, a disorder referred to as Food

Avoidance Emotional Disorder (FAED) warrants mention due to increasing data supporting the appearance of this symptom constellation in several laboratories. Children with FAED exhibit wide heterogeneity in presentation; however, they share food avoidance with unhealthy weight loss. FAED delineates a syndrome in which severe food refusal and weight loss are present; nonetheless, the desire to be thin is not the stated motivational goal. Rather, some children and young adolescents in this group appear to be exquisitely sensitive to somatic sensations of fullness or changing bodily states and their food avoidance may be intended to avoid these perceptions of somatic discomfort. Although the body of evidence to date has not warranted inclusion of this diagnosis in a formalized diagnostic system, the increasing body of evidence certainly necessitates that clinicians be aware and sensitive to this symptom expression (Cooper et al., 2002).

Food neophobia, the fear of trying new foods, may manifest as extreme selectivity that affects the range of food variety (Galloway, Lee, & Birch, 2003). Researchers have highlighted the dispositional nature of this eating pattern as many children exhibit this style of eating from early childhood. High trait anxiety is often reported in both children with food neophobia and their mothers (Galloway et al., 2003). In contrast, children with food selectivity may demonstrate similar limitations in food variety, nonetheless the association to dispositional factors is less clear and has been hypothesized to be more sensitive to environmental factors (Galloway et al., 2003); that is, the child will eat more variety at school than at home. Unlike the food avoidance seen in AN, weight and shape concerns are not the initial motivating factors for food avoidance and extreme weight loss is often not part of the clinical picture.

Notwithstanding, self-imposed limitations on food variety may threaten health. Chatoor and Ganiban (2003) suggest guidelines for the point at which food selectivity or neophobia demands intervention. Treatment may be necessary if adequate nutrition can not be sustained without supplementation (i.e., even if weight is in a healthy range, vitamin supplementation is necessary for the child to avoid disorders caused by vitamin deficiencies). Abrupt food refusal and corresponding weight loss may occur in children who experience a choking incident or other traumatic incident. The clinical picture may be captured by the diagnosis of simple phobia. Extreme concerns about weight or shape are absent and unlike the clinical picture of AN, symptoms are aversive for the child or adolescent. Food refusal and corresponding weight loss are often witnessed in response to more pervasive traumatic reactions to harmful life events. Symptoms are related temporally to the onset of this trauma, however, food refusal may be seen as part of a more pervasive pattern of developmental regression (Workgroup for the Classification of Eating Disorders in Children and Adolescents, 2007).

CASE EXAMPLE: ASSESSMENT OF WEIGHT HISTORY FROM PARENTS

Therapist: I want to learn about your daughter's pattern of growth and weight gain. I have looked over her medical chart, however, I would like to hear your view of your daughter's weight history.

Mother: Lucy has always been thin and has always been a picky eater. Our pediatrician never seemed to be very concerned by this as she ate enough to grow; it's just that her range of foods was rather limited. She always ate decent amounts of the foods she liked. Last fall, a number of her friends decided to become vegetarian and Lucy decided to follow. We thought we were doing the right thing, took her to a nutritionist to make sure she met all of her nutritional requirements. At first, she adhered to recommendations but had trouble eating enough to maintain weight. I admit she had to eat a lot of food and it seemed like she was doing a good job. However, I noticed her choices became a bit more limited with time. I wasn't overly concerned until her gym teacher called me noticing a change in both her weight and an unusual intensity in the manner in which she pursued activities at gym. I brought her to the doctor, and again he wasn't overly concerned. She had lost some weight and had fallen below her previous height percentage but just recommended we return in several months for follow-up. I was worried however as something seemed different. That's why I brought her here.

We present this excerpt to highlight a challenging circumstance that clinicians often face in the determination of clinical severity: when parents suspect a problem, clinical indices may not be sensitive enough to pick up on significant, but subtle clinical changes. Given the potentially severe consequences of eating disturbance, the prognostic benefit conferred by early intervention, and the value of parental input into their child's normative state of functioning, intervention should be undertaken when there is parental concern. Indeed, if not of clinical significance, weight loss that raises parental concern may be a key window of opportunity to intervene very early in the illness trajectory. There is no empirical data that we are aware of to support the notion that early intervention can do harm.

Food Restriction: Definition and Significance of Construct

It is important to note that although inadequate energy intake is usually a necessary prerequisite for extreme weight loss, specific patterns of food restriction are not specified in the diagnostic criteria for an eating disorder. Despite this, deliberate food restriction has both clinical and empirical significance in both AN and BN. Given that weight loss is a result of energy imbalance, deliberate food restriction is a frequent clinical feature. However, this is not always the case as energy imbalance can also be achieved via increased physical activity without any changes in previous food intake, although, in the latter case, eating failed to increase in response to increased energy demands. Dietary restriction may take several forms including limits on total energy (e.g., eating only a certain number of calories), limits on the variety of foodstuffs (e.g., no longer eating any fried foods), or limitations on temporal patterns of consumption (e.g., no eating after 7 PM; Cooper & Fairburn, 1987). To be of clinical significance, these patterns of food restriction must interfere with nutritional or psychological health.

Further investigation of the potentially deleterious consequences of food restriction has highlighted that it is not dietary restriction, per se, but the manner of dietary restriction that is clinically significant. To illustrate, Stice, Presnell, Groenz, and Shaw (2005) experimentally manipulated dietary restriction in a group of adolescents evidencing symptoms of BN. The experimental group was provided strategies to promote healthy eating via gradual lifestyle changes such as increasing fruit and vegetable consumption while decreasing intake of high-calorie foods of low nutrient density (Stice et al., 2005). No specific calorie limit was applied and no calorie counting was completed. Engaging in this moderate gradual form of healthy lifestyle eating was reported to decrease symptoms of BN including binge eating.

The authors argue that these findings challenge the etiological role of dietary restriction on subsequent eating disorder development and raise the possibility that it is the rigid manner of restriction that is problematic. This interpretation supports the clinical strategies employed in the most empirically validated treatment for BN, cognitive behavior therapy (Fairburn, 1996), a treatment that specifically targets rigid approaches to dietary intake. In short, it is not just the amount of food consumed that is important, but rather the manner in which decisions about the range, timing, and quality of nutritional habits are established and maintained that is crucial to assess.

Developmental Considerations

The assessment of restrictive eating practices in children and adolescents is complicated by a potential lack of insight into behavioral motives, the child's lack of control over the food environment, and their literal interpretation of assessment questions. The ability to forecast temporally distant outcomes such as risk evolves throughout the adolescent period (Boyer, 2006). Similarly, limited insight into the motivational consequences of eating may cause children to answer in ways that mask the true nature of their relationship to food. For example, on learning that a child no longer eats cake, an interviewer may ask, "Why don't you eat cake?" A child would be likely to reply, "Because I don't like it." It requires perceptive querying to ascertain that, in fact, the child used to enjoy the taste of cake, but now feels "bad" after eating it and thus "doesn't like it."

Limitations on abstract reasoning may further preclude understanding of the specific relation between a pattern of dietary intake, subsequent energy imbalance, and weight loss (Marini & Case, 1994). Rather, children may learn rigid rules about food intake (e.g., cake is bad) or, more severely, "Food is bad," thus precipitating an unhealthy period of severe food restriction. However, given the reciprocal nature of the feeding relationship (i.e., parental influence on the home food environment) combined with the child's dependence on parents for the type of food at home, any assessment of dietary restriction must incorporate normative family patterns.

Finally, children or adolescents may interpret assessment questions in an overly literal manner, a style of response that may mask serious food restriction. For example, the question, "What did you have for lunch?" could be answered by the child according to what was in her lunch bag and not according to what she actually consumed. Thus, assessors must be very specific and concrete and judiciously incorporate collateral reports in trying to understand patterns of dietary intake.

Assessment Strategies

The goal of dietary assessment is determination of the adequacy of current nutrition intake and the presence of dietary rigidity. The assessment of dietary intake has been investigated extensively with current consensus questioning the validity and accuracy of dietary food records relative to interview-assisted dietary recalls. Although the former method has an individual record of their food intake for a number of days, the latter approach uses food records as the basis for subsequent probing regarding food intake during the previous 24 hours (Cullen et al., 2004).

Nutritionist-assisted dietary recalls may utilize visual food models to illustrate portion sizes (Godwin, Chambers, & Cleveland, 2004) a strategy that may be particularly apt for the assessment of dietary intake in children and adolescents as it provides concrete examples to facilitate the visualization of quantity. Such models can be ordered from nutrition education companies. Assessment of nutritional intake in children and adolescents is best facilitated by short time intervals and concrete examples of food quantity.

Attitudes regarding dietary intake and strategies to facilitate reduced caloric intake have been most reliably assessed in children and adolescents by clinician-administered structured interviews. For example, the Eating Disorder Examination for Children (EDE-C) is a clinician-administered structured interview frequently used in studies aimed to characterize disordered eating in children and adolescents (Watkins, Frampton, Lask, & Bryant-Waugh, 2005). Recently, researchers examining the use of the EDE with adolescents suggest that the inclusion of new supplementary items created by the authors may capture a more accurate picture of pathology when assessing adolescents with AN (Couturier & Lock, 2006). This measure provides detailed questions regarding the past 28 days, has items that assess the prior three months, and provides continuous measures of ED symptoms as well as items that specifically assess *DSM–IV* diagnostic criteria (American Psychiatric Association, 1994).

The EDE is comprised of four subscales that assess eating disorder symptoms related to shape concern, weight concern, eating concern, and dietary restraint (Fairburn, & Cooper, 1993). The child version is adapted from the adult version by providing more age-appropriate language and by using concrete examples to explain abstract concepts. Advantages to this measure are its previous use in studies of eating pathology in children and adolescents (Tanofsky-Kraff et al., 2003).

In regard to food restriction, the child version of the EDE (chEDE) assesses specific food rules (e.g., food types the individual does not permit herself to eat) and periods of fasting or deliberate food restriction. Researchers have challenged the sensitivity of this measure to the features of minimization or poor insight in children (Couturier & Lock, 2006). An additional challenge with this measure is the length, approximately an hour. A shortened, semi-structured interview based on the EDE was developed by Field et al. (2004) to be used as a screening tool for eating pathology and takes approximately 15–20 minutes (Field, Taylor, Celio, & Colditz, 2004). Thus, the goals of the assessment should dictate whether a more extensive review of disordered eating patterns is required.

Some self-report measures assessing eating disorder symptoms exist, and although these measurement tools certainly represent developmentally sensitive advances to adult measures, studies that assess correspondence between child- and parent-report highlight the importance of integrating both perspectives into the interpretation of clinical data. Table 14.1 provides a summary of self-report measures and the advantages and disadvantages of these measures. In each symptom section, we highlight measures within this table.

For screening purposes, the most validated screening measure for adolescents is the five-item Weight Concerns Scale (Shisslak et al., 1999). The Eating Disorder Inventory (EDI), one of the most frequently used measures of attitudes frequently reported in individuals with ED, has extensive normative data and has the clinical advantage of providing a graphic profile of attitudes that may facilitate assessment feedback (Garner, 1991). A child version of this measure has been published with initial normative data reported using a representative community sample of adolescents (Franko et al., 2004). Its use as a treatment outcome measure has not been thoroughly explored.

The Kids Eating Disorder Survey (KEDS) is a screening tool designed for children and adolescents (Childress, Brewerton, Hodges, & Jarrell, 1993). Acceptable psychometric data exist although some authors have challenged the absence of certain key constructs (e.g., loss of control in the assessment of binge eating). For clinical purposes, measures that can provide graphic feedback (such as plotted profiles) may have utility in engaging the family about the serious nature of current symptoms, particularly when plotted in respect to typically functioning individuals.

Differential Diagnosis

In addition to disorders associated with potential weight loss, there are several disorders of childhood associated with food selectivity or food refusal. Children diagnosed with an autism spectrum disorder often manifest rigid patterns of eating and/or sensitivity with food taste and texture (Ahearn, Castine, Nault, & Green, 2001). Although rigid, these patterns are often interpreted as a manifestation of the child's insistence on sameness, a part of the diagnostic profile for these disorders (Kanner, 1943). Importantly, the stated intent of these behaviors is not weight and shape concerns and weight loss is often not present.

SAMPLE QUESTIONS FOR ASSESSMENT

Are there any foods that you do not let yourself eat? For example, if I had a piece of candy, and you were hungry, could you eat it? Did you ever eat candy? Why did you stop? What if I told you that this was a magical piece of candy and if you ate it, it would make you lose weight? Could you eat it then? Do you have any rules about eating? For example, are there certain good foods that you are only allowed to eat or bad foods that you are not allowed to eat? Can you ever eat the "bad foods" or do you just try to eat less of them than other foods?

Binge Eating: Definition and Significance

Binge eating behavior may be the most highly prevalent eating disorder symptom in childhood and adolescence due, in part, to its association with pediatric obesity. Studies in both treatment-seeking and community samples support that a significant proportion of overweight children and adolescents endorse this pathological eating pattern (Decaluwe & Braet, 2003). Of importance, overweight children who endorse binge eating often exhibit higher levels of affective symptoms such as anxiety and depression and those who endorse disordered eating attitudes have elevated BMIs relative to overweight children without this pattern (Tanofsky-Kraff, Faden, Yanovski, Wilfley, & Yanovski, 2005). Furthermore, adults who report binge eating often date adolescence as the origin of this pattern, highlighting the potential chronicity of this feature.

Binge eating requires the experience of subjective distress. Individuals who binge eat, by definition, are uncomfortable and distressed by this pattern of eating. Beyond subjective experiences, binge eating is differentiated into subtypes (objective vs. subjective) based on the amount of food consumed. Across both subtypes, a feeling of loss of control, that is, a feeling that one cannot stop eating even though a part of the individual would like to stop, is present. However, in objective binge eating, the amount of food consumed is considered excessive given the eating context (American Psychiatric Association, 2000). There is currently no consensus on the size of binge necessary to be considered excessive, and an individual who eats an extremely large meal would not be considered to be binge eating unless accompanied by a sense of loss of control.

Several ways to operationalize excessive food consumption have been attempted. In the Structured Interview for Anorexia and Bulimia Nervosa (Fichter & Quadflieg, 2001), quantity of food is assessed using cut-points, with marked episodes considered 1000–3000 kcalories of energy whereas severe episodes are >5,000 kcalories. However, the importance of the context in which the eating occurs is also important. Eating a fast-food double cheeseburger, an extra large order of French fries, and a milkshake, although providing an arguably marked amount of energy (i.e., approximately 1,500 kcalories) would not be considered a binge eating episode if this person felt comfortable with this pattern, it was during the lunch meal, and the meal was enjoyed in the presence of friends. However, this same amount, eaten late at night, hiding this eating due to embarrassment, telling oneself not to finish the fried potatoes but doing so anyway, and feeling distress about the event would be considered a binge eating episode (Goldfein, Devlin, & Kamenetz, 2005).

In contrast, in a subjective binge eating episode, the individual experiences subjective distress, however, he does not consume an amount of food deemed excessive (e.g., having a sandwich and chips for lunch when one told oneself not to eat the chips). Given these complicated issues, researchers have taken great care in accurately defining binge eating in children (Marcus & Kalarchian, 2003).

The setting events that increase the likelihood of subsequent binge eating may highlight different strategies for intervention. A dual pathway model of subsequent bulimic symptoms has been described in adolescents (Stice, 2001). Binge eating episodes triggered by affective symptoms fall into one arm of this model. Given the relationship to negative affect, several hypotheses regarding the function of binge eating have been proposed. Binge eating may contribute to a temporary elevation in affect possibly due to the effects of foodstuffs on levels of neurotransmitters implicated in affective regulation such as serotonin and dopamine (Steiger & Bruce, 2007).

For some, binge eating may function as a temporary distraction from aversive experiences (Heatherton & Baumeister, 1991). Individuals often describe a decreased level of self-awareness while binge eating using phrases such as "being in a daze" or "feeling robotic." In an oft-cited theoretical paper, Heatherton and Baumeister (1991) propose that binge eating may narrow attention to the immediate presence of food thereby capturing attentional resources that would be otherwise allocated to provocative stimuli. Indeed, individuals who binge eat often describe these periods as the one time during their day in which "The rules disappear, and I can do anything I want." Subsequent to this escape, however, often occur feelings of guilt, shame, and associated depressive symptoms.

The dietary restraint pathway to binge eating highlights rigid, untenable dietary rules combined with maladaptive reactions to rule violation, that is, an abstinence violation effect. According to this model, deviation from dietary rules may occur because the amount of food prescribed is not sustainable due to true biologic needs (Polivy, 1998). Entering an eating occasion overly hungry is proposed to increase the difficulty with meal termination leading to consuming more food than intended. The subsequent breaking of the standard is posited to increase negative affect, seemingly ironically promoting overeating via a "What the heck, I've already blown it" mentality (Urbszat, Herman, & Polivy, 2002). Assessment thus involves the nature of the dietary rules (see previous section) and the consequences of rule violation.

Researchers have supported this distinction demonstrating that a subgroup of individuals describe a pattern of dietary restriction preceding the first binge eating episode in adolescents (Stice, 2001). In a study of overweight children, however, 2/3 reported that the experience of loss of control eating preceded any form of dietary restriction for weight loss (Tanofsky-Kraff et al., 2005). As such, historical dietary influences on binge eating may aid in case formulation in addition to more proximal functional analyses.

Developmental Considerations

There are unique behavioral patterns associated with binge eating in children and adolescents relative to adults (Marcus & Kalarchian, 2003). Parent reports appear to be particularly necessary in the assessment of this feature as comparisons of child-/adolescent- to parent-reports indicated that parental reports had greater clinical validity (Steinberg et al., 2004). Of interest, the experience of loss of control appears to be more clinically valid than the amount of food consumed for children and adolescents (Marcus & Kalarchian, 2003). This may reasonably be due to the environmental reality that children and adolescents do not have as much control over the home food environment as adults and thus may have less ability to buy food to fuel a binge eating episode. It is perhaps not surprising then that Marcus and Kalarchian (2003) recommend provisional criteria for the diagnosis of binge eating in children that includes associated clinical features such as secretive eating or food hoarding. These features may reflect the pragmatic reality of behavioral adaptations that occur when one engages in a self-perceived embarrassing pattern of behavior (i.e., binge eating) while living with family.

Assessment Methods

The chEDE is the most researched tool for the assessment of binge eating in children and adolescents (see previous section). Content related to binge eating in this measure utilizes more concrete examples to assess rather vague concepts such as excessive food consumption such as asking whether someone watching the eating would think it was too much. Self-report assessments of binge eating demonstrate less sensitivity to the differentiation of subjective relative to objective binge eating. For example, the Questionnaire of Eating and Weight Patterns-Adolescent Version (QWEP-A), a self-report measure designed to assess the presence of binge eating disorder, was found to exhibit acceptable specificity (91%) but limited sensitivity (17%) to objective relative to subjective binge eating episodes (Tanofsky-Kraff et al., 2003).

Comparison of a parent relative to the adolescent version indicates that although this measure is concordant when symptoms are absent, parent reports are more aligned with other clinical indicators such as BMI, associated eating disorder cognitions, and general problems (Tanofsky-Kraff et al., 2003). A more recent measure, the Child Binge Eating Scale, was designed to be a more convenient clinical screening tool administered by a clinician (Shapiro et al., 2007). This measure was reported to correspond with a well-validated structured clinician administered clinical interview (SCID) and to be more sensitive to subsyndromal presentations.

Examples of Assessment Questions Include:

Do you ever have times when you eat a large amount of food, more than other people would eat if they were in the same situation? Do you think other people would think it was too much food? Would you be embarrassed if I saw you eating during those times? Do you ever eat in private because you are embarrassed by what you are eating? During those times when you feel like you eat a lot of food, do you feel like you can stop eating? Do you ever try to stop? What happens when you try to stop? When you are finished eating, do you feel bad about what you have just eaten? What do you tell yourself after this period of eating is over?

Weight Control: Significance of the Construct

Weight control strategies such as exercise are often considered a healthy lifestyle behavior, however, it is the extreme use of unhealthy weight loss strategies that distinguish individuals with an ED. Of importance, extreme weight loss strategies are undertaken with the specific intent to facilitate weight loss, irrespective of the effectiveness of these strategies. In both AN and BN, a purging subtype is distinguished by the presence of self-induced vomiting; abuse of laxatives, diet pills, enemas, diuretics; or use of syrup of ipecac whereas the practice of excessive exercise is distinguished by a nonpurging subtype of both disorders (American Psychiatric Association, 1994). The significance of this distinction is reinforced by research supporting the phenotypic consistency in the presentation of the restricting subtype of AN (Wonderlich, Lilenfeld, Riso, Engel, & Mitchell, 2005), reports partially supported by increasing neurobiological evidence among individuals with this specific subtype (Bailer et al., 2005). It is the severe impact of these behaviors on health combined with often secretive nature of these behavioral patterns that increase challenges to their assessment.

Of concern, population-based surveys indicate that not only are unhealthy weight loss strategies practiced in a significant percentage of the population, but also these behaviors are appearing in demographic groups that were previously thought protected. For example, findings from two large adolescent self report surveys reveal that 10% to 30% of males and 26% to 56% of females report engaging in one or more unhealthy weight control strategies (Croll at al., 2002; Forman-Hoffman, 2004).

Neumark-Stzainer et al. (2006) examined the prevalence of extreme weight control strategies in a cohort of 2,516 adolescents at two key developmental transitions: early to middle adolescence (junior high to high school) and middle to late adolescence (high school to post high school). The use of extreme weight control behaviors nearly doubled during the early to middle adolescent transitions from a prevalence of 9.4% to 17.9%; and a second increase occurred during the later adolescent transition (14.5% to 23.9%). Although the overall prevalence of these behaviors was lower in males, the trends were the same, demonstrating a near doubling of prevalence during key developmental transitions (Neumark-Sztainer, Wall, Eisenberg, Story, & Hannan, 2006). These patterns should alert clinicians to the importance of life transitions and their assessment for the presence of eating pathology.

Developmental Considerations

Research indicates behaviors that comprise the purging subtype are less likely to appear in children below the age of 13 years of age relative to middle to late adolescence (Peebles et al., 2006). However, given the lower fat stores reported in childhood relative to adulthood, a lower threshold of symptom frequency may result in more deleterious health consequences, a fact that strengthens the importance of a thorough medical assessment to determine level of treatment intensity.

Additionally, involvement in extracurricular activities may also mask the onset of eating disordered behaviors. First, adolescents may use excessive participation in organized sports as a way to mask eating pathology. For example, a not infrequent clinical presentation is for an adolescent to be engaged in multiple sports simultaneously. Although there is nothing inherently pathological in this practice, it is the attitude the adolescent has towards this participation that is problematic. For example, a typically developing individual may engage in sports because he or she enjoys sports participation, can take days off when needing rest, and follows the coach's directions regarding intensity of practice. In contrast, an individual with an eating disorder will often experience sports participation as a way to relieve guilt (e.g., burning calories associated with physical activity), may exhibit a level of intensity towards the sport that may be counterproductive for sports conditioning, may have difficulty responding or noticing bodily fatigue, and may exercise above and beyond that instructed by coaches.

Sports participation may also be a clandestine way for the adolescent to skip meals. Involvement in extracurricular activities is often exceedingly time intensive and often occurs during the evening meal. Unfortunately, an adolescent with an eating disorder may capitalize on this opportunity, using it is a way to mask food restriction (e.g., telling her parents she has eaten with the team when she really hasn't). To assess these nuances, assessment of the child's or adolescent's activity schedule, number of sports and number hours spent practicing each sport, and involvement in other extracurricular activities such as clubs or organizations is extremely important in gaining an understanding of how and when certain weight control behaviors may be used. Another factor to consider is access to resources. If the adolescent is using laxatives or taking diet pills or smoking, inquiring as to their means of obtaining these items is an important factor for assessment.

Assessment Methods

There are several questionnaires that assess weight loss strategies and attitudes about eating and weight loss. The most commonly used of these self-report measures is the questionnaire version of the Eating Disorder Examination or EDE-Q. Although the EDE-Q has not been as extensively studied as the interview format, there is some evidence for correspondence between the two forms. While support has been found for the internal consistency of the self-report version, recent studies propose changes to the factor structure that may improve the measure's psychometric properties (Peterson et. al, 2007). Notwithstanding these limitations, the questionnaire format of this measure provides a more convenient form of assessment than the structured clinical interview.

The eating attitudes test or EAT is a self-report measure developed as a screening tool for the assessment of anorexic beliefs, attitudes, and behaviors (Garner & Garfinkel, 1979). Some authors have questioned the specificity of this measure to particular forms of eating disorder pathology (Mintz & O'Halloran, 2000). Despite the need for further inquiry, there is evidence that the EAT does serve as the first stage screening to highlight individuals who may need more extensive assessment. A child version of this measure has been developed, the ChEAT (Maloney, McGuire, Daniels, & Specter, 1988). Research on the ChEAT has also shown it to be a valid screening measure for nonclinical samples of children (Anton et al., 2006).

The Bulimia Test-Revised or BULIT-R (Thelen, Farmer, Wonderlich, & Smith, 1991) was developed to assess symptoms of bulimia, many of which are inappropriate compensatory or weight loss behaviors. Though originally developed and tested on adults, it is often used to assess adolescents. Research into the use of this measure with adolescents shows that four factors emerge (bingeing, control, normative weight loss behaviors, and extreme weight loss behaviors) that are similar to the five factors that emerge for adults. In addition, this work has found that the BULIT-R displays acceptable reliability and validity in adolescent samples (Vincent, McCabe, & Ricciardelli, 1999).

Self-monitoring through the use of diary cards or food records is also a key part of assessing the nature and degree of weight control measures. These records usually track strategies such as dietary restriction, exercise, and other compensatory weight loss strategies, as well as when and where they occurred, whether there were any identifiable environmental triggers, and any thoughts or feelings that arose before, during, and after engaging in the behavior in question. Having patients and their family provide detailed accounts of strategies used, and how often they are used each day will provide even greater depth into the degree of severity and open a discussion of the functions these behaviors serve in the patient's daily living.

Differential Diagnosis

As mentioned previously, weight loss strategies range in severity and are not necessarily indicative of an eating disorder. It is important to assess whether these behaviors are taken to extremes, which often rests on the judgment of the clinician. For instance, in adolescents who are involved in athletic activities, it is important to assess whether their exercise is in excess of what is required for a sport, distress if activity is not available, and the presence of fear of weight gain or desire to lose weight. Children may exhibit vomiting in response to extreme anxiety. In such cases, the vomiting is usually not intentional but rather in reaction to an environmental trigger. Weight loss is also a symptom of depression, however, in this case, the change in body mass is due to loss of appetite rather than deliberate attempts at food restriction for weight loss.

BODY IMAGE DISTURBANCE

Significance of the Construct

Body image disturbance, first described by Hilde Bruch in 1962 (Bruch, 1962), is currently recognized as a central feature of eating disorders (Garner, & Garfinkel, 1997). The *DSM–IV–TR* identifies two primary manifestations of body image disturbance in the diagnostic criteria for AN and BN: distortion in the way in which one's body weight or shape is experienced, and distortion in the significance of body shape and weight, such that it is seen as largely determining one's self-worth or has undue influence on one's self-evaluation (American Psychiatric Association, 2000). In the case of AN, body image disturbance may also include a failure to appreciate the seriousness of the current low body weight. As of yet, the DSM does not make a distinction between the body image (BI) disturbance seen in adults and that experienced by children and adolescents.

A thorough assessment of BI is necessary for diagnostic decision-making; however, it also has clinical relevance. Research suggests that BI disturbance has a role in the etiology and maintenance of eating pathology (Stice, 2002; Stice, & Shaw, 2002), a finding further substantiated by longitudinal research that has indicated negative body image among children increases the risk of developing an eating or weight-related disorder (Cattarin & Thompson, 1994; Eisenberg, Neumark-Sztainer, Haines, & Wall, 2006). In addition, several studies have found that body image provides some indication of long-term prognosis. Clinical outcome research has found that severely disturbed body image is related to poorer outcome and greater risk of relapse following treatment (Keel, Dorer, Franko, Jackson, & Herzog, 2005).

The BI disturbance identified in the diagnostic criteria for AN and BN is not to be confused with the normative discontent that plagues industrialized societies in which there is an emphasis on the thin ideal in an environment of plenty (Kostanski & Gullone,1999; Rodin, Silberstein, & Striegel-Moore, 1984). Indeed, ED prevalence rates range from 0.5% to 3%, whereas the rate of body dissatisfaction among children and adolescents in the general population is much higher (Ricciardelli & McCabe, 2001). Misinterpreting normative body dissatisfaction as pathological can be avoided by carefully assessing the severity of the BI disturbance and examining the impact of body concerns on functioning. Body image concerns that are clinically significant interfere with social, occupational, or academic functioning by producing behavioral deficits (e.g., avoidance of particular people, places, or activities because of one's body, concentration difficulties), behavioral excesses (e.g., body checking, eating or exercise rituals), or extreme distress.

The multidimensional nature of body image necessitates assessment strategies that accommodate both the unique and interacting contributions of each domain. Body image is a complex construct connoting perceptual (e.g., body size estimation), cognitive-evaluative, (e.g., attitudes or feelings toward one's body), experiential (i.e., the ability to accurately sense and tolerate the constantly changing state of the body habitus), and behavioral (e.g., body checking) components (Thompson & Smolak, 2001). There is wide variability in the research knowledge base and reliability of measures to assess each of these domains. Although the cognitive and perceptual aspects of body image have been the most studied to date, there is not wide acceptance on the nature of perceptual aspects of body image disturbance, a knowledge gap that necessarily interferes with reliable assessment (Fernandez, Probst, Meermann, & Vandereycken, 1994; Gardner & Bokenkamp, 1996). The experiential deficits associated with body image disturbance are also poorly understood and perhaps best captured by measures of alexithymia (Lane et al., 1996) or poor interoceptive awareness (Sim & Zeman, 2004), measures that assess an individual's ability to differentiate emotional from somatic bodily signals. The cognitive and, more recently, behavioral aspects of body image have been associated with the most reliable assessment strategies although little work has been done in children. Strategies in these domains are briefly summarized.

In regard to perceptual aspects of body image, there continues to be controversy regarding the extent to which individuals with disordered eating actually overestimate the size of their bodies (Fernandez et al., 1994; Gardner, & Bokenkamp, 1996; Skrzypek, Wehmeier, & Remschmidt, 2001). For example, in one study, individuals with AN were presented with a life-size image of their body that was distorted to either over- or underestimate their actual size. Participants were asked to adjust the image accordingly. Results indicated no consistent pattern of misperception. Individuals with AN under, over, and accurately estimated their body size. The authors note that the 20% of AN individuals who overestimated tended to have a more neurotic profile and negative body attitude (Probst, Vandereycken, Coppenolle, & Pieters, 1998). This latter finding is consistent with recent research that has suggested the perceptual and attitudinal aspects of body image may not be as distinct as once thought (Thompson, & Gardner, 2002).

Historically, the prevailing hypothesis for the lack of consistent findings regarding the perceptual aspect of BI has been that discrepancies reflect the inadequacy of current assessment methods. This has led to more ecologically valid approaches that are less confounded by issues such as memory (e.g., having to conjure a mental image of one's appearance). For example, researchers have asked participants to adjust a digital image to match what is being seen in the mirror thus precluding reliance on memory (Shafran & Fairburn, 2002). The relevance of whole body versus body part estimation (Farrell, Lee, & Shafran, 2005), ordered versus random presentation of body estimation stimuli (e.g., figure drawings) (Doll, Ball, & Willows, 2004), and variability in the way in which body perception accuracy is calculated have also been questioned (Farrell et al., 2005).

The stability of body image disturbance has also been challenged. Researchers propose that inconsistent findings may result from approaching BI disturbance as a trait when perhaps it is better understood as a state phenomenon (Cash, 2002a). They point to data that indicate the accuracy of body size estimation is influenced by a number of internal and external factors such as manipulation of experimental instruction (Thompson, & Dolce, 1989), mood state (Carter, Bulik, Lawson, Sullivan, & Wilson, 1996), hunger (Pietrowsky, Staub, & Hachl, 2003), demand characteristics or response bias (Gardner, & Bokenkamp, 1996), and other contextual factors (Haimovitz, Lansky, & Reilly, 1993). Perhaps the most likely scenario is a synthesis of these opposing views in which the perception of one's body is a function of trait factors (e.g., way in which direct sensory input is processed) and state factors (e.g., fluctuating internal processes such as emotion and cognition and environmental factors).

There is less controversy regarding the cognitive-evaluative components of body image. This may be attributable to the fact that assessment of body-related thoughts and feelings necessarily rely more heavily on questionnaires that are far less complicated methodologically. In any case, studies examining body attitudes have found a strong and consistent relationship between body dissatisfaction and disordered eating (Stice & Shaw, 2002). Although body dissatisfaction is a more robust predictor of BN than AN (Stice, 2002), extreme body dissatisfaction may be more dangerous or have a different meaning for those who are already emaciated. Furthermore, there is wide within-participant variability in ratings of body part satisfaction (i.e., individuals can rank-order body parts from most to least desired). Thus, assessment strategies that are sensitive to these evaluative nuances and incorporate measurement of an individual's ability to decipher somatic signals (such as interoceptive awareness) may elucidate the phenomenological experience of body image disturbance and may highlight novel hypotheses regarding disorder pathogenesis.

Developmental Considerations

Assessing BI in children and adolescents requires sensitivity to developmental factors that may affect the manifestation of the disturbance or the ability to report body-related thoughts, feelings, or experience. For example, children and young adolescents may lack the capacity to appreciate abstract concepts such as self-worth or to describe the experience of their bodies in other than concrete terms. Furthermore, children and adolescents may not have the cognitive capacity or experience to articulate fear of fatness. As a result, they may present BI concerns much differently than adults.

Although abstract reasoning and other cognitive skills are not fully developed in young children and adolescents, there has been some research indicating that even young children can differentiate body size. In fact, studies have shown that very young children are able to do so with relative accuracy (Gardner, Stark, Friedman, & Jackson, 2000). In terms of developmental trajectory for body dissatisfaction, however, studies have indicated that dissatisfaction begins early and, without intervention, tends to increase over time. Researchers have found that overweight children as young as 6 and 7 years old are aware of weight prejudice and want to be thinner (Kostanski & Gullone, 1999; Tiggemann & Wilson-Barrett, 1998). Furthermore, as they get older, they typically endorse a thinner ideal body size (Gardner, Sorter, & Friedman, 1997). This progression is especially pronounced in young girls whose body satisfaction decreases beginning at age 7, becomes a significant predictor of ED symptoms by age 10–11, and continues to decline through age 14 (Gardner et al., 2000), perhaps as females become more aware of cultural ideals and experience an increase in body fat associated with puberty.

Data that suggest a relationship between physical development and body satisfaction highlight the importance of assessing weight history and rate of maturation among children and adolescents presenting with an ED. Indeed, BMI (McCabe, Ricciardelli, & Holt, 2005) and atypical rates of sexual development have been identified as risk factors for disordered eating and BI disturbance (McCabe, & Ricciardelli, 2004). However, physical development does not occur in a vacuum, and BI may be greatly influenced by sociocultural context. Contextual factors may include parents, peers, and broader culture.

Children are constantly receiving direct and indirect messages about the importance of weight, body size and shape, and appearance from other people. Parents may reinforce attention to physical features, make comments about the child's weight or body, model maladaptive attention to particular body parts, and remark on their own body. Studies have confirmed the influence of parents on their children's body satisfaction (Annus, Smith, Fischer, Hendricks, & Williams, 2007; Davidson & Birch, 2001) and some researchers have suggested that daughters are particularly susceptible to comments made by their mothers. Peers may also influence body satisfaction via social comparison (Krones, Stice, Batres, & Orjada, 2005), appearance-related teasing (Eisenberg, 2006), and the adoption of unhealthy group norms (Shroff & Thompson, 2006). Furthermore, participation in sports or other activities that require a particular body size or shape may increase exposure to social comparison, rejection, and body-related teasing (e.g., Ravaldi et al., 2006). However, it is important to note that perception of exposure is sufficient, regardless of accuracy (Stice, 2002).

Body image may also be affected by significant historical events such as sexual trauma that function as potent learning experiences about the boundaries, use or worth of one's body, and the importance of controlling bodily urges (e.g., Preti, Icani, Camboni, Petretto, & Masala, 2006). The relationship of previous trauma to BI is complex as highlighted by recent genetic studies emphasizing the interaction of temperament (e.g., interpersonal sensitivity, perfectionism, fear responsivity), or other general psychiatric risk factors, such as impulsivity, to cause clinically significant eating disorder symptoms (Steiger & Bruce, 2007).

Assessment Methods

A comprehensive assessment of body image would elucidate the nature and severity of the disturbance, provide indication of impact on functioning, and identify factors that contributed to the development of the disturbance or are currently functioning to maintain it. Below is a sample of the types of questions addressed by a thorough BI assessment:

Nature of the Disturbance

Are there thoughts that you have about your body that really bother you? What about sensations that you have in your body? Do any really bother you? Are there any parts of your body that you really do not like looking at? What is your favorite part of your body? What is your least favorite?

Impact on Functioning

Do you ever avoid doing things because you don't like the way you look? Do you have any routines that you have to do every day to make sure you look okay? For example, some people have to keep looking in the mirror again and again, or touch a certain part of their body to make sure it hasn't changed.

Developmental Factors

What is the child or adolescent's weight history? What is or was his or her experience of body maturation or puberty? What have the parents and other significant people in the child's life communicated in terms of the importance of body weight and shape? Has the child or adolescent experienced a significant life event or trauma that may have impacted experience of his or her body?

Current Contextual Factors

Are there situations in which the BI thoughts/feelings are more intense? What internal or external factors function as triggers for distressing BI thoughts/feelings? Is the child or adolescent engaging in any behaviors that exacerbate disturbance (e.g., focusing attention on problem areas when looking in the mirror)? How do peers, parents, and teachers respond when the child or adolescent engages in BI-related behaviors? Do others compliment the child or adolescent for the current weight/shape of their body? Does a certain body type allow him to participate and/or perform well in a sport or other activity? Does focusing on BI thoughts allow the child or adolescent to avoid other things that are more difficult or distressing? Does the child or adolescent believe that changing her body will lead to a particular desired outcome?

Methods for assessing the severity of body image disturbance and the impact it has on functioning include dynamic assessment techniques, self-report measures, self-monitoring, and structured interviews. The appropriate assessment method, or combination of methods, depends on the purpose of assessment (e.g., differential diagnosis, research, treatment planning).

Dynamic assessment techniques (see Table 14.1) focus on body size estimation and include analogue scales such as adjusting two points of light to show width of various body parts, image marking methods such as drawing one's body on a vertically mounted piece of paper, and optical distortion methods in which individuals are presented with distorted image of self that must be adjusted to the appropriate size. The most commonly and easily administered dynamic assessment technique consists of presenting schematic or figure drawings of different body sizes and asking the individual to identify the one that best approximates his or her current and ideal body size. Some of these assessments, such as the Contour Drawing Rating Scale (Thompson & Gray, 1995), are fairly precise with body sizes increasing incrementally. There have also been computer-adapted versions to assist with ease of administration (e.g., Body Image Testing System; Schlundt & Bell, 1993). Figure drawings have been used effectively with younger children and because of their brevity they tend to circumvent attention problems that sometimes interfere with the administration of other assessment techniques. There are also some scales that have been specifically designed for, and standardized with, younger children. These include the Body Image Assessment-Children (Veron-Guidry & Williamson, 1996), the Body Rating Scale (Sherman et al., 1995), and the Children's Body Image Scale (Truby & Praxton, 2002), among others.

Although most of the child-specific scales include male figure stimuli and male children in the standardization sample, some have argued that traditional measures that have figures ranging from thin to obese are not sensitive to the primary manifestation of BI disturbance in males (Kostanski, Fischer, & Gullone, 2004; Smolak, 2004). They state evidence that males are often concerned with being "too small" rather than "too big," a phenomenon often referred to as muscularity (Lynch & Zellner, 1999). Proponents of this viewpoint maintain that figures should not only be varied in terms of adiposity but also muscularity. Cafri and colleagues have proposed a somatomorphic matrix that takes into account these different aspects of body composition (Cafri & Thompson, 2004).

Self-report measures are useful for quantifying the extent to which body size and shape determines one's self-worth, level of distress regarding the size or shape of one's body, and resulting impairment in functioning. They have the advantage of being easily administered and readily available. Some of the most commonly used self-report measures include the shape and weight concern subscales of the EDE (adolescent and child versions available) (Fairburn, & Cooper, 1993; Peterson et al., 2007), the Body Dissatisfaction Subscale of the EDI (Garner, Olmstead, & Polivy, 1983), the Body Esteem Scale (Mendelson & White, 1982), and the Body Shape Questionnaire (Cooper, Taylor, Cooper, & Fairburn, 1987; Rosen, Jones, Ramirez, & Waxman, 1996). Although behavioral manifestations of BI disturbance are included in some of the aforementioned scales, there are measures that focus specifically on this aspect of BI (e.g., Body Checking Questionnaire (Reas & Grilo, 2004). State measures of body image assess body-related affect in particular contexts and include the Situational Inventory of Body Image Dysphoria and the Body Image States Scale (Cash, Fleming, Alindogan, Steadman, & Whitehead, 2002), among others. However, there is little information on whether these latter measures are appropriate for children.

There is some discussion in the literature about whether traditional BI scales capture the essence of male body concerns. In contrast to female BI issues, which focus on the thin ideal and the size and shape of the hips, thighs, and stomach, male BI concerns tend to be more centered around muscular appearance and the torso (McCreary & Sasse, 2000). Data regarding whether traditional measures are in fact inadequate are somewhat mixed. For example, although studies using the Body Esteem Scale have found no gender differences in overall score, research using the Body Dissatisfaction subscale of the EDI has found that females score higher than males generally. In effort to deal with this issue, male-specific BI measures have been developed including the Drive for Muscularity Scale which has acceptable validity and test–retest reliability (Cafri & Thompson, 2004).

Self-monitoring can be used to identify relevant contextual factors supporting BI disturbance. This is typically done by asking the individual to complete the body image diary when they note a change in BI experience (i.e., exacerbation or attenuation of body distress) or when they engage in a body-relevant target behavior. Children or adolescents who have particular difficulty detecting change or are less aware of their internal experience or behavior may be asked to complete the diary at scheduled intervals. Body image diaries may vary considerably in complexity. The more comprehensive diary may involve recording: (1) time/place, (2) activators/triggers, (3) body-relevant thoughts and feelings, (4) rating of bodily discomfort, (5) responses or overt behaviors to these internal events, and (6) consequences (i.e., change in internal state or external environment). What is perhaps the most challenging with this type of assessment is that it requires a willingness and ability to tolerate the negative affect that inevitably comes with thinking about the BI experience for the additional time needed to complete the recording. There are also some unique challenges to using self-monitoring forms with younger children who may not be able to read, write, and therefore record. There are some creative solutions to this problem; however, such as using pictorials, providing multiple choice responses, and having a parent record.

Differential Diagnosis

Preoccupation with a particular body part and exaggeration of a perceived defect in appearance may reflect Body Dysmorphic Disorder (BDD) rather than an ED. Eating disorders and BDD are considered by some authors to form part of the obsessive compulsive disorder spectrum (Hollander & Benzaquen, 1997). The continua that comprise this spectrum remain to be adjudicated, advances that will help to better differentiate BDD from ED (Lochner et al., 2005). Despite these caveats, individuals with BDD demonstrate patterns unique to this diagnostic class. BDD differs from ED in that individuals with BDD often focus on a physical defect, often in the head or neck region. Belief in the hideousness of the imagined or exaggerated defect is so great that it may result in extreme behaviors attempted to correct the imagined deficits (e.g,. attempts at repeated cosmetic surgeries). In contrast, ED patients are largely focused on concerns with body weight or shape. There is behavioral overlap. For example, both individuals with BDD and ED may exercise excessively, frequently seek reassurance from others, and check mirrors. However, individuals with BDD do so to correct their imagined or exaggerated flaw whereas individuals EDs do so due to prevent a feared outcome (i.e., weight gain) or to achieve a desired weight. Advances in the neurobiology, genetics, and developmental course of these illnesses will assist in understanding their relative position on the obsessive compulsive disorder spectrum.

FUNCTIONAL ASSESSMENT OF EATING DISORDER SYMPTOMS

Significance of the Construct

Clinicians who are new to the treatment of eating disorders may be perplexed by the extent to which eating disorder patients struggle to relinquish their symptoms. Why is the anorexic patient who is emaciated, lethargic, and losing hair unable to let go of restriction? Why is the bulimic patient who experiences incredible shame regarding her bingeing unable to stop engaging in this behavior? Identifying contextual factors that function to maintain the symptoms can shed light on such confusing patterns of behavior and provide invaluable information for case conceptualization and treatment.

Many agree that an eating disorder serves an important psychological function. Some have gone so far as to conceptualize eating disorders as coping strategies; however, critics of the coping-strategy formulation maintain that eating pathology may emerge for a variety of other reasons (e.g., as an attempt to force a body type that conforms to cultural ideals regarding attractiveness) and acquire deeper meaning and psychological functions only over time (Vitousek, Watson, & Wilson, 1998). Whether ED behaviors function as a coping strategy from the onset is an important theoretical issue that can have bearing on disorder pathophysiology. Regardless, it does not change the likelihood that the identification of factors currently maintaining the behaviors may allow for effective intervention.

Functional assessment is most often talked about in the context of binge eating, perhaps because the utility of stimulus control in decreasing overeating has a long history of support (Stuart, 1967). For example, one hypothesis is that binge eating functions to alleviate negative mood states by temporarily directing attention toward the immediate stimulus environment. Of interest, negative affect is actually exacerbated as a result of the episode, and patients often feel worse rather than better after they binge. However, the fact that increased negative affect which inevitably follows a binge episode is insufficient to decrease the behavior more likely speaks to the potency of temporary relief from dysphoria as a negative reinforcer. Indeed, the more effective binge eating is for even a brief escape from negative affective states, aversive self-awareness (especially among perfectionistic, low-esteem individuals), or physical distress from hunger related to restriction, the more likely it is to continue despite the more long-term negative consequences.

Purging may similarly have the capacity to regulate affect. Individuals with ED often express decreased guilt following subjective or objective binges following an episode of purgative behavior. Other individuals describe purging habits, such as self-induced vomiting, initiate a feeling of calmness. Others describe the feeling of emptiness following abuse of laxatives to be soothing.

Researchers interested in understanding the psychological functions of restriction, which may be less circumscribed temporally than bingeing and purging, have employed a variety of narrative and interview approaches. For example, Serpell, Treasure, and colleagues (1999) asked AN patients to write a letter to their illness. Content analyses revealed common themes regarding the needs satisfied by AN. Almost all the participants in the study endorsed what the authors described as a "guardian" theme. That is, AN patients reported that the illness keeps them safe and protected, that it is dependable, consistent, and looks after them. Other themes that emerged included attractiveness, control (provides structure, tells her how to eat, offers simplicity and certainty), difference (makes her feel superior or special), confidence/skill (provides her with something that she does well), avoidance (helps her hide away from emotions or things that are too difficult to deal with, reduces feelings of ineffectiveness), and communication (allows her to communicate distress to the outside world).

This body of research, along with data that describe personality traits of individuals with AN, suggests that restrictive AN behaviors are negatively reinforced by avoidance or escape from chaos, uncertainty, and aversive arousal states that often accompany particular developmental stages and are experienced as intolerable to individuals with a high need for control, order, and predictability. This work also indicates positive reinforcement for AN behaviors. Most notably, research suggests that individuals with AN, who tend to be self-critical and feel generally ineffective, experience a sense of accomplishment, pride, and self-control when they are able to overcome bodily urges and maintain low weight.

Developmental Considerations

It is not uncommon for there to be a lack of insight regarding the relationship between ED symptoms and situational events or life stressors. This may be especially pronounced among children and young people who may not have developed the cognitive abilities to fully understand cause and effect, or the metacognitive abilities to report internal experience or describe thought processes. Very young children may also be unable to complete recording forms. In order to overcome these challenges, it may be necessary to provide multiple examplars, shape reporting of thoughts and feelings, simplify recording devices, adjust language to the appropriate level, use pictorials, gather collateral information from parents or teachers, or directly observe the child.

Assessment Methods

Conducting a functional analysis requires that the target behavior be clearly defined. A thorough functional assessment identifies both internal (e.g., thoughts, feelings, bodily sensations) and external (e.g., environmental or situational factors) events that reliably precede or follow a target behavior. Methods include event or time-based recording, retrospective recall in session, and expressive techniques such as letter writing.

Event or time-based recording is the most common functional assessment method. It requires that a recording form be completed whenever the target behavior is performed or at regularly scheduled intervals. For older children and adolescents, this typically takes the form of self-monitoring. Traditionally, recording forms have resembled the thought record used in Beck-style Cognitive-Behavioral Therapy. However, more recently researchers and clinicians have begun to use diary cards like those employed in Dialectical Behavior Therapy (DBT) that have individuals check off prelisted options of maladaptive behaviors and targeted therapeutic strategies. More recently, the use of electronic recording options, such as Palm Pilots, cell phones, and interactive voice response technology has been explored. Thus far, the electronic format has been found to facilitate more complete and accurate recall than retrospective reporting, at least for binge–purge behavior (Bardone, Krahn, Goodman, & Searles, 2000).

Accurate recall is essential in the identification of antecedent and consequential events and it is not uncommon to have to shape awareness and reporting of relevant thoughts, feelings, and situational factors. It is not uncommon for ED patients to initially have difficulty reporting thoughts and feelings other than eating or body-related talk. A sample entry from a 16-year-old female with anorexia is provided in Figure 14.1. This particular patient had been in treatment for three months at the time of the entry. Initially, she reported only awareness of food, eating, and exercise concerns. However, over time, she became aware of a fuller range of thoughts and

Figure 14.1. Sample diary card entry used to identify relevant contextual factors for eating disorder symptoms.

Date Time	Situation	Thoughts	Feelings; Identify and rate intensity (1–10)	Bodily sensations; Identify and rate discomfort (1–10)	Response	Consequences: Change in thoughts, feelings, bodily comfort; Change in situation or other's behavior.
Monday 11:00 am	Sitting alone in library, studying chemistry. Notice other girls sitting together, talking.	Why don't I have anyone to sit with? ... why don't I understand this new material? No one else seems confused. Start to think about how I can't do anything well anymore... Remember that I ate 2 apple slices that I did not plan on having and I didn't do any extra laps to make up for it...I am so lazy. Spent the next several minutes thinking about how worthless I am.	Shame 7 Disgust 9	Heavy, fat, stomach tight, uncomfort-able 9	Left library to go for a run. Ran for 3 hours,	Felt better about self. Able to concentrate on assignment when I got home. Studied in my dorm room rather than at the library.

feelings. The result of this was an acknowledgment of the extent to which she was feeling lonely, isolated, and ineffective, and using problematic eating and exercise behavior to decrease contact this experience and increase her sense of mastery.

Functional analytic techniques can also be employed in session in the form of retrospective recall. Therapists may ask patients to describe a time over the past week in which they engaged in the target ED behavior or noticed exacerbation of ED thoughts and feelings. The therapist then helps the patient work forward and backward in from this time point to identify antecedents and consequences of the ED behavior. A sample of dialogue from a session using retrospective reporting is provided below.

Therapist: Based on your food log, it looks like you restricted on Thursday ...

Patient: Yeah ... well, I was drinking my Boost and my stomach started to hurt, so I skipped breakfast and lunch. I don't think that I should be expected to drink Boost and eat breakfast. It's too much.

Therapist: ... And yet that is what's necessary in order for you to be healthy enough to stay at school....

Patient: It just felt so out of control ... my stomach felt bloated and fat. It was overwhelming ... to have to drink the Boost. I wasn't even hungry.

Therapist: You know how we have been talking about things that may prompt ED thoughts and feelings? Let's spend a little time thinking about what was going on right before you had the Boost....

Patient: I was studying for my exam in public policy.

Therapist: You have been struggling with that class all semester....

Patient: Yeah, and I don't understand why. I should be able to do the work. ... If I can't do the work in that class, how will I ever be successful? This is the most important year of my life. Then my dad calls and asks if I was practicing my Fox Trot. The debutante ball is in two weeks, you know.

Therapist: How are you feeling about it?

Patient: Well ... I want to go. ... My grandmother would be crushed if I didn't. Everyone expects me to be there too. I think my dad was kidding, but that was the last thing I wanted to think about. ... Other people seem so relaxed about it. I haven't even asked anyone to go with me. I want to be 99.9% sure that they'll say "Yes" before I ask. Otherwise, it's not worth it. It just feels like so many things are coming at me at once ... and then the treatment team wants me to eat all of this food! If I didn't have to eat this much, I would be okay. It's my body that is the problem. I feel so fat.

Therapist: Could it be that pressure to do well on the exam and represent your family at debutante ball ... and maybe even anxiety about asking someone to escort you, contributed to you feeling uncomfortable in your body ...?

Patient: Hmmm I guess so. ... I had not thought about all the things that were going through my mind until now. At the time, all I could think about was the fact that I was drinking Boost and my stomach was tight and uncomfortable. So I didn't eat breakfast and lunch....

Therapist: And what was the result of not finishing your Boost or eating your meals?

Patient: ... Well, I felt better. A lot better, actually—after I put down the Boost I started strategizing how I was going to avoid lunch with my mom ... and then I went to the gym. I don't think about anything when I'm at the gym.

CONCLUDING REMARKS

Understanding the phenomenology of an eating disorder requires that a clinician try to appreciate a child or adolescent's experience of his or her body. Being uncomfortable in one's own body and having difficulty reading the signals conveyed by the body has profound impact on self-knowledge, self-trust, and goal-directed actions. A therapist must employ strategies that facilitate a child or adolescent's ability to explore responses that may fit her experience as she may not be able to decipher her current state. Indeed, sometimes not knowing the answer is often the most revealing answer. Thus, believing that individuals with eating disorders just wish to be thin for the sake of being thin misses the true nature of these disorders. Symptoms are a means, they are not the end. Appreciating that is the beginning of a very thorough assessment.

REFERENCES

Abidin, R. R. (2004). *Stress Index for Parents of Adolescents* (3rd ed.). Lutz, FL: Psychological Assessment Resources.

Ackard, D. M., & Neumark-Sztainer, D. (2001). Family mealtime while growing up: Associations with symptoms of bulimia nervosa. *Eating Disorders, 16*(1), 239–249.

Ahearn, W. H., Castine, T., Nault, K., & Green, G. (2001). An assessment of food acceptance in children with autism or pervasive developmental disorder-not otherwise specified. *Journal of Autism and Developmental Disorders, 31*(5), 505–511.

American Psychiatric Association. (1994). Diagnostic and Statistical Manual of Mental Disorders, 4th ed. Washington, DC.

Andreasen, N. C., Endicott, J., Spitzer, R. L., & Winokur, G. (1977). The family history method using diagnostic criteria. *Archives of General Psychiatry, 34*, 1229–1235.

Annus, A. M., Smith, G.T., Fischer, S., Hendricks, M., Williams, S.F. (2007). Associations among family-of-origin food-related experiences, expectancies, and disordered eating. *International Journal of Eating Disorders, 40*(2), 179–186.

Anton, S. D. et al. (2006). Reformulation of the Children's Eating Attitudes Test (ChEAT): Factor structure and scoring method in a non-clinical population. *Eating and Weight Disorders, 11*, 201–210.

Association, A. P. (2000). *Diagnostic and statistical manual of mental disorders* (4th ed.). American Psychiatric Association.

Bailer, U. F., Frank, G. K., Henry, S. E., Price, J. C., Meltzer, C. C., Weissfeld, L., et al. (2005). Altered brain serotonin 5-HT1A receptor binding after recovery from anorexia nervosa measured by positron emission tomography and [carbonyl11C]WAY-100635. *Archives of General Psychiatry, 62*(9), 1032–1041.

Bardone, A. M., Krahn, D. D., Goodman, B. M., & Searles, J. S. (2000). Using interactive voice response technology and timeline follow-back methodology in studying binge-eating and drinking behavior: Different answers to different forms of the same question. *Addictive Behaviors, 25*(1), 1–11.

Beaumont, P. J. V., Garner, D. M., & Touyz, S. W. (1994). Diagnoses of eating or dieting disorders - What may we learn from past mistakes. *International Journal of Eating Disorders, 16*(4), 349–362.

Bettelheim, B. (1967). The empty fortress: Infantile autism and the birth of the self. New York: Free Press.

Boyer, T. W. (2006). The development of risk-taking: A multi-perspective review. *Developmental Review, 26*(3), 291–345.

Bray, G. A. (1998). Definitions and proposed current classification of obesity. In G. A. Bray, C. Bouchard, & W. P. T. Jame (Eds.), *Handbook of obesity* (pp. 31–40). New York: Marcel Decker.

Bruch, H. (1962). Perceptual and conceptual disturbances in anorexia nervosa. *Psychosomatic Medicine, 24*(2), 187–194.

Bulik, C. M. (1995). Anxiety disorders and eating disorders: A review of their relationship. *New Zealand Journal of Psychology, 24*(2), 51–62.

Cafri, G., & Thompson, J. K. (2004). Measuring male body image: A review of the current methodology. *Psychology of Men and Masculinity, 5*(1), 18–29.

Carter, F. A., Bulik, C. M., Lawson, R. H., Sullivan, P. F. & Wilson, J.S. (1996). Effect of mood and food cues on body image concerns of women with bulimia and normal controls. *International Journal of Eating Disorders, 20*(1), 65–76.

Cash, T. F. (2002a). Beyond traits: Assessing body image states. In T. F. Cash & T. Pruzinsky (Eds.), *Body Images: A Handbook of Theory Research, and Clinical Practice* (pp. 163–170). NY: Guilford Press.

Cash, T. F. (2002b). The situational inventory of body-image dysphoria: Psychometric evidence and development of the short form. *International Journal of Eating Disorders, 32* 362–366.

Cash, T. F., Fleming, E. C., Alindogan, J., Steadman, L., & Whitehead, A. (2002). Beyond body image as a trait: The development and validation of the body image states scale. *Eating Disorders, 10*, 103–113.

Cattarin, J. A., & Thompson, J. K. (1994). A three-year longitudinal study of body image, eating disturbance, and general psychological functioning in adoelscent females. *Eating Disorders: Journal of Prevention and Treatment, 2*, 114–125.

Center for Disease Control. (2002). 2000 CDC Growth Charts for the United States: Development and Methods. In H. a. H. Services (Ed.) (Vol. 11). Center for Disease Control.

Chatoor, I., & Ganiban, J. (2003). Food refusal by infants and young children: Diagnosis and treatment. *Cognitive and Behavioral Practice, 10*(2), 138–146.

Childress, A. C., Brewerton, T. D., Hodges, E. L., & Jarrell, M. P. (1993). The Kids Eating Disorders Survey (Keds) - A study of middle school students. *Journal of the American Academy of Child and Adolescent Psychiatry, 32*(4), 843–850.

Colton, P., Olmsted, M., Daneman, D., Rydall, A., & Rodin, G. (2004). Disturbed eating disorders behavior and eating disorders in preteen and early teenage girls with type 1 diabetes - A case-controlled study. *Diabetes Care, 27*(7), 1654–1659.

Cooper, P. J., Taylor, M. J., Cooper, Z., & Fairburn, C. G. (1987). The development and validation of the Body Shape Questionnaire. *International Journal of Eating Disorders, 6*, 485–494.

Cooper, P. J., Watkins, B., Bryant-Waugh, R., & Lask, B. (2002). The nosological status of early onset anorexia nervosa. *Psychological Medicine, 32*(5), 873–880.

Cooper, Z., & Fairburn, C. (1987). The eating disorder examination - A semistructured interview for the assessment of the specific psychopathology of eating disorders. *International Journal of Eating Disorders, 6*(1), 1–8.

Couturier, J. L., & Lock, J. (2006). Denial and minimization in adolescents with anorexia nervosa. *International Journal of Eating Disorders, 39*(3), 212–216.

Croll, J., Neumark-Sztainer, D., Story, M., & Ireland, M. (2002). Prevalence and risk and protective factors related to disordered eating behaviors among adolescents: Relationship to gender and ethnicity. *Journal of Adolescent Health, 31*, 166–175.

Crow, S. J., Agras, W. S., Halmi, K., Mitchell, J. E., & Kraemer, H. C. (2002). Full syndromal versus subthreshold anorexia nervosa, bulimia nervosa, and binge eating disorder: A multicenter study. *International Journal of Eating Disorders, 32*(3), 309–318.

Cullen, K. W., Watson, K., Himes, J. H., Baranowski, T., Rochon, J., Waclawiw, M., et al. (2004). Evaluation of quality control procedures for 24-h dietary recalls: results from the Girls health Enrichment Multisite Studies. *Preventive Medicine, 38*, S14–S23.

Davidson, K. K., & Birch, L. L. (2001). Weight status, parent reaction, and self-concept in five-year-old girls. *Pediatrics, 107*, 46–53.

Decaluwe, V., & Braet, C. (2003). Prevalence of binge-eating disorder in obese children and adolescents seeking weight-loss treatment. *International Journal of Obesity & Related Metabolic Disorders: Journal of the International Association for the Study of Obesity., 27*(3), 404–409.

Dixon, R., Adair, V., & O'Connor, S. (1996). Parental influences on the dieting beliefs and behaviors of adolescent females in New Zealand. *Journal of Adolescent Health, 19*(4), 303–307.

Doll, M., Ball, G. D. C., & Willows, N. D. (2004). Rating of figures for body image assessment varies depending on the method of figure presentation. *International Journal of Eating Disorders, 35*, 109–114.

Eisenbarth, G. S., Polonsky, K. S., & Buse, J. B. (2003). Type I Diabetes Mellitus. In P. R. Larsen, H. M. Kronenberg, S. Melmed, & K. S. Polonsky (Eds.), *Williams textbook of endocrinology* (10th ed.). Philadelphia: Elsevier Science.

Eisenberg, M. E., Neumark-Sztainer, D., Haines, J. & Wall, M. (2006). Weight-teasing and emotional well-being in adolescents: Longitudinal findings from Project EAT. *Journal of Adolescent Health, 38*(6), 675–683.

Eisler, I., Dare, C., Russell, G. F., Szmukler, G., le Grange, D., & Dodge, E. (1997). Family and individual therapy in anorexia nervosa. A 5-year follow-up. *Archives of General Psychiatry., 54*(11), 1025–1030.

Eklund, K., Paavonen, E. J., & Almqvist, F. (2005). Factor structure of the Eating Disorder Inventory-C. *International Journal of Eating Disorders, 37*, 330–341.

Fairburn, C. G. (1996). *Binge eating: Nature, assessment, and treatment.* New York: Guilford Press.

Fairburn, C. G., & Cooper, Z. (1993). *The Eating Disorder Examination* (12 ed.). New York: Guilford Press.

Fairburn, C. G., Cooper, Z., & Shafran, R. (2003). Cognitive behaviour therapy for eating disorders: a "transdiagnostic" theory and treatment. *Behaviour Research and Therapy, 41*(5), 509–528.

Farrell, C., Lee, M., & Shafran, R. (2005). Assessment of body size estimation: A review. *European Eating Disorders Review, 13*, 75–88.

Fassino, S., Piero, A., Gramaglia, C., & Abbate-Daga, G. (2004). Clinical, psychopathological and personality correlates of interoceptive awareness in anorexia nervosa, bulimia nervosa and obesity. *Psychopathology, 37*(4), 168–174.

Fernandez, F., Probst, M., Meermann, R., & Vandereycken, W. (1994). Body size estimation and body dissatisfaction in eating disorder patients and normal controls *International Journal of Eating Disorders, 16*(3), 307–310.

Fichter, M., & Quadflieg, N. (2001). The structured interview (SIAB-EX) and questionnaire (SIAB-S) for anorexic and bulimic eating disorders for *DSM–IV* and ICD–10. *Verhaltenstherapie, 11*(4), 314–325.

Field, A. E., Taylor, C. B., Celio, A., & Colditz, G. A. (2004). Comparison of self-report to interview assessment of bulimic behaviors among preadolescent and adolescent girls and boys. *International Journal of Eating Disorders, 35*(1), 86–92.

Forman-Hoffman, V. (2004). High prevalence of abnormal eating and weight control practices among U.S. high-school students. *Eating Behaviors, 5*, 325–336.

Franko, D. L., Striegel-Moore, R. H., Barton, B. A., Schumann, B. C., Garner, D. M., Daniels, S. R., et al. (2004). Measuring eating concerns in Black and White adolescent girls. *International Journal of Eating Disorders, 35*(2), 179–189.

Galloway, A. T., Lee, Y., & Birch, L. L. (2003). Predictors and consequences of food neophobia and pickiness in young girls. *Journal of the American Dietetic Association, 103*(6), 692–698.

Gardner, R. M., & Bokenkamp, E. D. (1996). The role of sensory and nonsensory factors in body size estimations of eating disorder subjects. *Journal of Clinical Psychology, 52*(1).

Gardner, R. M., Sorter, R. G., & Friedman, B. N. (1997). Developmental changes in children's body images. *Journal of Social Behavior and Personality, 12*, 1019–1037.

Gardner, R. M., Stark, K., Friedman, B. N., & Jackson, N. A. (2000). Predictors of eating disorder scores in children 6 through 14: A longitudinal study. *Journal of Psychosomatic Research, 49*, 199–205.

Garner, D. M. (1991). *Eating Disorder Inventory-2 (EDI-2) Professional Manual.* Lutz, FL: Psychological Assessment Resources.

Garner, D. M., & Garfinkel, P. E. (Ed.). (1997). *Handbook of treatment for eating disorders* (2nd ed.). New York: Guilford Press.

Garner, D. M., & Garfinkel, P. E. (1979). The Eating Attitudes Test: An index of the symptoms of anorexia nervosa. *Psychological Medicine., 9*(2), 273–279.

Garner, D. M., Olmstead, M. P., & Polivy, J. (1983). Development and validation of a multidimensional Eating Disorder Inventory for anorexia nervosa and bulimia nervosa. *International Journal of Eating Disorders, 2,* 15–34.

Godwin, S. L., Chambers, E., & Cleveland, L. (2004). Accuracy of reporting dietary intake using various portion-size aids in-person and via telephone. *Journal of the American Dietetic Association, 104*(4), 585–594.

Goldfein, J. A., Devlin, M. J., & Kamenetz, C. (2005). Eating Disorder Examination-Questionnaire with and without instruction to assess binge eating in patients with binge eating disorder. *International Journal of Eating Disorders, 37*(2), 107–111.

Haimovitz, D., Lansky, L., & Reilly, P. (1993). Fluctuation in body satisfaction across situations. *International Journal of Eating Disorders, 13,* 77–83.

Hartwell, C. E. (1996). The schizophrenogenic mother concept in American psychiatry. *Psychiatry-Interpersonal and Biological Processes, 59*(3), 274–297.

Haworth-Hoeppner, S. (2000). The critical shapes of body image: the role of culture and family in the production of eating disorders. *Journal of Marriage and Family, 62*(1), 212–227.

Heatherton, T. F., & Baumeister, R. F. (1991). Binge eating as escape from self-awareness. *Psychological Bulletin, 110*(1), 86–108.

Hebebrand, J., Casper, R., Treasure, J., & Schweiger, U. (2004). The need to revise the diagnostic criteria for anorexia nervosa. *Journal of Neural Transmission, 111*(7), 827–840.

Hollander, E., & Benzaquen, S. D. (1997). The obsessive-compulsive spectrum disorders. *International Review of Psychiatry, 9*(1), 99–109.

Kanner, L. (1943). Autistic disturbances of affective content. *Nervous Child, 2,* 217–250.

Keel, P. K., Dorer, D. J., Franko, D. L., Jackson, S. C., & Herzog, D. B. (2005). Postremission predictors of relapse in women with eating disorders. *American Journal of Psychiatry, 162*(12), 2263–2268.

Kostanski, M., & Gullone, E. (1999). Dieting and body image in the child's world: Conceptualization and behavior. *Journal of Genetic Psychology, 160,* 488–499.

Kostanski, M., Fischer, A., & Gullone, E. (2004). Current conceptualization of body image dissatisfaction: Have we got it wrong? *Journal of Child Psychology and Psychiatry, and Allied Disciplines, 45,* 1317–1325.

Krones, P. G., Stice, E., Batres, C., & Orjada, K. (2005). In vivi social comparison to a thin-ideal peer promotes body dissatisfaction: A randomized experiment. *International Journal of Eating Disorders, 38*(38), 134–142.

Lane, R. D., Sechrest, L., Reidel, R., Weldon, V., Kaszniak, A., & Schwartz, G. E. (1996). Impaired verbal and nonverbal emotion recognition in alexithymia. *Psychosomatic Medicine, 58*(3), 203–210.

Le Grange, D., Eisler, I., Dare, C., & Hodes, M. (1992). Family criticism and self-starvation: A study of expressed emotion. *Journal of Family Therapy, 14*(2), 177–192.

Lilenfeld, L. R., Kaye, W. H., Greeno, C. G., Merikangas, K. R., Plotnicov, K., Pollice, C., et al. (1998). A controlled family study of anorexia nervosa and bulimia nervosa: psychiatric disorders in first-degree relatives and effects of proband comorbidity. *Archives of General Psychiatry., 55*(7), 603–610.

Lochner, C., Hemmings, S. M. J., Kinnear, C. J., Niehaus, D. J. H., Nel, D. G., Corfield, V. A., et al. (2005). Cluster analysis of obsessive-compulsive spectrum disorders in patients with obsessive-compulsive disorder: Clinical and genetic correlates. *Comprehensive Psychiatry, 46*(1), 14–19.

Lock, J., Le Grange, D., Agras, W. S., & Dare, C. (2001). *Treatment manual for Anorexia Nervosa: A family-based approach.* New York: Guilford Press.

Lynch, S. M., & Zellner, D. A. Figure preferences in two generations of men: The use of figure drawings illustrating differences in muscle mass. *Sex Roles, 40,* 833–843.

Maloney, M., McGuire, J., Daniels, S., & Specter, S. (1988). Reliability testing of a children's version of the Eating Attitudes Test. *Journal of the American Academy of Child and Adolescent Psychiatry, 5,* 541–543.

Marcus, M. D., & Kalarchian, M. A. (2003). Binge eating in children and adolescents. *International Journal of Eating Disorders, 34 Suppl,* S47–57.

Marini, Z., & Case, R. (1994). The development of abstract reasoning about the physical and social world. *Child Development, 65*(1), 147–159.

McCabe, M. P., & Ricciardelli, L. A. (2004). A longitudinal study of pubertal timing and extreme body change behaviors among adolescent boys and girls. *Adolescence, 39*(153), 145–166.

McCabe, M. P., Ricciardelli, L. A., & Holt, K. (2005). A longitudinal study to explain strategies to change weight and muscles among normal and overweight children. *Appetite, 45*, 225–234.

McCreary, D. R., & Sasse, D. K. (2000). An exploration of the drive for muscularity in adolescent boys and girls. *Journal of American College Health, 48*(6), 297–304.

McIntosh, V. W., Jordan, J., Carter, F. A., McKenzie, J. M., Luty, S. E., Bulik, C. M., et al. (2004). Strict versus lenient weight criterion in anorexia nervosa. *European Eating Disorders Review, 12*(1), 51–60.

Mendelson, B. K., & White, D. R. (1982). Relation between body-esteem and self-esteem of obese and normal weight children. *Perceptual and Motor Skills, 54*, 899–905.

Mintz, L. B., & O'Halloran, M. S. (2000). The Eating Attitudes Test: Validation with *DSM–IV* eating disorder criteria. *Journal of Personality Assessment, 74*, 489–503.

Minuchin, S., Rosman, B. L., & Baker, L. (1978). *Psychosomatic families: Anorexia nervosa in context*, Cambridge, MA: Harvard University Press.

Mitchell, J. E., & Crow, S. (2006). Medical complications of anorexia nervosa and bulimia nervosa. *Current Opinion in Psychiatry, 19*(4), 438–443.

Mitchell, J. E., Pomeroy, C., & Adson, D. E. (1997). Managing medical complications. In D. M. Garner & P. E. Garfinkel (Eds.), *Handbook of treatment for eating disorders*. New York: Guilford Press.

Neumark-Sztainer, D., Wall, M., Eisenberg, M. E., Story, M., & Hannan, P. J. (2006). Overweight status and weight control behaviors in adolescents: Longitudinal and secular trends from 1999 to 2004. *Preventive Medicine, 43*(1), 52–59.

Nicholls, D., Chater, R., & Lask, B. (2000). Children into *DSM* don't go: A comparison of classification systems for eating disorders in childhood and early adolescence. *International Journal of Eating Disorders, 28*(3), 317–324.

Olson, D. H. (2000). Circumplex model of marital and family systems. *Journal of Family Therapy, 22*(2), 144–167.

Oninla, S. O., Owa, J. A., Onayade, A. A., & Taiwo, O. (2007). Comparative study of nutritional status of urban and rural Nigerian school children. *Journal of Tropical Pediatrics, 53*(1), 39–43.

Peebles, R., Wilson, J. L., & Lock, J. D. (2006). How do children with eating disorders differ from adolescents with eating disorders at initial evaluation? *Journal of Adolescent Health, 39*(6), 800–805.

Peterson, C. B. et al. (2007). Psychometric properties of the eating disorder examination-questionnaire: Factor structure and internal consistency. *International Journal of Eating Disorders, 40*, 386–389.

Pietrowsky, R., Staub, K., & Hachl, P. (2003). Body dissatisfacrion in female restrained eaters depends on food deprivation. *Appetite, 40*(3), 285–290.

Polivy, J. (1998). The effects of behavioral inhibition: Integrating internal cues, cognition, behavior, and affect. *Psychological Inquiry, 9*(3), 181–204.

Preti, A., Icani, E., Camboni, M. V., Petretto, D. R., Masala, C. (2006). Sexual abuse and eating disorder symptoms: The mediator role of bodily dissatisfaction. *Comprehensive Psychiatry, 46*(7), 475–481.

Probst, M., Vandereycken, W., Coppenolle, H. V. & Pieters, G. (1998). Body size estimation in anorexia nervosa patients: The significance of overestimation. *Journal of Psychosomatic Research, 44*, 451–456.

Ravaldi, C., Vannacci, A., Bolognesi, E., Mancini, S., Faravelli, C. & Ricca, V. (2006). Gender role, eating disorder symptoms, and body image concern in ballet dancers. *Journal of Psychosomatic Research, 61*(4), 529–535.

Reas, D. L., & Grilo, C. M. (2004). Cognitive-behavioral assessment of body image disturbances. *Journal of Psychiatric Practice, 10*(5), 314–322.

Ricciardelli, L. A., & McCabe, M. P. (2001). Children's body image concerns and eating disturbance: A review of the literature *Clinical Psychology Review, 21*(3), 325–344.

Rieger, E., & Touyz, S. (2006). An investigation of the factorial structure of motivation to recover in anorexia nervosa using the Anorexia Nervosa Stages of Change Questionnaire. *European Eating Disorders Review, 14*(4), 269–275.

Rodin, J., Silberstein, L., & Striegel-Moore, R. (1984). Women and weight: A normative discontent. *Nebraska Symposium on Motivation, 32,* 267–307.

Rome, E. S., Ammerman, S., Rosen, D. S., Keller, R. J., Lock, J., Mammel, K. A., et al. (2003). Children and adolescents with eating disorders: the state of the art. *Pediatrics, 111*(1), e98–108.

Rosen, J. C., Jones, A., Ramirez, E., & Waxman, S. (1996). Body shape questionnaire: Studies of validity and reliability. *International Journal of Eating Disorders, 20*(3), 315–319.

Schlundt, D. G., & Bell, C. (1993). Body image testing system: A microcomputer program for assessing body image. *Journal of Psychopathology and Behavioral Assessment, 15*(3), 267–285.

Schmidt, U., Tiller, J., Blanchard, M., Andrews, B., & Treasure, J. (1997). Is there a specific trauma precipitating anorexia nervosa? *Psychological Medicine, 27*(3), 523–530.

Serpell, L., Treasure, J., Teasdale, J., & Sullivan, V. (1999). Anorexia nervosa: Friend or foe? *International Journal of Eating Disorders, 25,* 177–186.

Shafran, R., & Fairburn, C. G. (2002). A new ecologically valid method to assess body size estimation and body size satisfaction. *International Journal of Eating Disorders, 32,* 458–465.

Shapiro, J. R., Woolson, S. L., Hamer, R. M., Kalarchian, M. A., Marcus, M. D., & Bulik, C. M. (2007). Evaluating binge eating disorder in children: Development of the Children's Binge Eating Disorder Scale (C-BEDS). *International Journal of Eating Disorders, 40*(1), 82–89.

Sherman, D. K., Iacono, W. G., & Donnelly, J. M. (1995). Development and validation of body rating scales for adolescent females. *International Journal of Eating Disorders, 18*(4), 327–333.

Shisslak, C. M., Renger, R., Sharpe, T., Crago, M., McKnight, K. M., Gray, N., et al. (1999). Development and evaluation of the McKnight Risk Factor Survey for assessing potential risk and protective factors for disordered eating in preadolescent and adolescent girls. *International Journal of Eating Disorders, 25*(2), 195–214.

Shroff, H., & Thompson, K.J. (2006). Peer influences, body-image dissatisfaction, eating dysfunction and self-esteem in adolescent girls. *Journal of Health Psychology, 11*(4), 533–551.

Sim, L., & Zeman, J. (2004). Emotion awareness and identification skills in adolescent girls with bulimia nervosa. *Journal of Clinical Child and Adolescent Psychology, 33*(4), 760–771.

Skinner, H. A., Steinhauer, P. D., & Santa-Barbara, J. (2003). *Family Assessment Measure, Version III (FAM-III).* Lutz, FL: Psychological Assessment Resources

Skrzypek, S., Wehmeier, P. M., & Remschmidt, H. (2001). Body image assessment using body size estimation in recent studies on anorexia nervosa. A brief review. *European Child and Adolescent Psychiatry, 10,* 215–221.

Smolak, L. (2004). Body image in children and adolescents: Where do we go from here?. *Body Image, 1,* 15–28.

Steiger, H., & Bruce, K. R. (2007). Phenotypes, endophenotypes, and genotypes in bulimia spectrum eating disorders. *Canadian Journal of Psychiatry-Revue Canadienne De Psychiatrie, 52*(4), 220–227.

Steinberg, E., Tanofsky-Kraff, M., Cohen, M. L., Elberg, J., Freedman, R. J., Semega-Janneh, M., et al. (2004). Comparison of the child and parent forms of the questionnaire on eating and weight patterns in the assessment of children's eating-disordered behaviors. *International Journal of Eating Disorders, 36*(2), 183–194.

Steiner, H., & Lock, J. (1998). Anorexia nervosa and bulimia nervosa in children and adolescents: A review of the past 10 years. *Journal of the American Academy of Child and Adolescent Psychiatry, 37*(4), 352–359.

Stice, E. (2001). A prospective test of the dual-pathway model of bulimic pathology: Mediating effects of dieting and negative affect. *Journal of Abnormal Psychology, 110*(1), 124–135.

Stice, E. (2002). Risk and maintenance factors for eating pathology: A meta-analytic review. *Psychological Bulletin, 128,* 825–848.

Stice, E., & Shaw, H. E. (2002). Role of body dissatisfaction in the onset and maintenance of eating pathology: A synthesis of research findings *Journal of Psychosomatic
Research, 53,* 985–993.

Stice, E., Presnell, K., Groesz, L., & Shaw, H. (2005). Effects of a weight maintenance
diet on bulimic symptoms in adolescent girls: An experimental test of the dietary
restraint theory. *Health Psychology, 24*(4), 402–412.

Strober, M., Freeman, R., Lampert, C., Diamond, J., & Kaye, W. (2000). Controlled
family study of anorexia nervosa and bulimia nervosa: evidence of shared liability and transmission of partial syndromes. *American Journal of Psychiatry, 157*(3),
393–401.

Stuart, R. B. (1967). Behavioral control of overeating. *Behaviour Research and Therapy,
5*(4), 357–365.

Szmukler, G. I., Eisler, I., Russell, G., & Dare, C. (1985). Anorexia nervosa, parental
"expressed emotion" and dropping out of treatment. *British Journal of Psychiatry Vol
147 Sep 1985, 265–271 Royal College of Psychiatrists.*

Tanofsky-Kraff, M., Faden, D., Yanovski, S. Z., Wilfley, D. E., & Yanovski, J. A. (2005).
The perceived onset of dieting and loss of control eating behaviors in overweight
children. *International Journal of Eating Disorders, 38*(2), 112–122.

Tanofsky-Kraff, M., Morgan, C. M., Yanovski, S. Z., Marmarosh, C., Wilfley, D. E., &
Yanovski, J. A. (2003). Comparison of assessments of children's eating-disordered
behaviors by interview and questionnaire. *International Journal of Eating Disorders,
33*(2), 213–224.

Thelen, M. H., Farmer, J., Wonderlich, S, & Smith, M. (1991). A revision of the Bulimia-
Test: The BULIT-R. *Psychological Assessment, 3,* 119–124.

Thompson, J. K., & Dolce, J. (1989). The discrepancy between emotional vs. rational
estimates of body size, actual size, and ideal body ratings: Theoretical and clinical
implications. *Journal of Clinical Psychology, 45,* 473–478.

Thompson, J. K., & Gardner, D.M.. (2002). *Measuring perceptual body image among
adolescents and adults.* New York Guilford Press.

Thompson, J. K., & Smolak, L. (Ed.). (2001). *Body image, eating disorders, and obesity in
youth: Assessment, prevention, and treatment.* Washington DC: American Psychological
Association.

Thompson, M. A., & Gray, J. J. (1995). Development and validation of a new body-
image assessment scale. *Journal of Personality Assessment, 64*(2), 258–269.

Tiggemann, M., & Wilson-Barrett, E. (1998). Children's figure ratings: Relationship to
self-esteem and negative stereotyping. *International Journal of Eating Disorders,
23,* 83–88.

Truby, H., & Paxton, S. J. (2002). Development of the children's body image scale.
British Journal of Clinical Psychology, 41, 185–203.

Turner, H., & Bryant-Waugh, R. (2004). Eating disorder not otherwise specified (EDNOS):
Profiles of clients presenting at a Community Eating Disorder Service. *European
Eating Disorders Review, 12*(1), 18–26.

Urbszat, D., Herman, C. P., & Polivy, J. (2002). Eat, drink, and be merry, for tomorrow
we diet: Effects of anticipated deprivation on food intake in restrained and unre-
strained eaters. *Journal of Abnormal Psychology, 111*(2), 396–401.

van Furth, E. F., van Strien, D. C., Martina, L. M., van Son, M. J., Hendrickx, J. J., &
van Engeland, H. (1996). Expressed emotion and the prediction of outcome in adolescent eating disorders. *International Journal of Eating Disorders, 20*(1), 19–31.

Vaughn, C., & Leff, J. (1976). Measurement of Expressed Emotion in Families of
Psychiatric-Patients. *British Journal of Social and Clinical Psychology, 15*(JUN),
157–165.

Veron-Guidry, S., & Williamson, D.A. (1996). Development of a body image assessment procedure for children and preadolescents. *International Journal of Eating
Disorders, 20*(3), 287–293.

Vincent, M. A., McCabe, M. P., & Ricciardelli, L. A. (1999). Factorial validity of the
Bulimia Test-Revised in adolescent boys and girls. *Behaviour Research and Therapy,
37,* 1129–1140.

Vitousek, K., Watson, S., Wilson, T.G. (1998). Enhancing motivation for change in treat-
ment-resistant eating disorders. *Clinical Psychology Review, 18*(4), 391–420.

Vitousek, K. B. (2002). Cognitive-behavioral therapy for anorexia nervosa. In C. G. Fairburn & K. D. Brownell (Eds.), *Eating disorders and obesity: A comprehensive handbook.* New York: Guilford Press.

Wade, T. D., Crosby, R. D., & Martin, N. G. (2006). Use of latent profile analysis to identify eating disorder phenotypes in an adult Australian twin cohort. *Archives of General Psychiatry, 63*(12), 1377–1384.

Walsh, J. M., Wheat, M. E., & Freund, K. (2000). Detection, evaluation, and treatment of eating disorders the role of the primary care physician. *Journal of General Internal Medicine., 15*(8), 577–590.

Watkins, B., Frampton, I., Lask, B., & Bryant-Waugh, R. (2005). Reliability and validity of the child version of the eating disorder examination: A preliminary investigation. *International Journal of Eating Disorders, 38*(2), 183–187.

Whitney, J., & Eisler, I. (2005). Theoretical and empirical models around caring for someone with an eating disorder: The reorganization of family life and inter-personal maintenance factors. *Journal of Mental Health, 14*(6), 575–585.

Wonderlich, S. A., Joiner, T. E., Keel, P. K., Williamson, D. A., & Crosby, R. D. (2007). Eating disorder diagnoses - Empirical approaches to classification. *American Psychologist, 62*(3), 167–180.

Wonderlich, S. A., Lilenfeld, L. R., Riso, L. P., Engel, S., & Mitchell, J. E. (2005). Personality and anorexia nervosa. *International Journal of Eating Disorders, 37 Suppl,* S68–71; discussion S87–69.

Workgroup for the Classification of Eating Disorders in Children and Adolescents. (2007)). Classification of Child and Adolescent Eating Disturbances. *International Journal of Eating Disorders,* 40, suppl: S117–122.

Zonnevylle-Bender, M. J. S., van Goozen, S. H. M., Cohen-Kettenis, P. T., van Elburg, A., de Wildt, M., Stevelmans, E., et al. (2004). Emotional functioning in anorexia nervosa patients: Adolescents compared to adults. *Depression and Anxiety, 19*(1), 35–42.

15

Pain Assessment

FRANK ANDRASIK and CARLA RIME

INTRODUCTION

In adults, pain is one of the most common physical complaints. For example, a comprehensive review of available epidemiological studies yielded a median point prevalence of chronic benign pain of 15% in adults, with individual study values ranging from 2–40% (Verhaak, Kerssens, Dekker, Sorbi, & Bensing, 1998). Unfortunately, pain is not limited to the adult years, as estimates of pain complaints in childhood and adolescence typically range from 15–20% (Goodman & McGrath, 1991), a level surprisingly similar to that for adults. The pain experienced by children and adolescents is sufficiently intense to require medical consultations by a large percentage of those so affected. Of the 25% of individuals aged up to 18 years studied by Perquin, Hazebroek-Kampschreur, Hunfeld, van Suijlekom-Smit, Passchier, and van der Wouden (2000) who had complaints of chronic pain (defined as continuous or recurrent pain occurring longer than three months), 57% had visited a physician and almost 40% had taken medication. The major types of pain experienced by children and adolescents are listed in Table 15.1, although in practice the pain presentations often overlap, with boundaries being less distinct (McGrath & Finley, 1999).

In the not too distant past pain was not viewed as a serious problem in children and adolescents. However, it is now clear that pain is a significant condition in childhood and adolescence and, when it is chronic or recurrent, it is unlikely to be outgrown (McGrath & Finley, 1999). Several findings highlight the seriousness of pain in children and adolescents.

FRANK ANDRASIK AND CARLA RIME • Department of Psychology University of West Florida 11000 University Parkway Pensacola, FL 32514.

J.L. Matson et al. (eds.), *Assessing Childhood Psychopathology and Developmental Disabilities*, DOI: 10.1007/978-0-387-09528-8,
© Springer Science+Business Media, LLC 2009

Table 15.1. Recurrent and chronic pain
conditions in children and adolescents.

Pain associated with chronic illness
  Juvenile rheumatoid arthritis
  Cancer
  Sickle cell disease
Pain resulting from trauma
  Complex regional pain syndrome
  Phantom limb pain
Chronic, but nonspecific pain
  Musculoskeletal pain
  Dysmenorrhea
Recurrent pain
  Migraine headache
  Tension-type headache
  Recurrent abdominal pain
Pain related to a mental health condition
  Psychogenic pain disorder
  Somatization disorder

The pathways that are responsible for perception and transmission of pain
are developed very early in life. Inadequate analgesia for pain experienced
early in life can disrupt the person's ability to effectively manage later
episodes of pain (primarily due to sensitization effects within the periph-
eral and central nervous system; c.f., Baccei & Fitzgerald, 2006; Fitzgerald
& Walker, 2006; Flor & Andrasik, 2006; Hermann, Hohmesiter, Demirakca,
Zohsel, & Flor, 2006; Woolf & Salter, 2000). Thus, successful intervention
during childhood and adolescence may, in addition to providing needed
symptom relief at the moment, serve preventive functions for later adult
life and restore normal pain nociception.

Recognition of the widespread occurrence and the personal, social,
and economic impact of pain led the Joint Commission on Accreditation
of Healthcare Organizations in the summer of 1999 to mandate regular
assessment of pain and require establishment of policies and procedures
that support the appropriate use of pain medication. Henceforth, pain has
become known as the "fifth vital sign" (being added to the list that already
includes heart rate, blood pressure, temperature, and respiration). U.S.
readers certainly have noticed the heightened awareness of assessing for
pain during routine physician office visits, where questions about pain now
routinely appear on intake/history forms and scales for assessing pain
intensity are prominently placed on the walls in all examination rooms.

PAIN: THE BIOPSYCHOSOCIAL MODEL

The dominant model for understanding and describing chronic pain
is best thought of as the "biomedical model." This model views pain as
resulting from the direct transmission of impulses from the periphery
to structures within the central nervous system (Turk & Flor, 1999).
This unidirectional model has led to a number of important insights

about important pathophysiological mechanisms and the development of pharmacological treatments directed at modifying these identified aberrant aspects. At the same time, this model has certain limitations and is unable to account for certain phenomena, such as pain that continues in the absence of identifiable pathology, pathology that exists in the absence of pain, varied individual responses of individuals to seemingly identical treatments, the failure of potent medications to provide consistent pain relief, and the absence of a strong relationship among pain, impairment, and disability.

A competing, more compelling model, termed the "biopsychosocial model," has arisen as a result. This model takes into account the varied psychological and sociological factors that can play an important role in the genesis and maintenance of recurrent pain conditions and, thus, provides a more complete understanding (Turk & Flor, 1999). This model also incorporates emotional aspects that were more formally acknowledged in the definition of pain provided by the International Association for the Study of Pain (IASP) (1986). Pain, according to the IASP, is "an unpleasant sensory and emotional experience associated with actual and potential tissue damage, or described in terms of such damage." Elsewhere, the following is mentioned, "It is unquestionably a sensation in a part or parts of the body, but it is also always unpleasant and therefore also an emotional experience."

This model views pain (and any chronic illness, for that matter) as originating from a complex interaction of biological, psychological, and social variables. From this viewpoint, the observed diversity in illness expression (including severity, duration, and consequences to the individual) can be accounted for by the complex interrelationships among predispositional, biological, and psychological characteristics (e.g., genetics, prior learning history), biological changes, psychological status, and the social and cultural contexts that shape the individual's perceptions and response to illness. This model contrasts sharply with the biomedical perspective that conceptualizes illness in terms of more narrowly defined physiochemical dimensions. This alternative model differs in other important respects as well, in that it is dynamic (as opposed to static) and recognizes the reciprocal influences and the changing nature of multiple factors over time. Although much is to be gained by application of this model, it has not been fully exploited within the realm of children, adolescents, and in particular with respect to those individuals experiencing developmental disabilities.

PAIN: AS IT APPLIES TO PERSONS WITH DEVELOPMENTAL DISABILITIES

Although pain is common, prevalent throughout the world, and respects no demographic or intellectual borders, minimal attention has been devoted to its study among people who are experiencing developmental disabilities (this is true for adults as well as child and adolescent populations). Many reasons account for this dearth of information and the lack of recognition of the serious nature of pain (Bottos & Chambers, 2006).

One of the chief reasons has been the prevalent but erroneous assumption that individuals with developmental disabilities are either indifferent or are less sensitive to pain (i.e., they have a heightened threshold for pain). Laboratory studies that have monitored pain behaviors of persons with disabilities and those without help shed light on why these false perceptions have endured. As just one example, Hennequin, Morin, and Feine (2000) assessed thresholds for cold-pain among individuals diagnosed with Down syndrome and those without Down syndrome (controls). To assess pain thresholds, an ice cube was applied directly to the skin while the experimenters noted the time lapse to the first verbal or behavioral reaction. Both groups showed similar reactions, but the latencies to respond were much longer for persons with Down syndrome.

Compounding the problem is the finding that persons with developmental disabilities often express their pain in a manner different from those who do not have such disabilities. When examining the typical everyday pains experienced in a child care setting (e.g., bumps and bruises), children with developmental disabilities, in comparison to children without such a diagnosis, were less likely to cry or seek out help and more likely to be devoid of any observable reaction (Gilbert-MacLeod, Craig, Rocha, & Mathias, 2000). However, an attenuated behavioral response is not the rule. For example, observations made on children with autism while they were undergoing venipuncture suggested the presence of a heightened sensitivity to acute pain, as evidenced by the intense facial expressions that occurred (Nader, Oberlander, Chambers, & Craig, 2004). Results from these and other studies call into the question the notion that persons with developmental disabilities are insensitive or indifferent to pain. It is more accurate to say that persons with developmental disabilities display pain behaviors that are different from those exhibited by their nondevelopmentally disabled counterparts and that these behaviors may be attenuated in certain circumstances.

Some have claimed that pain may be much less frequent overall in people with developmental disabilities. Here, too, the limited available evidence suggests otherwise. One can argue, in fact, that the opposite is true: that individuals with developmental disabilities may be at increased risk for experiencing pain. This may be true for two chief reasons. First, persons with developmental disabilities are more likely to undergo surgical or medical procedures that are painful, such as corrective surgeries, treatment for irritations resulting from protheses, and intravenous needle placements. Second, the higher presence of comorbid medical conditions can increment pain. As an example, Table 15.2 provides a listing of the varied associated conditions that can contribute to pain in persons with cerebral palsy (Bottos & Chambers, 2006).

Available research reveals that many children and adolescents with developmental disabilities exhibit high levels of pain persistently. During a one-month period, caregivers reported that nearly 80% of their cognitively impaired children experienced at least one episode of pain; between one-third and one-half were reported as experiencing pain on a weekly basis (Breau, Camfield, McGrath, & Finley, 2003). Similar findings have been reported by Stallard, Williams, Lenton, and Velleman (2001) and Stallard,

Table 15.2. Conditions contributing to pain in persons with cerebral palsy.

Placement of gastric feeding devices	Gastroesophagel reflux
Release of muscular contractures	Constipation
Needle injections	Abdominal gas
Blood pressure tests	Muscle spasms
Surgeries	Joint problems
Medical examinations	Headaches
Enemas	Earaches
Dental procedures	Seizures
Dislocated hips	Position/posture changes
Spontaneous pain	

Williams, Velleman, Lenton, and McGrath (2002). Looking more closely at the causes of pain, pain from nonaccidental sources has been found to occur at a rate double that for pain resulting from accidents (Breau et al., 2003) and the former type of pain is typically judged to be more severe in nature. These rates of pain exceed those for children absent of disabilities. Pain knows no boundaries within developmentally disabled populations, being highly prevalent in persons with Down Syndrome, Autism, and Cerebral Palsy (see review by Bottos & Chambers, 2006).

Assessment Approaches

In 2002, a landmark meeting was held for the purpose of developing consensus reviews and making recommendations that would improve the design, execution, and interpretation of clinical trials for pain assessment and treatment. This "Initiative on Methods, Measurement, and Pain Assessment in Clinical Trials" (IMMPACT) grew from a recognition that many patients with recurring pain conditions often were not obtaining adequate relief and/or were experiencing significant untoward side effects from extant treatments. At this first IMMPACT meeting (November 2002), a distinguished group of experts (drawn from academia, regulatory agencies: U.S. Food and Drug Administration and the European Agency for the evaluation of Medicinal Products, the U.S. National Institutes of Health, U.S. Veterans Administration, consumer support and advocacy groups, and industry) set out to develop core and supplemental measurement domains critical for assessing initial problem severity and subsequent response to treatment in clinical trials.

They (Turk et al., 2003) recommended that all treatment trials consider incorporating measures for six key domains: (1) pain itself, (2) physical functioning, (3) emotional functioning, (4) participant evaluations of improvement and treatment satisfaction, (5) symptoms and adverse events, and (6) participant disposition. A followup article from the IMMPACT group (Dworkin et al., 2005) offered more specificity regarding these core domains, for trials with adults.

To date, eight IMMPACT consensus meetings have been held, with six focusing on chronic pain in adults, one addressing acute pain in adults, with the remaining one examining pediatric acute and chronic pain (see www.immpact.org/index.html for further information about this initiative and resulting publications). The latter group, named the "Pediatric Initiative on Methods, Measurement, and Pain Assessment in Clinical Trials" (Ped-IMMPACT) (McGrath, Turk, Dworkin, Brown, Davidson, Eccleston, et al., 2008) identified the following eight core outcome domains for recurrent pain in children and adolescents, some of which overlap those identified by the adult working group: (1) pain, (2) physical functioning, (3) emotional functioning, (4) role functioning, (5) symptoms and adverse events, (6) global judgment of satisfaction, (7) sleep, and (8) economic factors.

To date, two comprehensive reviews of pain measures specific to children and adolescents (age range of 3 to 18) have appeared. Recommendations from these two reports (Stinson, Kavanagh, Yamada, Gill, & Stevens, 2006; von Baeyer & Spagrud, 2007) are discussed in the next section, where appropriate. Although these efforts are notable, minimal attention was directed at concerns unique to persons with developmental disabilities. This is unfortunate as pain assessment with individuals who are experiencing developmental disabilities poses a special challenge for healthcare professionals, as the ability to comprehend and translate a pain sensation is compromised for those with cognitive deficits. In cases where there are language deficits, nonverbal communication needs to be explored in relation to pain expression (Anand & Craig, 1996; Davies & Evans, 2001).

We now turn our attention to review of issues when utilizing self-report, proxy report, observational tools, and physiological responses, as these are the domains that have been the chief focus to date.

SELF-REPORT

Despite recognition of the multidimensional nature of pain and the recommendations from the Ped-IMMPACT working group to include multiple domains, self-report of pain intensity has long served as the main measure (referred to by some as the "gold standard") in pain assessment even though problems with this approach are acknowledged (Anand & Craig, 1996; Bodfish, Harper, Deacon, Deacon, & Symons, 2006; Foley & McCutcheon, 2004; Hodgins, 2002; McGrath & Unruh, 2006; Williams, Davies, & Chadury, 2000). This method, although widely used, is undermined when patients are unable to verbalize the characteristics of their pain. Even if an individual can signify the presence of pain, she or he may have trouble quantifying (Cook, Niven, & Downs, 1999), specifying the location, or describing the pain experience (Foley & McCutcheon, 2004).

With this and related issues in mind, Stinson et al. (2006) were charged with reviewing extant self-report measures of pain intensity, with regard to psychometric integrity (reliability, validity, and responsivity), interpretability (meaningfulness of the obtained score values), and feasibility (ease of scoring and interpretation). Their systematic literature search revealed 34 single-item measures designed for use across pain disorders (they specifically ignored measures developed for specific pain diagnoses or disorders, such as headache and sickle cell disease), of which 6 were judged to be adequate. These consisted of the Pieces of Hurt Tool (Hester, 1979), Faces Pain Scale and Faces Pain Scale-Revised (Bieri, Reeve, Champion, Addicoat, & Ziegler, 1990; Hicks, von Baeyer, Spafford, van Korlaar, & Goodenough, 2001), Wong-Baker FACES Pain Scale (Wong & Baker, 1988), Oucher (Beyer & Aradine, 1986), and Visual Analogue Scales (Scott, Ansell, & Huskisson, 1977). Table 15.3 summarizes the key features of these measures, which are discussed in brief below.

Pieces of Hurt Tool

This scale consists of four red plastic poker chips, with the first representing "a little hurt" and the last "the most hurt you could ever have." The child is instructed to select the chip that best represents the current pain intensity, with scores ranging from "0" (no chip) to "4" (most hurt). This measure has a number of advantages (used successfully with children as young as three, easy to understand, shown useful in various settings). Disadvantages range from those of a minor nature (such as the need to sanitize the chips between use, misplacement of chips) to those that are more major (limited use with recurrent pain conditions).

Faces Pain Scale/Faces Pain Scale-Revised

The original version utilized seven gender-neutral faces, with expressions ranging from "no pain" to "most pain possible," arranged at equal intervals. The child respondent was asked simply to point to the face showing how much pain was being felt. Score values ranged from 0 to 6. The revised scale uses six faces, with score values ranging from 0 to 5, as this enhanced comparability with other measures that more commonly use score values ranging in multiples of 5 (0 to 5 or 0 to 10). Both versions have good psychometric support and are quick and easy to administer. However, given the way they are anchored, ratings tend to skew towards the "no pain" end of the scale. Less is known about interpretability and acceptability.

Versions of the Faces Pain Scale (FPS) now include 3, 5, 6, or 7 pain face intensities. Another feature that deviates for each version is whether the first, "no pain" face is neutral or smiling, or whether tears are included in the higher intensity pain faces. The FPS (Bieri et al., 1990) and FPS-R (Hicks et al., 2001) have neutral "no pain" faces and tears are not present. These variations have sparked some debate as to whether the different versions of the FPS measure pain intensity or pain distress. One study reported consistently higher pain ratings from both children and parents with versions that included smiling, "no pain" faces, even though children and parents preferred scales with "happy" and cartoonlike faces (Chambers, Giesbrecht, Craig, Bennett, & Huntsman, 1999). A similar bias was found in a study investigating ratings provided by nurses (Chambers, Hardial, Craig, Court, & Montgomery, 2005). These factors, in addition to age and mental capabilities, need to be taken into consideration when obtaining pain intensity ratings.

Table 15.3. Summary of psychometric properties, interpretability and feasibility of self-report pain intensity measures.

Name of Scale (Acronym) Author (year)	Age range	Type of Pain	Reliability	Validity	Responsivity	Interpretability	Feasibility
Pieces of Hurt tool; Hester (1979)	I: 4–7 years S: 3–18 years	Acute procedural, hospital-based	Test-retest (+) Inter-rater reliability (+)	Construct (+++)	Yes(+)	No	Moderate
Faces Pain Scale (FPS); Bieri et al. (1990)	I: 4+ years	Acute procedural, post-op, disease-related	Test-retest (+)	Content (+) Construct (+++)	Yes (++)	Yes	High
Faces Pain Scale-Revised (FPS-R); Hicks et al. (2001)	S: 4–12 years	Acute procedural, post-op, disease related	Test-retest (+)	Content (+) Construct (+)	Yes(+)	No	High
Oucher-Photographic; Beyer and Aradine (1986)	I: 3–7 years S: 3–18 years	Acute procedural, post-op, disease-related disease-related	Test-retest (+)	Content (+) Construct (+++)	Yes (++)	Yes	Moderate
Oucher-NRS; Beyer and Aradine (1986)	I: 3–12 years S: 3–18 years	Acute procedural, post-op, disease-related	Test-retest (+)	Content (+) Construct (++)	Yes (++)	Yes	Moderate
Wong-Baker FACES Pain Scale; Wong and Baker (1988)	I: 3–18 years S: 9 months-18 years	Acute procedural, post-op, disease-related	Test-retest (++)	Content (+) Construct (+++)	Yes(++)	Yes	High
Visual Analogue Scale; Scott et al. (1977)	I: 2–17 years S: 3–20 years	Acute, procedural, disease-related, recurrent/chronic	Test-retest (+)	Construct (+++)	Yes (++)	Yes	Moderate

Note: + = 1–3 studies; ++ = 3–6 studies; +++ = >6 studies; I = Intended. S = studied.
Source: Reprinted from Stinson et al., 2006.

Wong-Baker FACES Pain Scale

This measure consists of six hand-drawn faces, ranging from smiling ("no hurt") to crying ("hurts worst"), with scores ranging from 0 to 5. Ease of administration and cost-effectiveness are among the advantages. Disadvantages discussed in the literature include tendencies for children to select faces at the extreme end when experiencing procedural pain, avoidance of the face depicting crying by children who do not want to admit to actually crying, and questions about whether it might be confounding varied dimensions of pain (affective/reactive dimension versus the sensory/intensity dimension).

Oucher

This scale combines two separate scales, a photographic faces scale, consisting of six pictures of culturally sensitive faces (Afro-American, Caucasian, and Hispanic) that are scored from 0 to 5, with a numerical rating scale, ranging from 0 to 100mm in a vertical array. As with other measures, most research has been conducted with acute pain conditions and with children/adolescents of an older age.

Visual Analogue Scales

These types of measures have long been used in research and practice with adult pain patients. They consist of continuous vertical or horizontal lines (with some believing that children have an easier time with vertical lines as they can more easily assess intensities with a going up or going down analogy), of a predetermined length, anchored at each end by the extreme limits of pain intensity. There are a number of variations on this basic approach, with some using different line lengths and some adding hash or division marks. These types of measures have good psychometric support in general for children eight and above, and they are quick and easy to administer. The varied ways they have been displayed and the differing anchors that have been used have hampered development (by precluding standardization) and complicate comparisons across studies and conditions.

The Coloured Analogue Scale (CAS) (McGrath, Seifert, Speechley, Booth, Stitt, & Gibson, 1996) is an alternative to the standard VAS and was designed to aid young children in self-reporting the degree of their pain. As such, it may be appropriate as well for those who have mild cognitive impairment. The CAS is a vertical scale, much like a thermometer, with progressively darker shades of red moving upward on the scale to illustrate increased pain intensity. Children move a marker on the scale to the point where the gradation of color best reflects their pain intensity. Numerical values are printed on the backside for clinicians to document the child's response. McGrath and colleagues (1996) found the CAS to be a simple, practical tool with preliminary validity to assess pain in those ages 5–16. Although the CAS may facilitate the self-report for pain in children, it has some limitations for individuals with developmental disabilities (LaChapelle, Hadjistavropoulos, & Craig, 1999).

Despite some of the shortcomings with self-report measures, it is still worthwhile to attempt obtaining such reports from young children (Stanford, Chambers, & Craig, 2006) and individuals with developmental disabilities who possess appropriate understanding (Hadjistavropoulos, von Baeyer, & Craig, 2001). When self-reports are not an option or are suspected to be unreliable, healthcare professionals may turn to proxy reports of parents and other caregivers for pain details. Proxy reports are discussed in the next section.

Upon completing their review, Stinson et al. (2006), noting that no single scale was preferred for all ages, developmental levels, and clinical conditions, offered a number of recommendations to help guide selection of self-report measures of pain intensity in clinical trials. These are reproduced in Table 15.4. They concluded their review by pointing out the need to continue developing, testing, and standardizing existing as well as new measures, focusing increased efforts on younger children, and determining how much of a change is needed for claiming clinically significant effects (which they termed as the "minimally clinically significant difference").

Daily Pain Diaries

Although not reviewed by Stinson et al. (2006), when treating children and adolescents with ongoing pain problems it is a common practice to require participants to monitor some aspects of their condition on a systematic basis, most typically using diaries or logs that are completed on a daily basis. In fact, this has become the standard when working with pediatric headache (Andrasik & Schwartz, 2006; McGrath & Unruh, 2006), when patients have sufficient cognitive capacity to do so. The exact type and form vary as a function of age and intervention intent. For example, if attempts are made to alter antecedents and consequence as a part of treatment, then these aspects are typically monitored daily. These diaries, thus, can help guide treatment as well as assess outcome, and they may additionally be useful for tracking specific pain characteristics when

Table 15.4. Summary of recommendations of self-report pain intensity measures for clinical trials in children 3–18 years of age.

- In most clinical trials, a single-item self-report measure of pain intensity is the appropriate primary outcome dimension for children 3 years of age and older.
- Pieces of Hurt tool is recommended for acute procedure-related and post-operative pain in young children between 3 and 4 years of age.
- Given the wide variability in young children's ability to use self-report measures especially between the ages of 3 and 7 years of age, it would be prudent to consider using a behavioral observational measure as a secondary outcome in this age group.
- Faces Pain Scale-Revised is recommend for acute procedure-related, post-operative, and disease-related pain in children between 4 and 12 years of age.
- A 100 mm visual analogue scale is recommended for acute procedure-related, post-operative, and disease-related pain in children over the age of 8 years of age and adolescents.
- For children between the ages of 8 and 12 years it might be useful to use the Faces Pain Scale-Revised as a secondary outcome measure with the visual analogue scale.

Source: Reprinted from Stinson et al., 2006 (Permission granted by the International Association for the Study of Pain).

diagnoses are complicated or unclear (Metsähonkala, Sillanpää, & Tuominen, 1997). The approaches typically involve monitoring intensity, frequency, and duration of pain.

Sample diary approaches and comparisons of them may be found in Andrasik, Burke, Attanasio, and Rosenblum (1985) and Richardson, McGrath, Cunningham, and Humphreys (1983). The most recent innovation involves electronic forms, using either the Internet or personal digital assistants (Palermo, Valenzuela, & Stork, 2004). Various committees have drafted guidelines for measures to use with headache patients (Andrasik, Lipchik, McCrory, & Wittrock, 2005; Penzien et al., 2005). Although developed largely with adult patients in mind, they should be applicable with pediatric headache patients as well as other recurrent pain conditions.

PROXY REPORT

Parents and other caregivers can be most helpful in corroborating self-reports of pain and speaking on behalf of those who cannot "speak for themselves." A survey administered to physicians and nurses indicated they preferred self-report measures for children who were absent of or only mildly affected by cognitive impairments, whereas proxy reports were preferred for children who have moderate or severe cognitive impairments (Fanurik, Koh, Schmitz, Harrison, Roberson, & Killebrew, 1999). Parents and other caregivers who are familiar with a child's routine behaviors thus can provide valuable information. Fanurik, Koh, Schmitz, Harrison, and Conrad (1999) found it helpful to divide the pain expressions of children having cognitive impairments into direct or indirect behaviors.

Direct pain expressions include the child's efforts to communicate the pain and its location, to verbalize the presence of pain without localization, and to localize the pain with nonverbal behavior. In contrast, indirect pain expressions include inferences about pain, as judged by crying, certain facial movements, physical or emotional changes, and engaging in self-injurious behaviors. Sixty-six percent (66%) of parents who have children who are mild to moderately impaired report an ability to determine pain in their child through direct expression, whereas 90% of parents with children who are severely to profoundly impaired infer the presence of pain through indirect pain expressions. If someone is unfamiliar with a child who has a cognitive impairment, such as a healthcare professional, pain behaviors thus may be misinterpreted.

Pain assessment is further complicated in individuals with developmental disabilities, as they may display atypical pain patterns (McGrath, Rosmus, Camfield, Campbell, & Hennigar, 1998). Caregivers may be in a position to distinguish unique behaviors that may be suggestive of the presence of pain. For instance, parents have reported that cries of a certain tone, laughing, seizures, self-abusive behaviors, particular postures, and changes in eating, sleeping, and socializing patterns may be indicative of pain (Carter, McArthur, & Cunliffe, 2002; Hadden & von Baeyer, 2002). These pain behaviors may not be obvious to someone other than the caregiver.

The potential relationship between self-injurious behavior (SIB) and pain merits further consideration. SIB is a serious, complex, multidetermined behavior that can serve varied functions (attention, escape, nonsocial, physical, tangible). We (Baldridge & Andrasik, 2008) and others (Bosch, Van Dyke, Smith, & Poulton, 1997), however, have found instances where such behavior has been indicative of an underlying pain condition, as illustrated by the following case. DG, a person seen at a developmental center, had a long-standing history of pulling and pounding on his ears, which produced ear sores that would not heal and, as a result, gave his ears a cauliflower appearance (Baldridge & Andrasik, 2008). At times, he remained in bed, in a fetal position, crying and displaying a furrowed brow. At other times, he moved about freely. Prior medical evaluations all proved to be negative.

When a detailed functional analysis performed by his treating psychologist failed to identify controlling environmental factors, our thoughts turned to the possibility of an underlying pain condition (noticing his behavior being similar to that of a colicky infant). In further discussions with direct care staff they mentioned that DG simply did not look comfortable at the times when SIB was in evidence. Closer observations revealed him to have excessive flatus. A review of his medications indicated that he was receiving Lactulose, a medicine known to promote abdominal cramping and gas. The Lactulose was discontinued, and he was then placed on Miralax, a medication whose different mechanism of action lessens these particular side effects. Within a few days, DG was noted to appear much more comfortable, as he was now able to rest quietly and he no longer whined or drew up his legs. A short time later his ears began to heal. A year later, staff reported his SIB as occurring very infrequently.

Isolated cases of ours and those reported in the literature by others (Bosch et al., 1997) do not inform us of the co-occurrence of pain and SIB. Rather, they serve to remind us of the importance of utilizing a multidisciplinary team approach when evaluating and treating persons suspected of having an underlying pain disorder. In cases where SIB is present, measures such as the Questions About Behavioral Function (Applegate, Matson, & Cherry, 1999; Paclawskyj, Matson, Rush, Smalls, & Vollmer, 2000) can be invaluable in guiding assessment and treatment efforts.

Fanurik, Koh, Schmitz, Harrison, and Conrad (1999) found that several parents of children with cognitive impairment believe that pain is often underestimated and undertreated in their child. Parents (Chambers, Reid, Craig, McGrath, & Finley, 1998) and nurses (Romsing, Moller-Sonnergaard, Hertel, & Rasmussen, 1996) have even been found to underestimate pain in children absent of cognitive impairments. Overall, it seems as though pain intensity can be miscalculated in all children, those with and those without cognitive impairment. Although parents may be able to detect subtle pain behaviors, certain factors may influence the accuracy of their proxy report.

Breau, MacLaren, McGrath, Camfield, and Finley (2003) reported that some caregivers have a pre-existing belief that children with cognitive impairment are less sensitive to pain as compared to children who are not impaired. The investigators speculate that this belief may arise by healthcare professionals shaping parent's beliefs on their child's sensitivity to pain. Another explanation is that this belief may be adaptive or serve a protective function because parents often have to witness their child undergoing a number of painful procedures. Regardless of how the belief was formed, it can lead to caregivers underestimating pain. This same study noted an important relationship between a child's cognitive level and reaction to pain. It was believed that children with mild or moderate impairment were prone to overreact to pain compared to nonimpaired children. In opposite fashion, it was believed that an extreme reaction from children with severe or profound impairments was associated with a greater amount of pain. The basis of these beliefs is unclear, but they can interfere with an accurate assessment of pain by parents and caregivers.

Caregivers are in a unique position to identify expressions and behaviors that can predict the presence of pain that otherwise would be undetectable to a person not familiar with the individual. Even so, caregiver pre-existing beliefs and attitudes can affect the accuracy of such reports, as shown in the study by Nader, Oberlander, Chambers, and Craig (2004), who investigated parent reports of venipuncture pain in children with autism and children who were unimpaired. The facial activity of the children in both groups was found to be similar during the venipuncture. Parent reports of pain for the nonimpaired children showed greater concordance with facial activity than the parental reports of pain for the autistic children. In fact, the children who were autistic had greater facial activity but were judged to be less sensitive and reactive by their parents. It is unclear as to why the parents of autistic children underestimated their child's pain. Although self-report and proxy reports are subjective in nature, observational methods are more objective. Caregivers, nurses, and physicians have assisted in the development of various observational assessment tools, which are next reviewed.

OBSERVATIONAL METHODS

The second systematic measurement review commissioned by the Ped-IMMPACT group focused on observational (behavioral) measures of pain, for children and adolescents aged 3 to 18 years (von Baeyer & Spagrud, 2007). Their initial search of the literature (employing methodologies similar to those of Stinson et al., 2006) uncovered 20 observational pain scales that included behavior checklists, behavior rating scales, and global rating scales. It needs to be pointed out that all of the scales included in this review pertained to acute pain conditions, medical procedures, and other relatively brief painful events (post-op). None were recommended for assessing recurrent or chronic forms of pain, the authors pointed out, because behavioral displays of pain tend to dissipate or habituate with time, making it quite difficult to obtain reliable ratings. The authors pointed out several situations where observational measures may be of particular value. These are when children are too young, upset, distressed, or cognitively impaired; are lacking in communication abilities; are restricted by the treatment procedures themselves (e.g., bandaged, on ventilators, recipient of paralyzing medications, etc.); or are likely to be unreliable in reporting (e.g., tendencies to distort by exaggeration or minimization, etc.).

Using a grading system, four scales were categorized as meeting the highest level of evidence (I, well-established assessment), and three were judged as approaching the well-established level (Level II). These scales, along with their key characteristics, are listed in Table 15.5. These and a few other scales are discussed further below, with a particular focus on applications with special populations.

Facial expressions are a nonverbal cue that can signify pain, and they figure prominently in pain assessment measures. Both the frequency and intensity of facial activity can convey an expression of pain. LaChapelle et al. (1999) found that the frequency of chin raises in addition to the intensity of brow lowering and chin raises were significant in indicating pain during a vaccination. Prkachin (2005) asserts that brow-lowering, eyelid tightening with raised cheeks, nose wrinkling, and eyes closing are facial movements commonly associated with pain.

One of the first studies on common observable pain behaviors asked physicians to list all behaviors indicative of pain in those with a developmental disability (cerebral palsy; Giusiano, Jimeno, Collignon, & Chau, 1995). McGrath et al. (1998), who asked caregivers to provide a similar list, developed a 31-item checklist, which came to be known as the Non-Communicating Children's Pain Checklist (NCCPC). It consists of seven categories of behaviors: vocal, eating/sleeping, social/personality, facial expression of pain, activity, body and limbs, and physiological. The NCCPC has been demonstrated to be reliable and valid when evaluating pain in nonverbal children (Breau, McGrath, Camfield, Rosmus, & Finley, 2000).

Breau, Camfield, McGrath, Rosmus, and Finley (2001) conducted an item analysis of the NCCPC (which excluded the eating/sleeping category) and found that seven of the items are particularly reliable for pain as compared to distress. Two of these items, cranky and seeks comfort, were from the social category. One item, change in eyes (squeezing eyes, eyes wide open, eyes frown), was from the facial expression category. Another item, less active, was from the activity category. One item, gestures to body part that hurts, was from the body and limb category. The last two items, tears and sharp intake of breath or gasping, were from the physiological category. Although the entire checklist may offer an overall picture of pain, this subgroup of items could be utilized as an abbreviated assessment method when limited displays are of interest. A series of other studies have used modified versions of the NCCPC and in the process have replicated its validity (Breau, Finley, McGrath, & Camfield, 2002; Breau, McGrath, Camfield, & Finley, 2002).

Stallard et al. (2002) extended this work to behaviors associated with chronic pain. Caregivers of noncommunicating children were interviewed and a total of 203 pain cues were identified. The researchers then categorized these behaviors into 11 categories: vocal, facial, physical, withdrawal, seeks comfort, physiological, agitation, tense, inconsolable, pain sites, and anger/irritability. Three of these categories—vocal, facial, and inconsolable—were determined to signify definite and severe pain. Six specific cues from five of the categories were deemed significant in denoting the presence of pain: cries, screams/yells, face screwed up, flinches from contact, appears tense, unable to be comforted. In a subsequent study,

Table 15.5. Scales recommended by intended context of measurement, with source, age of child for which each tool is intended, metric, rationale, and level of evidence.

Recommended context of measurement	Acronym Name of tool	First author (year)	Age range[a]	Metric	Comments	Level of evidence
Procedural pain; brief painful events	FLACC Face, Legs, Arms, Cry, Consolability	Merkel et al. (1997)	I: 4–18 years S: 0–18 years	0–10. 5 items scored 0 to 2	Uses items similar to well-established CHEOPS but with a readily understood 0–10 metric. Low burden. Excellent inter-rater reliability. Moderate concurrent validity with FACES and good with VAS. Inconsistent responsiveness data. Has been used in studies of post-operative pain, minor non-invasive procedures, ear-nose–throat operations	I
	CHEOPS Chilldren's Hospital of Eastern Ontario Pain Scale	McGrath et al. (1985)	I: 1–7 years S: 4 months– 17 years	4–13: 6 items second 0 to 3	Well-established reliability and validity in many studies. Scores range from 4 to 13, with scores 4–6 indicating no pain Good indications of inter-rater and test–retest reliability. Good evidence for construct and concurrent validity, and responsiveness. Has been used in studies of general surgery; myringotomy and ear tube insertion; bladder nerve stimulation; closed fracture reduction; intravenous cannulation; sickle cell episodes; circumcision, and immunizations	I
Post-operative pain in hospital	FLACC Face, Legs, Arms, Cry, Consolability	Merkel et al. (1997)	I: 4–18 years S: 0–18 years	0–10: 5 items scored 0 to 2	See above	I
Post-operative pain at home (parent assessment)	PPPM Parents' Post-operative Pain Measure	Chambers et al. (1996)	I: 2–12 years S: 1–12 years	0–15: 15 items scored 0 or 1	Well-established assessment. High inter-rater reliability and internal consistency. Good construct validity with the FPS, sensitivity, specificity, content validity. Good responsiveness data. Has been used in studies of post-operative pain (many kinds) and hernia repair	I

(continued)

Table 15.5. (continued)

On ventilator or in critical care	COMFORT COMFORT Scale	Ambuel et al. (1992)	I: Newborn–17 years S: Newborn–17 years	8–40: 8 items scored 1 to 5	Only validated instrument available for this purpose. Good inter-rater reliability and internal consistency. Inconsistent responsiveness data. Has been used in studies of heart surgery; switching position to improve oxygenation; medical ventilation	II
Distress; pain-related fear or anxiety (not necessarily pain intensity; may be observed before as well as after a painful procedure)	PBCL Procedure Behavior Check List	LeBaron and Zeltzer (1984)	I: 6–17 years S: 0.1 year–19 years	Original 8–40: 8 items scored 1 to 5. Various revisions.	Good inter-rater reliability. Good construct validity and responsiveness data. Has been used in studies of bone marrow aspirations, lumbar punctures, radiation therapy, and immunization. Contains 1 unusual item	II+ (as measure of pain)
	PBRS-R Procedure Behavioral Rating Scale – Revised	Katz et al. (1980)	I: 8 months–17 years S: 3 years–10 years	0–11: 11 items scored 0 or 1	Good inter-rater, inter-item reliability. More investigation of validity and responsiveness is needed. Has been used in studies of bone marrow aspirations, immunizations and venipuncture	III+ (as measure of pain)

For level of evidence, see Table 1 and Sections 2.6 and 2.7.

[a]I = intended age range when the scale was first published; S = age range studies in subsequent research.

Source: Reprinted from von Baeyer & Spagrud, 2007. (Permission granted by the International Association for the Study of Pain).

Stallard, Williams, Velleman, Lenton, McGrath, and Taylor (2002) termed these six behaviors as the Pain Indicator for Communicatively Impaired Children (PICIC). The behavior of screwed up/distressed face was shown to be the strongest predictor of the presence of pain. The five other cues were also significant when taken together, but they were more likely to indicate "possible pain".

Terstegen, Koot, de Boer, and Tibboel (2003) studied pain behaviors before and after surgery in children who had profound cognitive impairments. The frequency of 134 potential pain behaviors categorized as facial expressions, motor behaviors, social behaviors/mood, attitude towards sore body part, vocalization, and physiological were observed. Twenty-three of these behaviors were found to be distinct in signifying pain. Four of these items on the checklist that were not present before surgery, but appeared after surgery were trembling chin, protecting sore body part, crying hard/loudly, and breath holding. Moreover, the behaviors "eyes squeezed" and "trembling chin" reflected pain intensity.

Zwakhalen, van Dongen, Hamers, and Abu-Saad (2004) surveyed nurses who work at institutions for profound intellectually disabled persons. Nurses were instructed to rate 158 pain indicators on a scale of 1–10 based on observations they use in assessing pain in their patients. More than half of the nurses deemed seven of the following pain cues as important: moaning during manipulation, crying during manipulation, painful facial expression during manipulation, swelling, screaming during manipulation, not using the sore body part, and moving the body in a specific way.

It appears as though a number of common pain behaviors can be detected from the diverse population of cognitively impaired individuals. There are, however, some internal contradictions. For instance, in the various versions of the NCCPC items such as "tense" and "floppy", "less active" and "jumping around", and "seeks comfort" and "inconsolable" are opposing behaviors. This suggests that in addition to common pain expressions, there are also behaviors that are distinctive for each individual. Even though a person may react differently to pain compared to another person, parents have reported that their children respond to pain in a predictable manner (Carter et al., 2002). Observational methods coupled with proxy reports may provide a more accurate means of detecting pain.

An assessment tool involving observation and proxy reports is the Face Legs Activity Cry and Consolability (FLACC), so named because the method reflects the categories contained within it (Malviya, Voepel-Lewis, Burke, Merkel, & Tait, 2006). A rating of 0–2 is assigned to each of the five categories, where 0 is usual behavior, 1 is occasional pain behaviors associated with each category, and 2 is more intense pain behaviors (see Table 15.6). In addition to these general ratings, caregivers also give input about idiosyncratic pain behaviors expressed by the cognitively impaired child. This tool is an individualized approach to assessment, where both common and unique pain behaviors are observed and rated. We have found great utility with this measure at our work at a developmental center, modifying categories to track behaviors specific to individuals being treated and even omitting categories that do not apply.

Table 15.6. FLACC.

Category	Scoring		
	1	2	3
Face	No particular expression or smile	Occasional grimace or frown, withdrawn, disinterested	Frequent to constant quivering chin, clenched jaw
Legs	Normal position or relaxed	Uneasy, restless, tense	Kicking, or legs drawn up
Activity	Lying quietly, normal position, moves easily	Squirming, shifting back and forth, tense	Arched, rigid or jerking
Cry	No cry (awake or asleep)	Moans or whimpers; occasional complaint	Crying steadily, screams or sobs, frequent complaints
Consolability	Content, relaxed	Reassured by occasional touching, hugging or being talked to, distractible	Difficult to console or comfort

Observational instruments can be of great assistance to caregivers, physicians, and nurses in assessing pain in cognitively impaired individuals. A majority of the research has focused on pain behaviors associated with acute pain, such as postoperative pain and needle injections (Stallard et al., 2001). It is unclear whether the same behaviors for acute pain would apply to chronic pain or if the cues are more subtle and difficult to detect (Stallard et al., 2002). Answers must come from future research investigations.

PHYSIOLOGICAL MEASURES

The Royal College of Paediatrics and Child Health (1997, as cited in Davies & Evans, 2001) contends that physiological responses to pain vary between children and adults and between individuals who are cognitively impaired and individuals who are unimpaired. Although some individuals who are cognitively impaired may have a reduced physiological response to pain, this does not generalize to all individuals with cognitive impairment. Defrin, Pick, Peretz, and Carmeli (2004) found that individuals with developmental disabilities were actually more sensitive to pain than a nonimpaired comparison group, but that there was a delayed reaction to pain. It is not fully known how pain sensation, perception, and cognitive processes affect physiological responses. Due to these inconsistent findings, physiological measures in cognitively impaired individuals are not recommended as a sole pain assessment technique (Breau, McGrath, & Zabialia, 2006).

In the previously described survey conducted by Zwakhalen et al. (2004), nurses rated physiological measures as a source for determining pain in their patients. They identified turning red in the face, vomiting, gasping for breath, holding one's breath, or marked changes in respiration or heart rate. The various adaptations of the NCCPC contain a physiological category, including items such as shivering, change in color/

pallor, sweating, tears, sharp intake of breath/gasping, and breath-holding (Breau, Finley, et al., 2002; Breau, McGrath, et al., 2002; McGrath et al., 1998). These cues are attributed to distress (Hadjistavropoulos et al., 2001) and possible symptoms of pain (Zwakhalen et al., 2004), rather than pain directly. Of available physiological/biological measures, McGrath and Unruh (2006) judge the evidence as sufficient to warrant considering using heart rate, transcutaneous oxygen, electrodermal activity, and aspects of the stress response when assessing pain. Research with endorphins, respiration, and blood pressure is limited, but worthy of continued pursuit.

In summary, presumed insensitivity to pain in certain child and adolescent groups may be a consequence of communication barriers. In a study with children who were developmentally delayed, the older children were found to respond to pain with more anger (Gilbert-MacLeod, Craig, Rocha, & Mathias, 2000). This may be a learned behavior for gaining attention to communicate the presence of pain. If an individual displays atypical pain behaviors and reacts differently to pain, it cannot be concluded that she is not experiencing pain (refer to the earlier described case of DG). In order to understand pain, the assessment tools of self-report, proxy report, observational methods, and physiological measures can be employed. Each of these methods has its advantages and disadvantages. A multidimensional approach in combining these evaluative tools would be more likely to reveal an overall, accurate picture of pain.

Far and away, the majority of measures reviewed here have been designed for assessment of acute pain states and they have focused on a limited domain of pain: intensity and frequency of pain. Other important aspects of the pain experience—affective and evaluative—have all but been ignored. Initial work by Wilkie, Holzemer, Tesler, Ward, Paul, and Savedra (1990) has shown it is possible to distinguish these dimensions, at least with children above the age of eight. The other domains identified for assessment by the Peds-IMMPACT group are only now beginning to be explored (Eccleston, Jordan, & Crombez, 2006; Gauntlett-Gilbert & Eccleston, 2007; Goubert, Eccleston, Vervoort, Jordan, & Crombez, 2006; Hermann et al., 2007; Sleed, Eccleston, Beecham, Knap, & Jordan, 2005; Tsao, Meldrum, Kim, & Zeltzer, 2007). These aspects, plus a greater focus on measures appropriate for chronic forms of pain in children and adolescents, with and without developmental disabilities, all merit further study.

Prediction of Chronic Pediatric Pain and Disability

The procedures reviewed above constitute the approaches, empirically researched, typically taken when assessing the presence and quantifying its amount. Most recently Miró, Huguet, and Nieto (2007) approached this measurement issue from a somewhat unique perspective. Noting the methodological problems that plague extant research (i.e., small sample sizes, varied and narrowed definitions of pain, and inadequate designs, data collection methods, and data analytic strategies), they sought to poll experts about the factors that were most important to consider.

Drawing upon the Delphi method, the sought opinions from participants who met either of two inclusion criteria: having conducted prior clinical research on the topic (as judged by serving as first or second author of at least two peer-reviewed journal articles, published between 1995–2005, addressing prediction of chronic pain and pain-related disability), or prior involvement in pain clinical work (as judged by having at least two years of experience in a pediatric pain program/service, with names initially drawn from the subscriber pain lists of the IASP Special Interest Group on Pain in Childhood and the Pediatric-Pain list serve). Participants identified at this level were asked to indicate others who might be approached (to see if they met either of the above criteria). The participants came from diverse professions (60% physicians, 25% psychologists, 13% nurses, with the remaining 2% coming from varied groups). Furthermore, there was considerable variability within their professional groupings, with participants coming from research and clinical practice settings, anesthesiology, epidemiology, nursing, oncology, rheumatology, rehabilitation, and so on.

A list of potential predictive factors was initially developed by reviewing the extant literature and then asking a small international multidisciplinary group of experts to add important items not yet included. This yielded 28 potential general predictors of chronic pain and/or pain-related disability, all operationalized to the extent possible. A larger list (in excess of 100) was then generated to best describe the 28 potential predictors, with these being re-examined by the expert panelists. Additional items and potential predictive factors were added at this step, and one item included earlier was omitted. A number of other iterations ensued (pilot and actual), consistent with the Delphi approach (wherein participation continues until there is stability in responding or there is no further appreciable gain in understanding, the point of diminishing returns, in economic terms), with the goal of identifying items that predicted chronicity, disability, both, or neither and the direction (positive or negative) and magnitude (value from 0 to 100) of the effect.

Although a number of items were rated as having value, in order to narrow the array of variables the authors compiled a final list of items most likely to determine pain persistence and disability. Items additionally had to meet the following criteria: the item had to be identified as important by more than three-quarters of the participants, the mean score assigned to the item had to be above the 75th percentile, and the coefficient of variation for the item had to be below the 25th percentile (as the lower the coefficient, the less the variation among respondents). The items that resulted from this analysis are reproduced in Table 15.7. Although the authors sought to identify "protective" factors in addition to factors having a negative influence, surprisingly only one positive influence surfaced: parental coping skills. It is important to note that this variable has not been addressed in the literature to date.

The factors exerting a negative influence on pain and disability fell within five groupings: (1) psychological characteristics of the child, (2) psychological characteristics of the parents, (3) characteristics of the pain experience itself, (4) characteristics of pain management, and (5) psychological factors related to the child's pain experience. Factors within groups 1, 3, and 5 have been the chief focus of research. Increasing the focus on

Table 15.7. Items considered as the most important ones to predict chronic pain and disability problems.

Unit of Analysis	Predictor Factors	Relationship with Chronic Pain	Items
Chronic pain Child	Traits of personality	R	20. The child has a tendency to somatize.
		R	34. The child has a depressive personality.
		R	1. The child has an anxious personality.
	Individual history	R	73. The child has a family history of chronic pain.
	Pain catastro-phizing	R	71. The child tends to dwell on the pain and magnify or exaggerate its threat or serious-ness. He/she is incapable of dealing with it.
	Pain attitudes	R	108. The child believes that his/her pain will persist over time.
	Characteristics of pain problem	R	42. The child's pain is constant.
Parents (or family)	Traits of personality	R	23. The parents are emotionally unstable.
	Pain catastro-phizing	R	109. The parents tend to dwell on and mag-nify or exaggerate the threat or seriousness of their child's pain. They are incapable of dealing with the child's pain.
Environ-ment	Characteristics of pain treatment	R	7. The child uses the health care services excessively for his pain complaints.
		R	30. The child's consumption of medicaments to relieve the pain is not appropriate. 77. Compliance with the therapy prescribed to treat the pain is low.
		R	123. The child and his/her parents have consulted numerous doctors about the pain but no one has found anything wrong.
	Consequences to pain behaviors	R	68. The child receives attention and/or other privileges immediately after expressing pain.
	Stressful environment	R	16. The child is subject to stress in his/her immediate environment (for example: family difficulties, problems at school).
Disability Child	Traits of personality	R	20. The child has a tendency to somatize.
		R	34. The child has a depressive personality.
	Pain coping skills	R	110. The child constantly avoids activities that involve moving the part of the body that hurts through fear of experiencing more pain.
	Pain catastro-phizing	R	71. The child tends to dwell on the pain and magnify or exaggerate its threat or serious-ness. He/she is incapable of dealing with it.
	Pain attitudes	R	66. The child believes he/she is disabled by the pain. 106. The child believes that pain means he is damaging him/herself and that he/she should avoid exercise.

(continued)

Table 15.7. (continued)

Unit of Analysis	Predictor Factors	Relationship with Chronic Pain	Items
Parents (or family)	Traits of personality	R	117. Parental anxiety is high.
	Pain coping skills	P	116. The parents are able to identify, assess and alleviate the child's pain.
	Pain catastrophizing	R	109. The parents tend to dwell on and magnify or exaggerate the threat or seriousness of their child's pain. They are incapable of dealing with the child's pain.
	Pain attitudes	R	5. The parents believe that pain incapacitates.
		R	91. When the child's parents are in pain they believe that they are in danger and that they should avoid exercise as much as possible.
	Disability	R	61. The parents are disabled as a result of their pain.

Abbreviations: R, Risk factor; P, protective factor.
NOTE: Items included in this table comply with the following criteria: 75% of participants agreement on the predictive nature of the item, the predictive power value attributed to the item lies above 75th percentile, and variation coefficient lies below 25th percentile.
Source: Reprinted from Miró et al., 2007. (Permission granted by American Pain Society)

factors within groups 2 and 4 may lead to enhanced understanding and pain outcomes. These and other directions pointed out within the body of this chapter all seem worthy of pursuit in the future. Finally, although it is not known whether these factors will apply uniformly across pain conditions, this is judged unlikely. Thus, future researchers need to examine applicability of these factors for varied pain disorders.

REFERENCES

Ambuel, B., Hamlett, K. W., Marx, C. M., & Blumer, J. L. (1992). Assessing distress in pediatric intensive care environments: The COMFORT scale. *Journal of Pediatric Psychology, 17*, 95–109.

Anand, K. J. S, & Craig, K. D. (1996). New perspectives on the definition of pain. *Pain, 67*, 3–6.

Andrasik, F., Burke, E. J., Attanasio, V., & Rosenblum, E. L. (1985). Child, parent, and physician reports of a child's headache pain: Relationships prior to and following treatment. *Headache, 25*, 421–425.

Andrasik, F., Lipchik, G. L., McCrory, D. C., & Wittrock, A. A. (2005). Outcome measurement in behavioral headache research: Headache parameters and psychosocial outcomes. *Headache, 45*, 429–437.

Andrasik, F., & Schwartz, M. S. (2006). Behavioral assessment and treatment of pediatric headache. *Behavior Modification, 30*, 93–113.

Applegate, H., Matson, J. M., & Cherry, K. E. (1999). An evaluation of functional variables affecting severe problem behaviors in adults with mental retardation by using the Questions about Behavioral Function Scale (QABF). *Research in Developmental Disabilities, 20,* 229–237.

Baccei, M., & Fitzgerald, M. (2006). Development of pain pathways and mechanisms. In S.B. McMahon & M. Koltzenburg (Eds.), *Wall and Melzack's textbook of pain* (5th ed., pp. 143–158). Amsterdam: Elsevier.

Baldridge, K., & Andrasik, F. (2008). Barriers to effective pain management in people with intellectual/developmental delays. Manuscript submitted for publication.

Beyer, J., & Aradine, C. (1986). Content validity of an instrument to measure young children's perceptions of the intensity of their pain. *Journal of Pediatric Nursing, 1,* 386–395.

Bieri, D., Reeve, R. A., Champion, D., Addicoat, L., & Ziegler, J. B. (1990). The Faces Pain Scale for the self-assessment of the severity of pain experienced by children: development, initial validation, and preliminary investigation for ratio scale properties. *Pain, 41,*139–150.

Bodfish, J. W., Harper, V. N., Deacon, J. M., Deacon, J. R., & Symons, F. J. (2006). Issues in pain assessment for adults with severe to profound mental retardation. In T. F. Oberlander & F. J. Symons (Eds.), *Pain in children and adults with developmental disabilities* (pp. 173–192). Baltimore, MD: Paul H. Brookes.

Bosch, J., Van Dyke, D. C., Smith, S. M., & Poulton, S. (1997). Role of medical conditions in the exacerbation of self-injurious behavior: An exploratory study. *Mental Retardation, 35,* 124–130.

Bottos, S., & Chambers, C. T. (2006). The epidemiology of pain in developmental disabilities. In T. F. Oberlander & F. J. Symons (Eds.), *Pain in children and adults with developmental disabilities* (pp. 67–87). Baltimore, MD: Paul H. Brookes.

Breau, L. M., Camfield, C. S., McGrath, P. J., & Finley, G. A. (2003). The incidence of pain in children with severe cognitive impairments. *Archives of Pediatric and Adolescent Medicine, 157,* 1219–1226.

Breau, L. M., Finley, G. A., McGrath, P. J., & Camfield, C. S. (2002). Validation of the non-communicating children's pain checklist-postoperative version. *Anesthesiology, 96,* 528–535.

Breau, L. M., MacLaren, J., McGrath, P. J., Camfield, C. S, & Finley, A. F. (2003). Caregivers' beliefs regarding pain in children with cognitive impairment: Relation between pain sensation and reaction increases with severity of impairment. *The Clinical Journal of Pain, 19,* 335–344.

Breau, L. M., McGrath, P. J., Camfield, C. S., & Finley, G. A. (2002). Psychometric properties of the non-communicating children's pain checklist-revised. *Pain, 99,* 349–357.

Breau, L. M., McGrath, P. J., Camfield, C., Rosmus, C., & Finley, G. A. (2000). Preliminary validation of an observational pain checklist for persons with cognitive impairments and inability to communicate verbally. *Developmental Medicine & Child Neurology, 42,* 609–616.

Breau, L. M., McGrath, P. J., & Zabalia, M. (2006). Assessing pediatric pain and developmental disabilities. In T. F. Oberlander & F. J. Symons (Eds.), *Pain in children and adults with developmental disabilities* (pp. 149–172). Baltimore, MD: Paul H. Brookes.

Carter, B., McArthur, E., & Cunliffe, M. (2002). Dealing with uncertainty: Parental assessment of pain in their children with profound special needs. *Journal of Advanced Nursing, 38,* 449–457.

Chambers, C. T., Giesbrecht, K., Craig, K. D., Bennett, S. M., & Huntsman, E. (1999). A comparison of faces scales for the measurement of pediatric pain: Children's and parents' ratings. *Pain, 83,* 25–35.

Chambers, C. T., Hardial, J., Craig, K. D., Court, C., & Montgomery, C. (2005). Faces scales for the measurement of postoperative pain intensity in children following minor surgery. *The Clinical Journal of Pain, 21,* 277–285.

Chambers, C. T., Reid, G. J., McGrath, P. J., & Finley, G. A. (1996). Development and preliminary validation of a postoperative pain measure for parents. *Pain, 68,* 307–313.

Cook, A. K. R., Niven, C. A., & Downs, M. G. (1999). Assessing the pain of people with cognitive impairment. *International Journal of Geriatric Psychiatry, 14,* 421–425.

Davies, D., & Evans, L. (2001). Assessing pain in people with profound learning disabilities. *British Journal of Nursing, 10,* 513–516.

Defrin, R., Pick, C. G., Peretz, C., & Carmeli, E. (2004). A quantitative somatosensory testing of pain threshold in individuals with mental retardation. *Pain, 108*, 58–66.

Dworkin, R. H., et al. (2005). Core outcome measures for chronic pain clinical trials: IMMPACT recommendations. *Pain, 113*, 9–19.

Eccleston C., Jordan, A. L., & Crombez, G. (2006). The impact of chronic pain on adolescents: A review of previously used measures. *Journal of Pediatric Psychology, 31*, 684–697.

Fanurik, D., Koh, J. L., Schmitz, M. L., Harrison, R. D., & Conrad, T. M. (1999). Children with cognitive impairment: Parent report of pain and coping. *Journal of Developmental and Behavioral Pediatrics, 20*, 228–234.

Fanurik, D., Koh, J. L., Schmitz, M. L., Harrison, R. D., Roberson, P. K., & Killebrew, P. (1999). Pain assessment and treatment in children with cognitive impairment: A survey of nurses' and physicians' beliefs. *The Clinical Journal of Pain, 15*, 304–312.

Fitzgerald, M., & Walker, S. (2006). Infant pain traces. *Pain, 125*, 204–205.

Flor, H., & Andrasik, F. (2006). Chronic pain. In M. E. Selzer, S. Clarke, L. G. Cohen, P. W. Duncan, & F. H. Gage (Eds.). *Textbook of neural repair and rehabilitation: Volume II: Medical rehabilitation* (pp. 219–230). NY: Cambridge University Press.

Foley, D. C., & McCutcheon, H. (2004). Detecting pain in people with an intellectual disability. *Accident and Emergency Nursing, 12*, 196–200.

Gauntlett-Gilbert, J., & Eccleston, C. (2007). Disability in adolescents with chronic pain: Patterns and predictors across different domains of functioning. *Pain, 131*, 132–141.

Gilbert-MacLeod, C. A., Craig, K. D., Rocha, E. M., & Mathias, M. D. (2000). Everyday pain responses in children with and without developmental delays. *Journal of Pediatric Psychology, 25*, 301–308.

Giusiano, B., Jimeno, M. T., Collignon, P., & Chau, Y. (1995). Utilization of a neural network in the elaboration of an evaluation scale for pain in cerebral palsy. *Methods Information in Medicine, 34*, 498–502.

Goodman, J. E., & McGrath, P. J. (1991). The epidemiology of pain in children and adolescents: A review. *Pain, 46*, 247–264.

Goubert, L., Eccleston, C., Vervoort, T., Jordan, A., & Crombez, G. (2006). Parental catastrophizing about their child's pain. The parent version of the Pain Catastrophizing Scale (PCS-P): A preliminary validation. *Pain, 123*, 254–263.

Hadden, K. L., & von Baeyer, C. L. (2002). Pain in children with cerebral palsy: Common triggers and expressive behaviors. *Pain, 99*, 281–288.

Hadjistavropoulos, T., von Baeyer, C., & Craig, K. D. (2001). Pain assessment in persons with limited ability to communicate. In D. C. Turk & R. Melzack (Eds.), *Handbook of pain assessment* (2nd ed., pp. 134–148). New York: Guilford Press.

Hennequin, M., Morin, C., & Feine, J. S. (2000). Pain expression and stimulus localization in individuals with Down's syndrome. *Lancet, 356*, 1882–1887.

Hermann, C., Hohmeister, J., Demirakca, S., Zohsel, K., & Flor, H. (2006). Long-term alteration of pain sensitivity in school-aged children with early pain experiences. *Pain, 125*, 278–285.

Hester, N. (1979). The preoperational child's reaction to immunization. *Nursing Research, 28*, 250–255.

Hicks, C. L., von Baeyer, C. L., Spafford, P. A., van Korlaar, I., & Goodenough, B. (2001). The Faces Pain Scale-Revised: Toward a common metric in pediatric pain measurement. *Pain, 93*, 173–183.

Hodgins, M. J. (2002). Interpreting the meaning of pain severity scores. *Pain and Research Management, 7*, 192–198.

International Association for the Study of Pain. (1986). Classification of chronic pain: descriptions of chronic pain syndromes and definitions of pain terms. *Pain (Suppl. 3)*, S1–S225.

Katz, E. R., Kellerman, J., & Siegel, S. E. (1980). Behavioral distress in children with cancer undergoing medical procedures: Developmental considerations. *Journal of Consulting and Clinical Psychology, 48*, 356–365.

Katz, J. N. (2006). Lumbar disc disorders and low-back pain: Socioeconomic factors and consequences. *Journal of Bone and Joint Surgery, 88-A (Suppl)*, 21–24.

LaChapelle, D. L., Hadjistavropoulos, T, & Craig, K. D. (1999). Pain measurement in persons with intellectual disabilities. *The Clinical Journal of Pain, 15,* 13–23.

LeBaron, S., & Zeltzer, L. (1984). Assessment of acute pain and anxiety in children and adolescents by self-reports, observer reports, and a behavior checklist. *Journal of Consulting and Clinical Psychology, 52,* 729–738.

Malviya, S., Voepel-Lewis, T., Burke, C., Merkel, S., & Tait, A. R. (2006). The revised FLACC observational pain tool: Improved reliability and validity for pain assessment in children with cognitive impairment. *Pediatric Anesthesia, 16,* 258–265.

McGrath, P. A., Seifert, C. E., Speechley, K. N., Booth, J. C., Stitt, L., & Gibson, M. C. (1996). A new analogue scale for assessing children's pain: An initial validation study. *Pain, 64,* 435–443.

McGrath, P. A. (1999). Chronic pain in children. In I. K. Crombie, P. R. Croft, S. J. Linton, L. LeResche, & M. Von Korff (Eds.), *Epidemiology of pain* (pp. 81–101). Seattle: IASP Press.

McGrath, P. J., & Finley, G. A. (1999). Chronic and recurrent pain in children and adolescents. In P. J. McGrath & G. A. Finely (Eds.), *Chronic and recurrent pain in children and adolescents: Progress in pain research and management* (Vol. 13; pp. 1–4). Seattle: IASP Press.

McGrath, P. J., Johnson, G., Goodman, J. T., Schillinger, J., Dunn, J., & Chapman, J. (1985). CHEOPS: A behavioral scale for rating postoperative pain in children. In H. L. Fields, R. Dubner, & F. Cervero (Eds.), *Advances in pain research and therapy* (Vol. 9; pp. 395–402). New York: Raven Press.

McGrath, P. J., Rosmus, C., Camfield, C., Campbell, M. A., & Hennigar, A. (1998). Behaviours caregivers use to determine pain in non-verbal, cognitively impaired individuals. *Developmental Medicine & Child Neurology, 40,* 340–343.

McGrath, P. J., & Unruh, A. M. (2006). Measurement and assessment of paediatric pain. In S. B. McMahon & M. Koltzenburg (Eds.), *Wall and Melzack's textbook of pain* (5th ed.; pp. 305–315). London: Churchill Livingstone.

McGrath, P. J., Walco, G. A., Turk, D. C., Dworkin, R. H., Brown, M. T., Davidson, K., Eccleston, C., Finely, G. A., Goldschneider, K., Haverkos, L., Hertz, S. H., Ljungman, G, Palermo, T., Rappaport, B. A., Rhodes, T., Schechter, N., Scott, J., Sethna, N., Svensson, O. K., Stinson, J., von Baeyer, C. L., Walker, L., Weisman, S., White, R. E., Zajicek, A., & Zeltzer, L. (2008). Core outcome domains and mearures for pediatric acute and chronic/recuurrent pain clinical trials: PedIMMPACT recommendations. *Journal of Pain, 9,* 771–783.

Merkel, S. I., Voepel-Lewis, T., Shayevitz, J. R., & Malviya, S. (1997). The FLACC: A behavioral scale for scoring postoperative pain in young children. *Pediatric Nursing, 23,* 293–297.

Metsähonkala, L., Sillanpää, M., & Tuominen, J. (1997). Headache diary in diagnosis of childhood migraine. *Headache, 37,* 240–244.

Miró, J., Huguet, A., & Nieto, R. (2007). Predictive factors of chronic pediatric pain and disability: A Delphi poll. *Journal of Pain, 8,* 774–792.

Nader, R., Oberlander, T. F., Chambers, C. T., & Craig, K. D. (2004). Expression of pain in children with autism. *The Clinical Journal of Pain, 20,* 88–97.

Paclawskyj, T. R., Matson, J. L., Rush, K. S., Smalls, Y., & Vollmer, T. R. (2000). Questions about Behavioral Function (QABF): A behavioral checklist for functional assessment of aberrant behavior. *Research in Developmental Disabilities, 21,* 223–229.

Palermo, T. M., Valenzuela, D., & Stork, P. P. (2004). A randomized trial of electronic versus paper pain diaries in children: Impact on compliance, accuracy, and acceptability. *Pain, 107,* 213–219.

Penzien, D. B., Andrasik, F., Freidenberg, B. M., Houle, T. T., Lake, A. E., 3rd, Lipchik, G. L., Holroyd, K. A., Lipton, R. B., McCrory, D. C., Nash, J. M., Nicholson, R. A., Powers, S. W., Rains, J. C., & Wittrock, D. A. (2005). Guidelines for trials of behavioral treatments for recurrent headache, first edition: American Headache Society Behavioral Clinical Trials Workgroup. *Headache, 45,* S110–S132.

Perquin, C. W., Hazebroek-Kampschreur, A. A., Hunfeld, J. A., van Suijlekom-Smit, L. W., Passchier, J., & van der Wouden, J. C. (2000). Chronic pain among children and adolescents: Physician consultation and medication use. *Clinical Journal of Pain, 16,* 229–235.

Prkachin, K. M. (2005). The consistency of facial expressions in pain. In P. Ekman & E. L. Rosenberg (Eds.), What the face reveals: Basic and applied studies of spontaneous expression using the Facial Action Coding System (FACS) (2nd ed., pp. 181–197). New York: Oxford University Press.

Richardson, G. M., McGrath, P. J., Cunningham, S. J., & Humphreys, P. (1983). Validity of the headache diary for children. *Headache, 23*, 184–187.

Scott, P., Ansell, B., & Huskisson, E. (1977). Measurement of pain in juvenile chronic polyarthritis. *Annals of the Rheumatic Diseases, 36*, 186–187.

Sleed, M., Eccleston, C., Beecham, J., Knapp, M., & Jordan, A. (2005). The economic impact of chronic pain in adolescence: Methodological considerations and a preliminary costs-of-illness study. *Pain, 119*, 183–190.

Stallard, P., Williams, L., Lenton, S., & Velleman, R. (2001). Pain in cognitively impaired, non-communicating children. *Archives of Disease in Childhood, 85*, 460–462.

Stallard, P., Williams, L., Velleman, R., Lenton, S., & McGrath, P. J. (2002). Brief report: Behaviors identified by caregivers to detect pain in noncommunicating children. *Journal of Pediatric Psychology, 27*, 209–214.

Stallard, P., Williams, L., Velleman, R., Lenton, S., McGrath, P. J., & Taylor, G. (2002). The development and evaluation of the pain indicator for communicatively impaired children (PICIC). *Pain, 98*, 145–149.

Stanford, E. A., Chambers, C. T., & Craig, K. D. (2006). The role of developmental factors in predicting young children's use of a self-report scale for pain. *Pain, 120*, 16–23.

Stinson, J. N., Kavanagh T., Yamada, J., Gill, N., & Stevens, B. (2006). Systematic review of the psychometric properties, interpretability and feasibility of self-report pain intensity measures for use in clinical trials in children and adolescents. *Pain, 125*, 143–157.

Terstegen, C., Koot, H. M., de Boer, J. B., & Tibboel, D. (2003). Measuring pain in children with cognitive impairment: Pain response to surgical procedures. *Pain, 103*, 187–198.

Tsao, J. C. I., Meldrum, M., Kim, S. C., & Zeltzer, L. K. (2007). Anxiety sensitivity and health-related qualify of life in children with chronic pain. *The Journal of Pain, 8*, 814–823.

Turk, D., & Flor, H. (1999) Chronic pain: A biobehavioral perspective. R. J. Gatchel & D. C. Turk (Eds.), *Psychosocial factors in pain*. New York: Guilford Press.

Turk, D., et al. (2003). Core outcome domains for chronic pain clinical trials: IMMPACT recommendations. *Pain, 106*, 337–345.

Verhaak, P. F. M., Kerssens, J. J., Dekker, J., Sorbi, M. J., & Bensing, J. M. (1998). Prevalence of chronic benign pain disorder among adults: A review of the literature. *Pain, 77*, 231–239.

von Baeyer, C. L., & Spagrud, L. J. (2007). Systematic review of observational (behavioral) measures of pain for children and adolescents aged 3 to 18 years. *Pain, 127*, 140–150.

Williams, A. C., Davies, H. T., & Chadury, Y. (2000). Simple pain rating scales hide complex idiosyncratic meanings. *Pain, 85*, 457–463.

Wong, D., & Baker, C. (1988). Pain in children: Comparison of assessment scales. *Pediatric Nursing, 14*, 9–17.

Woolf, C. J., & Salter, M. W. (2000). Neuronal plasticity: Increasing the gain in pain. *Science, 288*, 1765–1769.

Zwakhalen, S. M. G., van Dongen, K. A. J., Hamers, J. P. H., & Abu-Saad, H. H. (2004). Pain assessment in intellectually disabled people: Non-verbal indicators. *Journal of Advanced Nursing, 45*, 236–245.

16

Assessment of Pediatric Feeding Disorders

CATHLEEN C. PIAZZA and HENRY S. ROANE

Eating is a genetically programmed behavior that is necessary for survival. But eating has a larger role in human behavior in that it forms the back-drop for many of the social interactions individuals have with one another. In fact, most of our major life events (e.g., birthdays, anniversaries, retire-ment) are marked in the context of food, and food often dominates our cultural (e.g., Thanksgiving) and religious (e.g., Christmas, Bar Mitzvah) celebrations (Ivanovic et al., 2004). But what happens when eating is dysfunctional? How does disordered eating affect both the physiological and socioemotional functioning of humans, particularly when those prob-lems emerge in infancy? The purpose of this chapter is to describe the various eating problems that occur in children and discuss how eating problems are assessed in children.

The term *feeding disorder* is used to describe dysfunctional eating that occurs in childhood. By contrast, *eating disorder* is the diagnostic label for dysfunctional eating in adolescents and young adults (which is covered elsewhere in this volume). The characteristics of a feeding disorder are heterogeneous, which has made the development of a diagnostic nosology difficult. That is, children with feeding disorders may display a wide variety of behaviors such as refusal to eat, refusal to eat certain types or textures of food, dependence on a limited or developmentally inappropriate source of nutrition (e.g., bottle dependence in a three-year-old), and skill deficits

CATHELEEN C. PIAZZA and HENRY S. ROANE • Munroe–Meyer Institute for Genetics and Rehabilitation and University of Nebraska Medical Cent

J.L. Matson et al. (eds.), *Assessing Childhood Psychopathology and Developmental Disabilities*, DOI: 10.1007/978-0-387-09528-8, © Springer Science+Business Media, LLC 2009 such as inability to self-feed. Problematic feeding behavior may occur in isolation or in combination with a variety of medical (gastroesophageal reflux disease), oral motor (apraxia), or behavioral (tantrums) issues.

PREVALENCE AND ETIOLOGY

Prevalence

The prevalence of feeding disorders is difficult to estimate due in part to the heterogeneity of the problem. Esparo et al. (2004) estimated that the prevalence of nonmedically related feeding problems was 4.8%, based on questionnaires completed with caregivers of 851 Spanish school-aged children. Other estimates suggest that approximately 25% to 35% of typically developing children and approximately 33% to 80% of children with developmental delays exhibit feeding problems of varying severity (Gouge & Ekvall, 1975; Palmer & Horn, 1978). In fact, most children will exhibit difficulties during meals at some point during infancy or childhood (Wilson, 1994). Some of these problems resolve in the absence of intervention (the child will "grow out of it"). But for a small number of children, feeding difficulties result in a number of negative consequences such as malnutrition, dehydration, and long-term cognitive and behavioral disabilities (Dobbing, 1985; Ivanovic et al., 2004; Ivanovic et al., 2000; Lanes, 2004; Levitsky, 1995; Morgan, 1990; Winick, 1969). For these children, feeding problems are not likely to resolve in the absence of intervention and may be related to life-long struggles with eating (Dahl, 1987; Dahl & Kristiansson, 1987; Dahl & Sundelin, 1992; Rydell, Dahl, & Sundelin, 2001).

Etiology

Recent studies have suggested that the etiology of feeding disorders is complex and multifactorial, and attempts have been made to construct classification systems that account for a wider range of feeding problems and the potential complex etiology of these problems (Burklow, McGrath, Allred, & Rudolph, 2002; Field, Garland, & Williams, 2003; Rommel, De Meyer, Feenstra, & Veereman-Wauters, 2003). For example, Rommel et al. (2003) reviewed the medical records of 700 children under the age of ten years referred for the assessment and treatment of severe feeding difficulties. The authors classified the feeding problems as medical ("specific diagnoses in the field of pediatrics or pediatric subspecialties based on clinical findings and confirmed by diagnostic examinations when indicated") for 86% of children, oral-motor ("any oropharyngeal functional abnormality diagnosed by the feeding specialist") for 61% of children, and/or behavioral ("behavior that crossed current norms and rules in specific situations in which the severity was determined by the frequency, duration, extent, and way in which the behavior harmed the patient and his or her environment psychologically") for 18% of children. Combined causes of the feeding problem (e.g., medical–behavioral) occurred in over 60% of children.

The most frequently identified medical problem was gastrointestinal conditions diagnosed for 54.3% of children with 33% of this group diagnosed with gastroesophageal reflux disease (GERD).

Field, Garland, and Williams (2003) examined the records of 349 children ages 1 month to 12 years who had been evaluated by an interdisciplinary team for a feeding disorder and classified children according to topography of feeding problem. Their data suggested that 34% of children exhibited food refusal (refusal to eat all or most foods, such that the child failed to meet his or her caloric or nutritional needs), 21% exhibited selectivity by type (eating a narrow range of food that was nutritionally inappropriate), 26% exhibited selectivity by texture (refusal to eat food textures that were developmentally appropriate), 44% exhibited oral motor problems (problems with chewing, tongue movement, lip closure or other oral motor areas as determined by a speech and/or occupational therapist), and 23% exhibited dysphagia (problems with swallowing, documented by a history of aspiration pneumonia, and/or barium swallow study). Similar to the findings of Rommel et al. (2003), the most commonly identified medical problem was GERD (51%).

Burklow, Phelps, Schultz, McConnell, and Rudolph (1998) evaluated data from 103 children seen in an interdisciplinary clinic for children with feeding disorders. They categorized children as having structural abnormalities (anatomic abnormalities of the structures associated with eating and feeding, such as micrognathia, cleft palate), neurological abnormalities (feeding problems associated with central nervous system insult or musculoskeletal disorders such as cerebral palsy or pervasive developmental disorder), behavior issues (feeding difficulties from psychosocial factors such as poor environmental stimulation, lack of available food, phobias, negative feeding behaviors shaped and/or maintained by reinforcement), cardiorespiratory problems (feeding difficulties associated with diseases and symptoms that compromise the cardiovascular and respiratory systems such as bronchopulmonary dysplasia), and metabolic dysfunction (feeding difficulties associated with metabolic diseases and syndromes such as hereditary fructose intolerance).

The majority of children had multicategorical feeding problems with 30% categorized as structural–neurological–behavioral, 27% as neurological–behavioral, 12% as behavioral, 9% as structural–behavioral, and 8% as structural–neurological. The results of these studies confirm that multiple factors contribute to the development of feeding problems, including medical, oral-motor, and behavioral difficulties. These findings also indicate that biological factors play an important role in the etiology of feeding disorders. In fact, the high prevalence of chronic medical problems that affect the gastrointestinal system directly (e.g., GERD, food allergies, malabsorption) suggests that these problems may cause feeding disorders. For example, GERD causes the release of excess acid into the stomach or esophagus and often worsens after a meal. Thus, a child with GERD may learn to associate eating with vomiting and pain.

Chronic medical problems also may contribute to the onset or maintenance of feeding problems because infants with complex medical histories are subjected to numerous invasive diagnostic tests and procedures that may involve manipulation of the face and mouth (e.g., laryngoscopy). To illustrate, from the child's perspective a spoon may be indistinguishable from a laryngoscope or other devices, which are used during invasive tests and procedures and which may be associated with discomfort or pain. Parents of chronically hospitalized and medically fragile children often report "oral aversions" that affect feeding and other activities associated with the face and mouth (e.g., tooth brushing, face washing). A number of studies have shown a relation between feeding difficulties and medical problems such as intraventricular hemorrhage and central nervous system damage (Braun & Palmer, 1985), fetal alcohol syndrome (Van Dyke, Mackay, & Ziaylek, 1982), prematurity (Braun & Palmer, 1985; Dodrill, McMahon, Ward, Weir, Donovan, & Riddle, 2004), bronchopulmonary dysplasia and respiratory problems, enteral or parenteral feedings (Bazyk, 1990; Benoit, Wang, & Zlotkin, 2000; Blackman & Nelson, 1985; Geertsma, Hyams, Pelletier, & Reiter, 1985), and cardiac problems (D'Antonio, 1979).

The high prevalence of oral-motor dysfunction also appears to contribute to the development of feeding problems. Children with oral-motor dysfunction have difficulties with the motor component of eating (e.g., swallowing, inability to lateralization of food, tongue thrust, and sucking), which may preclude eating altogether or may cause eating to be effortful or uncomfortable (e.g., due to choking or gagging). Pre-existing oral-motor dysfunction may be exacerbated when the child refuses to eat, which contributes further to the child's failure to develop appropriate oral motor skills. That is, the child does not have the opportunity to practice the skill of eating and does not develop the oral motor skills to become a competent eater. Furthermore, refusal to eat may lead to failure to thrive (FTT), and undernourished children lack the energy to become competent eaters (Troughton & Hill, 2001).

Refusal behavior (e.g., batting at the spoon, crying, head turning) may emerge when eating is paired with an aversive experience (e.g., pain, discomfort), but feeding problems also occur in children who have no identifiable medical or oral motor difficulties. Studies by Dahl and colleagues (Dahl, 1987; Dahl & Kristiansson, 1987; Dahl & Sundelin, 1992) suggest that feeding problems can be identified in early infancy, feeding problems in infancy are related to poor growth at age two, and feeding problems in infancy may persist for up to four years if left untreated.

One puzzling question is why some children grow out of their feeding problems and some do not. Some authors have hypothesized that children with no known organic cause of their eating problem have underlying dysfunctions of appetite regulation. Drewer, Kasese-Hara, and Wright (2002) showed that children with FTT ate less total food than age and sex-matched controls, although the foods consumed tended to be equivalent in caloric density. In addition, caregivers of the FTT children offered as much food and spent as much or more time feeding their child as did the controls, suggesting that the FTT was not a function of neglect or insufficient provision of calories.

Kasese-Hara, Wright, and Drewett (2002) tested the hypothesis that children with FTT lack a normal sensitivity to hunger and satiation cues by comparing energy compensation in children with FTT and age and sex-matched controls with normal weight. Children who ate typically altered their energy intake in response to their energy intake in a previous meal, whereas children with FTT did not. The authors suggested that these results supported the hypothesis that children with FTT lack the normal responses to hunger and satiety cues that would allow them to effectively regulate their energy intake.

Taken together, these results suggest that a small number of children will exhibit feeding problems that are severe and may not resolve without treatment, and the presence of feeding problems early on is correlated with eating disorders in adolescence and adulthood. There are a number of medical problems that increase a child's risk for the development of feeding problems. In addition, some children without diagnosed medical problems will display persistent, severe feeding problems. Disorders of appetite regulation may play a role in these problems.

Diagnostic Considerations in the Assessment of Feeding Disorders

Early attempts to classify feeding problems focused on a dichotomy between so-called organic (OFTT) and nonorganic failure to thrive (NOFTT). NOFTT was a diagnosis of exclusion in this classification system in that it was applied when no medical cause could be identified for growth failure (Powell, Low, & Speers, 1987). One underlying assumption was that NOFTT was the result of the failure of the mother to provide adequate nutrition to the child (Skuse, 1985). A typical workup to distinguish OFTT from NOFTT was to conduct numerous tests to ascertain if there was an underlying medical problem that may account for the FTT. If the medical tests were negative, then a typical second step would be to feed the child (often during an inpatient hospitalization) to determine if the child could gain weight under controlled and structured conditions. The child would be diagnosed with NOFTT if he or she gained weight under these circumstances. However, the dichotomy of organic and nonorganic FTT is inadequate for a number of reasons.

First, the dichotomy of organic and nonorganic FTT is not prescriptive. Identification of an organic etiology for the FTT may define a set of medical interventions that would treat the identified physiological problem. However, the presence or absence of an organic cause of a feeding problem does not inform a method of feeding the child that will result necessarily in weight gain. That is, many children continue to refuse food or demonstrate inadequate caloric intake even when medical causes of FTT are treated (e.g., an acid blocker to treat reflux disease). Children who experience negative consequences during eating (e.g., when vomiting is paired with intake as a result of reflux) often continue to refuse food even after the medical problem resolves.

Second, demonstrating that the child gains weight in the hospital may be useful in determining that the child can gain weight from a physiological standpoint (e.g., the child does not have a metabolic disease that negatively affects weight gain). However, the demonstration that the child gains weight in the hospital does not identify the variables that contributed to the child's poor weight gain outside the hospital. In some cases, a child's failure to gain weight in the home may be a function of inadequate provision of calories. On the other hand, a child's failure to gain weight in the home may have other causes (e.g., oral motor dysfunction, refusal behavior). Weight gain in the hospital does not result in a discrimination among these various causes that contribute to poor weight gain at home. In contrast, studies have not shown a consistent association between psychosocial factors (e.g., provision of inadequate calories, dysfunctional family) and nonorganic FTT (Pollitt, Eichler, & Chan, 1975; Ramsay, Gisel, & Boutry, 1993; Singer, Song, Hill, & Jaffe, 1990).

Third, organic and nonorganic classifications apply only to children whose growth is affected by the feeding problem. Some children evince feeding problems in the absence of growth failure. For example, children with severe food selectivity (e.g., child eats only French fries) may gain weight adequately due to the high caloric density of consumed foods. Nevertheless, a child with severe selectivity still would be at risk for nutritional (as opposed to caloric) deficits. Organic and inorganic dichotomies fail to capture the wide variety and complexity of problems that may be characteristic of a feeding disorder (Burklow, Phelps, Schultz, McConnell, & Rudolph, 1998; Rommel, 2003).

More recent classification systems such as the *Diagnostic and Statistical Manual of Mental Disorders, 4th Edition* (*DSM–IV–TR*) also are limited in terms of capturing the heterogeneity of feeding problems. The *DSM–IV–TR* diagnosis of Feeding Disorder of Infancy and Childhood (307.59) is described as a "persistent failure to eat adequately, as reflected in significant failure to gain weight or significant weight loss over at least 1 month" with an onset prior to age six (American Psychiatric Association, 2000). *DSM–IV–TR* criteria for diagnosis of a feeding disorder exclude children with a medical condition severe enough to account for the feeding disturbance. The diagnostic criteria also specify that the feeding problem cannot be accounted for by another mental disorder or lack of available food. Thus, this diagnosis only applies to a small percentage of children with feeding disorders; those who fail to gain weight but have no other concomitant medical condition.

Yet, a large number of children with feeding problems present with concomitant medical conditions (Rommel et al., 2003) and some children with significant feeding problems do not have problems with growth failure, yet do not consume any calories by mouth (e.g., a child who is gastrostomy -tube dependent). The *DSM* diagnosis suffers from some of the same shortcomings as the organic/inorganic classification in that the diagnosis does not inform treatment. Finally, the *DSM* diagnosis lacks specificity with respect to some of the essential features of the diagnosis, such as defining the parameters of a "lack of weight gain" or a "significant" weight loss. Thus, determination of inadequate growth is left up to the judgment of the clinician. Likewise, the criteria also do not specify what constitutes a "medical condition severe enough to account for the feeding disorder."

The term "feeding difficulties and mismanagement" (783.3) is used in the *International Classification of Diseases, 10th Revision* (World Health Organization, 1993). In this classification system, feeding problems of an inorganic nature are excluded from the diagnosis. Again, this classification system suffers from the same shortcomings described for *DSM–IV–TR* with even less information for the clinician to use to apply the diagnosis.

In sum, existing classification systems are inadequate with respect to the spectrum that includes many children with feeding disorders. These systems do not provide criteria that reflect the heterogeneity of potential feeding problems, do not account for the complex etiology of feeding problems, and they lack sufficient specificity in terms of operationally defining the criteria for the diagnosis. Most important, the extant classification systems are not prescriptive for treatment development. That is, these systems provide clinicians with a limited categorization of feeding disorders and offer no support for developing interventions based on the presenting problem.

One method that can be used to evaluate the extent to which a child's eating behavior is inappropriate is to compare the child's behavior to developmental norms for eating (Carruth, 2002; Gisel, 1988; Young, 2000). For example, Carruth and Skinner (2002) interviewed mothers of 98 healthy children at one- to four-month intervals. Mothers reported child intake for the previous 24 hours and also provided information about the emergence of a number of feeding-related behaviors. The mean ages and ranges when each skill emerged are described in Table 16.1.

Reau, Senturia, Lebailly, and Kaufer-Christoffel (1996) conducted a survey of the feeding patterns of infants and toddlers, using a questionnaire developed by the authors. The results of the survey suggested that the average meal length was less than 30 minutes for 90% of the participants. Parents who reported problematic feeding behaviors (e.g., "Is not always hungry at mealtime, does not always enjoy a feeding, has strong food preferences") at both 6 and 12 months had children who ate more

Table 16.1. Fine motor and oral-motor development related to feeding behaviors.

SKILL	MEAN AGE (Months)	RANGE (Months)
Opens mouth when spoon approaches lips	4.46	0.5–9.0
Tongue moves gently back and forth as food enters mouth	4.85	2.0–10.0
Keeps food in moth and is not re-fed	5.72	0.5–10.5
Reaches for spoon when hungry	5.47	2.5–9.5
Feeds self cookies or crackers	7.7	4.0–14.0
Brings top lip down on spoon to remove food	7.73	4.0–16.0
Eats foods without gagging	8.44	6.0–12.0
Uses finger to rake food toward self	8.67	5.0–20.0
Eats food with tiny lumps without gagging	8.7	4.8–15.5
Puts finger in mouth to move food and keep it in	9.3	4.0–18.0
Chews softer foods, keeps most in mouth	9.42	6.0–14.0
Chews firmer foods, keeps most in mouth	10.53	4.0–16.0
Chews and swallows firmer foods without choking	12.17	7.5–20.0
Uses fingers to self-feed soft, chopped food	13.52	9.5–20.0
Brings side of spoon to mouth	14.37	9.0–20.0
Chews foods that produce juice	15.28	9.5–23.0
Picks up, dips foods, and brings to mouth	16.42	10.0–23.0
Scoops puddings and brings to mouth	17.05	11.0–24.0

Source: Adapted from Carruth, B. R., & Skinner, J. D. (2002).

slowly than the other toddlers without reported feeding difficulties at those ages. The finding that meal length is correlated with feeding problems has been replicated in other studies (Powers et al., 2002, 2005; Stark et al., 1997; Young, 2000). Therefore, meal length may be a useful screening tool for the identification of feeding problems.

METHODS OF ASSESSING OF FEEDING DISORDERS

Questionnaires

Several authors have developed and used questionnaires and rating scales (Archer, Rosenbaum, & Streiner, 1991; Crist, & Napier-Phillips, A., 2001; Matson & Kuhn, 2001; Powers et al., 2002) to assess child behavior at mealtimes. For example, the Behavioral Pediatric Feeding Assessment Scale (BPFAS; Crist, McDonnell, Beck, Gillespie, Barrett, & Mathews, 1994) consists of 25 items that describe the child's behavior (e.g., "My child will try new foods") and 10 items that describe parents' feelings about or strategies for dealing with feeding problems (e.g., "I disagree with other adults about how to feed my child"), which caregivers rate on a 5-point-Likert scale (ranging from "never" to "always"). The caregiver also indicates if the behavior in question is a problem by circling yes or no.

Crist and Napier-Phillips (2001) used the BPFAS to evaluate the feeding behavior of children with and without feeding problems. The results showed that parents of children with a feeding disorder rated feeding problems as occurring more frequently (i.e., based on Likert-scale scores) and rated more behaviors as problems (i.e., yes/no rating) relative to parents of children in the normative sample. Powers et al., (2002) used the BPFAS and found significant differences between parental report of mealtime behavior (frequency and number of problems) in children diagnosed with Type 1 diabetes relative to healthy controls. Powers et al. (2005) also found the same significant differences for parent-report of mealtime behavior when comparing a group of children diagnosed with cystic fibrosis (CF) relative to a healthy control group on the BPFAS.

The Children's Eating Behavior Inventory (CEBI; Archer, Rosenbaum, & Streiner, 1991) assesses child, parent, and family variables related to eating and mealtime problems across a broad age span, and a variety of developmental and medical conditions. The inventory consists of 40 items related to eating and mealtime problems in children, with 28 items in the "child domain" (e.g., "My child enjoys eating, my child vomits at mealtimes") and 12 items in the "parent domain" (e.g., "I get upset when my child doesn't eat", "I feel confident my child eats enough"). The items are rated on a 5-point Likert scale indicating how often the behavior occurs, and parents also indicate whether any individual issue is a problem (yes/no).

Archer et al. (1991) compared the ratings of 206 mothers of nonclinic children (typically developing children recruited from community pediatricians) with the ratings of 110 mothers of clinic-referred children (children presenting for services in outpatient pediatric and mental health clinics). The comparison of the Likert ratings was significant, and mothers of children in the clinic group endorsed more items as problematic than those in the nonclinic group. Archer and Szatmari (1990) further showed that scores on the CEBI changed following intervention for the feeding disorder for one child undergoing treatment.

The Screening Tool of Feeding Problems (STEP; Matson & Kuhn, 2001) was developed to identify feeding problems in individuals with mental retardation. The scale consists of 23 items within five categories (aspiration risk, selectivity, feeding skills, food refusal related behavior problems, nutrition-related behavior problems) that describe feeding problems common to individuals with mental retardation. Items are rated for frequency and severity, using a Likert scale. Matson and Kuhn (2001) used the STEP to assess the feeding behavior of 570 individuals diagnosed with mental retardation. The test–retest reliability of the STEP was 0.72.

Questionnaires such as the ones reviewed above have the advantage of being relatively easy to use and time efficient. However, the use of questionnaires is less consistent with a behavioral model of assessment, which relies more often on direct observation of behavior (Fernandez-Ballesteros, 2004). By contrast, questionnaires may include items that refer to constructs or that describe behavior more broadly. Thus, questionnaires may not provide specificity with respect to identification, description, and quantification of target behaviors and their respective antecedents and consequences. For example, a questionnaire may identify that the child exhibits refusal behavior (e.g., parent endorses an item such as "My child refuses to eat") but endorsement of this item does not indicate how often refusal occurs, what the specific behaviors are that constitute refusal (e.g., child clenches teeth, says "No", turns head), and what the antecedents and consequences are for the target behavior.

Furthermore, the use of information derived from questionnaires for treatment prescription has not been tested and the sensitivity of questionnaires to changes that occur following intervention is unclear. For example, a treatment that produces a reduction in refusal from 100% of bites to 50% of bites may not be reflected in an item such as "My child refuses to eat" inasmuch as refusal behavior continues to occur at some level. Nevertheless, questionnaires may be useful in some situations, particularly when efficiency is of primary concern (e.g., screening a large group of children).

Direct Observation

Direct observation provides the most specificity in term of describing and quantifying behavior (Freeman & Miller, 2002). For example, Powers et al. (2005) compared the behavior of 34 infants and toddlers with cystic fibrosis to a matched community sample of same-aged peers. The dependent variables coded during the direct observation were parent behaviors (i.e., direct commands, indirect commands, coaxes, parent talks, reinforcement, physical prompts, feeds) and child's eating behaviors (i.e., noncompliance to direct commands, food refusals/complaints, requests for food, child talks, child away from table/food). There were no differences with respect to child behaviors for the CF and community sample; however, parents of children with CF gave more direct commands to eat relative to the parents of the children in the community sample.

Young and Drewett (2000) collected direct observation data at four mealtimes for 30 children ages 50–57 weeks to describe mealtime behavior in one-year-old children. The dependent variables were feeds self (child grasps spoon/fork, brings it toward the mouth without assistance, and places it in the mouth), accept (child takes spoon/food into mouth after caregiver has placed it in or near the child's mouth), refuse (child fails to open mouth to allow food to enter), reject (child expels spoon or food from mouth), drink (child has a drink of liquid from a cup or bottle), give (caregiver brings spoon/food to child's mouth), and retract (caregiver withdraws spoon/food/cup after failure to gain child's attention or child refuses bite/drink). The results of the study showed that there was a high level of variability for child feeding behavior, and the authors suggested that more than one meal should be observed to obtain an accurate representation of feeding behavior in young children.

Sanders (1993) observed the mealtime behavior of toddlers and preschool-aged children with and without feeding problems. The observed behaviors included 11 disruptive child feeding behaviors (e.g., noncompliance, complaint, refuses food, spits/vomits), six appropriate child feeding behaviors (e.g., requests food, chews), six aversive parent behaviors (e.g., aversive contact, aversive vague instruction), and nine nonaversive parent behaviors (e.g., praise, social attention). Analysis of behavior of the two groups showed that the children identified as problem feeders had significantly higher levels of disruptive behavior, food refusal, noncompliance, complaining, oppositional behavior, and playing with food, and lower rates of chewing. Parents of children with a feeding disorder had higher levels of negative and positive vague instructions, negative physical contact, negative prompting, negative eating comments, and negative social attention.

Direct observation provides a more precise quantification of child and parent behavior during mealtimes than those obtained from questionnaires. Even though the specific dependent variables differed from study to study, there are some commonalities to the variables of interest. Most studies identify a series of child inappropriate behavior related directly to the food (e.g., refusal or expulsion of food), other inappropriate behavior (e.g., disruption), and appropriate behavior (e.g., acceptance of food). Likewise, these studies identified classes of behavior related to caregivers, including caregiver inappropriate behavior (e.g., removal of a bite) and caregiver appropriate behavior (e.g., praise for acceptance). Descriptive categorizations of child and caregiver feeding behaviors, such as those described above, permit the quantification of variables of interest when studying the course of a child's feeding difficulty. Thus, as compared to information obtained from questionnaires, the information obtained from direct observation should result in the development of a more precise measurement system for identifying the behaviors of interest during mealtimes and should be sensitive to changes behavior following intervention.

Functional Assessment

The term functional assessment refers to a specific type of direct observation. The functional assessment of behavior provides an even more specific method of identifying the environmental correlates of inappropriate mealtime behavior. Traditional functional assessment procedures manipulate antecedent and/or consequent events associated with a behavior problem (Iwata, Dorsey, Slifer, Bauman, & Richman, 1994). For example, Munk and Repp (1994) conducted a functional assessment to identify the specific characteristics that were associated with the limited intake of five individuals. The authors presented 10 to 12 foods at different textures to each participant. The assessed textures included junior (blended into a puree), ground (blended to a semisolid consistency like ground beef), chopped fine (.25-in. pieces), and regular (.5-in. pieces or larger). The dependent variables for the assessment were acceptance, rejection, expulsion, and other negative behaviors. The results of the assessment showed that one participant's limited intake was characterized by selectivity by texture, one by selectivity by type, two by selectivity by type and texture, and one participant had total refusal.

Piazza, Fisher et al. (2003) directly tested the role of reinforcement in the maintenance of the feeding problems of 15 children. First, the authors conducted descriptive assessments of child and parent behavior during meals. The results of the descriptive assessments suggested that parents responded to child inappropriate behavior with one or more of the following consequences: (a) allowing escape from bites of food or the meal, (b) coaxing or reprimanding (e.g., "Eat your peas, they are good for you"), or (c) providing the child with a toy or preferred food. The effects of these consequences on child behavior then were tested systematically using analogue functional analyses.

During the analogue assessment, sessions were 5 min in length and a therapist presented bites approximately once every 30 s. Acceptance (the child opens his or her mouth and the entire bite is deposited within 5 s of the initial bite presentation) and mouth clean (no food or drink larger than the size of a pea visible in the child's mouth within 30 s of initial acceptance) resulted in brief praise ("Good job"). In the control condition, preferred toys based on the results of a preference assessment (Fisher et al., 1992) and adult attention were available continuously and inappropriate behavior resulted in no differential consequence. In the attention condition, inappropriate behavior resulted in 20 s of attention and the therapist removed the bite at the end of the 20-s interval. In the escape condition, inappropriate behavior resulted in 20 s of escape (i.e., the therapist removed the spoon). Lastly, in the tangible condition, inappropriate behavior resulted in 20 s of access to a tangible item and the therapist removed the bite at the end of the 20-s interval.

Functional analyses were useful for identifying the maintaining variables for inappropriate mealtime behavior for some children. Most of the children in the study (67%) showed differential responding during one or more functional analysis conditions. Piazza, Fisher et al. (2003) found negative reinforcement (in the form of escape from bites of food) as the most frequently identified (90%) maintaining variable for the inappropriate mealtime behavior exhibited by children who had differentiated functional analyses in the study; a finding consistent with prior research (Ahearn, Kerwin, Eicher, Shantz, & Swearingin, 1996a; Cooper et al., 1995b; Hoch, Babbitt, Coe, Krell, & Hackbert, 1994b; Piazza, Patel, Gulotta, Sevin, & Layer, 2003a; Reed et al., 2004a), which suggested the importance of the role of negative reinforcement in the maintenance of feeding disorders. However, multiple functions (i.e., access to adult attention or tangible items) also were identified for a significant number (80%) of the children who showed differential responding during functional analyses.

In subsequent unpublished investigation, Piazza and colleagues analyzed functional analysis data from 38 children who were admitted to an intensive day treatment program for the assessment and treatment of a pediatric feeding disorder. For all participants, the analogue functional analysis was conducted using the procedures described by in Piazza et al. (2003) within a pairwise design (Iwata, Duncan, Zarcone, Lerman, & Shore, 1994), which we found to be more time efficient. The results of the analyses are depicted in Figure 16.1. Ninety-eight percent (98%) of the functional analyses were differentiated; 2% of children had undifferentiated (undif) results.

Consistent with the results of Piazza, Fisher et al. (2003), negative reinforcement in the form of escape from bites, was identified as a reinforcer for 100% of children whose functional analyses were differentiated.

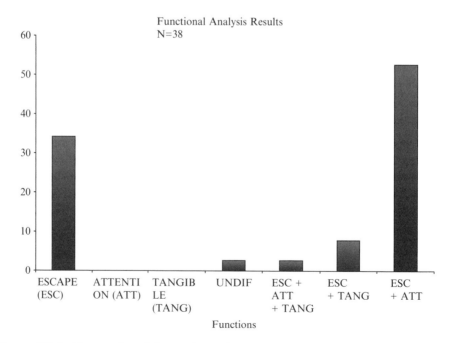

Figure 16.1. The results of the analogue functional analyses of 38 children admitted to an intensive day treatment program for the assessment and treatment of a pediatric feeding disorder.

Multiple functions in the form of escape, attention and tangible (esc + att + tang); escape and tangible (esc + tang); and escape and attention (esc + att) were identified for 2%, 9%, and 53% of participants, respectively. No children demonstrated sensitivity to attention only (att) or tangible (tang) only. The results of the study by Piazza, Fisher et al. (2003) and our additional pilot work suggested that negative reinforcement plays a primary role in the maintenance of feeding problems, and that a significant number of children with feeding disorders also may be sensitive to positive reinforcement.

Interdisciplinary Assessment

Functional assessment should play a primary role in the evaluation of feeding problems as noted above. However, the complexity of feeding problems necessitates a comprehensive interdisciplinary approach to understand all of the factors that may contribute to the problem. A thorough medical evaluation is necessary to rule out potential medical causes of the feeding problem. Aggressive behavioral treatment in the context of an ongoing medical problem may worsen the feeding problem. For example, behavioral treatment of a child who aspirates or feeding a child textures of foods that are inappropriate for the child's oral motor skills can cause life-threatening complications.

A thorough evaluation by a speech and language pathologist and/ or an occupational therapist is necessary to assess the adequacy of the child's oral motor skills and to assess the child's safety for oral feeding. In addition, speech and language pathologists and/or occupational therapists have the expertise necessary to identify textures of foods to present that are appropriate for the child's oral motor skills. In addition, some children present with medical disorders that necessitate highly specialized diets. Failure to follow these specialized diets can cause severe illness and sometimes death. Thus, a thorough evaluation by a dietitian also is critical to determine the child's caloric and nutritional needs.

Example of an Interdisciplinary Evaluation

The following is a brief example of an interdisciplinary evaluation as conducted in the Pediatric Feeding Disorders Program at the University of Nebraska Medical Center's Munroe–Meyer Institute. The intent of this case example is to provide an overview of an interdisciplinary evaluation and should not be considered a recommendation for discipline-specific evaluation of a feeding disorder. Individual professionals in each discipline always should determine the specificity and scope of their own evaluation. The Pediatric Feeding Disorders' interdisciplinary team consists of professionals who have specialized expertise and interest in the assessment and treatment of pediatric feeding disorders. Our interdisciplinary team consists of a dietician, occupational therapist, physician, behavioral psychologist, speech and language pathologist, and social worker.

Major goals for the physician's assessment are to (1) identify or rule out any underlying medical causes for the child's feeding problems, (2) assess the child's current level of nutrition, hydration, and growth, and (3) assess the child's safety for oral feeding. During the assessment, the physician conducts a comprehensive history and physical examination. Referrals may need to be made to specialists if a specific condition (e.g., referral to a geneticist for assessment of Silver–Russell syndrome) or disease (e.g., referral to an allergist for assessment of food allergy) is suspected and laboratory workups are completed as indicated. The physician obtains the child's height and weight, plots the child's growth parameters on a growth chart (Center for Disease Control and Prevention, 2000), and evaluates the adequacy of the child's growth, nutrition, and hydration. The physician generally will recommend necessary therapy related to the findings of the workup (e.g., prescribe Prevacid® for GERD). The physician also obtains information about current and previous medications, illnesses, surgeries, and hospitalizations. The physician provides a specific recommendation regarding the appropriateness of initiating feeding therapy.

Major goals for the dietitian are to (1) document the child's current level of caloric and nutritional intake, (2) document the timing and volume of feeds, (3) evaluate the adequacy of the child's intake with respect to calories, nutrition, and hydration, (4) evaluate the adequacy of the child's growth, and (5) identify any special dietary needs. We obtain a three-day food diary from the caregiver, which is brought to the initial evaluation. The dietician then can calculate the child's current level of calories, nutrients, and fluids based on the three-day food records.

Major goals for the occupational and/or speech therapist are to (1) assess the adequacy of the child's oral motor skills, (2) evaluate the child's ability to manage different types and textures of food and liquid, (3) identify any behaviors that may affect the child's intake such as choking or gagging, and (4) evaluate the child's safety for oral feeding. The evaluation of the child's safety for oral feeding cannot be overemphasized, and it is critical that evaluation of safety for oral feeding play a prominent role in the assessment.

In our program, we consider the social worker a critical member of the team. The social worker evaluates the family's ability and resources to participate in treatment. The social worker also can assist the family in understanding the child's diagnosis, treatment program, and prognosis, and expectations for the family during assessment, treatment, and follow-up.

Major goals of the assessment for the behavioral psychologist are to (1) identify, prioritize, and operationally define problem behaviors, (2) determine the onset and history of the feeding problem, (3) identify significant dimensions of the problem (e.g., frequency, duration, intensity), (4) delineate environmental antecedents and consequences associated with the behavior, (5) review previous behavioral interventions, and (6) define the goals of treatment.

In our program the behavioral psychologist conducts a structured interview to obtain information about the child's past and current feeding behavior and other information as indicated above for specific disciplines. We then observe the caregiver feeding the child a meal. We ask the caregivers to bring foods to the evaluation that he or she typically feeds the child at home and any materials (e.g., plates, spoons) that are used at home. We instruct the caregiver to feed the child as he or she would at home and to use the same strategies that he or she uses at home during the meals. During these meals, we record data on both child and caregiver behavior.

Examples of dependent variables for child behavior may include acceptance (child allows the food or liquid to be deposited in his or her mouth within 5s of the presentation), mouth clean (no visible food or liquid in the child's mouth 30s after the bite entered the child's mouth), inappropriate behavior (head turns, batting or blocking the spoon or cup), negative vocalizations (crying, saying "No"), and expels (any solid or liquid greater than the size of a pea outside the plane of the lips after the bite or drink has entered the child's mouth).

Examples of dependent variables for caregiver behavior may include allows escape (removal of the spoon or cup greater than 4cm from the child's mouth), incorrect attention (any verbal statement to or physical contact with the child within 5s of the child engaging in an inappropriate behavior), and correct praise (positive verbal statement to or physical contact with the child 5s after child appropriate behavior). We also weigh the food and liquid before and after the meal and subtract any spill and/or vomit from the total to obtain a measure of grams consumed.

Children who are admitted to our program for day treatment, intensive outpatient, or outpatient services participate in additional assessment of their feeding problems. Children with high levels of inappropriate behavior during caregiver-fed meals would participate in a functional assessment (FA) to determine how specific environmental events affect child behavior (Piazza, Fisher et al., 2003a). The assessment may be conducted by the caregiver or a clinician who has received extensive in vivo training in the application of FA methods and other behavioral procedures. The FA typically consists of three or four conditions, which allow us to observe the child's behavior when inappropriate behavior results in (1) adult attention, (2) breaks from presentations of liquids or solids, (3) access to a tangible item (e.g., preferred toy or food), or (4) no differential consequence (control). We conduct these conditions in a pairwise fashion in which levels of acceptance and inappropriate behavior in each test condition (attention, escape, tangible) are compared to those in the control condition. This analysis provides us with information regarding possible ways we can alter the mealtime environment to improve the child's eating. That is, the results of the FA result in a specific prescribed treatment for the child.

Children with high levels of inappropriate behavior in the presence of specific foods would participate in a food preference assessment (Munk & Repp, 1994a). During the preference assessment the caregiver nominates 8 to 16 foods (2 to 4 foods in each of the food groups of protein, starch, fruit, vegetable) that the child refuses to eat, but that the caregiver would like the child to eat. We present these 8 to 16 items, along with other items that the child eats willingly. Foods items are presented in pairs and each food item is presented with every other food item once. We ask the child to "pick one." We can develop a hierarchy of food preferences for the child based on the results of this assessment. The results of the assessment then are used to develop treatment to increase the child's acceptance of foods that are less preferred.

Children with high levels of inappropriate behavior in the presence of specific textures of foods would participate in a food texture preference assessment (Munk & Repp, 1994a; Patel, Piazza, Layer, Coleman, & Swartzwelder, 2005; Patel, Piazza, Santana, & Volkert, 2002). Again, the caregiver nominates 8 to 16 foods (2 to 4 foods in each of the food groups of protein, starch, fruit, vegetable) that the child refuses to eat, but that the caregiver would like the child to eat. We present these 8 to 16 items in different textures to assess which textures and foods the child will eat and which textures and foods that child refuses. Food items are presented in pairs and each food item is presented with every other food item once. We ask the child to "pick one." We can develop a hierarchy of food preferences for the child based on the results of this assessment. The results of the assessment then are used to develop treatment to increase the child's acceptance of a variety of textures of foods.

We often conduct preference assessments to identify preferred items to use as reinforcement (Fisher et al., 1992). Parents identify approximately 16 items that the child appears to prefer. During the preference assessment, items are presented to the child in pairs, and each item is paired with every other item. The child is asked to "pick one" of the pair of items. A hierarchy of child preferences can be constructed based on the results of the assessment. We use the most highly preferred items based on the results of the preference assessment during treatment (Mueller et al., 2003b; Mueller, Piazza, Patel, Kelley, & Pruett, 2004; Patel, Piazza, Kelly, Ochsner, & Santana, 2001; Patel et al., 2005; Patel, Piazza, Martinez, Volkert, & Christine, 2002; Patel, Piazza, Santana et al., 2002; Patel et al., 2006; Piazza, Anderson, & Fisher, 1993; Piazza, Carroll-Hernandez, 2004; Piazza, Fisher et al., 2003a; Piazza, Patel et al., 2003a; Piazza et al., 2002a; Reed et al., 2004a).

We work cooperatively with the speech and/or occupational therapist to evaluate oral motor skills such as tongue lateralization, chewing, and swallowing. We take the same, systematic data-based approach with these problems as we do with all other feeding problems. Assessment of chewing and swallowing necessitates careful consideration of the types of solids and/or liquids that can be presented to the child to assess the skill without placing the child at risk for choking or aspiration. Finally, the complexity and heterogeneity of feeding problems often necessitates that we develop other assessments specific to individual children and idiosyncratic problems.

SUMMARY

Feeding disorders of some type are fairly common throughout childhood, particularly among children with developmental disabilities. Given this prevalence, the topography of feeding disorders includes a variety of maladaptive mealtime behaviors. Likewise, the etiology of feeding disorders may differ greatly across children. These issues combine to make the diagnosis of pediatric feeding disorders difficult, which affects the utility of existing diagnostic taxonomies. Thus, a comprehensive assessment is necessary to describe the physical conditions that gave rise to the development of the disorder as well as the environmental conditions that serve to maintain the occurrence of these problems.

Although a number of questionnaires have been developed to assess the feeding disorders, these measures tend to be limited in the specificity of information obtained on an individual. As an alternative, direct observation of a child's feeding behavior (including functional assessment) may yield more detailed information on the occurrence and maintenance of feeding disorders. However, most children with feeding disorders benefit from a multifaceted team assessment consisting of individuals from the medical, psychology, social work, and nutrition disciplines. An interdisciplinary approach allows for the evaluation and incorporation of physical, oral, and psychological factors that may lead to the development of effective treatments for pediatric feeding disorders.

REFERENCES

Ahearn, W. H., Kerwin, M. L., Eicher, P. S., Shantz, J., & Swearingin, W. (1996). An alternating treatments comparison of two intensive interventions for food refusal. *Journal of Applied Behavior Analysis, 29*(3), 321–332.

American Psychiatric Association (2000). *Diagnostic and statistical manual of mental disorders,* fourth edition text revision. Washington, DC: Author.

Archer, L. A., Rosenbaum, P. L., & Streiner, D. L. (1991). The children's eating behavior inventory: Reliability and validity results. *Journal of Pediatric Psychology, 16*(5), 629–642.

Archer, L. A., & Szatmari, P. (1990). Assessment and treatment of food aversion in a four year old boy: A multidimensional approach. *Canadian Journal of Psychiatry, 35*(6), 501–505.

Bazyk, S. (1990). Factors associated with the transition to oral feeding in infants fed by nasogastric tubes. *American Journal of Occupational Therapy, 44*(12), 1070–1078.

Benoit, D., Wang, E. E. L., & Zlotkin, S. H. (2000). Discontinuation of enterostomy tube feeding by behavioral treatment in early childhood: A randomized controlled trial *The Journal of Pediatrics, 137*(4), 498–503.

Blackman, J. A., & Nelson, C. L. (1985). Reinstituting oral feedings in children fed by gastrostomy tube. *Clinical Pediatrics, 24*(8), 434–438.

Braun, M. A., & Palmer, M. M. (1985). A pilot study of oral-motor dysfunction in 'at-risk' infants. *Physical and Occupational Therapy in Pediatrics, 5*(4), 13–25.

Burklow, K. A., McGrath, A. M., Valerius, K. S., & Ruldolph, C. (2002). Relationship between feeding difficulties, medical complexity, and gestational age. *Nutrition in Clinical Practice, 17*(6), 373–378.

Burklow, K. A., Phelps, A. N., Schultz, J. R., McConnell, K., Rudolph, C. (1998). Classifying complex pediatric feeding disorders. *Journal of Pediatric Gastroenterology and Nutrition,* 27(2), 143–147.

Carruth, B. R., & Skinner, J. D. (2002). Feeding behaviors and other motor development in healthy children (2–24 months). *Journal of the American College of Nutrition, 21*(2), 88–96.

Centers for Disease Control and Prevention. (2000). *Clinical growth charts.* Retrieved August 20, 2007 from http://www.cdc.gov/nchs/about/major/nhanes/growth-charts/clinical_charts.htm.

Cooper, L. J., Wacker, D. P., McComas, J. J., Brown, K., Peck, S. M., Richman, D., et al. (1995). Use of component analyses to identify active variables in treatment packages for children with feeding disorders. *Journal of Applied Behavior Analysis, 28*(2), 139–153.

Crist, W., McDonnell, P., Beck, M., Gillespie, C. T., Barrett, P., & Mathews, J. (1994). Behavior at mealtimes of young children with cystic fibrosis. *Journal of Developmental and Behavioral Pediatrics, 15*, 157–161.

Crist, W., & Napier-Phillips, A. (2001). Mealtime behaviors of young children: A comparison of normative and clinical data. *Developmental and Behavioral Pediatrics, 22*(5), 279–286.

Dahl, M. (1987). Early feeding problems in an affluent society. III. Follow-up at two years: Natural course, health, behaviour and development. *Acta Paediatrics Scandanavia, 76*(6), 872–880.

Dahl, M., & Kristiansson, B. (1987). Early feeding problems in an affluent society. IV. Impact on growth up to two years of age. *Acta Paediatrics Scandanavia, 76*(6), 881–888.

Dahl, M., & Sundelin, C. (1992). Feeding problems in an affluent society. Follow-up at four years of age in children with early refusal to eat. *Acta Paediatrics, 81*(8), 575–579.

D'Antonio, I. G. (1979). Cardiac infant's feeding difficulties. *Western Journal of Nursing Research, 1*(1), 53–55.

Dobbing, J. (1985). Infant nutrition and later achievement. *The American Journal of Clinical Nutrition, 41,* 477–484.

Dodrill, P., McMahon, S., Ward, E., Weir, K., Donovan, T., & Riddle, B. (2004). Long-term oral sensitivity and feeding skills of low-risk pre-term infants. *Early Human Development, 76,* 23–37.

Drewett, R. F., Kasese-Hara, M., & Wright, C. (2002). Feeding behaviour in young children who fail to thrive. *Appetite, 40,* 55–60.

Esparo, G., Canals, J., Jane, C., Ballespi', S., Vinas, F., & Domenech, E. (2004). Feeding problems in nursery children: Prevalence and psychosocial factors. *Acta Paediatrics, 93,* 663–668.

Fernandez-Ballesteros, R. (2004). Self-report questionnaires. In S. N. Haynes & E. M. Heiby (Eds.), *Comprehensive handbook of psychological assessment, Vol. 3: Behavioral assessment.* New York: John Wiley & Sons.

Field, D., Garland, M., & Williams, K. (2003). Correlates of specific childhood feeding problems. *Journal of Paediatric Child Health, 39,* 299–304.

Fisher, W., Piazza, C. C., Bowman, L. G., Hagopian, L. P., Owens, J. C., & Slevin, I. (1992). A comparison of two approaches for identifying reinforcers for persons with severe and profound disabilities. *Journal of Applied Behavior Analysis, 25*(2), 491–498.

Freeman, K. A. & Miller, C. A. (2002). Behavioral case conceptualization for children and adolescents. In M. Hersen (Ed.), *Clinical behavior therapy: Adults and children.* New York: John Wiley & Sons.

Geertsma, M. A., Hyams, J. S., Pelletier, J. M., & Reiter, S. (1985). Feeding resistance after parenteral hyperalimentation. *American Journal of Diseases of Children, 139*(3), 255–256.

Gisel, E. G. (1988). Chewing cycles in 2 to 8-year-old normal children: A developmental profile. *American Journal of Occupational Therapy, 42*(6), 41–45.

Gouge, A. L., & Ekvall, S. W. (1975). Diets of handicapped children: Physical, psychological, and socioeconomic correlations. *American Journal of Mental Deficiency, 80*(2), 149–157.

Hoch, T., Babbitt, R. L., Coe, D. A., Krell, D. M., & Hackbert, L. (1994). Contingency contacting. Combining positive reinforcement and escape extinction procedures to treat persistent food refusal. *Behavior Modification, 18*(1), 106–128.

Ivanovic, D. M., Leiva, B. P., Perez, H. T., Inzunza, N. B., Almagia, A. F., Toro, T. D., Urrutia, M. S. C., Cervilla, J. O., & Bosch E. O. (2000). Long-term effects of severe undernutrition during the first year of life on brain development and learning in Chilean high-school graduates. *Nutrition, 16*(11–12), 1056–1063.

Ivanovic, D. M., Leiva, B. P., Perez, H. T., Olivares, M. G., Diaz, N. S., Urrutia, M. S., et al. (2004). Head size and intelligence, learning, nutritional status and brain development. Head, IQ, learning, nutrition and brain. *Neuropsychologia, 42*(8), 1118–1131.

Iwata, B. A., Dorsey, M. F., Slifer, K. J., Bauman, K. E., & Richman, G. S. (1994). Toward a functional analysis of self-injury. *Journal of Applied Behavior Analysis, 27*(2), 197–209.

Iwata, B. A., Duncan, B. A., Zarcone, J. R., Lerman, D. C., & Shore, B. A. (1994). A sequential, test-control methodology for conducting functional analyses of self-injurious behavior. *Behavior Modification, 18*(3), 289–306.

Kasese-Hara, M., Wright, C., & Drewett, R. (2002). Energy consumption in young children who fail to thrive. *Journal of Child Psychology and Psychiatry, 43*(4), 449–456.

Levitsky, D. A., & Strupp, B. J. (1995). Malnutrition and the brain: Changing concepts, changing concerns. *Journal of Nutrition 125*, 2212S–2220S.

Matson, J. L., & Kuhn, D. E. (2001). Identifying feeding problems in mentally retarded persons: development and reliability of the screening tool of feeding problems (STEP). *Research in Developmental Disabilities, 22*(2), 165–172.

Morgan, B. L. G. (1990). Nutritional requirements for normative development of the brain and behavior. *Annals New York Academy of Sciences, 602*, 127–132.

Mueller, M. M., Piazza, C. C., Moore, J. W., Kelley, M. E., Bethke, S. A., Pruett, A. E., et al. (2003). Training parents to implement pediatric feeding protocols. *Journal of Applied Behavior Analysis, 36*(4), 545–562.

Mueller, M. M., Piazza, C. C., Patel, M. R., Kelley, M. E., & Pruett, A. (2004). Increasing variety of foods consumed by blending nonpreferred foods into preferred foods. *Journal of Applied Behavior Analysis, 37*(2), 159–170.

Munk, D. D., & Repp, A. C. (1994). Behavioral assessment of feeding problems of individuals with severe disabilities. *Journal of Applied Behavior Analysis, 27*(2), 241–250.

Palmer, S., & Horn, S. (1978). Feeding problems in children. In S. Palmer & S. W. Ekvall (Eds.), *Pediatric nutrition in developmental disorders.*

Patel, M. R., Piazza, C. C., Kelly, L., Ochsner, C. A., & Santana, C. M. (2001). Using a fading procedure to increase fluid consumption in a child with feeding problems. *Journal of Applied Behavior Analysis, 34*(3), 357–360.

Patel, M. R., Piazza, C. C., Layer, S. A., Coleman, R., & Swartzwelder, D. M. (2005). A systematic evaluation of food textures to decrease packing and increase oral intake in children with pediatric feeding disorders. *Journal of Applied Behavior Analysis, 38*(1), 89–100.

Patel, M. R., Piazza, C. C., Martinez, C. J., Volkert, V. M., & Christine, M. S. (2002). An evaluation of two differential reinforcement procedures with escape extinction to treat food refusal. *Journal of Applied Behavior Analysis, 35*(4), 363–374.

Patel, M. R., Piazza, C. C., Santana, C. M., & Volkert, V. M. (2002). An evaluation of food type and texture in the treatment of a feeding problem. *Journal of Applied Behavior Analysis, 35*(2), 183–186.

Patel, M. R., Reed, G. K., Piazza, C. C., Bachmeyer, M. H., Layer, S. A., & Pabico, R. S. (2006). An evaluation of a high-probability instructional sequence to increase acceptance of food and decrease inappropriate behavior in children with pediatric feeding disorders. *Research in Developmental Disabilities, 27*(4), 430–442.

Piazza, C. C., Anderson, C., & Fisher, W. (1993). Teaching self-feeding skills to patients with Rett syndrome. *Develpmental Medicine and Child Neurology, 35*(11), 991–996.

Piazza, C. C. & Carroll-Hernandez, T. A. (2004). *Assessment and treatment of pediatric feeding disorders.* Retrieved August 31, 2005, from http://www.excellence-earlychildhood.ca/documents/Piazza-Carroll-HernandezANGxp.pdf.

Piazza, C. C., Fisher, W. W., Brown, K. A., Shore, B. A., Patel, M. R., Katz, R. M., et al. (2003). Functional analysis of inappropriate mealtime behaviors. *Journal of Applied Behavior Analysis, 36*(2), 187–204.

Piazza, C. C., Patel, M. R., Gulotta, C. S., Sevin, B. M., & Layer, S. A. (2003). On the relative contributions of positive reinforcement and escape extinction in the treatment of food refusal. *Journal of Applied Behavior Analysis, 36*(3), 309–324.

Piazza, C. C., Patel, M. R., Santana, C. M., Goh, H. L., Delia, M. D., & Lancaster, B. M. (2002). An evaluation of simultaneous and sequential presentation of preferred and nonpreferred food to treat food selectivity. *Journal of Applied Behavior Analysis, 35*(3), 259–270.

Pollitt, E., Eichler, A. W., & Chan, C. K. (1975). Psychosocial development and behavior of mothers of failure-to-thrive children. *The American Journal of Orthopsychiatry, 45*(4), 525–537.

Powell, G. F., Low, J. F., & Speers, M. A. (1987). Behavior as a diagnostic aid in failure-to-thrive. *Developmental and Behavioral Pediatrics, 8*(1), 18–24.

Powers, S. W., Byars, K. C., Mitchell, M. J., Patton, S. R., Standiford, D. A., & Dolan, L. M. (2002). Parent report of mealtime behavior and parenting stress in young children with type 1 diabetes and in healthy control subjects. *Diabetes Care, 25*(2), 313–318.

Powers, S. W., Mitchell, M. J., Patton, S. R., Byars, K. C., Jelalian, E., Mulvihill, M. M., et al. (2005). Mealtime behaviors in families of infants and toddlers with cystic fibrosis. *Journal of Cystic Fibrosis, 4*(3), 175–182.

Ramsay, M., Gisel, E. G., & Boutry, M. (1993). Non-organic failure to thrive: Growth failure secondary to feeding-skills disorder. *Developmental Medicine and Child Neurology, 35*(4), 285–297.

Reau, N. R., Senturia, Y. D., Lebailly, S. A., & Kaufer Christoffel, K. (1996). Infant and toddler feeding patterns and problems: Normative data and a new direction. *Developmental and Behavioral Pediatrics, 17*(3), 149–153.

Reed, G. K., Piazza, C. C., Patel, M. R., Layer, S. A., Bachmeyer, M. H., Bethke, S. D., et al. (2004). On the relative contributions of noncontingent reinforcement and escape extinction in the treatment of food refusal. *Journal of Applied Behavior Analysis, 37*(1), 27–42.

Rommel, N., De Meyer, A. M., Feenstra, L., & Veereman-Wauters, G. (2003). The complexity of feeding problems in 700 infants and young children presenting to a tertiary care institution. *Journal of Pediatric Gastroenterology and Nutrition, 37*, 75–84.

Rydell, A. M., Dahl, M., & Sundelin, C. (2001). Characteristics of school children who are choosy eaters. *The Journal of Genetic Psychology, 156*, 217–229.

Sanders, M. R., Patel, R. K., Le Grice, B., & Shepherd, R. W. (1993). Children with persistent feeding difficulties: An observational analysis of the feeding interactions of problem and non-problem eaters. *Health Psychology, 12*(1), 64–73.

Singer, L. T., Song, L. Y., Hill, B. P., & Jaffe, A. C. (1990). Stress and depression in mothers of failure-to-thrive children. *Journal of Pediatric Psychology, 15*(6), 711–720.

Skuse, D. H. (1985). Non-organic failure to thrive: A reappraisal. *Archives of Disease in Childhood, 60*(2), 173–178.

Stark, L. J., Mulvihill, M. M., Jelalian, E., Bowen, A. M., Powers, S. W., Tao, S., et al. (1997). Descriptive analysis of eating behavior in school-age children with cystic fibrosis and healthy control children. *Pediatrics, 99*(5), 665–671.

Troughton, K. E., & Hill, A. E. (2001). Relation between objectively measured feeding competence and nutrition in children with cerebral palsy. *Developmental Medicine and Child Neurology, 43*(3), 187–190.

Van Dyke, D. C., Mackay, L., & Ziaylek, E. N. (1982). Management of severe feeding dysfunction in children with fetal alcohol syndrome. *Clinical Pediatrics, 21*(6), 336–339.

Wilson, M. H. (1994). Feeding the healthy child. In F. A. Oski, C. D. DeAngelis, R. D. Feigin, J. A. McMillan, & J. B. Warshaw (Eds.), *Principles and practice of pediatrics*. Philadelphia: J. B. Lippincott.

Winick, M. (1969). Malnutrition and brain development. *The Journal of Pediatrics, 74*(5), 667–679.

World Health Organization (1993). *International classification of diseases* (10th ed.). Geneva: Author.

Young, B., & Drewett, R. (2000). Eating behavior and its variability in 1-year-old children. *Appetite, 35*(2), 171–177.

Index

Printed in the United States of America